2nd edition

# pediatrics

*The National Medical Series for Independent Study*

# 2nd edition
# pediatrics

**Editor**
## Paul H. Dworkin, M.D.

*Professor and Vice-Chairman of Pediatrics*
*Head, Division of General*
*Pediatrics*
*University of Connecticut*
*School of Medicine*
*Farmington, Connecticut*

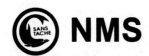

National Medical Series from Williams & Wilkins
Baltimore, Hong Kong, London, Sydney

*Harwal Publishing Company, Malvern, Pennsylvania*

**Williams & Wilkins**

Managing Editor: Debra Dreger
Project Editor: Debra Dreger
Production: Laurie Forsyth
Illustration: Wieslawa B. Langenfeld
Composition and Layout: TeleComposition, Inc.

**Library of Congress Cataloging-in-Publication Data**

Pediatrics / Paul H. Dworkin. — 2nd ed.
    p.    cm. — (The National medical series for independent study)
   Includes bibliographical references and index.
   ISBN 0-683-06246-8 (pbk. : alk. paper)
   1. Pediatrics—Outlines, syllabi, etc.   2. Pediatrics—
Examinations, questions, etc.    I. Dworkin, Paul H.   II. Series.
   [DNLM: 1. Pediatrics—examination questions.    WS 18 P3702]
  RJ48.3.P44   1992
  618.92—dc20
  DNLM/DLC
  for Library of Congress                    91-15343
                                    CIP

ISBN 0-683-06246-8

©1992 Williams & Wilkins

10 9 8 7 6 5 4 3 2

# Contents

# Contributors

**Arnold J. Altman, M.D.**
Hartford Whalers Professor of Childhood
   Cancer
Chief, Division of Pediatric Hematology
   and Oncology
University of Connecticut School
   of Medicine
Farmington, Connecticut

**Mark Ballow, M.D.**
Professor of Pediatrics
State University of New York at Buffalo
Chief, Division of Allergy/Immunology
Department of Pediatrics
Children's Hospital of Buffalo
Buffalo, New York

**Leonard I. Banco, M.D.**
Associate Professor of Pediatrics
University of Connecticut School
   of Medicine
Farmington, Connecticut
Director, Pediatric Ambulatory Services
Associate Director, Department
   of Pediatrics
Hartford Hospital
Hartford, Connecticut

**Suzanne B. Cassidy, M.D.**
Associate Professor of Pediatrics
Section of Genetics/Dysmorphology
University of Arizona College
   of Medicine
Tucson, Arizona

**Leon Chameides, M.D.**
Clinical Professor of Pediatrics
Head, Division of Pediatric Cardiology
University of Connecticut School
   of Medicine
Farmington, Connecticut
Director, Pediatric Cardiology
Hartford Hospital
Hartford, Connecticut

**Michelle M. Cloutier, M.D.**
Professor of Pediatrics
Chief, Division of Pediatric Pulmonology
University of Connecticut School
   of Medicine
Farmington, Connecticut

**Daniel J. Diana, M.D.**
Assistant Clinical Professor of Pediatrics
University of Connecticut School
   of Medicine
Farmington, Connecticut
Pediatric Cardiologist
Hartford Hospital
Hartford, Connecticut

**Paul H. Dworkin, M.D.**
Professor and Vice-Chairman of Pediatrics
Head, Division of General Pediatrics
University of Connecticut School
   of Medicine
Farmington, Connecticut

**Henry M. Feder, Jr., M.D.**
Professor of Pediatrics and Family Medicine
University of Connecticut School
  of Medicine
Farmington, Connecticut

**Jeffrey S. Hyams, M.D.**
Professor of Pediatrics
Head, Division of Pediatric
  Gastroenterology and Nutrition
University of Connecticut School
  of Medicine
Farmington, Connecticut
Director, Pediatric Gastroenterology
  and Nutrition
Hartford Hospital
Hartford, Connecticut

**Thomas L. Kennedy, M.D.**
Associate Clinical Professor of Pediatrics
Yale School of Medicine
New Haven, Connecticut
Chairman, Department of Pediatrics
Bridgeport Hospital
Bridgeport, Connecticut

**Peter J. Krause, M.D.**
Professor of Pediatrics
University of Connecticut School
  of Medicine
Farmington, Connecticut
Chief, Division of Pediatric Infectious
  Diseases
Hartford Hospital
Hartford, Connecticut

**Daniel A. Kveselis, M.D.**
Assistant Professor of Pediatrics
State University of New York
  Health Science Center
Syracuse, New York

**Harris B. Leopold, M.D.**
Assistant Clinical Professor of Pediatrics
University of Connecticut School
  of Medicine
Farmington, Connecticut
Pediatric Cardiologist
Hartford Hospital
Hartford, Connecticut

**Milton Markowitz, M.D.**
Associate Dean, Student Affairs
Professor of Pediatrics
University of Connecticut School
  of Medicine
Farmington, Connecticut

**John J. Quinn, M.D.**
Professor of Pediatrics
Director, Pediatric Clerkship
Pediatric Director, Bone Marrow
  Transplant Unit
University of Connecticut School
  of Medicine
Farmington, Connecticut

**Susan K. Ratzan, M.D.**
Chase/Freedman Associate Professor
  of Pediatrics
Clinical Director, Connecticut Program
  for Children with Diabetes
University of Connecticut School
  of Medicine
Farmington, Connecticut

**Ted S. Rosenkrantz, M.D.**
Associate Professor of Pediatrics
  and Obstetrics and Gynecology
Associate Director of Newborn Services
University of Connecticut School
  of Medicine
Farmington, Connecticut

**Barry S. Russman, M.D.**
Professor of Pediatrics and Neurology
Chief, Division of Pediatric Neurology
University of Connecticut School
  of Medicine
Farmington, Connecticut
Chief, Pediatric Neurology
Newington Children's Hospital
Newington, Connecticut

**David A. Schaeffer, M.D.**
Assistant Professor of Pediatrics
University of Connecticut School
  of Medicine
Farmington, Connecticut

**Neil L. Schechter, M.D.**
Associate Professor of Pediatrics
Head, Division of Developmental
  and Behavioral Pediatrics
University of Connecticut School
  of Medicine
Farmington, Connecticut
Director, Section of Developmental
  and Behavioral Pediatrics
St. Francis Hospital and Medical Center
Hartford, Connecticut


**Aric Schichor, M.D.**
Assistant Professor of Pediatrics
Head, Division of Adolescent Medicine
University of Connecticut School
  of Medicine
Farmington, Connecticut
Director, Adolescent Medicine
St. Francis Hospital and Medical Center
Hartford, Connecticut

**Betty S. Spivack, M.D.**
Assistant Professor of Pediatrics
Head, Division of Pediatric Intensive Care
University of Connecticut School
  of Medicine
Farmington, Connecticut
Director, Pediatric Intensive Care Unit
Hartford Hospital
Hartford, Connecticut

**William R. Treem, M.D.**
Assistant Professor of Pediatrics
University of Connecticut School of
  Medicine
Farmington, Connecticut
Associate Director, Pediatric
  Gastroenterology and Nutrition
Hartford Hospital
Hartford, Connecticut

**David A. H. Whiteman, M.D.**
Assistant in Medicine
Children's Hospital
Boston, Massachusetts

# Preface

Many helpful recommendations of medical students, pediatric residents, and medical educators are reflected in the second edition of NMS *Pediatrics*. All chapters have been updated to include new knowledge and to eliminate outdated and incorrect material. Several chapters have been extensively rewritten. A new chapter by Dr. Betty S. Spivack integrates pathophysiology with an overview of assessment and intervention techniques in the critical care of children. The addition of nearly 200 new questions and explanations offers additional opportunity for self-evaluation.

This book reflects the continued emphasis placed on medical education by the Department of Pediatrics of the University of Connecticut School of Medicine. All authors are current or former members of this department. Our intent remains that this book not serve as a comprehensive pediatrics text, but rather as a useful tool for intensive review and self-evaluation.

Paul H. Dworkin

# Acknowledgments

The editor and contributing authors thank the staff at Harwal—in particular, Matthew Harris and Debra Dreger—for their assistance in the preparation of this second edition. Katherine Kean performed meticulous and thoughtful copy editing. We are also grateful to Dr. John R. Raye, Professor and Chairman of the Department of Pediatrics at the University of Connecticut School of Medicine, for his continued support and encouragement of this project. We also thank the many medical students, pediatric residents, and medical educators for their invaluable feedback in response to the first edition of this text.

# To the Reader

Since 1984, the *National Medical Series for Independent Study* has been helping medical students meet the challenge of education and clinical training. In this climate of burgeoning knowledge and complex clinical issues, a medical career is more demanding than ever. Increasingly, medical training must prepare physicians to seek and synthesize necessary information and to apply that information successfully.

The *National Medical Series* is designed to provide a logical framework for organizing, learning, reviewing, and applying the conceptual and factual information covered in basic and clinical sciences. Each book includes a comprehensive outline of the essential content of a discipline, with up to 500 study questions. The combination of an outlined text and tools for self-evaluation allows easy retrieval of salient information.

All study questions are accompanied by the correct answer, a paragraph-length explanation, and specific reference to the text where the topic is discussed. Study questions that follow each chapter use current National Board format to reinforce the chapter content. Study questions appearing at the end of the text in the Comprehensive Exam vary in format depending on the book. Wherever possible, Comprehensive Exam questions are presented as a clinical case or scenario intended to simulate real-life application of medical knowledge. The goal of this exam is to challenge the student to draw from information presented throughout the book.

All of the books in the *National Medical Series* are constantly being updated and revised. The authors and editors devote considerable time and effort to ensure that the information required by all medical school curricula is included. Strict editorial attention is given to accuracy, organization, and consistency. Further shaping of the series occurs in response to biannual discussions held with a panel of medical student advisors drawn from schools throughout the United States. At these meetings, the editorial staff considers the needs of medical students to learn how the *National Medical Series* can better serve them. In this regard, the NMS staff welcomes all comments and suggestions.

# Child Health Supervision

Paul H. Dworkin

**I. GOAL AND SCOPE OF PEDIATRIC PRACTICE.** The goal of child health supervision is the optimal growth and development of children. In general, the practice of pediatrics divides as follows.

**A. Well-child care and child health supervision** account for about 30% of practice time.

**B. Infectious diseases** represent about 50% of practice time, and the most common problems are upper respiratory tract illnesses and otitis media.

**C. Other disorders** that account for the remainder of practice time include injuries and trauma, skin disorders, and behavioral and developmental disorders.

**D. Recent trends.** The scope of pediatric practice has changed significantly over the past decade. Pediatricians today are more concerned with problems relating to allergies, functioning in school, child behavior, and child health supervision than with life-threatening problems or with caring for hospitalized children.

**II. WELL-CHILD VISITS**

**A. Components**

1. **History.** An initial history should be taken at the first visit, and an interval history should be obtained at each subsequent visit. Parents should be encouraged to express any problems or concerns.

2. **Anticipatory guidance** is the process by which pediatric health care providers offer **counseling during child health supervision** (e.g., on such topics as nutrition, safety and injury prevention, child behavior and development, parent-child interaction, various medical issues). Through such counseling, the pediatrician helps parents foresee normal deviations in children's behavior, thereby alleviating undue parental anxiety and concern (Figure 1-1).

3. **Physical examination.** A complete physical examination should be performed during each visit. Particular areas should receive emphasis, depending on the age of the child. For example, the newborn examination must include a careful search for congenital anomalies, while assessment of an adolescent should include a determination of pubertal stage and screening for scoliosis.

4. **Developmental monitoring** should be performed during each well-child visit.
   a. Ideally, such monitoring should be performed by the process of **developmental surveillance**. During developmental surveillance, emphasis is placed on the following:
      (1) Eliciting and attending to parental concerns
      (2) Making accurate and informative observations of children
      (3) Obtaining a relevant developmental history
   b. A variety of **techniques** may be used by the pediatric provider during developmental surveillance to make observations of children.
      (1) The pediatrician may use an informal collection of age-appropriate tasks.
      (2) The provider may administer a specific screening instrument (e.g., Denver Developmental Screening Test, Goodenough Draw-A-Man Test, Preschool Readiness Experimental Screening Scale).

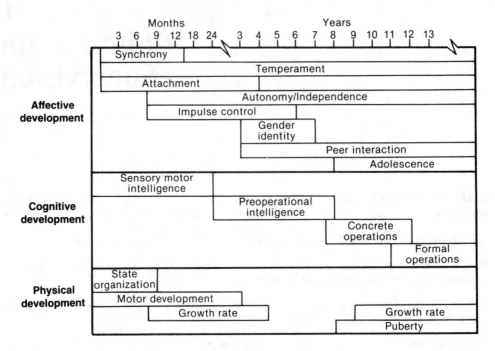

**Figure 1-1.** Agenda for discussion of developmental stages during anticipatory guidance. (Adapted from Telzrow RW: Anticipatory guidance in pediatric practice. *J Cont Educ Pediatr* 20:14–27, 1978.)

      **(a)** The well-recognized limitations of such tools must be considered when interpreting results. Whenever possible, efforts should be made to compare findings with the opinions of the child's parents, day care provider, preschool teacher, social worker, or public health nurse.

      **(b)** A developmental screening test must not be considered equivalent to intelligence quotient (IQ) testing or as a definite predictor of current or future abilities. **Screening merely identifies children at risk for possible developmental problems** and confirms subjective suspicions of delay.

      **(c)** Accurate screening for developmental delays must be based on more than just a history of developmental milestones, a few motor development landmarks, general observations of speech and language ability, or a child's behavior within the office setting.

  **5. Procedures**

    **a. Measurements.** All measurements should be plotted on an appropriate growth chart.

      **(1) Height** (length during infancy) **and weight** should be ascertained at each visit.

      **(2) Head circumference** should be measured at each visit during the first year of life.

      **(3) Blood pressure** measurements are recommended for children who are age 3 years and older.

    **b. Metabolic screening** is performed during the newborn period.

      **(1)** This screening must be part of a comprehensive program ensuring effective treatment for problems that are disclosed.

      **(2)** Cost-effectiveness is greatly improved by a screening program that encompasses multiple disorders (e.g., the phenylketonuria and hypothyroidism screening performed through state laboratories).

    **c. Sensory screening** is subjectively performed by the examiner during infancy and early childhood. A standard testing method in the preschool years may be used to screen vision and hearing objectively.

    **d. Laboratory procedures** should be performed selectively. The individual needs of the child should determine the frequency of such tests as urinalysis, urine culture, and hemoglobin and hematocrit measurements as well as tests for lead poisoning, sickle cell disease, and tuberculosis.

    **e. Immunizations.** At present, children are routinely immunized against diphtheria, pertussis, tetanus, polio, measles, mumps, rubella, and infections due to *Hemophilus influenzae* type b

(Hib). Routine immunization against hepatitis B and varicella is anticipated. Other vaccines (e.g., pneumococcal and influenza vaccines) are administered to certain high-risk groups.

(1) **Factors determining the usefulness of a vaccine** include:
   (a) Current risk of the disease
   (b) Benefit of disease prevention to the individual and society
   (c) Efficacy, safety, cost, and availability
   (d) Alternatives regarding prevention
   (e) Special needs and characteristics of the individual or group to be immunized

(2) **Types of vaccines** include:
   (a) **Bacterial**
      (i) Killed, whole organisms (e.g., for pertussis)
      (ii) Toxoids (e.g., for tetanus and diphtheria)
      (iii) Specific portions of organisms (e.g., the pneumococcal polysaccharide vaccine and the Hib conjugate vaccines, in which capsular polysaccharide or oligosaccharide is covalently linked to a carrier protein to enhance immunogenicity)
   (b) **Viral**
      (i) Live, attenuated strains (e.g., for polio, measles, mumps, and rubella)
      (ii) Killed organisms (e.g., for influenza)
      (iii) Genetically engineered material (e.g., yeast recombinant-derived antigen for hepatitis B)

(3) **Combination and spacing recommendations** are empiric.
   (a) **Antigenic combinations** are recommended for general use when investigation has shown that they are effective and safe. An adequate immune response to each antigen must develop, and there must be no enhancement of side effects from any component (i.e., from the interaction of one antigen with another).
   (b) **Spacing recommendations** depend on the type of vaccine.
      (i) Live viral vaccines should be administered at least 1 month apart.
      (ii) An interval of 2 or preferably 4 weeks is recommended between an inactivated vaccine [e.g., diphtheria and tetanus toxoids with pertussis (DTP)] and an unrelated live viral vaccine.

(4) **Immunization schedule** (Table 1-1)

(5) **Adverse reactions and contraindications** (Table 1-2)

**B. Recommended schedule for well-child visits** (Table 1-3)

## III. THE PRENATAL VISIT

**A. History.** Information to be reviewed should include:

**1. Maternal health**
   **a.** Nutritional status

**Table 1-1.** Recommended Schedule for Active Immunization of Normal Infants and Children

| Age | Vaccine* |
|---|---|
| 2 months | DTP, TOPV, Hib |
| 4 months | DTP, TOPV, Hib |
| 6 months | DTP, Hib[†] |
| 15 months | MMR, Hib[†] |
| 18 months | DTP, TOPV |
| 4–6 years | DTP, TOPV |
| 11–12 years | MMR |
| 14–16 years | Td |

DTP = diphtheria and tetanus toxoids with pertussis; TOPV = oral, attenuated poliovirus with poliovirus types 1, 2, and 3; MMR = live, attenuated measles-mumps-rubella; Hib = *Hemophilus influenzae* type b conjugate vaccine; Td = adult tetanus toxoid and reduced-dose diphtheria toxoid.
*Recommendations for routine immunizations against hepatitis B and varicella are anticipated.
[†]Specific schedule will vary, depending upon preparation used.

**Table 1-2.** Adverse Reactions and Contraindications to Immunization

| Local reactions | Systemic reactions | Contraindications |
|---|---|---|
| Mild | Mild | Acute, febrile illness |
|   Slight induration |   Fever | Immunosuppressive therapy, immunodeficiency |
|   Tenderness |   Rash |   disorders and malignancies (only immuniza- |
|   Heat |   Fussiness |   tion with live vaccine contraindicated) |
|   Erythema |   Arthralgia | Recent (within 8 weeks) gamma globulin, |
| Severe |   Malaise |   plasma, or blood transfusion |
|   Marked edema |   Headache | Prior allergic or severe reaction to same or re- |
|   Induration |   Fainting |   lated vaccine or vaccine component |
|   Erythema | Severe[†] | Evolving or changing neurologic status (pertussis |
|   Pain |   High fever |   vaccine should be withheld); history of con- |
| **Allergic reactions*** |   Chills |   vulsion may indicate deferring pertussis vac- |
| Urticaria |   Extreme irritability |   cine |
| Erythema multiforme |   Seizure | |
| Bronchospasm |   Collapse | |

*Allergic reactions are rare.
[†]Rarely, paralytic poliomyelitis after live, oral polio vaccine, and rarely, if ever, postimmunization encephalomyelitis associated with pertussis vaccine.

    **b.** Illnesses and chronic disorders
    **c.** Previous childbirth experiences

  **2. Pregnancy**
    **a.** Bleeding
    **b.** Weight gain
    **c.** Illnesses during pregnancy and exposure to infectious diseases
    **d.** Use of drugs, alcohol, and tobacco

  **3. Family history.** Risk factors include any familial and inherited disorders.

  **4. Social history.** Support for the parents, including extended family and financial resources, should be determined.

**B. Anticipatory guidance**

  **1. Physician-parent relationship.** Information to be discussed may include the pediatrician's schedule of availability, provisions for after-hours coverage, telephone arrangements (e.g., call hours), appointment procedures, and the schedule for health maintenance visits.

  **2. Parental readiness** for the arrival of the baby may be suggested by parental expectations concerning changes in home life, paternal involvement, and attendance at prenatal classes.

  **3. Delivery room and nursery procedures.** Routine procedures and personnel should be reviewed as well as issues such as rooming-in, natural childbirth, and circumcision.

  **4. Infant feeding.** Does the mother plan to breast-feed or bottle-feed?

  **5. Care arrangements.** Parents may have questions regarding equipment, clothing, and sleeping arrangements. Parents must have access to an approved infant car seat.

  **6. Economics.** The cost of medical care for delivery and the postpartum period should be reviewed. Do parents have adequate medical insurance?

  **7. Newborn behavior.** The pediatrician's interest in infant development and behavior should be stressed from the beginning. A preliminary discussion of newborn behavior, with an explanation of **state organization** (see IV B 6 a) and **synchrony** (see IV B 6 b) will set the stage for future discussions.

**IV. NEWBORN CARE** (see also Ch 5 IV)

  **A. History.** Important details include the mother's parity, age, and blood type, as well as the length of gestation, duration of labor, timing of rupture of the membranes, evidence of vaginal bleeding, the infant's Apgar score (see Ch 5 III D), and the type of infant resuscitation required.

**Table 1-3.** General Guidelines for Well-Child Visits and Child Health Supervision

| | Infancy | | | | | | Early Childhood | | | | | | Late Childhood | | | | Adolescence | | | |
|---|---|---|---|---|---|---|---|---|---|---|---|---|---|---|---|---|---|---|---|---|
| | 2–4 wks | 2 mos | 4 mos | 6 mos | 9–10 mos | 12 mos | 15 mos | 18 mos | 2 yrs | 3 yrs | 4 yrs | 5 yrs | 6 yrs | 8 yrs | 10 yrs | 12 yrs | 14 yrs | 16 yrs | 18 yrs | 20 yrs |
| History | x | x | x | x | x | x | x | x | x | x | x | x | x | x | x | x | x | x | x | x |
| Anticipatory guidance | x | x | x | x | x | x | x | x | x | x | x | x | x | x | x | x | x | x | x | x |
| Physical examination | x | x | x | x | x | x | x | x | x | x | x | x | x | x | x | x | x | x | x | x |
| Developmental monitoring | x | x | x | x | x | x | x | x | x | x | x | x | x | x | x | x | x | x | x | x |
| Measurements: | | | | | | | | | | | | | | | | | | | | |
| Height | x | x | x | x | x | x | x | x | x | x | x | x | x | x | x | x | x | x | x | x |
| Weight | x | x | x | x | x | x | x | x | x | x | x | x | x | x | x | x | x | x | x | x |
| Head circumference | x | x | x | x | x | x | | | | | | | | | | | | | | |
| Blood pressure | | | | | | | | | | x | x | x | x | x | x | x | x | x | x | x |
| Procedures: | | | | | | | | | | | | | | | | | | | | |
| Metabolic screening | x | | | | | | | | | | | | | | | | | | | |
| Sensory screening | x | x | x | x | x | x | x | x | x | x | x | x | x | x | x | x | x | x | x | x |
| Hemoglobin/hematocrit | | | | | x | | | | | | | x | | | | | x | | | |
| Urinalysis | | | | | | | | x | | | | x | | | | | x | | | |
| Tuberculin test | | | | | | x | | | | | | | | | | | | | | |
| Lead screening | | | | | | x | | x | | | | | | | | | | | | |
| Immunization | | x | x | x | | | x | x | | | | x | | | | | x | | | |

Guidelines are based on the recommendations of the Committee on Practice and Ambulatory Medicine of the American Academy of Pediatrics.

**B. Anticipatory guidance.** Areas for discussion with parents during the postpartum period include the following.

1. **Physical status.** During the immediate postpartum period, concerns for the baby's well-being are of highest priority for parents.

2. **General care.** Issues include bathing, dressing, skin care, and cord care.

3. **Feeding**
   a. **Breast-feeding** is facilitated by a hospital rooming-in policy, which permits a demand-feeding schedule of every 2–4 hours. The routine dietary supplementation with either formula or water should be discouraged for breast-fed babies. Nursing and medical staff must provide consistent, accurate advice about breast-feeding.
   b. **Commercial infant formula** is a satisfactory substitute for human milk. For most newborns, a lactose-containing modified cow's milk formula is well tolerated. Rarely, infants who are intolerant of lactose or of cow's milk protein may require a formula containing alternative carbohydrates (e.g., sucrose, dextrose, maltose, dextrins) or an alternative protein source (e.g., soy isolate, casein hydrolysate).

4. **Safety and injury prevention**
   a. **Crib safety.** Crib bars should be no further than 2⅜ inches apart. Bumpers should be used to avoid suffocation from mattresses and to prevent injury from head banging. To avoid suffocation, objects such as pacifiers and mobiles should not be hung within the crib.
   b. Setting the **water-heater temperature** below 120° F (49° C) will help to prevent accidental scalding.
   c. An approved **car seat** should be used to transport infants in automobiles.

5. **Elimination.** Infants vary considerably in their patterns of elimination. A pattern of urinating six times within 24 hours suggests adequate fluid intake. Infants may have a bowel movement as frequently as after every feeding or as infrequently as once every 4–5 days. Breast-fed babies tend to have loose stools with small curds, and the bowel movements may be explosive.

6. **Developmental issues**
   a. **State organization.** The normal variability in infant behavior is vividly demonstrated by the newborn's frequent changes in state of consciousness. The newborn is able to shut out disturbing aspects of the new environment and has the capacity to choose to respond to certain stimuli.
   b. **Synchrony.** From the outset, the nature of the parent-infant relationship is one of mutual awareness, with parents and newborn each responding to one another via cues.
   c. **Attachment.** The unique relationship between parent and child is being established as early as the postpartum period.
   d. **Temperament.** Individual differences in behavior style are evident as early as the newborn period.

**C. The physical examination** must be thorough to assess the newborn's gestational age, any congenital anomalies, birth trauma, and specific neonatal problems.

1. **Gestational age** may be estimated by general physical characteristics at birth and by neurologic examination performed 24 hours after birth (Table 1-4).

2. **General appearance.** Important observations include body proportions, activity, color, gross abnormalities, and signs of respiratory distress.

3. **Skin**
   a. **Color** may suggest cyanosis, pallor, or jaundice.
   b. Common **birthmarks** include vascular nevi, which may be either flat (e.g., a salmon patch nevus) or raised (e.g., a capillary or strawberry hemangioma, cavernous hemangioma), and mongolian spots.
   c. Benign **rashes** are common.
      (1) **Erythema toxicum** presents as small vesicles filled with eosinophils on a typically erythematous base.
      (2) **Milia** are fine, pinpoint white spots caused by retained sebum that typically cover the bridge of the nose, chin, and cheeks.
      (3) **Miliaria rubra** are red lesions that occur over sebaceous glands, typically from overheating.
   d. The presence of **edema** and **skin turgor** should be noted.

**Table 1-4.** Characteristics Suggesting Prematurity

**Physical characteristics**
  Thick layer of vernix
  Poorly defined incurving of pinna, with scant ear cartilage
  Smooth soles with few anterior creases
  Thin skin with short nails
  Lanugo
  Testes that are palpable in inguinal canal; widely separated, small labia
    majora with prominent clitoris
  Softness of skull bones
  Hypotonic or frog-like posture at rest, with limited recoil of arms and legs
  Absent breast buds

**Neurologic findings**
  Poor body tone, demonstrated by:
    Heel to ear maneuver (allows baby's heel to touch ear)
    Scarf sign (elbow easily crosses midline when baby's arm is pulled
      across chest)
    Head lag
  Increased flexion angles at wrist, ankle, and knee
  Poorly developed primitive reflexes, including:
    Sucking
    Rooting
    Grasping
    Moro
    Crossed extension
    Automatic walk

4. **Head and neck**
   a. The amount of overriding or spreading of the **sutures** and the size of the **fontanelles** should be noted.
   b. **Cephalhematomas** are subperiosteal hemorrhages resulting from the trauma of labor.
   c. **Caput succedaneum** is edema of the scalp due to the pressure caused during labor and delivery. In contrast to cephalhematomas, these lesions extend beyond suture lines.
   d. **Eyes.** Conjunctival or scleral hemorrhages are common and usually are of no clinical significance. The presence of a red reflex excludes the presence of lens opacities and retinoblastoma.
   e. Malformed or low-set **ears** may be associated with congenital anomalies or hearing loss.
   f. **Newborns are nose-breathers.** Obstruction of the nasal passages results in respiratory distress.
   g. The **mouth** should be examined by inspection and palpation. Common minor anomalies include small, white **epithelial pearls** along the gum margins; small, white cysts termed **Epstein's pearls** along the median raphe of the hard palate; and small, hard tumors within the gingiva, termed **epulis**. Palpation may reveal a submucosal bony cleft of the palate.
   h. **Neck masses** include goiter, cystic hygroma, branchial cleft cysts, and thyroglossal duct cysts.

5. **Chest**
   a. **Crepitations** along the length of the clavicle suggest a fracture resulting from a difficult delivery with shoulder dystocia.
   b. **Respiratory rate and pattern** and the presence of chest asymmetry, retractions, grunting, and nasal flaring must be determined.
   c. **Heart murmurs** are commonly heard in the newborn period and usually result from a closing ductus arteriosus or normal changes in pulmonary vascular resistance. **Femoral pulses** must always be palpated since diminished pulses suggest coarctation of the aorta.

6. **Abdominal examination** of the normal newborn usually allows palpation of the liver edge 1–2 cm below the right costal margin and palpation of the spleen tip 1 cm below the left costal margin. The lower portions of the kidneys are normally felt with deep palpation.

7. **Genitalia**
   a. Examination of **male genitalia** should include location of the testes, urethral meatus, and a search for hernia and hydrocele.

**b.** A careful inspection of the **clitoris and labia** should be performed on all female infants to exclude ambiguous genitalia, imperforate hymen, and vaginal atresia.

8. **Extremities.** Approximately 5% of all newborns have limb deformities due to either deformations from positional abnormalities and intrauterine posture or true malformations.
   **a. Congenital dislocation of the hip** occurs in 1 in 1000 live births and is much more common in girls. If the hips are flexed to 90°, the legs normally can be abducted fully to touch the examining table. "Telescoping" of the femoral head with the subluxation (Barlow) maneuver or a palpable "thump" with the Ortolani maneuver suggests dislocation.
   **b.** Trauma to the cervical nerves during delivery may result in asymmetrical arm movements indicating **Erb palsy** (C5 and C6 nerve roots) or **Klumpke palsy** (C8 to T2 nerve roots).
   **c. Metatarsus adductus** is a condition in which the fore part of the foot is adducted and usually supinated. It may result from intrauterine positional compression.

9. **Neurologic examination** (see Table 1-4)

**D. Developmental assessment** of the newborn involves observing activity and response to sensory stimuli and a neurologic examination.

**E. Procedures**

1. **Prophylaxis of gonococcal ophthalmia** is mandated for all newborns. Either a 1% silver nitrate solution in single-dose ampules or a sterile ophthalmic ointment containing 1% tetracycline or 0.5% erythromycin in single-use tubes is an acceptable regimen.

2. Every newborn should receive a single parenteral dose of 0.5–1.0 mg of natural **vitamin K₁ oxide** (phytonadione) within 1 hour of birth to prevent vitamin K–dependent hemorrhagic disease and coagulation disorders.

3. **Metabolic screening.** Prior to discharge, a blood sample should be obtained from every neonate for screening for the persistence of the **hyperphenylalaninemias,** including **phenylketonuria (PKU),** and for congenital **hypothyroidism.**
   **a.** Blood should be drawn from the heel to screen for PKU and the hyperphenylalaninemias as close as possible to the time of discharge. If an infant is discharged early and, as a result, is screened before 24 hours of age, he must be rescreened before the third week of life. Cases may be missed if screening is done too soon after delivery—before there is adequate protein input. Many states require repeat screening at 2 weeks of age.
   **b.** Cord blood at birth or heel blood at discharge may be used to screen for congenital hypothyroidism, and many states require rescreening for this disorder at 2 weeks.
   **c.** In some laboratories, screening is done for other inborn errors such as **homocystinuria, maple syrup urine disease, histidinemia, galactosemia,** and **cystic fibrosis.**

4. **Newborn circumcision** has potential medical benefits and advantages but also has risks and disadvantages. If parents are considering this procedure, benefits and risks should be carefully explained.
   **a. Benefits and advantages.** Properly performed circumcision prevents inflammation of the glans and prepuce of the penis and decreases the incidence of cancer of the penis among adults. It may reduce the incidence of urinary tract infections in male infants.
   **b. Risks and disadvantages.** The most common complications are local infection and bleeding. Newborns undergoing the procedure without anesthesia do experience pain.

**F. Common problems and concerns**

1. **Rashes** are very common during the newborn period. The benign nature of **erythema toxicum, milia,** and **miliaria rubra** has already been discussed (see IV C 3 c).
   **a. Acne neonatorum** resembles the adolescent form of acne vulgaris. It probably results from the hormonal stimulation of sebaceous glands that have not yet involuted to their childhood state of immaturity.
   **b. Transient neonatal pustular melanosis** is found in about 5% of black newborns and is characterized by the presence of papulovesicles at birth, which leave hyperpigmented maculae surrounded by fine white scales.
   **c. Cradle cap** is seborrheic dermatitis involving the scalp.

2. **Conjunctivitis. Ophthalmia neonatorum** is conjunctivitis occurring within the first 4 weeks of life. It may affect between 2% and 8% of all newborns.

a. **Chemical conjunctivitis** that is secondary to administration of silver nitrate drops usually appears within the first day of life and disappears within 3–4 days.

b. **Gonococcal ophthalmia** has decreased in frequency as a result of neonatal prophylaxis, with an annual incidence of 2–3 cases in 10,000 live births. The mean incubation period is about 6 days, with a range of 1–21 days.

c. ***Chlamydia trachomatis*** is the most prevalent identifiable infectious cause of neonatal conjunctivitis, accounting for 20%–30% of cases. The incubation period is 5–14 days.

   (1) Diagnosis is established by examining a Gram-stained conjunctival scraping for basophilic cytoplasmic inclusion bodies, by culturing the organism, or by a rapid test using fluorescent antibody staining or spectrometric evaluation.

   (2) Oral therapy with erythromycin is preferable, as topical therapy often is inadequate.

3. **Weight loss.** A normal newborn may lose 5%–8% of her birthweight during the first 3 days of life. A weight loss of up to 10% is acceptable if the infant's examination and behavior are normal.

4. **Jaundice** is very common among newborns, with 50% having serum bilirubin levels of at least 5–7 mg/dl.

   a. **Physiologic jaundice**—as opposed to pathologic jaundice—is characterized in term newborns by:

      (1) Clinical jaundice appearing after 24 hours

      (2) An increase in the total serum bilirubin concentration of less than 5 mg/dl/day

      (3) A total serum bilirubin concentration of less than 13 mg/dl and direct serum bilirubin concentration of less than 1.5–2.0 mg/dl

      (4) Persistence of clinical jaundice for less than 1 week

   b. **Breast-feeding jaundice** may have either an early onset (i.e., within 3–4 days of birth) or a late onset (i.e., within 4–5 days of birth, with a peak at 10–15 days). Peak bilirubin levels may reach 20–30 mg/dl, although kernicterus has never been reported. Temporarily discontinuing breast-feeding for 24–48 hours typically lowers bilirubin levels.

5. **Breast-feeding problems**

   a. Cracked and painful nipples may be helped by altering the nursing position of the infant, by airing the nipples after nursing, and by using a lanolin-based cream.

   b. Plugged milk ducts may be caused by improper breast emptying, a tight-fitting brassiere, or by sleeping prone.

6. **Vaginal bleeding.** White vaginal secretions as well as actual bleeding may occur in the female infant as a result of fetal stimulation by maternal hormones.

## V. EARLY INFANCY (2 weeks to 6 months)

A. **Interval history.** Parents' questions and concerns should be explored. How is the family functioning since the infant's arrival?

B. **Anticipatory guidance**

1. **Feeding.** Breast milk is the optimal source of infant nutrition, and commercially prepared formula is an acceptable alternative. Whole cow's milk is inappropriate for use during the first 6 months of life. The introduction of solid food should be deferred until the infant is 4–6 months of age.

   a. Infants receiving commercially prepared formula fortified with iron require no vitamin and mineral supplementation, with the possible exception of fluoride. If the formula is prepared with water from a nonfluoridated source, 0.25 mg of fluoride per day is recommended.

   b. Breast-fed infants either not drinking water or receiving nonfluoridated water should also receive 0.25 mg of fluoride per day. During the winter months, breast-fed infants may also benefit from receiving 400 IU of vitamin D per day. Iron supplementation is probably not required during this time because of the increased bioavailability of iron in breast milk.

2. **Safety and injury prevention.** Crib safety, the use of a car seat, and water temperature should be reviewed (see IV B 4). Other topics for review include the following.

   a. **Toys** should be soft and washable, without sharp edges or removable parts, and should be too large to fit within the infant's mouth.

   b. Parents must be alerted to the danger of the infant rolling off elevated surfaces.

   **3. Elimination.** Breast-fed infants tend to have thin, yellow, seedy stools with almost every feeding, while formula-fed infants tend to have stools with more form but less frequency. There is,
   however, considerable variation in elimination patterns.

   **4. Sleep habits.** Most infants sleep through the night by 4 months of age. The danger of a nighttime bottle causing milk-bottle caries should be stressed.

   **5. Immunization.** Benefits and risks should be reviewed at the time of each immunization, and
   any previous reactions or side effects should be documented (see Table 1-1).

   **6. Developmental issues**
   **a. State organization.** The "predictable unpredictability" of the newborn is followed by increasing regularity in demands when the infant is approximately 2 months of age. By this
   time, feeding and sleep schedules may be established.
   **b. Synchrony.** Parent-infant interaction is reciprocal in nature, and a sense of mutual awareness and expectations evolves during the first months of the infant's life.
   **c. Attachment** becomes the main affective issue by 2–3 months of age. By this time, the infant
   both recognizes and uniquely responds to parents.
   **d. Temperament.** The infant's behavioral style becomes increasingly evident during this time.
   The regular patterns, adaptability, and positive mood of the "easy" infant contrast with the
   irregularity, unpredictability, and intensely negative mood of the "difficult" infant. The
   wide range of normal behavior should be stressed.
   **e. Motor skills.** The infant's increasing mobility is usually evident by 4–6 months of age, as
   the infant rolls over, sits with support, grasps a rattle, and places objects within his mouth.

**C. Physical examination.** The following areas deserve special emphasis during the complete examination.

   **1. General appearance** should be noted, including body proportions and the measurement of the
   length, weight, and head circumference of the infant.

   **2. Skin**
   **a.** The infantile form of **atopic dermatitis** usually begins when the infant is 2–6 months of age
   and is characterized by erythema, papules, vesicles, crusting, and pruritus. The rash usually begins on the cheek, forehead, or scalp and extends to the trunk or extremities.
   **b. Infantile seborrheic dermatitis** involving the scalp is termed **cradle cap**.

   **3. Head and neck**
   **a. Sutures** usually are palpable as ridges until the infant is about 6 months of age. The **posterior fontanelle** closes by the second month of age, but the **anterior fontanelle** is patent
   for 1–2 years.
   **b. Vision** may be roughly assessed by noting the infant's response to a light or bright object.
   **c.** Examination of the **tympanic membranes** in infants is facilitated by pulling the auricle down,
   since the canal is directed upward. Mobility of the drum should be evaluated by pneumatic
   otoscopy. Parents should be queried as to their impression of the infant's hearing.
   **d.** Small white patches on the buccal mucosa that cannot be scraped off indicate **candidal
   infection (thrush)**.

   **4. Chest.** Cardiac auscultation during the first 6 months of life may reveal **functional murmurs**
   (i.e., physiologic sounds of turbulence) or murmurs of such disorders as patent ductus arteriosus, atrial septal defect, and ventricular septal defect [see also Ch 11 I B 5 c].

   **5. Abdomen. Umbilical hernias** are commonly noted in infants, often with **diastasis** of the rectus
   muscles.

   **6.** A **hydrocele** is frequently found during examination of the **male genitalia** during infancy. The
   presence of an accompanying hernia may be difficult to ascertain. Many hydroceles spontaneously resolve by the end of the first year.

   **7.** The **hips** of all infants must be carefully examined for **congenital dislocation,** even if the newborn examination was normal.

   **8. Neurologic examination.** Primitive reflexes elicited during the first months of life include
   Moro, grasping, and tonic neck reflexes. By the time the infant is 4–6 months of age, these
   reflexes diminish.

**D. Developmental assessment** is performed by a combination of direct observation and parent interview. Wide variations in normal development are the rule. The significance of an infant's failure to achieve a milestone must be interpreted with caution.

    **1. Vision.** Infants follow with their eyes first to and then past the midline by the age of 2 months, and then to a full 180° by the age of 4 months. From the newborn period on, infants fix transiently on faces and inanimate objects.

    **2. Hearing.** By 2 months of age, infants localize sounds by turning their head and eyes.

    **3. Language.** Vocalization during the first few months includes bubbles and coos. By 4–6 months of age, infants have begun to squeal.

    **4. Gross motor skills.** By 2 months of age, the prone infant may lift her head to 45°. The 4-month-old infant may be rolling over and sitting with support. The 6-month-old infant may be sitting alone and bearing some weight on her legs when held upright on a table with some support.

    **5. Fine motor skills.** The 4-month-old infant will typically grasp a rattle. By 6 months, the infant may reach out for a toy and even transfer an object such as a block from one hand to the other.

    **6. Personal-social interactions.** By 2 months of age, many infants smile responsively.

**E. Procedures**

    **1. Metabolic screening.** Some states require repeat screening at 2 weeks of age for PKU and hyperphenylalaninemias as well as congenital hypothyroidism (see IV E 3).

    **2. Immunizations.** Three doses of the DTP vaccine and 2 doses of the oral, attenuated poliovirus vaccine containing poliovirus types 1, 2, and 3 (TOPV) are routinely administered during the first 6 months of life (see II A 5 e). Recently, Hib conjugate vaccines (e.g., diphtheria CRM 197 protein conjugate; an outer membrane protein complex of *Neisseria meningitidis* conjugate) were licensed for use during infancy. Administration schedules vary, depending on the preparation used.

**F. Common problems and concerns**

    **1. Eye drainage,** typically from one eye, may indicate a blocked tear duct, or **dacryostenosis**. Swelling, erythema, and induration around the lacrimal sac may indicate an acquired infection, or **dacryocystitis**.

    **2. Diaper rash.** Common varieties of diaper dermatitis include the following.
        **a. Generic** diaper rash is erythematous, spares the skin folds, and produces dry, wrinkled skin.
        **b. Candidal** rash involves the deep skin folds and is characterized by satellite lesions and bright red erosions.
        **c.** The **nodulo-ulcerative** variety is suggested by nodules with central ulcers on the body prominences.
        **d. Impetigo** may involve any site, although usually not the deep skin folds.
        **e. Infantile seborrheic dermatitis** starts as erythema and satellite lesions in the diaper area and typically spreads to involve the face, scalp, and flexural areas.
        **f. Intertrigo** is a poorly understood dermatitis that is characterized by a white or yellow exudate involving the deep skin folds.

    **3. Colic.** Fussing is normal infant behavior. Many infants exhibit intermittent, unexplained crying, usually beginning in the first month and typically occurring in the late afternoon and evening hours. During this time, the infant is difficult to console. Formula intolerance, constipation, teething, illness, and so forth usually do not explain episodes of colic. Spontaneous resolution usually occurs by the age of 3 months.

    **4. Constipation.** Infants commonly may have a bowel movement only once every several days. Unless stools are hard and pellet-like, accompanied by significant infant distress, parents should be reassured. Few infants become constipated due to an iron-containing formula.

    **5. Teething.** Infants may begin teething by 6 months of age. Excessive drooling, rhinorrhea, mild diarrhea, irritability, and decreased appetite may be associated with teething. High fevers should not be attributed to teething.

## VI. LATE INFANCY (6 months to 2 years)

**A. Interval history.** Parents' questions and concerns should be explored.

1. Have parents returned to work outside the home?

2. What are the arrangements for child care?

**B. Anticipatory guidance**

1. **Feeding**
   a. By the end of the first year, a schedule of 3 meals per day is feasible.
   b. Table foods should be introduced slowly, adding one new food every several days while observing any adverse reactions. With increasing fine motor control, finger foods should be encouraged. Foods should be prepared without added salt.
   c. Weaning from bottle to cup should commence by the end of the first year. Beginning use of a spoon is possible by the age of 15 months.
   d. With physical growth slowing by the end of the first year of life, a normal decrease in appetite occurs.

2. **Safety and injury prevention**
   a. With increasing mobility, potential dangers for the child include stairways, open windows, electric sockets, hanging tablecloths, and electric cords. Proper use of a playpen, high chair, expandable gates, and covers for wall sockets reduces dangers.
   b. When the infant reaches 18–20 pounds, use of a forward-facing toddler car seat is appropriate.
   c. Due to the possible danger of accidental ingestion of poisonous substances, parents should obtain syrup of ipecac and the phone number of the poison control center.

3. **Sleep habits.** If night awakening does occur it is recommended that the child not be brought into the parents' bed nor offered a nighttime bottle. Rather, after the child's safety is ensured, he should be put back to sleep in a loving but firm manner (see VI F 2).

4. **Toilet training** should be child-oriented and deferred until at least 18 months of age. Signs of readiness include:
   a. A desire to please the parents
   b. Pleasure in imitating adults
   c. A desire to develop autonomy and to master primitive impulses
   d. Adequate motor development, including the ability to sit and walk

5. **Dental care.** Following eruption, teeth should be cleaned. Initially, gauze or a soft cloth may be used with the substitution of a soft brush during the second year of life.

6. **Immunization** (see II A 5 e; V B 5; and Table 1-1)

7. **Developmental issues**
   a. **Autonomy.** The struggle between dependence and independence now becomes the main affective issue. Manifestations may include the infant's refusal of passive spoon feedings and the appearance of temper tantrums. The toddler continually explores the limits of the environment. By 15–18 months of age, the child's negativism and resistant behavior dramatically reflect the struggle for autonomy.
   b. **Temperament** remains highly discernible and may allow parents to predict the child's responses to certain circumstances.
   c. **Attachment.** Behaviors reflecting the continued importance of attachment include clinging to parents, night awakening, and stranger and separation anxiety.
   d. **Motor skills.** Further refinement of motor skills parallels the development of autonomy. Increased motor development renders the environment a potentially greater threat to the child's safety.
   e. **Cognitive development**
      (1) **Object permanence** is reflected by the infant's ability that develops around 9–10 months of age to uncover a hidden toy.
      (2) Also around 9–10 months, the infant's interest in a wind-up toy relates to **an understanding of causality**.
      (3) Around 18 months of age, the toddler is able to represent mentally an object or action that is not perceptually present. Symbolic play is now possible, as the child is capable of **thought**.

**C. Physical examination.** The following areas deserve special emphasis during the complete examination.

1. **General appearance** (see V C 1)

2. **Ears.** Given the high incidence of middle ear disease that occurs during this age period, careful inspection of the tympanic membranes must include color, landmarks, and mobility as assessed by pneumatic otoscopy. Tympanometry may be used to detect middle ear effusions.

3. **Teeth.** Decay, particularly involving the upper central and lateral incisors, suggests milk-bottle caries resulting from inappropriate bedtime practices. Mottled, pitted teeth may suggest excessive fluoride ingestion.

4. **Genitalia.** If a hydrocele has not resolved by the age of 2 years, surgical referral is indicated.

5. **Extremities**
   a. As infants begin to cruise and then walk, torsional deformities may become evident. **In-toeing** may result from increased femoral anteversion, internal tibial torsion, or metatarsus adductus.
      (1) Normally, external rotation of the hips is close to 90° during infancy, resulting in out-toeing during early weight-bearing. Later, internal and external rotation become equal. **Increased femoral anteversion** resulting in in-toeing typically improves with age.
      (2) In-toeing may be due to **internal tibial torsion,** which is assessed using the "thigh-foot angle" (i.e., the angular difference between the axis of the thigh and foot as viewed directly down with the knee flexed at 90°).
      (3) **Metatarsus adductus** may be overlooked at birth and may not be detected until later infancy. When the foot is flexible, spontaneous resolution is the rule. A **rigid varus** deformity may require casting.
   b. Fat pads occurring normally under the arch of the feet create an impression of **flatfeet** during the early toddler years.

**D. Developmental assessment**

1. **Language.** By 9–10 months of age, most infants vocalize "mama" and "dada," although not specifically with reference to a parent; such specific use typically occurs between 12 and 15 months of age. By 18 months of age, toddlers will use several new words and are able to point to parts of the body such as eyes, mouth, and toes (see VII D 1 for comparison) when they are named. During the latter part of the second year of life, new words are constantly added, culminating at the age of 2 years in the use of pronouns and the ability to combine two words in short sentences.

2. **Gross motor skills.** By 9–10 months of age, most infants are able to sit alone well, sustain weight with their legs when pulled to a standing position, and rock and creep when prone. Over the next several months, crawling, cruising, and then walking occur, as the infant becomes a toddler. By 18 months, the toddler may descend stairs unaided. The 2-year-old child can walk up stairs unaided, and kick a ball.

3. **Fine motor skills.** By 9–10 months of age, infants can transfer an object such as a block from hand to hand and feed themselves finger food, such as crackers. By 15 months, a thumb-finger (pincer) grasp allows manipulation of small objects and food. The toddler may bang together toys held in each hand and may scribble if offered a crayon and paper. By 2 years of age, most children can stack four blocks and hold a cup securely.

4. **Personal-social interactions.** With increasing language skills, the toddler is able to indicate wants without crying. The child enjoys playing simple games such as peek-a-boo.

**E. Procedures**

1. **Immunizations** routinely administered from age 6 months through 2 years include the measles-mumps-rubella (MMR) and the DTP, TOPV, and Hib conjugate vaccine booster doses (see II A 5 e and Table 1-1).

2. **Anemia.** Screening for anemia should be done near the end of the first year of life, since depleted iron stores may result in iron deficiency anemia. Hemoglobin, hematocrit, red blood cell indices, or free erythrocyte protoporphyrin may be measured.

3. **Lead poisoning.** For children at environmental risk for lead intoxication, screening should be performed by fingerstick blood lead or free erythrocyte protoporphyrin determination (see Ch 2 IX E 5).

4. **Tuberculosis.** Due to a significant decline in the incidence of tuberculosis within the United States, the value of periodically screening all children with a tuberculin test is uncertain.
   a. For low-risk groups, acceptable alternatives include performing no screening or administering a multiple puncture test containing liquid old tuberculin (OT) every several years.
   b. For high-risk groups (e.g., children residing in inner city environments), the intracutaneous (Mantoux) test containing purified protein derivative (PPD) is preferred.

## F. Common problems and concerns

1. **Temper tantrums** are a normal manifestation of the toddler's struggle for autonomy while he is still dependent upon adults. Attempting to distract the child or ignoring his behavior after insuring the child's safety are reasonable approaches to a temper tantrum.

2. **Night crying.** Many infants 6–12 months of age abruptly awaken at night and cry, despite a previously good sleep pattern. Such awakening typically resolves within 1–4 weeks if parents provide brief positive interactions and avoid reinforcing the crying by picking up or feeding the child.

3. **Stranger and separation anxiety** are typical manifestations of attachment during the latter half of the first year of life.

4. Parents are frequently concerned about their child's **poor appetite**. In actuality, a decrease in appetite should be anticipated, since the child's slower physical growth demands fewer calories; in addition the child may refuse passive spoon feedings with increasing independence. The child's basic needs are met by a daily intake of a pint of milk, an ounce of fruit juice or a piece of fruit, 2 ounces of iron-containing protein, and possibly a multivitamin for the "picky" eater.

5. **Teething** (see V F 5)

## VII. THE PRESCHOOL YEARS (2–5 years)

**A. Interval history.** By the time that the child is 3–4 years old, a separate dialogue should be established with him during the visit.

## B. Anticipatory guidance

1. **Safety and injury prevention.** Topics for discussion include traffic and playground safety and the danger of serious bites from pets.

2. **Toilet training.** Maintaining a child-oriented approach is important (see VI B 4). Allowing the child to sit undressed on a potty-chair and dropping soiled diapers into the chair's bowl are helpful.

3. **Dental care.** The child should be instructed in the use of a toothbrush with a thin ribbon of toothpaste. Fluoride in a dose of 0.5 mg/day is administered to 2-year-olds requiring fluoride supplementation. The dosage increases to 1.0 mg/day at 3 years. By the age of 3 years, a referral for a dental check-up is indicated.

4. **Immunizations** (see V B 5 and Table 1-1)

5. **Play.** The 2-year-old child is not capable of sharing and engages in solitary, parallel play. During successive years, an interest in and the ability to engage in interactive play with peers emerge.

6. **Television.** Observing violence on television is believed to cause children to be more willing to harm others and to play more aggressively. Thus, monitoring a child's television viewing is appropriate.

7. **School readiness.** Attitudes concerning separation and readiness for school should be discussed with the parents and child.

8. **Developmental issues**
   a. **Autonomy.** Problematic behavior reflects the child's continuing negativism and may be encountered during such activities as eating, toilet training, and tooth care as well as in play groups.
   b. **Attachment.** The toddler's problems with separation continue to reflect the importance of attachment. As school entry approaches, the child's ability to separate is increasingly important.
   c. **Temperament.** The consistency of a child's behavior allows parents to predict the child's responses to certain situations. For example, responses to school entry may differ greatly for the "slow-to-warm-up" child as opposed to the "difficult" child.
   d. **Impulse control.** Wide variability in impulse control among children is apparent. Increasing demands are placed upon the child as school entry approaches.
   e. **Motor skills.** The "motor-minded" toddler enjoys rough-and-tumble play, whereas more passive activities are enjoyed by the calm child.
   f. **Cognitive development.** This age period is the preoperational period of cognitive development, and mastery of language is the major cognitive issue. The 2-year-old's incessant asking of "what's this" and "what's that" is followed by "why do I have to" at the age of 4 years. Rational thinking is not yet possible.
   g. **Gender identity.** The concept of gender as fixed and stable emerges around 4–5 years of age, reflecting the child's ability to establish a stable definition of physical concepts.
   h. **Peer interactions.** At 3–4 years of age, sharing and interactive play emerge. Sibling rivalry is typical at this age. As school entry nears, values and attitudes of those outside the family, particularly a child's peers, become increasingly important.

C. **Physical examination.** Areas deserving special emphasis during the complete examination include the following.

1. **Ears** (see VI C 2)

2. **Teeth.** The number and condition of the primary teeth and the type of occlusion should be noted.

3. **Blood pressure.** With the increasing cooperation of the child, around the age of 3 years, blood pressure measurements become routine.

4. **Extremities.** With ambulation, torsional deformities of the legs and flatfeet may be noted.
   a. **Increased femoral anteversion** is a relatively common cause of in-toeing in children 3–7 years of age.
   b. **Flatfeet.** Children who have a flatfoot when standing but an arch when sitting may benefit from an arch support. Constitutional flatfeet, which are flat whether or not they are bearing weight, do not benefit from correction.

D. **Developmental assessment**

1. **Language.** By the age of 3–4 years, children are able to point to such parts of the body as their waist, knee, nose, and heel as well as respond to questions with their name, age, and address.

2. **Gross motor skills.** The 3-year-old child may pedal a tricycle, while the 4-year-old child can typically heel walk a distance of 6 feet without difficulty.

3. **Fine motor skills.** By the age of 3 years, many children can imitate a vertical line and copy a circle. Over the next 2 years, the child masters a task of finger opposition in which thumb and forefinger are rapidly opposed; copies a cross, square, and diamond; and draws a person with three parts.

4. **Personal-social interactions.** The 3-year-old child begins to share playthings and begins to play interactive games. By the time of school entry, the child should easily separate from the mother.

E. **Procedures**

1. **Immunizations.** Children routinely receive booster doses of the DTP and TOPV at the age of 4–5 years (see Table 1-1 and II A 5 e).

2. **Vision screening.** By the age of 3–4 years, objective screening of visual acuity is possible using pictures, the "E" test, or other measures. Children's acuity should be 20/40 or better by the age of 3–4 years and 20/30 by the age of 5 years.

3. **Hearing** can be screened objectively at about the age of 4 years using a pure tone stimulus. Screening should be repeated every 2 years.

4. Once bladder control has been established, a **urinalysis** may be obtained every several years. Although its value as a screening test is uncertain, the urinalysis is relatively inexpensive and easy to perform.

5. **Tuberculosis screening** (see VI E 4)

6. **Screening for anemia** is typically performed prior to school entry (see VI E 2).

7. **Cholesterol testing.** The role of universal cholesterol screening is controversial. At present, screening of all children is not recommended. Rather, testing of children older than 2 years of age who have a family history of hyperlipidemia or early myocardial infarction is suggested (see Ch 16 II A 3). Such a strategy will not identify all children at risk.

**F. Common problems and concerns**

1. **Separation anxiety** (see VII B 8 b)

2. **Sibling rivalry** (see VII B 8 h)

3. **Night awakening** (see VI F 2). Parents must be careful not to reinforce the child's night awakening and crying by feeding the child or allowing the child to sleep in their bed.

4. **Stuttering.** Intermittent difficulty in producing a smooth flow of speech may begin 1 or 2 years after a child learns to speak. Between 2 and 5 years of age, many children experience normal dysfluency, which is characterized by repetitions of whole words and phrases. In contrast, stuttering is characterized by partial-word repetitions; multiple rather than single repetitions; irregular, rapid, or abrupt repetitions; and a high frequency of nonfluency. By late childhood, many children have recovered from stuttering.

## VIII. THE SCHOOL-AGE YEARS (5–12 years)

**A. Interval history.** The greater portion of the interview should now be conducted directly with the child.

**B. Anticipatory guidance**

1. **School progress.** Asking both parent and child about school performance is important.

2. **Safety and injury prevention.** Topics for review include the proper use of seat belts in the car, bicycle safety, protective equipment for sports, and water safety.

3. **Sex education.** With puberty approaching, topics to be discussed with parents include their attitudes toward sex education and plans for discussing sexuality with their children.

4. **Health habits.** With increasing autonomy and separation, the child is making decisions and developing his own health habits. The child should be encouraged to make wise decisions about diet, exercise, safety, and so forth.

5. **Developmental issues**
   a. **Autonomy.** The challenging of limits precedes the ability to make wise decisions and thus requires parental limit setting. By around 8 years of age, the child declares her independence by transferring allegiance to a peer group. Allowing the child to assume increasing responsibility may lessen family conflict. By early adolescence, the drive for autonomy culminates in the child's challenging long-standing beliefs.
   b. **Peer interaction.** Growing peer influence may represent a challenge to family values. Increasing segregation among peers occurs. The development of a "best friend" is a milestone in interpersonal growth.
   c. **Cognitive development**
      (1) **Concrete operations.** Around the age of 8 years, the child is able to focus on multiple aspects of a problem, establish hierarchies, use logic, and see the viewpoints of others.

       **(2) Formal operations.** By 12 years, the ability to use hypothetical and abstract reasoning emerges.

    **d. Physical development.** The physical changes heralding the onset of puberty may cause concern on the part of the parents or the child.

**C. Physical examination.** Areas deserving special emphasis during the complete examination include the following.

    **1. Skin.** With the onset of puberty, acne may develop (see Ch 4 VIII A).

    **2. Teeth.** The secondary teeth begin to erupt when the child is about 7–8 years of age.

    **3. Genitalia and breast development.** Documenting pubertal changes is important (see Ch 4 II C).

    **4. Back.** Screening for scoliosis is necessary during the rapid growth of puberty (see Ch 4 IX A).

**D. Developmental assessment.** School performance and classroom behavior are important indicators of developmental status.

    **1. Language** delays may result in difficulties with reading, spelling, and writing.

    **2. Gross motor skills.** Increasingly complex tasks are mastered such as skipping, hopping on one foot, and standing heel-toe with the eyes closed.

    **3. Fine motor skills.** The pencil grasp of the 5-year-old child allows writing and drawing, while the 6-year-old child is able to tie shoelaces. Increasing dexterity is indicated by mastery of tasks such as rapid sequential finger opposition and crumbling a piece of paper into a ball with one hand.

    **4. Visual motor performance** may be assessed by asking the child to draw a figure that is appropriate to the developmental age of the child.

**E. Procedures**

    **1. Vision screening** (see VII E 2). Objective screening every 2 years is recommended.

    **2. Hearing screening** (see VII E 3). Objective screening using a pure tone stimulus is recommended at the beginning and end of the school-age years and whenever history suggests a possible problem.

    **3. Urinalysis** (see VII E 4)

    **4. Tuberculosis screening** (see VI E 4)

    **5. Immunizations.** A booster dose of the MMR vaccine is recommended at 11–12 years of age [administration at age 5 is an acceptable alternative (see II A 5 e and Table 1-1)].

    **6. Cholesterol testing** (see VII E 7)

**F. Common problems and concerns**

    **1. Acting-out behavior.** With the child striving for independence, some challenging of limits is likely. With increasing peer influence, confrontations with authority figures (i.e., teachers, parents) occur.

    **2. Separation anxiety.** If the child is unsuccessful in securely achieving independence from home and family, school avoidance and school phobia may become problems (see Ch 3 III C).

    **3. Recurrent pains.** During the middle childhood years, children may have recurrent somatic complaints such as headache, abdominal pain, and limb pain. Pains of this sort typically have no clear-cut organic etiology. They are generally the consequence of environmental, temperamental, and constitutional factors (see Ch 3 VI).

    **4. Poor school performance.** School-related problems often are brought to the attention of the pediatric health care provider. The role of the provider includes helping the parents understand special education programs and services and the law requiring that school systems evaluate children experiencing difficulties in both learning and behavior. The pediatrician should also provide the names of local resources for help (see Ch 3 III A, B).

**IX. ADOLESCENCE** (see Ch 4). The pediatric health care provider must encourage the adolescent to express any concerns and to ask any questions, particularly those that he does not feel comfortable asking parents or friends. The pediatrician must be nonjudgmental in order to allow the adolescent to discuss emotion-laden topics.

## BIBLIOGRAPHY

American Academy of Pediatrics Committee on Standards of Child Health Care: *Standards of Child Health Care,* 4th edition. Evanston, IL, American Academy of Pediatrics, 1982.

Brazelton TB: Anticipatory guidance. *Pediatr Clin North Am* 22:533–544, 1975.

Casey P, Sharp M, Loda F: Child-health supervision for children under 2 years of age: a review of its content and effectiveness. *J Pediatr* 95:1–9, 1979.

Telzrow RW: Anticipatory guidance in pediatric practice. *J Cont Educ Pediatr* 20:14–27, 1978.

## STUDY QUESTIONS

**Directions:** Each of the numbered items or incomplete statements in this section is followed by answers or by completions of the statement. Select the **one** lettered answer or completion that is **best** in each case.

1. Children are routinely immunized against all of the following diseases EXCEPT

(A) pertussis
(B) pneumococcal infections
(C) mumps
(D) *Hemophilus influenzae* type b infections
(E) diphtheria

2. Which of the following physical characteristics does NOT suggest prematurity in a 1-day-old baby?

(A) A prominent diastasis of the rectus muscles
(B) Lanugo
(C) A thick layer of vernix
(D) Absent breast buds
(E) Scant ear cartilage

3. While examining a 2-day-old infant, small vesicles on an erythematous base are noted on the infant's face and chest. Wright's stain of the lesions reveals sheets of eosinophils. The diagnosis of this rash is

(A) miliaria rubra
(B) milia
(C) neonatal acne
(D) erythema toxicum
(E) neonatal pustular melanosis

4. A healthy newborn boy is discharged home with his mother at 24 hours of age. When he is seen in the pediatric office at 2 weeks of age, which of the following procedures must be performed?

(A) Prophylaxis for gonococcal ophthalmia
(B) Administration of vitamin $K_1$ oxide
(C) Blood sampling for PKU
(D) Blood sampling for congenital hypothyroidism
(E) Urine sampling for galactosemia

5. The most common explanation for colic in an infant is

(A) formula intolerance
(B) otitis media
(C) constipation
(D) teething
(E) none of the above

6. The preoperational period of cognitive development is most important for the development of

(A) object permanence
(B) causality
(C) language
(D) logic
(E) hypothetical reasoning

7. The concrete operations period of cognitive development is characterized by the ability to perform all of the following skills EXCEPT

(A) focusing on multiple aspects of a problem
(B) using hypothetical reasoning
(C) using logic
(D) establishing hierarchies
(E) appreciating the viewpoint of others

8. Findings that may be attributed to teething in an infant include all of the following EXCEPT

(A) rhinorrhea
(B) diarrhea
(C) decreased appetite
(D) irritability
(E) a fever of 39° C (102.2° F)

9. An 18-month-old child is found to have dental decay in the upper central and lateral incisors. This is most suggestive of

(A) excessive fluoride ingestion
(B) milk-bottle caries
(C) tetracycline exposure
(D) insufficient fluoride intake
(E) failure to brush the child's teeth properly

| | | |
|---|---|---|
| 1-B | 4-C | 7-B |
| 2-A | 5-E | 8-E |
| 3-D | 6-C | 9-B |

10. Readiness for toilet training includes all of the following signs EXCEPT

(A) the ability to sit and walk
(B) the achievement of impulse control
(C) a desire to please parents
(D) pleasure in imitating adults
(E) a desire to master primitive impulses

11. At the time of the 9-month well-child visit, the American Academy of Pediatrics recommends screening of all infants for

(A) lead poisoning
(B) tuberculosis
(C) urinary tract infection
(D) anemia
(E) hyperphenylalaninemia

**Directions:** Each question below contains four suggested answers of which **one or more** is correct. Choose the answer

    **A**  if **1, 2, and 3** are correct
    **B**  if **1 and 3** are correct
    **C**  if **2 and 4** are correct
    **D**  if **4** is correct
    **E**  if **1, 2, 3, and 4** are correct

12. Measurements to be recorded at all well-child visits include

(1) height/length
(2) head circumference
(3) weight
(4) blood pressure

13. Developmental issues appropriate for discussion at the 12-month well-child visit include

(1) state organization
(2) synchrony
(3) gender identity
(4) attachment

14. As infants begin to cruise and then walk, in-toeing may become apparent. Causes for in-toeing include

(1) increased femoral anteversion
(2) metatarsus adductus
(3) internal tibial torsion
(4) genu recurvatum

10-B        13-D
11-D        14-A
12-B

**Directions:** Each group of items in this section consists of lettered options followed by a set of numbered items. For each item, select the **one** lettered option that is most closely associated with it. Each lettered option may be selected once, more than once, or not at all.

**Questions 15–18**

For each aspect of physical examination, select the age period during which this should be emphasized.

(A) Newborn
(B) Early infancy (2 weeks to 6 months)
(C) Late infancy (6 months to 2 years)
(D) Preschool years (2–5 years)
(E) School-age years (5–12 years)

15. Measurement of the thigh-foot angle to determine tibial torsion

16. Elicitation of the tonic neck reflex

17. Examination of the permanent dentition for decay and occlusion

18. Fundoscopic determination of a bilateral red reflex

**Questions 19–22**

Particular types of vaccines are used to immunize children against specific diseases. Match the disease with the type of vaccine that is used in immunization.

(A) Killed, whole organism
(B) Live, attenuated strain
(C) Live, virulent strain
(D) Specific portions of organism
(E) Toxoid

19. Rubella

20. Pertussis

21. *Hemophilus influenzae* type b infections

22. Diphtheria

| | | |
|---|---|---|
| 15-C | 18-A | 21-D |
| 16-B | 19-B | 22-E |
| 17-E | 20-A | |

## ANSWERS AND EXPLANATIONS

**1. The answer is B** *[II A 5 e].*
Vaccines routinely recommended for all children include diphtheria, pertussis, tetanus, polio, measles, mumps, rubella, and *Hemophilus influenzae* type b (Hib). Other vaccines, such as those for pneumococcal infections and influenza, are administered only to certain high-risk groups. Factors determining the usefulness of a vaccine include the risk of the disease, benefits of prevention, efficacy, safety, cost, availability, alternatives to prevention, and the special needs of certain groups of individuals.

**2. The answer is A** *[IV C 1; Table 1-4].*
Findings suggesting prematurity include a thick layer of vernix, poorly defined incurving of the pinna with scant ear cartilage, smooth soles with few anterior creases, thin skin with short nails, lanugo, testes that are palpable in the inguinal canal, widely separated and small labia majora with a prominent clitoris, soft skull bones, a hypotonic posture at rest, and absent breast buds. Diastasis of the rectus muscles is a normal variant found in many term infants. Physical characteristics of the newborn are useful in estimating gestational age.

**3. The answer is D** *[IV C 3 c, F 1 a–b].*
Benign rashes often are noted during the newborn period. Common rashes include milia, miliaria rubra, erythema toxicum, neonatal acne, and transient neonatal pustular melanosis. The finding of eosinophils when the drainage from small vesicles is stained is diagnostic for erythema toxicum. These lesions are not of infectious etiology and require no treatment.

**4. The answer is C** *[IV E 1–3].*
Several procedures are routinely performed following delivery. Antibiotic prophylaxis for gonococcal ophthalmia and administration of vitamin $K_1$ oxide to prevent hemorrhagic disease of the newborn are performed immediately after birth. Blood sampling for congenital hypothyroidism may be performed using cord blood at birth or heel blood at discharge. If blood sampling for phenylketonuria (PKU) is performed before 24 hours of age as a result of early discharge, rescreening must be performed before the third week of life. Cases may otherwise be missed, since such early screening is performed before adequate protein intake. In some states, rescreening at 2 weeks for PKU is required for all newborns.

**5. The answer is E** *[V F 3].*
Many infants display intermittent, unexplained crying, typically beginning in the first month of life and occurring during the late afternoon and evening hours. Formula intolerance, constipation, teething, or illness usually do not account for such episodes. Spontaneous resolution by the age of 3 months usually occurs.

**6. The answer is C** *[VII B 8 f].*
During the preoperational period, the major cognitive issue is the mastery of language. Rational and logical thinking are not yet possible. Object permanence and causality are cognitive milestones during the sensory-motor period, which is around 9–10 months of age.

**7. The answer is B** *[VIII B 5 c 1].*
Around 8 years of age, the child enters the concrete operations period of cognitive development. At this stage, the child is able to focus on multiple aspects of a problem, establish hierarchies, use logic, and see the viewpoints of others. The ability to use hypothetical reasoning does not emerge until the formal operations period, around the age of 12.

**8. The answer is E** *[V F 5].*
Teething may begin by the age of 6 months and may be associated with excessive drooling, rhinorrhea, mild diarrhea, irritability, and decreased appetite. Whether teething may also be accompanied by fever is controversial. However, high fevers should not be attributed to teething.

**9. The answer is B** *[VI C 3].*
Inappropriate bedtime practices may result in several problems. The child who falls asleep with a propped bottle in his mouth may be predisposed to otitis media due to reflux through the eustachian tube. The bathing of teeth in milk while the child sleeps will cause decay. The upper central and lateral incisors are particularly susceptible, since the lower teeth are protected by the tongue.

**10. The answer is B** *[VI B 4]*.
Signs of readiness for toilet training include the child's desire to please parents, pleasure in imitating adults, desire to develop autonomy and to master primitive impulses, and adequate motor development with the ability to sit and walk. Achievement of impulse control is typically not accomplished until the age of school entry. Toilet training should be child-oriented and generally deferred until at least 18 months of age.

**11. The answer is D** *[VI E 2]*.
Around 9 months of age, depending on nutritional status, depleted body iron stores may result in anemia. Thus, screening for anemia by measuring hemoglobin, hematocrit, red blood cell indices, or free erythrocyte porphyrin is recommended. Screening for tuberculosis with a liquid old tuberculin (OT) multipuncture test is recommended at the age of 12 months and every 2–3 years thereafter. Urinalysis may be performed during the first year of life or deferred until toilet training is completed. Screening for lead poisoning should be performed at the discretion of the pediatrician, depending on the child's risk status. Screening for hyperphenylalaninemia must be completed by 2 weeks of age.

**12. The answer is B (1, 3)** *[II A 5 a]*.
During all health maintenance visits, height (length during infancy) and weight should be recorded on an appropriate growth chart. Head circumference should be measured during the first year of life. Measurements of blood pressure usually are feasible for children who are 3 years old and older.

**13. The answer is D (4)** *[VI B 7]*.
At the 12-month visit, appropriate developmental issues to discuss with parents include the toddler's struggle for autonomy and independence, the highly noticeable nature of the child's temperament, the continued importance of attachment, and the further refinement of the child's motor skills. Cognitive issues include object permanence and causality. State organization and synchrony are pertinent issues during early infancy, while gender identity is an important issue during the preschool years.

**14. The answer is A (1, 2, 3)** *[VI C 5]*.
In-toeing may occur from increased femoral anteversion, internal tibial torsion, or metatarsus adductus. Normally, external rotation of the hips is close to 90° during infancy, resulting in out-toeing during early weight bearing. Increased femoral anteversion resulting in in-toeing typically improves with age, as does in-toeing due to internal tibial torsion. Although flexible metatarsus adductus typically resolves spontaneously, a rigid deformity may require casting. Genu recurvatum refers to congenital dislocation of the knee and is not associated with in-toeing.

**15–18. The answers are: 15-C** *[VI C 5 a (2)]*, **16-B** *[V C 8]*, **17-E** *[VIII C 2]*, **18-A** *[IV C 4 d]*.
As the toddler begins to cruise and then walk, torsional deformities may become evident. In-toeing may result from increased femoral anteversion, metatarsus adductus, or internal tibial torsion. The latter may be measured by the thigh-foot angle (i.e., the angular difference between the axis of the thigh and foot as viewed directly down with the knee flexed at 90°).

Primitive reflexes (e.g., the Moro, grasp, and tonic neck reflexes) indicate the integrity of the central nervous system (CNS). In a term infant, such reflexes may be elicited within the first months of life, and they disappear around the age of 6 months. The absence or distortion of these reflexes may suggest prematurity or damage to the CNS. Similarly, persistence of such primitive reflexes beyond early infancy suggests neurologic dysfunction.

From the time of the initial eruption of the primary dentition, the teeth should be examined for decay and occlusion. Children should be referred for their initial dental examination around the age of 3 years. Secondary (permanent) dentition typically erupts around the age of 7–8 years.

Detailed fundoscopic examination typically is not performed during childhood unless it is specifically indicated. However, the determination of a red reflex bilaterally is an important part of the newborn examination because the presence of a red reflex excludes the presence of significant lens opacities or retinoblastoma.

**19–22. The answers are: 19-B** *[II A 5 e (2) (b)]*, **20-A** *[II A 5 e (2) (a)]*, **21-D** *[II A 5 e (2) (a)]*, **22-E** *[II A 5 e (2) (a)]*.
Attenuated strains of live viruses are used to prepare a number of vaccines, including polio, measles, mumps, and rubella. These vaccines tend to simulate natural immunity and require relatively few exposures to result in prolonged immunity. For example, two administrations of the measles-mumps-rubella (MMR) vaccine at the ages of 15 months and 11–12 years probably result in a life-long immunity.

Children are immunized against pertussis with a killed, whole organism vaccine. This type of vaccine is less effective than either natural disease or live, attenuated strain vaccines in producing immunity. Thus, multiple early exposures and periodic booster doses are required to maintain immunity. In addition, side effects and adverse reactions are common because the whole organism is administered rather than specific components of the organism.

Specific poly- or oligosaccharide portions of the capsules of organisms are used to immunize children against infections caused by the pneumococcus and *H. influenzae* type b. These vaccines produce immunity against certain strains of the organism that share antigenic similarities. The longevity of this immunity is uncertain.

Toxoids, or modified toxins, are used to immunize children against diphtheria and tetanus. These vaccines are less effective in producing immunity than either natural disease or live, attenuated strain vaccines. Multiple exposures during early infancy are required with periodic booster doses to maintain immunity.

# 2
# Injuries and Poisonings
Leonard I. Banco

## I. GENERAL CONSIDERATIONS

### A. Nomenclature

1. **Injury.** There are no basic scientific distinctions between injury and disease; therefore, injuries and poisonings should be viewed as being no more random or unexpected than disease. Use of the term **accident**—which implies unpredictability or fate—is gradually being replaced by the use of the term **injury,** which more accurately reflects the nature of the problem. Most childhood injuries are unintentional; however, intentional (inflicted) causes (e.g., abuse, homicide) must also be considered (see I E).

2. The **agent-host-environment model,** which is often used in reference to the epidemiology of infectious disease, can also be used to describe childhood injuries.
   a. The **agent** is the type of energy that causes damage, including:
      (1) **Kinetic energy** in collisions or falls
      (2) **Thermal energy** in burns
      (3) **Chemical energy** in poisonings
   b. The **host** is the injured child, who has particular attributes that can be used for description and categorization, such as:
      (1) **Age**
      (2) **Sex**
      (3) **Developmental level**
   c. The **environment** is the situation in which the injury occurs and comprises the:
      (1) **Physical environment,** such as the playground, automobile, or medicine cabinet
      (2) **Social environment,** such as familial stress and disorganization or parental absence

### B. Epidemiology

1. **Injuries** are recognized as **the leading cause of death in childhood** over the past 40 years.
   a. In the United States, over 20,000 children, ranging in age from birth to 19 years, die each year from injuries, for a death rate of 30.3 in 100,000.
   b. The number of childhood deaths from injuries is four times the number of childhood deaths due to any other cause.

2. **Death and morbidity** are two criteria by which the significance of childhood injuries can be measured. Although death is the worst outcome, injuries cause widespread morbidity, which results in the need for medical care as well as in the inability to perform normal daily activities.
   a. It is estimated that for each child who dies because of injury, 30 children are admitted to the hospital.
      (1) Each year in the United States, an estimated 600,000 children are hospitalized for injuries.
      (2) Injuries account for 17% of all hospitalizations of children, compared to 8% of hospitalizations of adults.
   b. For each death, 730 children are seen in hospital emergency rooms and are released. In the United States, over 16 million children per year are treated.
   c. For each death, many thousands of children are treated at home and many of them miss 1 or more days of school.

3. **Loss of working years of life** is a more powerful measure of outcome, since it places loss to society in perspective. As a consequence, the earlier in life one is debilitated or killed, the greater is the loss of working years of life. Pediatric injuries are shown by this measure to be a very significant problem to society at large.

C. **Relationship of child development to injuries.** The types of injuries that children experience at different ages can be explained and even predicted by age-specific development. Both motor and cognitive development play major roles.

1. **Infant: birth to 1 year**
   a. Motor development is key. In the first 6 months, infants squirm to the extent that they can fall from a changing table or adult bed even before they can roll over. The crib or playpen offers the safest environment.
   b. In the second half of the year, infants become more mobile. They can reach out for objects that they want and place them in their mouths with increasing efficiency. As a result, mechanical suffocation is a leading cause of death.

2. **Toddler: 1–2 years**
   a. First walking and then climbing allow toddlers mobility, reach, and speed. Fine motor control improves so that containers and closets previously inaccessible can now be investigated.
   b. Toddlers have no sense of danger; therefore, their motor activity is limited only by their physical ability.
   c. Toys must be safe; play must be supervised.

3. **Preschooler: 2–5 years**
   a. Running, climbing, and jumping are the mainstays of activity. Preschoolers can throw objects, ride tricycles, and interact with each other and their environment.
   b. Their thinking, however, remains illogical and egocentric. They are unable to appreciate cause and effect, and, as a result, injury to themselves or others may not prevent similar episodes in the future. However, children can be taught in a way that can develop their skills and alter their behavior.

4. **School-age child: 5–9 years**
   a. Fine and gross motor skills are refined. Organized games and rules are incorporated into play. Adventure and daring, including risk-taking without appreciation of the consequences, become the hallmarks of activity.
   b. Riding a bicycle becomes commonplace.
   c. Children begin to assume increasing responsibility for their own safety, often out of the sight of their parents and teachers.

5. **Preteenage and early teenage child: 10–14 years**
   a. Strenuous physical activity becomes common, and the incidence of sports-related injuries increases markedly.
   b. Hobbies and scientific activities are begun.
   c. Values and judgment become factors in decision-making and risk-taking.

6. **Adolescent: older than 14 years**
   a. Physical prowess is refined. Organized sports and part-time jobs make adolescents prone to sports- and work-related injuries.
   b. Decision-making becomes more logical but more abstract. Although there is knowledge of potential consequence, denial and a feeling of invulnerability often predominate in evaluating risks.
   c. Peer pressure and a need to feel comfortable in and accepted by a group may lead to potentially dangerous activities or to substance- or alcohol-related injury.
   d. Difficulty in finding one's role in peer groups, family, school, and society in general may lead to depression or acting out, which sometimes culminates in suicide gestures or attempts.

D. **The accident-prone child.** A subject of much discussion and some research is the attempt to define the characteristics of children at increased risk for recurrent injury. Characteristics include the following.

1. **Motor skills.** There is one group of children with immature or deficient skills. Another group of children with advanced skills attempt things that most children would not.

2. **Perception.** Deficits in visual-perceptual scanning exist such that attention is deployed differently than it is by children without these deficits.

3. **Behavior.** Increased impulsiveness, increased activity level, and emotional lability can lead to recurrent injury.

4. **Environment.** Some studies show that environment plays the major role in an increased risk for injury.
   a. Parents may need to be advised to monitor and modify the physical environment of the child.
   b. Factors such as family stress and disorganization also may contribute to more accidents in the home.
   c. The possibility that recurring accidents actually indicate child abuse must be considered.

E. **Recognition of intentional injury**

1. **Child abuse** (see Ch 3 VIII). Physically abused children usually present to physicians with an acute injury or a history of recurrent injury. A detailed history of the circumstances surrounding each episode of injury is essential to screen for the possibility of abuse or neglect. Red flags that should arouse suspicions of abuse include:
   a. **Recurrent injuries or ingestions.** Some "accident-prone" children are really abused children.
   b. **Injuries that are out of proportion to or atypical for a child's developmental stage:**
      (1) Head contusion in a child who cannot yet stand or walk
      (2) Back bruises in a child who cannot climb
      (3) Burns in a child who has no access to hot liquids or faucets
   c. **Evidence or marks of inflicted injury** (e.g., from a belt buckle)
   d. **Injuries that are known to have a high association with abuse:**
      (1) Scald burns of the buttocks
      (2) Cigarette burns
      (3) Spiral fracture of the femur
      (4) Retinal hemorrhage due to the "shaken baby syndrome"
      (5) Subdural hematoma
   e. **Parental supervision that is inadequate** for a child's age
   f. **Parental psychiatric disease,** including psychosis and depression
   g. **A history of the events surrounding the incident that is inconsistent** with the observed injury

2. **Suicide** primarily is an adolescent phenomenon (see Ch 4 VI B); it is the third leading cause of death for male adolescents and the fourth leading cause for female adolescents. Both injuries and poisonings are methods of suicide. Some episodes are straightforward (e.g., medication overdose, self-inflicted gunshot wound); others are less obvious (e.g., single-passenger automobile accidents, many of which are thought to be suicide attempts).
   a. The differentiation of a **suicide attempt**—a serious effort to end one's life—from a **suicide gesture**—a cry for help—is crucial in the management of adolescent injuries and poisonings. Attention must be paid to both cause and effect in each episode, including:
      (1) Acute management of the injury or ingestion
      (2) The motives and underlying problems that caused the adolescent to attempt to hurt herself
   b. **Hospitalization** may be necessary to:
      (1) Treat the effects of the injury or ingestion
      (2) Sort out the events leading to the attempt or gesture
      (3) Separate antagonistic individuals, especially within families, until problems can be identified
      (4) Demonstrate that attention is being paid to a patient's problems
      (5) Prevent a repeated attempt

3. **Homicide** rates for children of all age-groups have doubled over the past 25 years.
   a. In **children younger than 3 years,** homicide is primarily due to child abuse perpetrated by a parent or relative. The injury is often the result of blunt force, usually hitting or shaking.
   b. In **children age 4–12 years,** the pattern of homicide is mixed. Causes include injury inflicted by a parent or relative, risk-taking behaviors (e.g., playing with guns), and violence related to substance abuse.
   c. In **adolescents,** the injury is primarily inflicted by a friend or acquaintance after an argument and often is related to alcohol or drug abuse. The instrument usually is a handgun.

## II. MOTOR VEHICLE INJURIES

A. **Epidemiology.** Trauma to child passengers in motor vehicles is the **leading cause of death** between ages 6 months and 19 years.

1. There are 7500 deaths per year in child passenger–related events.
   a. The age-specific death rate peaks at 12 per 100,000 infants at 2 months, drops to 3 per 100,000 school-age children, and rises again in the teenage years.
   b. Nonfatal trauma is underestimated. Based on police reports, nonfatal trauma occurs at an annual rate of 186 per 100,000 children age 1–14 years, but many more incidents probably go unreported.

2. The epidemiology of motor vehicle injuries involving children is different from that involving adults.
   a. The most likely situation in adult injury involves a young, inebriated male driver at night on a wet road.
   b. An injury involving a child is most likely to occur with a sober female driver during the day on a dry road.

3. Adolescent drivers, as a group, are more likely than older drivers to be involved in a fatal automobile accident and are more likely to kill others in a collision.
   a. Drivers who are 16–18 years of age have a fatality rate per miles driven that is 8–10 times that of 30-year-old drivers.
   b. A study of Connecticut communities after state funding for public school driver education was ended revealed that the licensure, crash rate, and death rate for 16- to 17-year-old drivers declined significantly in towns that ended driver education programs compared to communities that continued them. This implies that the number of adolescents able to drive is directly proportional to their involvement in crashes, irrespective of level of education.
   c. Alcohol plays a significant role in adolescent vehicle-related death and morbidity.

B. **Most motor vehicle injuries are due to kinetic energy** resulting from movement of occupants either against the automobile, against other passengers, or against the outside environment, as in ejection. A much smaller number of injuries are due to **thermal energy** (i.e., burns).

1. The **nature and extent of injuries** depend on the:
   a. Mass of the victim
   b. Speed of travel
   c. Tolerance of impacted tissue to injury
   d. Degree of energy absorbed by impacting surfaces

2. An **unrestrained passenger becomes a projectile** during rapid deceleration.
   a. Since force of impact = mass × deceleration, a 20-lb infant involved in the crash of a car going 30 mph would generate 600 lbs of force in kinetic energy imparted or required for restraint.
   b. A child who is held on the lap of an unrestrained passenger may be crushed by the force of the passenger, which is much greater than the force imparted by the unrestrained child alone.

C. **Types of vehicle-related injuries**

1. **Passengers in automobiles.** In this case, injury may be due to collision or to an unrestrained passenger falling out of a moving vehicle.

2. **Pedestrians hit by vehicles.** In this case, injury may result from a pedestrian running in front of a car (this occurs more often in crowded urban areas, especially among the poor) or walking where sidewalks do not exist (e.g., in suburban and rural areas).

3. **Other vehicles** (e.g., all-terrain vehicles, bicycles, skateboards) also can cause injury.

D. **Prevention of injury**

1. **Restraints.** Use of **car seats** and **seat belts** is the most important strategy to prevent injury and death to children in automobile accidents involving passengers.
   a. Data in the United States, Canada, and the Scandinavian countries demonstrate a potential reduction of 90% in fatality rate and 50% in morbidity rate through use of restraints.

**b.** All states in the United States now have laws that mandate the use of car seats or seat belts for children in the first 5 years of life. While many of these laws are not optimum, early data demonstrate increased use of car seats.

   **(1)** The use of seat belts and car seats in Tennessee, the first state to enact restraint laws (1977), rose from 8% to 29% in the 2½ years after initiation of the law.

   **(2)** Rhode Island demonstrated an increase in use of 11%–23% upon initiation of the law.

   **(3)** Surveys have shown that seat belt use among all ages has increased up to 70% after states mandated use.

**c.** Numerous studies show that car seat availability for newborns, patient-consumer education programs, and reinforcement at health care visits all seem to increase car seat use significantly.

**d.** Improper installation and use of car seats have recently been recognized.

   **(1)** In one study of child restraint use, over 75% of seats were improperly anchored.

   **(2)** Of seats with tether attachments, 68% were not attached and 16% were attached incorrectly.

   **(3)** A seat that is easy to attach to the car via a seat belt and that allows easy seating and removal of the child is likely to yield the greatest success in correct, regular use.

**e.** It is likely that it will take a full generation of use before car seat restraint is the norm rather than the exception.

**2. Other safety factors**

**a. Safer cars.** Over the past 2 decades, federal law has mandated that new cars be equipped with seat belts, a padded dashboard, a padded steering wheel, and bumpers that minimize damage at 5–10 mph.

**b. Safer roads**

   **(1)** Dangerous roads should be identified and modified by changes in width, curve, and bank.

   **(2)** Breakaway signs and posts should be installed.

**c. Pedestrian safety**

   **(1)** Pedestrians should walk on sidewalks or, if sidewalks are not present, against the flow of traffic.

   **(2)** Bright, reflective clothing should be worn at night.

   **(3)** Supervision of small children should be increased, especially in congested areas.

   **(4)** Legal speed limits and observance of stop signs and traffic lights should be enforced, particularly in congested areas.

   **(5)** The effects of educational strategies on the frequency of pedestrian injuries have not been well evaluated.

**III. FALLS** are the most common injury requiring an emergency room visit. They also are the most common cause of injury in the home. Although a much greater cause of morbidity than mortality, falls are the fourth leading cause of death from injury in children.

**A. Epidemiology**

**1.** The **peak incidence** of falls occurs in the toddler period, with a relative decline throughout childhood. **Death due to falls** has two peaks, one in the toddler period and another in adolescence.

**2.** Falls are more common in boys than in girls. They occur twice as frequently in urban areas as in suburban and rural areas and are most prevalent in low socioeconomic groups.

**B. Sites of falls**

**1. The home** is the major site of falls for toddlers and preschoolers. Causes of falls in the home include:

**a. Structures,** such as:

   **(1)** Stairs and steps (related to the use of walkers in infancy and to poor footing in the toddler period)

   **(2)** Floors, porches, and windows

   **(3)** Bathtubs

**b. Furniture,** such as:

   **(1)** Beds

**(2)** Chairs and stools
**(3)** Tables, especially coffee tables, which children fall against
**(4)** Baby furniture
  c. **Toys,** such as:
    **(1)** Riding toys
    **(2)** Falls over toys
    **(3)** Broken toys

  **2. Nonhome sites** of falls include:
    **a.** Playground equipment and surfaces, which play a major role (grass, sand, and rubber are most desirable; concrete and asphalt, least)
    **b.** Baby carriages
    **c.** Bicycles
    **d.** Grocery carts

**C. Morbidity and mortality.** Only 3.3% of all injuries from falls seen at medical facilities require admission to the hospital. Death due to falls is infrequent and in 56% of cases is caused by head and neck trauma.

  **1. Head-related injuries** involve contusion, laceration, and fracture.
    **a.** Contusion is most common.
    **b.** Laceration is particularly common in toddlers.
    **c.** The fracture rate in children younger than 1 year is five times that in older children.

  **2. Nonfatal, nonhead-related falls** are associated with laceration in 38% of cases, sprains in 38%, and fractures (usually involving the extremities or clavicles) in 14%.

**D. Prevention of injury**

  **1. Housing codes.** Laws regarding safe housing standards should be created and strictly enforced.

  **2. Barriers**
    **a.** Gates on stairways should be used at both the top and bottom. These should be pressure gates, not the accordion type, which can cause head entrapment.
    **b.** Window guards should be used.

  **3. Behavior modification for parents**
    **a.** The mattress and siderails of the crib should be appropriately adjusted.
    **b.** Infants should not be left unattended, even briefly, on adult beds or changing tables.
    **c.** Tables with sharp edges and pointed corners should be removed.
    **d.** Doors to the basement should be kept closed.
    **e.** Use of infant walkers should be discouraged.

## IV. DROWNING (submersion injury)

**A. Epidemiology.** Drowning is the third most common cause of accidental death in children; it is second only to motor vehicle accidents as a cause of accidental death in adolescents.

  **1.** The male to female ratio is 5:1; the black to white ratio is 3:1. The **peak incidence** is 1–5 years of age for both sexes; the incidence peaks again at age 10–19 for boys only.

  **2.** Freshwater drownings outnumber saltwater drownings, even along the coast and in Hawaii. **Major sites of drowning** for children include:
    **a.** Pools and lakes, especially for toddlers who fall in and are unable to swim
    **b.** Streams, rivers, quarries, and oceans
    **c.** Bathtubs, which are the most common site of drowning in the first year of life

  **3.** There is a **high mortality to morbidity ratio;** however, many minor incidents are never brought to medical attention.
    **a.** In one survey, of 132 drownings and near drownings reported in individuals ranging in age from newborn to 21 years, 65 people died; among the 58 cases involving 1–3 year olds, there were 20 deaths.
    **b.** In another study, 25% of patients presenting to an emergency room with submersion injury were admitted.

**B. Pathophysiology**

1. **Hypoxemia** is the principal problem in submersion injuries.
   a. Aspiration occurs in 90% of cases, but less than 22 ml/kg of fluid are involved.
   b. There is no significant clinical difference between saltwater and freshwater drowning, and chlorine in the water is not a special problem in that it causes no injury beyond the submersion damage.

2. **Major organ system involvement**
   a. **Brain. Hypoxic brain injury** is most serious and life-threatening as well as being most likely to cause long-term damage. Full impact may not be known for days or weeks if the patient survives.
   b. **Lung. Pulmonary edema** occurs due to decreased surfactant and resulting atelectasis.
   c. **Kidney. Acute renal failure** occurs in most lengthy drownings and near drownings, but 80% of patients recover in 10 days.

**C. Prediction of outcome.** Certain variables can predict the likelihood of a good outcome after a submersion injury.

1. **Water temperature.** The outcome is better when the water is less than 70° F (21° C).

2. **Duration of submersion.** Submersion for more than 5 minutes in warm water leads to a major risk of damage.

3. **Fixed, dilated pupils and coma** result in a 100% incidence of serious deficit, damage, or fatal outcome.

4. **Need for cardiopulmonary resuscitation (CPR)** on arrival in the emergency room is the **major determinant of outcome**. In one study, of 21 patients requiring CPR on arrival at the hospital, 17 had a poor outcome; of 29 patients with spontaneous pulse and respiratory effort, all had a good outcome.

**D. Prevention of injury**

1. All children under 4 years of age should be supervised while in the bathtub.

2. A fence with a gate that closes should be used around in-ground pools, and a gate should be used at stairs or entries to above-ground pools.

3. All children should be supervised closely while swimming, especially those with known medical problems.

4. The depth of the pool should be checked before children and adolescents are allowed to dive.

5. A basic CPR course should be provided for all parents who own pools.

6. Children should be taught how to swim. This does not, however, negate the need for supervision.

**V. BURNS** rank third behind motor vehicle accidents and drownings as a cause of injury to children. They cause more than 1300 childhood deaths per year in the United States.

**A. Types of burns**

1. **Flame burns** most frequently result from house fires.
   a. **Etiology**
      (1) Smoking causes 30%–45% of all house fires.
      (2) Heating equipment and electrical malfunction (e.g., faulty extension cords, frayed wires) are the next most common cause.
      (3) Matches and fire-setting account for less than 5% of house fire deaths.
   b. **Epidemiology**
      (1) House fires in the United States occur most frequently in the East and Southeast.
      (2) They occur most frequently at night, in December through March.
      (3) Children are often alone when the event occurs.

   **c. Prevention of injury**
   **(1) Smoke detectors** provide early warning of house fires. Their use has increased from 5% in 1970 to 70% in 1989. They are particularly useful because:
   **(a)** Fatal residential fires more frequently occur when occupants are asleep.
   **(b)** Residential fires burn for a long time before detection.
   **(c)** Most deaths result from smoke inhalation.
   **(2) Sprinklers.** The use of sprinklers is mandated in commercial high-rise buildings. Thus far, they are neither required nor widely used in residential settings.
   **(3)** Increasingly **stringent sleepwear standards** have been implemented since 1967, and these have been responsible for a dramatic decrease in deaths. In 1968, 50 children reportedly died from night-clothing ignition; by 1980, only one death was reported.

**2. Scald burns**
   **a.** The **kitchen** is the major site of burns from water, beverages, and grease. Hot liquid in a cup or pot turned over in the kitchen is the most common scenario.
   **(1)** Of scald burns, 60% occur in the kitchen.
   **(2)** Hot liquids caused 44% of burn admissions to a children's hospital in one study.
   **(3)** In a study conducted in New Zealand in 1970, hot liquids accounted for 78% of burn injuries to children.
   **b. Tap water** causes one-fourth of all scald burns.
   **(1)** Half of all tap water burns occur in children less than 5 years old.
   **(2)** Tap water burns are most likely to occur in bathroom sinks and bathtubs.
   **(3)** Older siblings turning on hot water for younger children often causes scald burns.
   **(4)** This type of burn is a possible result of abuse.
   **c. Prevention of injury**
   **(1)** A child should not be held by an adult who is drinking a hot liquid.
   **(2)** Pot handles on the stove should be turned to the side. Cooking should be done on the back burner when possible.
   **(3)** Stable cups and coffee-making apparatus should be used.
   **(4)** Children should be in a safe area during food preparation.
   **(5)** Placemats should be used rather than tablecloths.
   **(6)** Children should be supervised in the bath and at the sink.
   **(7)** The temperature of the water heater should be reduced to 120° F (most water heaters are currently kept at approximately 150° F).

**3. Electrical burns.** Each year, over 4000 extension and appliance cord injuries require emergency room treatment. The majority occur in children under 5 years of age. Such injuries can result in disfiguring mouth burns, other skin burns, and electrocution.
   **a. Major causes of electrical burns**
   **(1)** Injuries are principally caused by a child sucking on the plug-receptor connection of an extension wire.
   **(2)** Another cause is a child inserting conducting objects into live wall sockets.
   **(3)** A less common cause is a child chewing on poorly insulated wire.
   **b. Prevention of injury**
   **(1)** Extension cords should be unplugged from wall sockets after use.
   **(2)** Safety plugs or caps should be used on unused wall sockets.
   **(3)** Appliance wires should be inspected for fraying.

**4. Contact burns.** Most injuries involve the extremities.
   **a. Sources** include:
   **(1)** Hot appliances, such as toasters and broilers (hands)
   **(2)** Wood-burning stoves (hands)
   **(3)** Heating register grates (feet)
   **b. Prevention of injury**
   **(1)** Hot appliances should be kept away from children and vice versa.
   **(2)** Toddlers should be kept away from a wood-burning stove.
   **(3)** Slippers or shoes should be worn in homes with floor heat grates.

**5. Chemical burns** in children often are related to ingestion of caustic agents.

**6. Ultraviolet radiation** primarily results from sun exposure.

**B. Acute therapy for fires and burns**

1. For an active flame burn, the victim should "drop and roll." Running only fans the flames that are already active.

2. For skin burns, cool water should be applied immediately. This will minimize active tissue damage.

3. In case of house fires, occupants should be instructed to know the evacuation route and to crawl under smoke.

4. For electrocution, the victim should be removed from contact by use of a nonconducting material such as wood or plastic. Cardiopulmonary resuscitation should be initiated as needed.

**VI. CHOKING AND FOREIGN BODY INJURY.** A foreign body is any substance that is not natural to the body passage in which it is found. The reasons why children ingest foreign objects range from normal infant behavior of putting everything into the mouth to a child trying to eat, run, and breathe at the same time. In addition, parents often have unrealistic expectations of what their children should be able to eat or do at a given age.

**A. Epidemiology.** Foreign body injury is the most common cause of injury-related death in children under 1 year of age. Twenty percent of all foreign body aspiration deaths in the United States occur in children under 4 years of age.

**B. Clinical findings.** Symptoms may be minimal, especially if the foreign body is small. Many (approximately 50%) of the episodes are unwitnessed.

1. **Factors involved in foreign body injury** include:
   a. **Size** and **composition** of the foreign body
   b. **Location.** The younger the age of the child, in general, the higher the involved anatomic site, which is directly a result of the relative size of the airway.
      (1) The **larynx** is the most common site in children younger than 1 year.
      (2) The **trachea** and **bronchi** are most commonly involved in children 1–4 years of age.
   c. **Degree** and **duration** of obstruction

2. **Upper airway obstruction** may cause asphyxiation and pose an immediate threat to life. It is manifested by gagging, choking, wheezing, cyanosis, and dysphonia or aphonia.

3. **Lower tract obstruction** may be tolerated for longer periods of time, especially the more distal the obstruction. It is usually manifested by wheezing or asymmetric or absent breath sounds.

**C. Acute management** of choking and foreign body ingestion consists of **nonintervention if the child can cough, breathe, or speak**. A natural cough is more effective than an artificial one.

1. Fingers should not be thrust blindly into the mouth to search for a foreign body. This might lodge the object in the airway.

2. Intervention for **upper airway asphyxiation** has been subject to much controversy (see Ch 6 II B 3).
   a. The American Heart Association recommends, as of 1990, abdominal thrusts (Heimlich maneuver) for children older than 1 year.
   b. Back blows and chest thrusts are recommended for children younger than 1 year because of the theoretical risk of abdominal viscus perforation with the Heimlich maneuver.
   c. As a general rule, if three or four attempts at each maneuver fail, the other should be tried.

3. If necessary, **rigid bronchoscopy** should be performed under general anesthesia. Occasionally, **thoracotomy** and **bronchotomy** may be required.

**D. Prevention of injury**

1. **Toys.** Infants should not have access to toys meant for older children. Dolls with button eyes and beanbag toys should not be given to infants.

2. **Food**
   a. Food should be cut, broken, or mashed into bite-sized pieces. Conversation and motor activity should be discouraged during eating.

   **b.** Nuts, hard beans, pretzels, gumballs, raw vegetables, and so forth should not be given to young children.

   **3. Chewable pills** should not be given to children younger than 3 years.

   **4. Small objects** (e.g., uninflated balloons, diaper pins, coins) should not be given to or left near small children. Children should be taught not to place these objects in their mouths.

**VII. TOYS.** Over 150,000 different toys are produced worldwide by 1500 toy manufacturers. Understanding the hazards peculiar to each developmental stage in childhood will aid in choosing appropriate toys and preventing injury.

**A. Aspiration and ingestion dangers**

   **1.** Toys should be large enough so that they cannot be swallowed, nor should they come apart or be easily shattered.

   **2.** Toys for small children should not have easily removable buttons or fillings (e.g., beans).

   **3.** Small children should not be given uninflated balloons. They can be aspirated, and they have caused death.

   **4.** Small plastic toys and parts of toys are not radiopaque and will rarely be visualized in x-rays of the trachea, chest, and abdomen.

**B. Burns and electric shock** can be caused by toys. Battery-operated toys are preferable to those with electric cords. Plug-in toys should not be used by children under the age of 8 years. Children should be taught how to use the toys and should be supervised when playing with them.

**C. Lacerations**

   **1.** Toys with sharp or poorly finished edges can cause lacerations.

   **2.** Glass toys should not be used by small children.

   **3.** Sharp points on toys should have protective covers.

**D. Projectile injuries.** The major site of projectile injury is the eye. BB guns, archery sets, and boomerangs should be restricted to use by older children with adult supervision.

**E. Skateboards** are associated with a high rate of injury because of the high speed attained (up to 35 mph) and the need for a high level of coordination.

   **1. Epidemiology.** The major group at risk are boys, age 10–14. Injuries include fractures, contusions and abrasions, and sprains and muscle injuries.

   **2. Recommendations for use** include:
      **a.** Use of protective equipment (e.g., helmets, gloves, elbow and knee pads)
      **b.** Prohibition of use on public streets
      **c.** Smooth skating surfaces free of traffic
      **d.** Skateboarding parks
      **e.** Safety rules

**F. Bicycles** are associated with significant injuries because they are used on streets and roads in competition with other vehicular traffic. Nationwide data indicate that there are 500 fatalities and over 40,000 injuries to bicyclists under 20 years of age per year.

   **1. Epidemiology**
      **a.** Most serious injuries involving bicycles are head injuries, and most deaths (93%) are motor-vehicle associated. The majority of these injuries and deaths involve traffic violations by the cyclist or driver.
      **b.** Boys are at higher risk than girls at all ages, although boys age 10–14 have the highest risk of death.
      **c.** Injuries are seasonal, with peak occurrence during May through September in the Northeast.

   **2. Recommendations for safety** include:
      **a.** Use of helmets

    **b.** Education concerning traffic regulations

    **c.** Shoulders on roads and bike paths.

**VIII. SPORTS INJURIES.** As children get older, participation in organized sports increases. Team and individual sports are commonplace for both boys and girls either in school or through organized leagues. In adolescence, physical maturity allows high proficiency at sports but also increases the risk of serious injury.

**A. Epidemiology**

  **1.** In a statewide study of accidents in Massachusetts, 1 in 7 school-age children visited an emergency room each year for sports-related injuries.

  **2.** In another study of high school students in Seattle, Washington, injury rates for different sports were monitored. Over 2 years, 82% of participants in football and 75% of participants in wrestling suffered injuries. Between 30% and 60% of all students in gym class were injured. Sports least likely to be associated with injury were tennis, swimming, and volleyball, each of which had no more than a 10% injury rate.

  **3. Most injuries occur during practice,** not competition.

    **a.** Most injuries are minor, primarily sprains, strains, and bruises.

      **(1)** Of injured children, 70% miss less than 1 week of participation, and 29% miss only 1 day.

      **(2)** Most children are treated initially by the coach, who must determine the general status of the child and if CPR is required (all coaches should be certified in CPR). If the injury is determined not to be severe, ice, compression, and elevation should be employed as necessary, as well as referral to a physician as appropriate.

    **b.** The use of medical resources is prevalent, however.

      **(1)** Of those injured, 42% are referred to a physician for care.

      **(2)** Of those seen by a physician, 91% have an x-ray and 2% are hospitalized, the majority of whom require surgical procedures.

**B. Types of injury.** Potentially life-threatening injuries include:

  **1.** Severe head or neck injury

  **2.** Cardiac or respiratory arrest

  **3.** Severe hemorrhage and shock

  **4.** Heat exposure

**C. Reinjury is a major problem,** both at the site of the original injury and at other sites. Causes of reinjury include resumption of sports too soon after the initial injury and inadequate rehabilitation.

## IX. POISONING

**A. Epidemiology**

  **1.** Poisoning involves 2 million children under 5 years of age each year. It is the third most common injury treated in emergency departments for all children under 16 years of age.

  **2.** There are two peak ages for poisonings: 1–5 years and adolescence. The former group is involved in involuntary, inadvertent poisonings. The latter group most often is involved in suicide gestures or attempts. While the developmental basis may be different, the initial treatment for a given agent remains the same regardless of the age and motivation of the victim.

**B. Environmental factors**

  **1. Circumstances that increase the risk of ingestion**

    **a.** Storing dangerous chemicals (e.g., cleaning agents, motor oil, pesticides) in drinking glasses, soda bottles, or unlabeled, open containers

    **b.** Changes in normal home routines (overall, 80% of ingestions occur at home)

    **(1)** These can occur during moving, preparation for vacation, spring cleaning, or periods of family stress.

    **(2)** Visiting friends and relatives may not be careful with their medications around children.

  **c.** Over-reliance on childproof caps on medicine containers

  **d.** Storing different medications in the same container

**2. Types of ingestions**

  **a.** Both over-the-counter and prescription medications (e.g., aspirin, acetaminophen, vitamins, antihistamines, tranquilizers, analgesics, cold and cough medicines, iron) are the cause of approximately 45% of all poisonings in children.

  **b.** Approximately 50% of ingestions involve cleaning agents, perfumes and toiletries, insecticides, paints, and paint solvents.

## C. Examination

**1.** A child who is behaving strangely or who is unresponsive must be considered to have ingested something, and a cause should be sought by taking a careful history and by screening blood and urine for toxic substances.

**2.** The level of consciousness should be documented and monitored frequently. Size and reactivity of pupils, odor of breath, cardiorespiratory status, and a careful neurologic examination are key points.

## D. Principles of therapy

**1. Removal of gastric contents.** In general, removal of toxic agents from the stomach as soon after ingestion as possible is the first step in therapy. Removal may be accomplished by induction of emesis or by gastric lavage.

  **a. Emesis.** In children, emesis is more effective and less traumatic than gastric lavage for most ingestions. Some toxic agents may have already caused spontaneous vomiting prior to consultation with a poison control center or physician. Emesis may be induced by ingestion of **syrup of ipecac,** a mixture of plant alkaloids. Ipecac induces vomiting by local gastric irritation as well as by central activity through the chemoreceptor trigger zone of the floor of the fourth ventricle of the brain. Ipecac can be given at home prior to transport to an emergency facility after telephone contact with a health care provider or poison control center.

    **(1) Dose.** Children between 6 months and 12 months of age should be administered 10 ml; children over 1 year of age should be given 15 ml. Either dose should be followed by fluids. Emesis results within 20 minutes in 90%–100% of children. The dose may be repeated once if no vomiting occurs.

    **(2) Contraindications**

      **(a)** Most authorities advise against use of ipecac in children under 6 months of age.

      **(b)** A depressed level of consciousness may result in lung aspiration.

      **(c)** Emesis is contraindicated when volatile hydrocarbons have been ingested, because aspiration into the lungs is possible due to the nature of the compound.

      **(d)** Corrosive substances will cause an increased risk of esophageal burn if vomited.

      **(e)** Emetics may not be effective if antiemetics or major tranquilizers of the chlorpromazine group are ingested.

  **b. Gastric lavage** should be reserved for use in children who cannot take ipecac, in whom the level of consciousness is depressed, and in whom there is no response to ipecac.

    **(1)** For children with severe depression of mental state, intubation with a cuffed endotracheal tube is required to prevent aspiration.

    **(2)** The largest bore tube that can be passed should be used since it will allow the removal of larger pill fragments. Lavage with normal saline should be continued until the return fluid is clear for two or three passes.

**2. Adsorption of poison.** The next step in therapy following the removal of poison from the stomach is binding the poison to inhibit gastrointestinal absorption. **Activated charcoal** adsorbs a variety of materials in the gastrointestinal tract. Adsorption occurs within the first few minutes and may be inhibited by food. Most toxins are adsorbed by activated charcoal; however, some agents [i.e., iron salts, boric acid, cyanide, mineral acids, strong bases (caustics), lithium, other small ionized molecules] are not.

    **a. Dose.** The completeness of adsorption depends on the amount of activated charcoal relative to toxin. Ideally, the amount of charcoal should be 5–12 times that of the ingested material. This often cannot be estimated accurately. The recommended pediatric dose is 15–30 g for children under 12 years of age and 50–100 g for children over 12. It is administered as a slurry in cold water. Poor palatability is a major drawback in its use in the pediatric population. Use of a nasogastric tube may be required.

    **b. Contraindications.** Since activated charcoal can bind with and render ipecac ineffective, charcoal should not be used until vomiting induced by ipecac is complete.

  **3. Intestinal cleansing. Cathartics** are routinely recommended following gastric emptying and adsorption. By decreasing transit time through the gastrointestinal tract, toxins are less available for absorption into the circulation.

    **a.** Magnesium sulfate administered at 250 mg/kg, sodium sulfate administered at 250 mg/kg, and magnesium citrate administered at 4 ml/kg are the most frequently used cathartics.

    **b.** The cathartic may be added to the activated charcoal for ease of administration without loss of efficacy for either substance.

**E. Specific poisonings**

  **1. Aspirin** is widely consumed by adults and children, and it is the **most common cause of drug poisoning** in children. It is generally not perceived as "medicine." Although the incidence has been decreasing over the past 20 years, aspirin poisoning still is a problem.

    **a. Pharmacology**

      **(1)** Aspirin is a weak acid that is absorbed rapidly from the stomach and small bowel into the circulation and is both freely ionized and protein-bound.

      **(2)** The drug is metabolized by the liver and excreted through the kidney.

      **(3)** The half-life is prolonged in overdoses to 18–36 hours, compared to 4–6 hours in therapeutic doses. When urine pH is greater than 7.4, most of the drug is ionized in the urine and not reabsorbed, thus shortening plasma half-life to 6–8 hours.

    **b. Pathogenesis**

      **(1)** There is increased sensitivity of the respiratory centers of the brain to changes in carbon dioxide and oxygen concentrations, leading to increased rate and depth of respiration, and resultant respiratory alkalosis. To compensate, hydrogen ions move from cells to the extracellular space.

      **(2)** Oxidative phosphorylation is uncoupled, increasing the metabolic rate and causing increased metabolism of glucose and oxygen, resulting in excess heat production. This causes tachycardia, tachypnea, fever, and hypoglycemia. Aspirin also inhibits the Krebs cycle, causing metabolic acidosis.

      **(3)** Aspirin damages hepatocytes, causing liver toxicity and prolonged prothrombin time. It also inhibits platelet organization, causing prolonged bleeding time.

    **c. Clinical features**

      **(1)** Clinical features include tinnitus and vomiting (the vomitus may be heme-positive); hyperpnea; fever, lethargy, and confusion; and convulsions, coma, and respiratory or cardiac failure.

      **(2)** In an acute overdose at 6 hours past ingestion, the serum level is predictive of the clinical course.

        **(a)** At less than 35 mg/L, there are no symptoms.

        **(b)** At 35–70 mg/L, symptoms are mild to moderate.

        **(c)** At 70–100 mg/L, symptoms are severe.

        **(d)** At over 120 mg/L, the outcome is potentially fatal.

    **d. Therapy** includes:

      **(1)** Ipecac-induced emesis, followed by administration of activated charcoal and cathartics

      **(2)** Alkalization with sodium bicarbonate given intravenously (a urinary pH of 8 is desired)

      **(3)** Adequate fluids to correct loss; colloid (as albumin or plasma) given to correct shock

      **(4)** Dialysis or hemofiltration, which should be considered in severe cases or when there is renal, hepatic, or cardiac failure

    **e. Prevention**

      **(1)** The number of baby aspirin is limited by regulation to thirty-six 75-mg tablets per bottle.

      **(2)** Safety closures (childproof caps) should be used on bottles.

      **(3)** It is likely that the association of Reye syndrome with aspirin will further curtail aspirin use in children and, as a result, decrease the number of poisonings.

2. **Acetaminophen** has replaced aspirin as an antipyretic/analgesic for use in children and is also widely used by adults. Consequently, the incidence of poisoning by this agent has markedly risen in recent years. In general, children under age 5 seem relatively resistant to severe toxic sequelae when compared to adults but still should be evaluated and managed aggressively.
   a. **Clinical features.** There are three main phases of acetaminophen poisoning.
      (1) **Phase I** usually begins 30–60 minutes after ingestion and may last for 12–24 hours.
         (a) Most patients with mild poisoning never progress beyond this stage and are asymptomatic.
         (b) In moderate to severe poisoning, gastrointestinal signs—anorexia, nausea, and vomiting—as well as pallor and diaphoresis predominate.
         (c) Changes in level of consciousness do not occur at this stage and if present suggest the ingestion of a different agent, perhaps in addition to acetaminophen.
      (2) **Phase II** occurs 24–48 hours after ingestion and may persist up to 4 days.
         (a) During this phase, the patient usually is clinically asymptomatic, although mild right upper quadrant tenderness relative to hepatic enlargement may occur.
         (b) Liver function tests—hepatic enzymes, serum bilirubin, and prothrombin time—rise as hepatic necrosis progresses.
         (c) Patients who are moderately poisoned do not progress beyond this point and gradually recover.
      (3) **Phase III** occurs 3–5 days after ingestion. Symptoms are related to hepatotoxicity.
         (a) Symptoms may be limited to anorexia, nausea, malaise, and abdominal pain.
         (b) More severe cases may progress to confusion and stupor as well as sequelae related to hepatic toxicity, including jaundice, coagulation defects, hypoglycemia, and encephalopathy. Renal failure and myocardiopathy also may occur.
         (c) Death occurs from irreversible hepatotoxicity.
   b. **Therapy**
      (1) **Assessment**
         (a) Maximum number of tablets or liquid missing from the container should be presumed ingested.
         (b) If the presumed ingested dose is less than 100 mg/kg of body weight, the ingestion is mild and need not be treated.
         (c) If the presumed dose is unknown or above 100 mg/kg, the child requires clinical evaluation and intervention.
      (2) **Intervention**
         (a) Syrup of ipecac should be given to empty the stomach; if a change in the level of consciousness is due to ingestion of another substance, gastric lavage should be performed.
         (b) Activated charcoal has generally not been advised, since it binds and inactivates N-acetylcysteine, the antidote for acetaminophen. Recent data suggest that a higher dose of N-acetylcysteine might overcome residual activated charcoal.
         (c) A loading dose of N-acetylcysteine (140 mg/kg body weight) should be given, followed by a maintenance dose (70 mg/kg) every 4 hours for 17 doses.
         (d) A serum sample for acetaminophen assay should be obtained 4 hours or more after ingestion and results compared to a published nomogram. Use of the nomogram will determine whether the full treatment course is needed or whether treatment can be stopped.
         (e) If the serum acetaminophen level is in the toxic range, the patient should be hospitalized, liver function tests performed, electrolyte, glucose, and creatinine concentrations obtained. Laboratory tests should be repeated daily while treatment is underway, until 4 days after ingestion.
         (f) Supportive care should be provided, depending on clinical observation and laboratory data.

3. **Iron.** Iron-containing products, such as ferrous salts alone or iron as part of multivitamin tablets, are a significant toxicologic hazard. Over 4000 cases of acute iron ingestion are reported to regional poison control centers annually, and iron is among the top 10 substances ingested by children under 5 years of age. Iron is widely available without prescription. It is formulated in large tablets that look like candy and is sold in containers of as many as 250 tablets. In addition, iron is commonly not appreciated by parents as potentially dangerous to their children.
   a. **Clinical features.** There are four main phases of iron poisoning.

(1) **Gastrointestinal symptoms.** Within 30–60 minutes, vomiting, colicky abdominal pain, gastrointestinal hemorrhage, and diarrhea occur. Iron acutely and directly damages the gastrointestinal tract, especially the gastric and small intestinal mucosa.

(2) There is a period of **relative stability** from 3–4 hours until 48 hours. It is marked by subtle changes and failure to recognize them. There is no evidence of change in the central nervous system (CNS).

(3) **Circulatory shock** occurs after 48 hours. It is caused by a combination of gastrointestinal fluid and blood loss, increased capillary permeability, and loss of vascular tone, which are all direct effects of excess iron. A secondary coagulopathy may result. Shock will result from absolute hypovolemia and the inability of the body to respond to it.

(4) **Late manifestations**
  (a) Gastric scarring occurs within 2–6 weeks. Since iron acts directly on the gastrointestinal tract as a corrosive, the healing process may result in areas of scarring and stenosis at both the pylorus and the small bowel.
  (b) Rarely, hepatic necrosis may result due to direct liver damage by iron.

b. **Therapy**
  (1) Potential risk must be determined.
    (a) It should be assumed that the maximum number of tablets missing were ingested by the child.
    (b) The weight of elemental iron in each preparation should be used to calculate the toxic dose ingested.
    (c) The toxic dose ingested (mg/kg) should be calculated, based on the child's weight. In general, less than 20 mg/kg of elemental iron poses little risk; 20–60 mg/kg requires syrup of ipecac–induced emesis and reevaluation if gastrointestinal pain or bleeding occurs; greater than 60 mg/kg requires examination by a physician.
  (2) Any patient with gastrointestinal or CNS symptoms must be evaluated, even if the calculated dose is nontoxic. Not only may the calculation be incorrect, but multiple ingestions may have occurred.
  (3) All adolescents with iron overdose should be seen by a physician since the ingestions must be regarded as intentional.
  (4) Serum iron levels should be measured 4–6 hours after ingestion. By that time, emesis and cathartics will have been given (activated charcoal has no effect).
    (a) If the concentration is less than 300 μg/dl, it is not significant.
    (b) If the iron concentration is 300–500 μg/dl, if it is greater than the total iron-binding capacity, or if the patient is symptomatic, the serum iron levels are considered to be significant.
    (c) If the concentration is greater than 500 μg/dl, it is toxic.
  (5) An abdominal x-ray might be helpful, since iron pills are radiopaque.
  (6) Deferoxamine, a chelating agent specific for iron, is recommended for intravenous use in patients with the significant or toxic levels noted above. It is given by slow continuous infusion at 15 mg/kg/hr. Its positive effect is noted when the urine turns pink, since the iron-chelate complex is excreted in the urine. Treatment is discontinued when the serum iron level is less than 300 μg/dl.

4. **Hydrocarbons—petroleum distillates.** Hydrocarbons are derivatives of crude petroleum and are mixtures of aromatic and aliphatic hydrocarbons. Naturally occurring derivatives extracted from plants, such as turpentine and pine oil, have similar properties and are included in this discussion. Common hydrocarbons include gasoline, kerosene, lighter fluid, paint thinner, turpentine, mineral seal oil (the major ingredient in furniture polish), and pine oil.

a. **Toxic effects**
  (1) **Aspiration** of the substance into the respiratory tract is the major danger. The more highly volatile the hydrocarbon, the more likely is aspiration. The major effect of aspiration is chemical irritation, which damages the alveolar lining and the capillaries, causing pneumonitis, atelectasis, or pulmonary edema. The degree of lung involvement is parallel to the degree of clinical compromise. Results are severe hypoxemia and ventilation-perfusion abnormalities, causing respiratory acidosis. Because of this risk, **emesis should not be induced** in management of volatile hydrocarbon ingestion.
  (2) **CNS depression.** All hydrocarbons will be absorbed to some degree. The amount absorbed will determine the degree of CNS depression. Aromatic distillates (e.g., toluene or xylene, turpentine, gasoline, mineral spirits) are most likely to cause a depressed sensorium.

**b. Clinical features**
   **(1)** Early on, there is burning in the mouth and throat, choking and gagging, coughing, nausea, vomiting, and hemoptysis.
   **(2)** Tachycardia and tachypnea reflect the degree of pulmonary insult. Often, a **chest x-ray** might show changes before the onset of significant clinical findings. The x-ray may reveal punctate, mottled densities of pneumonitis, atelectasis, or both, with findings tending to be more prominent in the dependent portion of the lung. X-ray findings peak at 72 hours and then begin to clear.
   **(3)** One hour after ingestion, symptoms of CNS depression occur (e.g., general weakness, hypotonia, dizziness, mental confusion, lethargy). Irritability, agitation, or convulsions may be seen.
   **(4)** There is a poor correlation between clinical symptoms, physical findings, and radiographic abnormalities.

**c. Therapy**
   **(1)** When a small amount—a mouthful or two—has been ingested, the child is best left without attempts at removal, in an upright position.
   **(2)** In large ingestions, spontaneous vomiting will usually occur. Comatose patients should be intubated with a cuffed endotracheal tube and lavaged.
   **(3)** All patients with respiratory or CNS symptoms should be admitted to the hospital, observed closely, and treated to support respiratory and fluid status. Oxygen, bronchodilators, and constant distending airway pressure should be employed.

**5. Lead poisoning (plumbism),** in contrast to the other acute poisonings discussed in this section, actually is a chronic disorder that may be punctuated by acute episodes. Studies indicate that 5%–15% of children in the United States have increased lead absorption. Most are asymptomatic.

**a. Sources** of increased lead absorption among children include:
   **(1)** Ingestion of paint and plaster chips in old, dilapidated buildings, which is the most important contributor to severe poisoning
      **(a)** The eating of nonfood items (pica) is common among infants and toddlers.
      **(b)** The combination of pica and living in old housing accounts for most cases of symptomatic poisoning.
   **(2)** Exposure to household dust in old houses
   **(3)** Living in close proximity to a lead smelter
   **(4)** Exposure to contaminated workclothes of parents
   **(5)** Lead-contaminated soil
   **(6)** Other, less common sources (e.g., contamination of acidic beverages and foods in lead-lined containers and lead-glazed ceramic pots, lead-painted furniture and toys, the burning of battery casings in fireplaces)
   **(7)** Leaded gasoline, formerly a major source of lead but used less frequently now (and soon unavailable in the United States)

**b. Clinical features.** The clinical diagnosis tends not to be suspected until the onset of CNS symptoms. The insidious nature of lead poisoning emphasizes the importance of screening for increased lead absorption during child health maintenance visits (see Ch 1 VI E 3).
   **(1)** General symptoms include apathy, decreased play, clumsiness, and intermittent vomiting.
   **(2)** Acute encephalopathy is manifested by vomiting, lethargy, stupor, and ataxia, followed by coma and seizures.
   **(3)** Chronic lead poisoning may present as nonspecific developmental delay, behavioral and attention disorders (see Ch 3 III B), seizures, or a peripheral neuropathy (see Ch 17 X B). Recent follow-up studies suggest that developmental abnormalities persist over a 10-year period.

**c. Laboratory findings**
   **(1) Biochemical evidence** of lead toxicity includes elevations of blood lead and signs of interference with hemoglobin synthesis, such as an increase in free erythrocyte protoporphyrin as well as increased lead excretion in the urine following administration of a chelating agent, such as calcium ethylenediaminetetraacetic acid (CaEDTA).
   **(2)** There may be evidence of a **sideroblastic anemia** (see Ch 14 III B 4).
   **(3) X-ray findings** may include lead lines at the metaphyses of the long bones and radiopaque foreign material within the small bowel.

**d. Therapy**
   **(1)** For children with symptomatic lead poisoning the **source of lead must be identified** and the child's intake immediately interrupted. This may require temporary housing for the child until the home is lead-free.
   **(2)** For such children, chelation therapy with agents such as CaEDTA, dimercaprol, and D-penicillamine is indicated.
      **(a)** Following an initial course of parenteral CaEDTA or CaEDTA-dimercaprol, oral D-penicillamine can be given for 2–6 months to prevent rebound increases in blood lead.
      **(b)** Supportive treatment may include control of increased intracranial pressure and seizure control as well as monitoring urine output.
      **(c)** Careful, long-term follow-up is essential since learning and behavioral problems are late sequelae.
   **(3)** The approach to asymptomatic children with evidence of increased lead absorption is controversial since no level of lead is acceptable in the human body.
      **(a)** Prompt identification of environment hazards is critical.
      **(b)** CaEDTA and D-penicillamine may be administered to children with persistent elevations of blood lead who also have biochemical evidence of adverse effects, such as marked elevation of free erythrocyte protoporphyrin or a positive CaEDTA challenge test.
**e. Prevention** is the key in eliminating this important source of morbidity.
   **(1)** Replacing or renovating old, substandard housing is the ultimate solution.
   **(2)** Avoidance of paints with lead additives is critical.
   **(3)** Screening of children in high-risk areas decreases the incidence of frank lead poisoning, although this will not eliminate increased lead absorption among children.
   **(4)** Decreased lead in gasoline will help reduce environmental exposure.
   **(5)** Pilot studies on decreasing other environmental sources (e.g., soil) are inconclusive.

## F. Prevention of poisonings

   **1. Preschool children.** Because developmental factors are the major issue, parents have the primary preventive role. Actions are aimed at physically preventing small children from ingesting toxic substances through:
   **a.** Use of childproof caps
   **b.** Dispensing a limited amount of medication
   **c.** Locking medicine cabinets
   **d.** Not combining different medications in the same container
   **e.** Not dispensing medications as candy

   **2. Adolescents.** Since the etiology of poisoning in this age-group may be experimentation or suicide-related, methods of passive prevention are not helpful. An attempt to identify adolescents with problems and to deal with them before they act out those problems is the best approach in suicide-related cases. Education about the hazards of drug and alcohol abuse may be helpful in avoiding the serious consequences of experimentation.

## G. Poison control centers. Because the number of potential poisons is immense and because the need to gather information about them is so time-consuming, statewide and regional poison control centers have been established.

   **1.** These centers may be accessed by the public as well as by health professionals.

   **2.** They serve not only to assist in recognition and management of potentially serious ingestions but also to provide reassurance regarding ingestion of or exposure to benign substances.
   **a.** One study found that inappropriate use of the emergency department could be reduced by up to 95% as a result of prior consultation by a parent with a poison control center.
   **b.** In another survey of poison control centers, 75% of calls concerned poisons with relatively low toxicity and required only reassurance, 20% required rapid removal of the ingested poison, and fewer than 5% required more intensive medical management.
   **c.** In a third study, only 3.6% of all calls regarding individuals 14 years of age and younger were referred to emergency departments.

## H. Telephone calls may come directly to health care providers or emergency departments instead of poison control centers. The person calling often is agitated, and it may be difficult to interpret the exact situation.

1. **Basic information** obtained via the telephone must include the:
   a. Patient's name, address, and telephone number (this information should be obtained first, since a hysterical person may hang up the phone prematurely)
   b. Patient's age and weight
   c. Type and amount of exposure or ingestion
   d. Clinical status and change in condition of the patient

2. Unfortunately, **telephone data are inaccurate half of the time,** and often a worst-case scenario must be invoked until it can be disproved or the patient can be examined.

## STUDY QUESTIONS

**Directions:** Each of the numbered items or incomplete statements in this section is followed by answers or by completions of the statement. Select the **one** lettered answer or completion that is **best** in each case.

**Questions 1–2**

A 2-year-old boy is brought to the emergency department 30 minutes after having ingested 20 of his mother's 325-mg ferrous sulfate tablets. Each tablet contains 65 mg of elemental iron. He has vomited once, but his behavior is otherwise normal. The child's physical examination is unremarkable. He weighs 13 kg.

1. Which of the following statements about this child's status is correct?

(A) The dose of iron that this child ingested should cause no clinical sequelae
(B) His single episode of vomiting is probably unrelated to the ingestion
(C) Although he has vomited once, ipecac should be administered
(D) Activated charcoal should be given to adsorb excess iron in the stomach
(E) Cathartics are ineffective in iron poisonings

2. With respect to further treatment and outcome, which of the following statements about this case is correct?

(A) The child should be observed over the next 4–6 hours, and if no further symptoms occur, he may be sent home and be followed up the next day
(B) A serum iron level should be drawn 4–6 hours after the ingestion, and if it exceeds 500 µg/dl, the child should be admitted and treated
(C) Treatment with deferoxamine will alter the outcome and should be begun immediately after vomiting has stopped
(D) An x-ray of the abdomen would be of no help in this case since pills generally are not radiopaque
(E) Had the parent of this child called a poison control center immediately after ingestion, an unnecessary emergency department visit could have been avoided

3. All of the following statements about child passenger restraints are true EXCEPT

(A) state laws mandating car seat use have resulted in increased frequency of use
(B) improper installation of car seats has been recognized as an important problem
(C) anticipatory guidance to parents is ineffective in increasing car seat use
(D) all states now mandate that car seats or seat belts be used for children under 5 years of age
(E) a potential 90% reduction in the fatality rate can be expected through use of child restraints

4. All of the following statements about the epidemiology of childhood injuries are true EXCEPT

(A) injuries are responsible for a greater percentage of hospital admissions among children than among adults
(B) death is the least likely outcome of childhood injuries
(C) respiratory diseases cause more deaths in children than do injuries
(D) most childhood injuries are treated at home
(E) "loss of working years of life" is a powerful measure of injury outcome

5. The most serious acute medical outcome of drowning is

(A) pulmonary edema
(B) acute renal failure
(C) hypoxic brain injury
(D) blood loss
(E) cardiac arrhythmia

6. According to the "agent-host-environment model," the agent most often responsible for motor vehicle injuries is

(A) chemical energy
(B) kinetic energy
(C) thermal energy
(D) electrical energy

| | |
|---|---|
| 1-C | 4-C |
| 2-B | 5-C |
| 3-C | 6-B |

7. Each of the following statements about adolescent drivers is true EXCEPT

(A) they are more likely than older drivers to be involved in a fatal automobile crash
(B) they are more likely than older drivers to kill others in a collision
(C) when corrected for miles driven, the adolescent death rate in automobile crashes is the same as that for older drivers
(D) in communities with driver education, death rate for adolescents in collisions is higher than that in communities without driver education
(E) alcohol plays a significant role in adolescent vehicle-related death and morbidity

8. The best initial treatment for scald burns is to

(A) débride the wound
(B) apply cool water
(C) apply butter or margarine
(D) cover the wound with a bandage
(E) apply pressure to the site of the burn

9. In a child who is poisoned, the most effective way to remove gastric contents is by the use of

(A) saline lavage with a wide-bore nasogastric tube
(B) tartar emetic
(C) syrup of ipecac
(D) manual induction of vomiting
(E) citrate of magnesia

10. Disfiguring mouth burns are most likely to occur as a result of

(A) an electrical burn
(B) a scald burn
(C) a contact burn
(D) ingestion of a caustic substance
(E) child abuse

11. Contraindications to induction of emesis in childhood poisoning include all of the following EXCEPT

(A) ingestion of turpentine
(B) rapidly increasing drowsiness
(C) ingestion of drain cleaner
(D) ingestion of acetaminophen
(E) ingestion by a child younger than 6 months

12. Which statement about sports injuries is correct?

(A) Most injuries occur during competition
(B) Most injuries require hospital-based care
(C) Football is the school sport most highly associated with risk of injury
(D) Reinjury is rarely a problem

13. Which of the following injuries accounts for the greatest number of emergency ward visits?

(A) An injury caused by a motor vehicle accident
(B) A burn
(C) An injury caused by a fall
(D) Poisoning
(E) Drowning

7-C   10-A   13-C
8-B   11-D
9-C   12-C

**Directions:** Each item below contains four suggested answers of which **one or more** is correct. Choose the answer

    **A**  if **1, 2, and 3** are correct
    **B**  if **1 and 3** are correct
    **C**  if **2 and 4** are correct
    **D**  if **4** is correct
    **E**  if **1, 2, 3, and 4** are correct

14. Which of the following signs and symptoms may be associated with foreign body aspiration?

(1) Cyanosis
(2) Wheezing
(3) Absent breath sounds
(4) Aphonia

15. Predictors of a good overall outcome in drowning include

(1) water temperature above 70° F
(2) submersion less than 5 minutes
(3) freshwater rather than saltwater
(4) spontaneous pulse and respiratory effort upon arrival in the emergency room

14-E
15-C

## ANSWERS AND EXPLANATIONS

**1–2. The answers are: 1-C** *[IX E 3]*, **2-B** *[IX E 3 b]*.
A single episode of vomiting does not empty the stomach sufficiently, and ipecac should be administered. The maximum dose of iron ingested by this child is 65 mg elemental iron × 20 pills ÷ 13 kg = 100 mg/kg, which is a potentially serious dose. Among the symptoms caused by serious iron ingestion is vomiting; therefore, in this case, the vomiting must be considered related to the ingestion. This implies potential serious sequelae. Activated charcoal does not adsorb iron and need not be given. Cathartics are helpful, once the stomach has been emptied.

Since this child has ingested a potentially serious dose of iron and has vomited spontaneously, observation alone is inadequate; the child requires evaluation in an acute care setting. Typically, there is a period of relative stability, during which the child may look well even after a serious ingestion. A serum iron level would always be drawn under such circumstances, and if it is 300–500 g/dl with clinical symptoms or over 500 g/dl without symptoms, in-hospital chelation therapy with deferoxamine should be initiated. Such treatment should not be begun empirically. An x-ray of the abdomen would be helpful since iron pills are radiopaque.

**3. The answer is C** *[II D 1]*.
Anticipatory guidance, both prenatally and as part of routine health care, has been shown to increase car seat use, although improper installation certainly lowers the effectiveness of the restraint. Laws mandating use of car seats and seat belts in children under age 5 have increased their use and recent studies have demonstrated reduction in fatalities in states requiring use of restraints.

**4. The answer is C** *[I B 1, 2, 3]*.
Prior to the mid-1940's respiratory disease was the most common cause of death; however, the widespread use of antibiotics has dramatically decreased childhood mortality due to pneumonia. Since the mid-1940's injuries have consistently been the most common cause of death in childhood, resulting in four times the number of childhood deaths due to any disease. Although children are responsible for a larger percentage of hospital admissions due to injury than are adults, most childhood injuries are treated at home and have death as their least likely outcome. "Loss of working years of life" is a powerful measure of injury outcome because it measures the loss to society.

**5. The answer is C** *[IV B 2 a]*.
Brain injury resulting from drowning may be severe, resistant to therapy or support, and is often permanent. The degree of hypoxia as part of the initial episode is probably the major determination with respect to outcome. Blood loss is rare in drownings. Arrhythmias are sometimes a secondary and possibly terminal event as a result of hypoxia, but the brain is severely damaged by the time an arrhythmia occurs. Pulmonary edema and acute renal failure, frequently associated with drowning, can be treated and supported during acute intensive therapy. Both will usually resolve.

**6. The answer is B** *[I A 2, II B]*.
The rapid deceleration that occurs as a result of motor vehicle collisions is responsible for massive changes in kinetic energy, and the transmission of kinetic energy to the human body is responsible for the severe tissue injuries that can be sustained. Thermal injury, such as that caused by a fire occurring as a result of a crash, is a much less common mode of injury. Electrocution can occur, although rarely, when a car hits a high-voltage pole.

**7. The answer is C** *[II A 3]*.
Adolescents are much more likely to die as a result of an automobile accident than adults, even when the rate is corrected for miles driven. Drivers who are 16–18 years of age have a fatality rate per miles driven that is 8–10 times that of 30-year-old drivers. Driver education has been shown to be associated with an increased incidence of motor vehicle-related death in communities where it is offered. This is probably due to the increased number of licensed adolescent drivers as a result of the program. Alcohol plays a major role in both adolescent and adult vehicular death but is a much less significant factor in child passenger deaths.

**8. The answer is B** *[V B 2]*.
Immediate application of cool water to a scald burn decreases the thermal injury to tissue. For many years, it was taught that warm water should be applied; however, warm water helps in frostbite but not in scald burns. The application of butter or margarine, a home remedy, is of no help. A large burn from which skin has sloughed should be covered with saline-soaked gauze but only as a second response after cooling. Pressure, although helpful for controlling bleeding, can increase tissue damage after a burn.

**9. The answer is C** *[IX D 1 a].*
Syrup of ipecac has been demonstrated to be a safe, efficient method to remove stomach contents in children. Nasogastric lavage is less apt to remove large pill fragments, given the limitation of the diameter of the tube in small children. In addition, many children vomit, with incomplete stomach evacuation, during attempts to place the tube. Nasogastric lavage is the method of choice, however, in unconscious patients. Manual induction of vomiting is an inefficient method. Citrate of magnesia is a good choice for catharsis but not for emesis.

**10. The answer is A** *[V A 3].*
Electrical burns most often occur when a child chews on extension cord receptacles or frayed wires. As a result, severe burns to the corner of the mouth may require extensive plastic surgery. Scald burns are more likely to be external. Caustic substances can cause mouth burns, but these usually heal spontaneously. Esophageal scarring, which leads to stricture, is the most serious outcome due to ingestion of caustics. While burns on a child with no access to hot liquids or faucets can indicate child abuse, disfiguring mouth burns are not a common indicator of abuse.

**11. The answer is D** *[IX D 1 a (2); E 2 b (2)].*
Acetaminophen can be removed by emesis without danger to the patient. Turpentine, which behaves as a volatile hydrocarbon, should not be removed by emesis due to the risk of lung aspiration. Drain cleaner, a corrosive, should not be removed due to risk of repeated burning of the esophagus, which will increase the risk of scarring. Emesis should not be induced in a child with a rapidly changing mental state since, in the 15–20 minutes it takes for ipecac to work, the child's alertness may become severely depressed, which can result in lung aspiration. Ipecac is safe for use in children over 6 months of age.

**12. The answer is C** *[VIII A 2].*
Not surprisingly, football is the school sport most likely to result in injury. In most cases, however, sports injuries are minor and treated at school or at home. In school-related sports injuries, hospital care is sought infrequently. However, when a physician is consulted, x-rays or other tests are frequently obtained. Most sports injuries occur during practice or recreation. Reinjury is a significant problem and is usually caused by full exertion too soon after the initial injury or by inadequate rehabilitation.

**13. The answer is C** *[III].*
Falls are responsible for the highest number of injury-related emergency ward visits. Head injuries and fractures are the most common serious diagnoses beyond bruises and sprains. While relatively few emergency ward visits are the result of drowning, a large percentage of these patients (25% in one study) are admitted to the hospital. Since the establishment of poison control centers with telephone hotlines, there has been a decrease in the number of poisonings seen in emergency wards.

**14. The answer is E (all)** *[VI B 2, 3].*
Cyanosis, aphonia, absence of breath sounds, and wheezing all may be associated with foreign body aspiration. The site at which the object lodges determines the specific signs or symptoms noted. Cyanosis is associated with major airway obstruction at the level of the glottis. Aphonia (absence of speech) is associated with either esophageal obstruction with external pressure on the larynx or direct obstruction of that area of the airway. Absence of breath sounds is due to obstruction of an entire lobe or lobar segment of the lung. Wheezing is caused by partial obstruction of the lower airway (bronchi and bronchioles), leading to a ball-valve effect that results in air-trapping.

**15. The answer is C (2, 4)** *[IV B, C].*
Spontaneous pulse and respiratory effort are favorable predictors of either complete recovery or minimal sequelae after a submersion injury. Conversely, absence of these factors (i.e., the necessity for complete cardiopulmonary resuscitation in the emergency room) is a predictor of very poor outcome (over 90% death rate or severe sequelae). Submersion for less than 5 minutes and water temperature under 70° F (40°–60° F is optimum) are associated with better overall outcome. The salinity of water is not a determinant of recovery.

# 3

# Developmental Disabilities and Behavioral Disorders

Neil L. Schechter

## I. NUTRITIONAL DISORDERS

### A. Failure to thrive

1. **Definition.** Failure to thrive is a term typically used to describe infants and young children whose weight is persistently below the third percentile for age on an appropriate standardized growth chart or less than 80% of ideal weight for age. It may also present as an acute weight loss or failure to gain weight at an expected rate.

2. **Etiology.** Failure to thrive is viewed as the final common pathway for multiple problems that result in an inadequate caloric intake or utilization. Etiologies include:
   a. Failure of the caretaker to provide adequate calories due to:
      (1) Poverty
      (2) Unusual dietary beliefs of the caretaker
      (3) Parental mental illness (e.g., depression)
      (4) Abuse
   b. Failure to ingest adequate calories due to:
      (1) Anatomic problems (e.g., gastroesophageal reflux)
      (2) Central nervous system (CNS) problems causing poor feeding (e.g., cerebral palsy)
      (3) Cardiorespiratory difficulties (e.g., congenital heart disease, bronchopulmonary dysplasia)
      (4) Interactive problems between parent and child
   c. Failure to utilize adequate calories due to:
      (1) Gastrointestinal disease (e.g., celiac disease, inflammatory bowel disease)
      (2) Renal disease (e.g., renal tubular acidosis)
      (3) Endocrine disease (e.g., hyperthyroidism, diabetes mellitus)
      (4) Metabolic disease (e.g., amino acid disorders, storage diseases)
      (5) Infectious disease [e.g., chronic inflammation, acquired immune deficiency syndrome (AIDS)]
      (6) Malignancies
      (7) Cardiac disease
      (8) Cystic fibrosis
      (9) Intrinsic deficits of cell numbers (e.g., fetal alcohol syndrome)
      (10) Severe psychosocial deprivation

3. **Assessment**
   a. A detailed **history and physical examination** often identify the etiology of failure to thrive. Observations of the mother-infant interaction may suggest a disordered relationship. In particular, the physician should gather:
      (1) A detailed history of the child's caloric intake (i.e., a 48-hour dietary recall)
      (2) Information about a typical mealtime experience
      (3) Information about poor feeding, drooling, distractibility, and bowel habits
   b. **Laboratory data** usually are not significant without positive findings in the history and physical examination.
      (1) Routine laboratory tests should include complete blood count, urine culture, urinalysis, blood urea nitrogen (BUN), and examination of stool for ova and parasites and for reducing substances. A sweat test and chest x-ray may be considered.
      (2) Additional laboratory investigation should be conducted based on information gathered in the history and physical examination.

### 4. Therapy

**a.** If any organic illness is identified, treatment specific for that disorder should be undertaken.

**b.** If the initial history and physical and laboratory data do not suggest an organic explanation for the failure to thrive, a high-calorie diet consisting of one and one-half to two times the child's daily caloric requirements should be devised.

**c.** Parents should keep a detailed diary of the child's caloric intake. If they are unable to get the child to take the high-calorie diet, then consultation with a dietitian may be helpful in creating a diet with increased calories but without increased volume.

**d.** If the parents cannot enforce the high-calorie diet and if no weight gain occurs, inpatient hospitalization should be considered so that intake and weight gain can be carefully monitored and further evaluation can take place. Parental involvement in feeding the child during the hospitalization is crucial.

**e.** Interactional issues must be addressed. An interdisciplinary team including social workers, psychologists, nurses, and developmental specialists is very helpful.

## B. Obesity

**1. Definition.** Obesity is defined as weight/height greater than 120% of standards for age and sex. Approximately 25% of children 6–17 years old are obese.

**2. Etiology.** Several factors may contribute to the development of obesity. **Exogenous obesity,** the most common reason for obesity, typically is viewed as the consequence of increased caloric intake and genetic predisposition.

**a. Genetic predisposition** is suggested by twin studies. Individuals with a propensity toward obesity may require fewer calories to maintain a normal weight.

**b. Increased caloric intake** may be secondary to a variety of psychosocial causes, such as anxiety and family modeling.

**c. Genetic disorders.** Prader-Willi syndrome [see Ch 7 IV D 1 d (2)] and Laurence-Moon-Biedl syndrome (now generally recognized as two distinct conditions, Laurence-Moon and Bardet-Biedl) are associated with obesity.

**d. Hormonal abnormalities** (e.g., hypothyroidism) are rare causes of obesity.

**3. Assessment**

**a. History.** Essential elements include:

**(1)** Family history (parental obesity is a strong predictor of childhood obesity)

**(2)** History of the child's weight and height gain over time

**(3)** A dietary diary to document eating patterns and caloric intake

**b. Physical examination**

**(1) Normal stature, sexual development, and intelligence** rule out most genetic disorders associated with obesity and strongly suggest exogenous obesity.

**(2) Triceps skin fold thickness** measurement may be helpful.

**(3) Blood pressure** should be obtained.

**c. Laboratory studies.** Total cholesterol, triglycerides, and high density lipoprotein cholesterol should be measured.

**4. Therapy**

**a.** A **reduced calorie diet** should be devised. A nutritionist often is helpful.

**b.** A formal **exercise program** should be encouraged.

**c.** Specific **weight goals** should be determined.

**d. Peer group support programs** are beneficial, if available.

**e. Mechanical approaches** such as jaw wiring, stomach stapling, and bypass procedures are not appropriate for growing children.

## C. Anorexia nervosa and bulimia (see Ch 4 VI D)

# II. CONTINENCE DISORDERS

## A. Enuresis

**1. Definition.** Enuresis is the involuntary discharge of urine at an age after continence has been reached by most children. Typically, this is age 5 years in girls and 6 years in boys. Two subclassifications of enuresis are important.

    **a. Primary versus secondary**

      **(1)** Children with **primary** enuresis have never been continent for a period of time lasting at least 3–6 months.

      **(2)** Children with **secondary** enuresis have had a prolonged period of bladder control but have resumed enuretic behavior.

    **b. Nocturnal versus diurnal**

      **(1) Nocturnal** enuresis occurs only at night and affects about 85% of all enuretic children.

      **(2) Diurnal** enuresis occurs during the day and affects about 5% of enuretic children.

      **(3)** Approximately 10% of enuretic children have a **mixed type** (nocturnal and diurnal) enuresis.

  **2. Etiology.** Enuresis is a symptom for which varying underlying causes have been implicated.

    **a. Maturation.** Because of high spontaneous remission rate (in approximately 10% of the enuretic population per year) and increased frequency in males, the level of physiologic maturity has been implicated as a cause of enuresis.

    **b. Sleep disorder.** Many enuretics are incontinent during stages 3 and 4 of the first sleep cycle, suggesting that enuresis is a non-rapid eye movement (non-REM) dyssomnia, like sleep walking and night terrors.

    **c. Genetics.** In 70% of families with an enuretic child, the symptom has occurred in at least one other family member.

    **d. Organic causes.** Urinary tract infections, obstructions of the outflow tract, lumbosacral disorders that affect bladder innervation (e.g., meningomyelocele), diabetes mellitus, diabetes insipidus, and sickle cell disease are all possible causes of incontinence but represent only 1%–5% of the causes of enuresis. Chronic stool retention also is a cause of enuresis.

    **e. Psychological factors** have been implicated in some children with enuresis. Stressors such as the birth of a sibling or a move may precipitate bedwetting in the susceptible child.

    **f. Abnormal antidiuretic hormone (ADH) cycles** have been suggested.

  **3. Assessment**

    **a. History.** Essential elements of the history include:

      **(1)** The family history of enuresis

      **(2)** The pattern of enuresis (primary versus secondary; nocturnal versus diurnal)

      **(3)** Defining urinary habits (frequency, urgency, dysuria, dribbling)

      **(4)** Identifying psychological stressors

    **b. Physical examination.** Essential elements include:

      **(1) Height and weight**

      **(2) Blood pressure**

      **(3)** A thorough **neurologic examination** emphasizing lower spinal vertebral function

      **(4)** Examination of the **external genitalia**

    **c. Laboratory and x-ray investigation**

      **(1)** A **urinalysis** should be obtained and should include specific gravity as well as determinations of glucose, protein, blood, and white cells. A **urine culture** should also be obtained.

      **(2)** Routine radiographic studies are not indicated for enuretic children with normal urinalysis, a normal physical examination, and no evidence of neurologic disease. Children with diurnal enuresis may require more extensive evaluation.

  **4. Therapy**

    **a. Behavioral approaches** include counseling, charting, hypnosis, bladder stretching exercises, night awakening by parents 1½ hours after sleep onset, and use of a buzzer alarm, which is the most successful treatment presently available.

    **b. Pharmacologic management**

      **(1) Tricyclic antidepressants** (e.g., imipramine) have a success rate of approximately 50% in reducing enuretic episodes, but the relapse rate on discontinuation is high. In addition, there are potentially serious side effects and marked toxicity in overdosage. Antidepressants are indicated only for rapid, short-term relief of symptoms (e.g., use prior to summer camp or vacation).

      **(2) Desmopressin** recently has been approved for use and may have a role in a subgroup of children with enuresis.

**B. Encopresis**

  **1. Definition.** Encopresis is involuntary fecal soiling at an age beyond which continence should have been achieved, which in most children is age 4 years. Approximately 1.5% of 7-year-old children have encopresis.

   a. **Primary versus secondary**
      (1) Primary encopresis occurs in children who have never been totally toilet trained.
      (2) Secondary encopresis occurs in children who have had at least 3–6 months of fecal continence.
   b. **Retentive versus nonretentive**
      (1) Most encopretic children suffer from chronic stool retention, with subsequent overflow incontinence.
      (2) Nonretentive encopretic children (i.e., nonconstipated children with encopresis) tend to have neurogenic sphincters or severe psychiatric illness.

2. **Etiology**
   a. **Developmental and behavioral factors.** Slower transit time, hyperactivity, the lack of school bathroom facilities, harsh toilet training, sexual abuse, and negative defecation experiences (e.g., those associated with prior gastroenteritis) have all been implicated as causing chronic stool retention, which can lead to encopresis.
   b. **Anatomic factors.** Hirschsprung's disease, anal stenosis, and anal fissures also are potential causes of chronic stool retention.
   c. **Metabolic factors.** Hypothyroidism, various endocrine neoplasms, and various drugs (e.g., opiates, phenothiazines) also can cause chronic constipation.

3. **Assessment**
   a. **History**
      (1) A detailed bowel history, including the age of the child at toilet training, the frequency of bowel movements, the history of constipation, and a description of the stools, is necessary to assess encopresis.
      (2) Also, gaining insight into the child's and the family's functioning can help determine if there are predisposing factors for encopresis.
   b. **Physical examination.** Essentials include:
      (1) Assessing **growth patterns**
      (2) A **neurologic examination** evaluating lower extremity deep tendon reflexes and the presence of anomalies
      (3) An **abdominal examination**
      (4) A **rectal examination,** which should reveal stool in the rectal ampulla within the reach of the examiner.
   c. **Laboratory and x-ray investigation**
      (1) Thyroid testing should take place if it is deemed necessary from physical findings.
      (2) An abdominal x-ray to determine the extent of fecal retention may be helpful if there is no response to initial therapy.
      (3) If Hirschsprung's disease is suspected, anal manometry or rectal biopsy is indicated.

4. **Therapy**
   a. **Initial catharsis** with a series of enemas and laxatives or stool softeners will remove retained stool.
   b. **Maintenance therapy** consists of:
      (1) Mineral oil (the typical course is a gradual decrease of mineral oil with discontinuation after approximately 4–6 months)
      (2) Bowel retraining by sitting on the toilet after meals to take advantage of the gastrocolic reflex
      (3) Dietary changes, which should emphasize increased roughage and liquid and decreased milk and milk products

## III. SCHOOL-RELATED PROBLEMS

A. **Specific learning disabilities**

1. **Definition**
   a. **The National Advisory Committee on Handicapped Children** states:

   > Children with specific learning disabilities exhibit a disorder in one or more of the basic psychological processes involved in understanding or using spoken or written language. These may be manifested in disorders of listening, thinking, talking, reading, writing, spelling, or arithmetic. . . . They do not include learning problems which are due primarily to visual, hearing, or motor handicaps, to mental retardation, emotional disturbance, or environmental disadvantage.

**b.** This definition is based on a recognized discrepancy between a child's academic performance and potential. This discrepancy is presumed to be secondary to subtle CNS dysfunction or subtle human variation.

**c.** These disabilities occasionally are described by reference to the academic function they affect (e.g., dyslexia for difficulty in reading, dyscalculia for difficulty in math).

**d.** These disabilities are found in 1%–10% of school-age children.

**2. Etiology.** No specific cause for learning disabilities is commonly accepted. Most likely, a number of subgroups of children with specific learning disabilities will be identified. Etiologic hypotheses at present include CNS damage, individual human variation, toxins, diet, and environmental factors.

**3. Assessment**

    **a. History.** Elements of the history should include:

        **(1)** A review of the perinatal course

        **(2)** Evidence of medical problems (e.g., persistent otitis media, seizure disorders)

        **(3)** The early developmental history, with an emphasis on language acquisition (there is often an uneven profile in the development of children with learning disabilities)

        **(4)** The history of other family members with learning problems

        **(5)** A review of school functioning

    **b. Physical examination** usually is normal.

        **(1)** An emphasis often is placed on a search for minor **neurologic indicators,** or "soft signs," which have been reported more frequently in learning-disabled children than in controls [e.g., synkinesis (mirror movements), dysdiadochokinesia (difficulty with rapid alternating movements), choreiform movements of the fingers]. The implications of these signs remain controversial.

        **(2)** Hearing and vision should be screened.

    **c. Laboratory investigation** is not called for unless it is suggested by the history or physical examination. CT scan and electroencephalogram (EEG) are not helpful.

    **d. Psychoeducational assessment** includes a battery of tests of intellectual functioning (IQ tests) as well as specific academic tests to profile a child's strengths and weaknesses. Usually these are performed by the public schools, which are mandated to test the child under federal public law 94-142. The psychoeducational profile is the basis on which a specific academic program is constructed. Public law 99-457 extends the mandate for special education assessment to the 3- to 5-year-old age-group.

**4. Therapy.** Many unorthodox therapies have been offered for children with learning problems, including dietary therapies, perceptual training, optometric training, and sensory integration training. None of these therapies has documented efficacy at this time.

    **a. Educational intervention is the mainstay of treatment** for learning disabilities. Typically, this occurs through a modification of the child's regular classroom experience or by varying degrees of special education, ranging from resource room support to a separate classroom. Educational intervention should identify specific goals (i.e., should be **individualized**) and should be monitored carefully.

    **b. Psychological counseling** is indicated for children with learning disabilities who suffer from diminished self-esteem that is not improved by a special education program. Children with learning disabilities can develop school phobia and avoidance (see III C), and this can be addressed in counseling.

    **c.** Various **support organizations** are helpful in providing parents and teachers with a forum to address the complex issues associated with these disabilities.

**B. Attention deficit-hyperactivity disorder (ADHD)**

**1. Definition.** ADHD involves an inadequate attention span, impulsiveness, and hyperactivity. The syndrome in general is marked by a lack of task performance and easy distractibility.

    **a.** This disorder has been plagued by vague and changing diagnostic criteria. This confusion is reflected in the numerous diagnostic labels for ADHD (minimal brain damage, minimal brain dysfunction, hyperkinetic impulse disorder, and most recently attention deficit disorder with or without hyperactivity), which reflect varying conceptual frameworks.

    **b.** Incidence figures suggest that 2%–4% of children may be affected, making ADHD the most common behavioral disorder of school-age children. Males are affected 10 times more frequently than females.

2. **Etiology.** No single etiology is presently accepted, and the cause of ADHD is thought to be multifactorial. The following may have a role:
   a. Genetic-temperamental factors
   b. Neurologic immaturity
   c. Biochemical aberration of dopamine production
   d. Toxins, such as lead, food dyes, and salicylates
   e. Psychological factors
   f. Perinatal adversity
   g. Inappropriate societal and teacher expectations

3. **Assessment**
   a. **History.** If possible, communication with teachers, special educators, and psychologists should take place. Essentials of the history include:
      (1) The perinatal history
      (2) The child's early temperament
      (3) A detailed preschool and school history
      (4) The family history of inattention or school problems
   b. **Physical examination.** Behavioral observations of the child during the physical examination should be cautiously interpreted, as anxiety may increase or decrease inattention. Elements of the physical examination that deserve emphasis are:
      (1) Evidence of minor physical anomalies that occasionally correlate with ADHD, such as:
         (a) Epicanthal folds and hypertelorism of the eyes
         (b) Low-set or malformed ears
         (c) High-arched palate
         (d) Clinodactyly (inward curvature) of the fifth finger
      (2) Head circumference
      (3) Neurologic examination, including soft signs [see III A 3 b (1)]
      (4) Hearing and vision assessment
   c. **Laboratory studies.** No single test establishes the diagnosis of ADHD. Hematocrit or hemoglobin concentration may be obtained to screen for anemia, blood lead or free erythrocyte protoporphyrin may be performed to look for evidence of lead toxicity, and thyroid studies may be obtained. ECG and CT scan appear to have no role in diagnosis at this time.

4. **Therapy**
   a. **Behavioral management** is the mainstay of treatment. Strategies include increasing structure in the environment, positive reinforcement, counseling, and a number of cognitive approaches that emphasize relaxation and/or self-control.
   b. **Special education.** Children with attention deficits often require highly structured classrooms with low student-teacher ratios to maximize their educational experience.
   c. **Medication** may have an adjuvant role in treatment but should only be considered after behavioral and educational interventions have been tried.
      (1) **Stimulants** (e.g., methylphenidate, dextroamphetamine, pemoline) are the drugs most commonly used to treat ADHD and should be the initial choice.
         (a) Stimulants primarily are intended to help with school performance, so they usually are given on school days rather than on vacation days.
         (b) **Side effects** of stimulants include anorexia, headache, sleep disturbances, and possible growth retardation. **Tourette syndrome** (see Ch 17 IX B 3) has been reported as a possible complication of stimulant therapy, so any child with tics or a family history of tics probably should not receive stimulants.
      (2) **Tricyclic antidepressants** (e.g., desipramine, imipramine) and **clonidine** have also been helpful in treating ADHD.
   d. **Alternative therapies.** Dietary restrictions, megavitamin therapy, and sensory motor integration training have all been suggested as treatment, but there is little evidence that they can alter hyperactive or inattentive behavior in the majority of affected children.

## C. School phobia

1. **Definition.** School phobia in a child is manifested by **poor school attendance** caused by unwarranted fear or by inappropriate anxiety about leaving home, or, in particular, the child's mother. The school-phobic child prefers to remain at home and avoid school. School phobia is seen in approximately 1.7% of school-age children per year. Typically, the phobic child has problems beginning school in the fall and returning to school after vacations.

**2. Etiology.** The reason for the development of school phobia in any given child depends on a variety of factors within the child and within the family. The typical scenario involves a passive and dependent child who encounters an additional stressor (e.g., illness, school problems, the death of a loved one).

**3. Assessment**
   **a.** School phobia has been described as "the great imitator." Typical findings are:
      **(1)** Vague physical symptoms
      **(2)** A normal physical examination and laboratory findings
      **(3)** Poor school attendance attributed to the somatic symptoms
   **b.** A thorough history and physical examination, in addition to select laboratory tests (e.g., complete blood count, erythrocyte sedimentation rate, urinalysis) often are necessary to assure parents that the child's symptoms are not secondary to organic disease. A symptom diary is also often helpful in this regard.

**4. Therapy**
   **a.** After the parents are assured that their child is well, the physician should insist on the **immediate return of the child to school**. The physician should then review with the parents what approach to use if the child reports that he or she is sick the next day.
   **b.** **Psychotherapy** may be indicated for the parents and child. Behavioral management techniques, such as desensitization, may be helpful.
   **c.** The short-term use of **antianxiety medications** may be necessary if the child's anxiety is overwhelming.

## IV. PROFOUND DEVELOPMENTAL DISORDERS

### A. Autism

**1. Definition.** Autism is characterized by profound deficits in interpersonal and communication skills. Specific symptoms include:
   **a.** Impaired social interaction (e.g., lack of awareness of existence of others, not seeking others for comfort)
   **b.** Impaired verbal and nonverbal communication (e.g., limited language, echolalia, limited eye contact)
   **c.** Restricted repertoire of activities and interests (e.g., stereotypic body movements, need for sameness in daily routines)
   **d.** Absence of hallucinations, delusion, and other features of schizophrenia
   **e.** Onset before 30 months of age

**2. Etiology.** Autism is believed to be caused by an as yet **unidentified brain dysfunction**. Prenatal complications, fragile X syndrome (as well as other genetic conditions), maternal rubella, phenylketonuria, meningitis, and encephalitis are thought to be predisposing factors to autism, although many autistic children have no known predisposing factors.

**3. Assessment**
   **a.** No specific biochemical or anatomic aberration has been consistently associated with autism, although abnormalities of serotonin and at the neocerebellum have been reported in some children with the disorder.
   **b.** Seventy percent of children with this disorder function in the retarded range, and this group is more prone to develop seizures in adolescence than the nonretarded group.
   **c.** Assessment of the autistic child should rule out other conditions that may present similarly, such as mental retardation, childhood schizophrenia, hearing impairment, developmental language disorders, genetic disorders, and the results of profound isolation and neglect.

**4. Therapy**
   **a.** **Medical management.** There is no proven medical treatment for autism at this time, although experimental treatment with drugs such as fenfluramine has been tried. If seizures are present, anticonvulsant agents should be used appropriately.
   **b.** **Special education.** The child should be in an educational program designed to address the complex needs of autistic children with a strong emphasis on communication and appropriate social interaction.
   **c.** **Psychological management.** The rearing of an autistic child is frustrating and emotionally draining, and parents should be offered professional support and exposure to other parents facing similar problems.

**B. Mental retardation**

1. **Definition.** Mental retardation is defined as significantly subaverage general intellectual functioning existing concurrently with deficits in adaptive behavior and manifested during the developmental period (i.e., prior to age 18 years).

2. **Incidence.** Approximately 3% of the population is affected.

3. **Classification.** Four subgroups of retardation have been designated.
   a. **Mild ("educable")—IQ levels of 55–70.** This group represents 80% of the retarded population. As adults, these people are able to live independently, marry, and be employed, and they have functional reading and writing skills. Their major deficits are in judgment.
   b. **Moderate ("trainable")—IQ levels of 40–55.** This group represents 12% of the retarded population. These people do not necessarily require custodial care, but they do require continuous supervision and economic support. They are capable of self-care and employment in a sheltered setting.
   c. **Severe—IQ levels of 20–40.** This group represents about 7% of the retarded population. These people are totally economically dependent and require close supervision. They may acquire language and can be trained in elementary self-care skills.
   d. **Profound—IQ levels of less than 20.** This group represents 1% of the retarded population. These people have limited communication and self-care skills and often have associated complex medical needs. They require a highly structured environment, with continuous care and supervision.

4. **Etiology.** The causes of mental retardation are varied and represent a wide variety of biologic and environmental factors. They are summarized in Table 3-1. Only a minority of cases of mental retardation can be attributed to known biologic factors. Mild retardation is more prevalent among lower socioeconomic groups and is rarely explained by biologic causes. Moderate and severe retardation are more evenly distributed throughout all socioeconomic groups and more frequently tend to have a biologic explanation.

5. **Assessment**
   a. **History.** The family's pedigree and details of the pregnancy, delivery, and the immediate postnatal period are critical.
   b. **Physical examination.** Attention should be given to the head circumference, to dysmorphic features and associated anomalies that might suggest a syndrome, and to the neurologic examination. As previously mentioned, children in the mildly retarded range rarely have evidence of biologic abnormalities.
   c. **Developmental testing**
      (1) Diagnosis of mental retardation can only be made with the use of standardized psychometric testing administered by a trained professional. It cannot be made with screening instruments, and it rarely is made in young children because of the lack of stability of the test scores of children younger than 5 years. Children under 5 with cognitive difficulties are considered to be developmentally delayed.
      (2) Developmental delay is a less specific term than mental retardation, because it implies only that the child's performance at the present time is delayed compared to peers of the same age. It does not predict future performance.

# V. SENSORY IMPAIRMENT

**A. Hearing impairment**

1. **Definitions**
   a. **Degree of impairment.** The designation **hearing-impaired** applies to any hearing disability within the mild to profound range.
      (1) **Mild** loss refers to a 20–40 dB loss.
      (2) **Moderate** (40–60 dB) or **severe** (60–80 dB) loss has significant impact on speech acquisition.
      (3) **Profound** loss (deafness) refers to a more than 80 dB loss in the speech frequency. A deaf child is unable to process language through audition, even with a hearing aid.
   b. **Functional subtypes of hearing loss**
      (1) **Conductive hearing loss** is defined as interference in the transmission of sound from the external auditory canal to the inner ear, most commonly due to otitis media or its sequelae. Most conductive loss can be corrected by medical treatment or surgery.

**Table 3-1.** Conditions Associated with Mental Retardation

| Period of Development | Type of Condition | Examples |
| --- | --- | --- |
| Pre- and periconceptual | Metabolic disorders | Mucopolysaccharidoses<br>Tay-Sachs disease |
| | Brain malformation | Encephalocele<br>Hydranencephaly |
| | Neurocutaneous disorders | Tuberous sclerosis<br>Neurofibromatosis |
| | Chromosomal abnormalities | Down syndrome<br>Cri du chat (5p-) syndrome |
| Prenatal | Teratogen exposure | Chemicals<br>Radiation<br>Alcohol |
| | Infection | Rubella<br>Cytomegalovirus |
| | Fetal malnutrition | Mother with high blood pressure or kidney disease |
| Perinatal | Prematurity | Complications such as poor oxygenation of the brain and intracranial hemorrhage |
| | Metabolic abnormalities | Asphyxia at birth<br>Hypoglycemia |
| | Infection | Herpes simplex encephalitis |
| Postnatal | Infection | Meningitis |
| | Trauma | Automobile accident<br>Child abuse |
| | Lack of oxygen | Near-drowning<br>Strangulation |
| | Severe nutritional deficiency | Kwashiorkor |
| | Environmental toxin exposure | Lead |
| | Environmental and social problems | Psychosocial deprivation<br>Parental psychiatric disorders |

Reprinted from: Blackman J (ed): *Medical Aspects of Developmental Disabilities in Children*. Rockville, MD, Aspen Publishers, 1984, p 148.

(2) **Sensorineural hearing loss** is hearing loss secondary to damage to the inner ear or auditory nerve. This type of hearing loss is nearly always irreversible, and treatment is usually amplification.
(3) A **mixed-type** of hearing loss involves both sensorineural and conductive loss simultaneously.

2. **Etiology**
   a. Causes of **conductive hearing loss** include:
      (1) Abnormalities of the external auditory canal or ossicles
      (2) Otitis media
      (3) Trauma
      (4) Foreign bodies
      (5) Otosclerosis
      (6) Cerumen in the ear canal
   b. Causes of **sensorineural hearing loss** include:
      (1) Rubella or another congenital infection
      (2) Mumps, meningitis, or another postnatal infection

       **(3)** Perinatal asphyxia or prematurity
       **(4)** Trauma
       **(5)** Kernicterus
       **(6)** Ototoxic drugs (e.g., aminoglycosides)
       **(7)** Genetic causes (e.g., Waardenburg syndrome, Alport syndrome, Usher syndrome, mucopolysaccharidosis, Pendred syndrome)
       **(8)** Environmental (noise-induced)

**3. Assessment**

  **a. History**

    **(1)** High-risk situations affecting **newborns** that should alert the physician to possible hearing loss include:

      **(a)** Familial hearing loss

      **(b)** Congenital rubella, cytomegalovirus, toxoplasmosis, or herpes

      **(c)** Low birth weight (less than 1500 g)

      **(d)** Hyperbilirubinemia

      **(e)** Congenital malformation of the pinna, skull, lip, or palate

      **(f)** Meningitis

      **(g)** Ototoxic drugs (e.g., aminoglycosides)

      **(h)** Significant perinatal asphyxia

    **(2)** The following should cause the physician to suspect a hearing loss in **infants and young children:**

      **(a)** Parental concern

      **(b)** A history of otitis media occuring under 6 months of age or recurrent otitis occurring under 2 years of age

      **(c)** Chronic serous otitis media

      **(d)** Failure on a school hearing test

      **(e)** Speech problems and language delay

  **b. Physical examination**

    **(1)** Abnormalities of and around the pinna, ear canal, or tympanic membrane should be noted. Pneumatic otoscopy should be performed.

    **(2)** Other abnormalities that may suggest a genetic explanation for hearing impairment should be identified.

  **c. Audiologic evaluation.** Depending on the age and cognitive abilities of the child, various audiologic evaluations are appropriate. These include behavioral and observational hearing assessments, pure tone audiometry, and evoked response audiometry.

**4. Therapy**

  **a. Medical management** may involve the antibiotic treatment of otitis media and the placement of tympanostomy tubes for chronic middle ear effusions. Surgical techniques (e.g., cochlear implants) are available for some children. Amplification may be necessary for sensorineural hearing loss.

  **b. Education.** The hearing-impaired child requires educational intervention to allow for maximal development.

    **(1) Alternate methods of communication.** Depending on the degree of impairment, signing may be required for effective education.

    **(2) Modification of curriculum** ranges from preferential seating in the front of the classroom to placement in a residential school. The degree of intervention is determined by the degree of hearing loss.

  **c. Genetic counseling** may be indicated, depending on the etiology of the hearing loss.

**B. Visual impairment**

**1. Definitions**

  **a. Visual impairment** is an educational term that implies that vision is impaired sufficiently enough to affect school functioning.

  **b.** A **partially sighted** individual has vision in the better eye between 20/70 and 20/200.

  **c. Blindness** is defined as vision of not more than 20/200 in the better eye, after correction, or as a defect in the visual field such that the widest diameter of vision subtends an angle of 10° or less.

**2. Etiology**

  **a. Congenital** etiologies include developmental malformations, perinatal infections (e.g., rubella, cytomegalovirus, toxoplasmosis), and genetic syndromes (e.g., albinism).

    **b. Neonatal** etiologies include birth asphyxia, prematurity, and infections.

    **c. Postnatal** etiologies include trauma, retinitis pigmentosa, demyelinating disease, neuro-degenerative disease, tumor, and increased intracranial pressure.

    **d. Functional** etiologies also are possible. For example, in cortical blindness the eye is structurally sound, but the cortex is unable to process visual information.

**3. Assessment**

    **a. History.** A number of risk factors should increase the suspicion of possible visual impairment in infants and young children, including:

      **(1)** A family history of visual defects

      **(2)** A history of congenital infections

      **(3)** A history of premature delivery or prolonged labor

      **(4)** Evidence of mental retardation, cerebral palsy, or hearing difficulty (40%–50% of partially sighted children have additional handicaps)

    **b. Physical examination**

      **(1)** In the **neonatal period,** the physical examination should assess the gross appearance of the eyes, the alignment of the eyes, brightness and clarity of the red reflex, and some funduscopic details.

      **(2)** In **older children,** the visual field should be assessed and more detailed funduscopic examinations should be performed. If more complicated assessments are required, or if there is a history of oxygen therapy or a family history of major visual defects, referral to an ophthalmologist is appropriate.

    **c. Visual assessment**

      **(1) Infancy.** By age 3 months, the child should be able to follow familiar objects. Optokinetic nystagmus should be assessed. **Visual evoked response testing** is a technique available for the assessment of vision in an infant.

      **(2) Preschool period.** Modified charts, such as the Stycar and the Random Dot E, can be used to assess visual acuity.

      **(3) School years.** Visual acuity is typically estimated using the Snellen E chart.

**4. Therapy**

    **a. Management** of visual impairment includes the correction of refraction errors with lenses, eye patching, as well as surgery for strabismus.

    **b. Developmental factors** should be considered when dealing with a visually impaired child.

      **(1)** Blind children require an extremely rich sensory environment to maximize the use of their other senses. Referral to an **early intervention** program is essential.

      **(2)** Blind children have a tendency to develop unusual movement patterns (**blindisms**), which can potentially isolate these children even further. Some of these behaviors can be easily extinguished using **behavior modification** techniques.

    **c. Education.** Many educational techniques are available to visually impaired children, including Optacon, which converts words to tactile print, as well as print to speech converters. Talking books, laser-guided canes, and other low-vision aids enable visually impaired individuals to function more independently in society.

    **d. Genetic counseling** is also necessary in many cases of visual impairment.

## VI. RECURRENT PAIN

**A. Introduction and definition.** Recurrent pain occurs frequently in children. The emphasis in this section is on those entities that are not due to organic disease—**recurrent abdominal pain syndrome, "psychogenic" headache,** and **limb pain**. These are pains that occur at least monthly for a 3-month period, in which no organic pathology is found; during the interval between episodes, the child is well. Because of similarities in the approach to assessing and treating these entities, they are discussed here as a group.

**B. Incidence.** Recurrent abdominal pain occurs in 10%–15% of school-age children, with a peak incidence at age 9 years. Growing pains occur in 15% of school-age children, with a peak incidence at age 11. Headache occurs in 15%–20% of school children with a peak incidence at age 12.

**C. Etiology.** Purely organic or purely emotional etiologic explanations account for only a minor percentage of recurrent pain. Current thinking regarding recurrent pain refutes the previous dichotomy of either an organic or a psychological explanation for these problems and substitutes a new category—**dysfunctional pain**. The pain is neither the result of pathophysiology nor obvious psychopathology but is the result of mild individual differences in physiology, which make the child vulnerable to pain and which may be exacerbated by stress. For example, in children with recurrent abdominal pain, there may be slower transit time resulting in constipation, lactose intolerance, or increased autonomic nervous system activity. The **differential diagnosis** for recurrent pain other than dysfunctional pain includes:

1. **Recurrent abdominal pain**
   a. Genitourinary problems (e.g., recurrent infections, lower tract obstruction, vulvovaginitis)
   b. Gastrointestinal disorders (e.g., inflammatory bowel disease, ulcer disease, hepatitis)
   c. Psychological causes (e.g., conversion reactions, somatoform disorders)
   d. Other disorders, including porphyria and trauma

2. **Headache**
   a. Medical causes (e.g., infection, increased blood pressure)
   b. Neurologic causes (e.g., migraine, increased intracranial pressure)
   c. Vascular abnormalities
   d. Psychological causes

3. **Limb pain** (growing pains)
   a. Orthopedic disorders (e.g., Osgood-Schlatter disease, Legg-Calvé-Perthes disease, trauma)
   b. Collagen vascular disease
   c. Infection
   d. Neoplastic disease

D. **Assessment**

1. **History.** Essentials include the following.
   a. Characteristics of the pain must be noted, such as onset, frequency, duration, and associated symptoms. Continuous pain, localized pain, pain that awakens the child from sleep, and pain associated with other symptoms (e.g., vomiting, fever, changes in stool color) suggest organic disease.
   b. Evidence of obvious psychopathology must be sought in the parents and in the child, and major stressors on the family should be identified. It is also important to identify whether other family members have symptoms similar to those of the patient.

2. **Physical examination** to rule out obvious organic explanations for the symptoms is essential. Normal growth and development are unlikely in the face of chronic organic disease.
   a. **Recurrent abdominal pain.** The further the pain is from the umbilicus, the more likely it is to be organic. A rectal examination is imperative.
   b. **Headache.** The more localized the pain, the less likely it is to be "psychogenic." Blood pressure determination, assessment of the visual field, and a thorough funduscopic examination are essential.
   c. **Limb pain.** The more localized the pain, the less likely it is to be growing pains. The physical examination should include assessment of the affected limb for evidence of atrophy, swelling, weakness, and effusion.

3. **Laboratory investigation.** Complete blood count, erythrocyte sedimentation rate, and urinalysis comprise a good screen. Further investigation should take place only if suggested by the history and physical examination.

E. **Therapy**

1. If **organic disease** is identified, it should be treated appropriately.

2. If there is a strong indication that **psychological factors** are responsible for the symptoms, the physician should provide appropriate counsel or referral to a mental health agency.

3. Most often, neither organic nor psychological factors appear responsible. If this is the case and if the characteristics fit the definition of **dysfunctional pain,** this type of pain should be explained to the family (see VI C). The long-term outlook for recurrent pain during childhood is promising.
   a. For dysfunctional pain, **normal activity should be encouraged,** and the pain should not be allowed to restrict the child significantly.
   b. A **symptom diary** should be kept by the parents and the child, detailing information regarding episodes of pain. Frequent visits to the physician with review of this diary are helpful.

    **c. Symptomatic relief** should be offered. Mild analgesics (e.g., acetaminophen) for pain episodes, dietary changes, exercise, and stress reduction may all be helpful.

## VII. EMOTIONAL DISORDERS

### A. Depression

  **1. Definition.** Depression is a clinical syndrome characterized by a persistent mood disorder and dysfunctional behavior. Although findings may differ at the various developmental stages, they generally include sadness or unhappiness, social withdrawal, eating problems, sleeping disorders, and a decreased ability to concentrate. The incidence of childhood depression in the general population is 2%, and depression accounts for 30% of childhood psychiatric disorders.

  **2. Etiology** is multifactorial. Genetic causes, chronic illness, as well as psychosocial stress have been implicated. Certain specific disease states are associated with depression (e.g., epilepsy, hypothyroidism, adrenal insufficiency, migraine), and a number of medical problems can mimic it (e.g., neuromuscular disease that affects facial expression, degenerative disease that causes psychomotor retardation).

  **3. Assessment**

    **a. History**

      **(1)** Details from home and school regarding the cause of the symptoms and the degree of dysfunction should be elicited.

      **(2)** Information about social withdrawal, mood, appetite, sleep patterns, and irritability should be obtained.

      **(3)** A history of family members with possible depressive illnesses who were hospitalized, who required electroconvulsive therapy, or who committed suicide is important to a complete assessment.

    **b. Physical examination**

      **(1)** In addition to the routine physical examination, funduscopic examination for evidence of increased intracranial pressure should be done.

      **(2)** Deep tendon reflexes should be carefully reviewed for evidence of hypothyroidism.

    **c. Laboratory and x-ray investigation**

      **(1)** If the cause of depression is not obviously psychosocial, complete blood count, erythrocyte sedimentation rate, and thyroid studies are helpful.

      **(2)** Evidence of drug abuse should be sought.

      **(3)** A CT scan is indicated if evidence of intracranial pathology is suspected.

      **(4)** A dexamethasone suppression test might be considered. Among adults with endogenous depression, hypersecretion of cortisol and failure to suppress cortisol secretion with dexamethasone have been reported in two-thirds of patients. The extent of such findings among depressed children is unclear.

  **4. Therapy**

    **a. Psychotherapy** for the child and family is indicated.

    **b. Antidepressant medication**—typically a tricyclic antidepressant—may be considered.

### B. Schizophrenia

  **1. Definition**

    **a.** Schizophrenia is a syndrome of grossly impaired behavior that is characterized by:

      **(1)** Characteristic disturbances of thought, perception, relationship to the external world, and motor activity

      **(2)** Deterioration from a previous level of functioning

      **(3)** A duration of at least 6 months

      **(4)** Often loose associations, delusions, and hallucinations

    **b.** Episodes of childhood schizophrenia typically occur after the age of 7 years and increase in frequency to adolescence.

  **2. Etiology**

    **a.** Many authorities suggest that the development of childhood schizophrenia is a multifactorial process involving **social and emotional stressors** in a child with a **genetic predisposition** or **a biologic vulnerability** or both.

   **b.** A number of **medical conditions** have been associated with childhood psychosis, including:
     **(1)** Wilson's disease
     **(2)** Thyroid disease
     **(3)** Systemic lupus erythematosus
     **(4)** Homocystinuria
     **(5)** Leukodystrophy
   **c.** Factors in the **differential diagnosis** include:
     **(1)** Brief reactive psychoses
     **(2)** Overwhelming anxiety
     **(3)** Depression
     **(4)** Imaginary friends and other normal developmental occurrences in childhood

**3. Assessment**
   **a. History.** The essential aspects of the patient's history to be determined include:
     **(1)** Whether the child's current problem represents a deterioration from a previous level of functioning or merely the continuation of a previous delay in development
     **(2)** Evidence of delusions and hallucinations
     **(3)** A family history with evidence of mental illness
   **b. Physical examination.** The focus of the physical examination should be on evidence of an organic explanation for the psychosis (e.g., drug ingestion, thyroid disease, Wilson's disease, increased intracranial pressure).
   **c. Laboratory investigation**
     **(1)** Urine should be tested for toxic substances.
     **(2)** Liver function tests should be performed, and serum levels of ceruloplasmin should be measured for evidence of Wilson's disease.
     **(3)** Psychometric testing might also be helpful.

**4. Therapy.** The course of childhood schizophrenia is usually chronic. A number of treatments should be considered, including:
   **a. Antipsychotic medication**
   **b. Psychotherapy** and support for the child and family (hospitalization during acute episodes may be necessary)
   **c. Education** (a specific educational program for the psychotic child is often necessary)

# VIII. CHILD ABUSE

**A. Definitions**

1. **Physical abuse** is the nonaccidental injury of a child (see Ch 2 I E 1).

2. **Sexual abuse** is any sexual activity between an adult and a child [assaultive or nonassaultive] (see Ch 4 VI E).

3. **Physical neglect** is failure to provide the necessities of life for the child (i.e., nourishment, clothing, shelter, supervision, and medical care).

4. **Emotional neglect** involves parental failure to provide an environment in which the child can thrive and develop.

5. **Munchausen syndrome by proxy** is defined as a syndrome in which the child becomes a victim of parentally induced or parentally fabricated illness, which often causes him to undergo unnecessary diagnostic and sometimes therapeutic interventions.

**B. Incidence.** Seven hundred new cases of child abuse occur per million people per year in the United States. The mortality rate is 3%, or 2000 deaths per year. Of children 1–6 months old, child abuse is second only to sudden infant death syndrome (SIDS) as a cause of child mortality. In the group 1–5 years old, it is second to injuries as a killer of children. One-third of the victims are less than 1 year old, one-third are 1–6 years old, and one-third are over age 6 years. Premature infants have a three times greater risk of abuse than full-term infants.

**C. Etiology.** The abuser is a related adult in 90% of cases of child abuse. Only 10% of abusers are seriously emotionally ill. The overwhelming majority are isolated and stressed individuals with limited social support.

### D. Assessment

1. **History.** Obtaining an accurate history is important. However, discussion with the child should be developmentally appropriate and nonthreatening. Repeated questioning or badgering is both inhumane and nonproductive. The parents should be interviewed in a nonconfrontational, nonjudgmental manner that is culturally sensitive. The physician should seek answers to the following questions.

   a. Are the circumstances surrounding the injury as documented by the parents consistent with the physical findings?

   b. Is the explanation of the injury plausible, given the child's age and developmental capabilities?

   c. Is there a history of previous trauma?

   d. Was there a delay in seeking care?

2. **Physical examination.** Photographs of the trauma should be obtained, if possible.

   a. A number of **cutaneous lesions** are frequently seen in abuse, including:

   (1) Linear bruising, which is caused by striking with a stick or rod

   (2) Loop marks, which occur when a belt, electric cord, or rope is used for striking

   (3) Binding injuries

   (4) Cigarette burns

   (5) Scald injuries, which are secondary to submersion in hot water, often having a stocking or glove distribution

   b. **Dating of bruises**

   (1) At 0–2 days, the area is swollen and tender.

   (2) At 0–5 days, it is red or blue.

   (3) At 5–7 days, it is green.

   (4) At 7–10 days, it is yellow.

   (5) At 10–14 days, it is brown.

   (6) At 2–4 weeks, the discoloration is gone.

   c. If **sexual abuse** is a concern, careful examination of the external genitalia and rectum is imperative. If available, colposcopic examination should be performed.

3. **Laboratory data**

   a. Coagulation studies to determine a bleeding disorder, urinalysis, and a long-bone survey should be performed.

   b. If sexual abuse is considered, cultures of the mouth, rectum, vagina, and urethra should be obtained. A Venereal Disease Research Laboratory (VDRL) test should be performed, and vaginal fluid should be aspirated to check for semen.

### E. Therapy

1. Children suspected of having been abused should be hospitalized for protection, evaluation, and treatment.

2. Notification of the appropriate state protective agency is vital. Physicians are mandated to report abuse in every state and are protected from liability. Failure to report abuse can lead to further harm to the child and prosecution of the physician.

3. The current trend is to provide services to the family to allow them to care for the child more adequately. Removal of the child from the home, or termination of parental rights, is usually a last resort and occurs usually only after serious abuse has occurred without response to treatment.

4. With treatment, most abusing families can provide adequate care for their children. Without intervention, 25% of these children will be repeatedly abused and 5% will be killed.

## STUDY QUESTIONS

**Directions:** Each of the numbered items or incomplete statements in this section is followed by answers or by completions of the statement. Select the **one** lettered answer or completion that is **best** in each case.

1. In the treatment of failure to thrive, if no organic problems are identified in the history or physical examination, the next step should be

(A) more extensive laboratory investigation

(B) hospitalization for further evaluation and observation

(C) provision of a high-calorie diet on an outpatient basis

(D) referral to a dietitian for dietary manipulation

(E) referral to a subspecialist

2. Which of the following symptoms would suggest a diagnosis of recurrent abdominal pain?

(A) Pain awakening a child from sleep

(B) Pain associated with vomiting

(C) Pain located periumbilically

(D) Pain radiating to the back

3. According to the definition given by the National Advisory Committee on Handicapped Children, which of the following conditions is NOT associated with a learning disability?

(A) Math difficulties

(B) Mental retardation

(C) Visual motor integration problems

(D) Sequential memory deficits

(E) Dyslexia

4. A 24-month-old child who has not yet begun to speak is brought to the pediatrician's office. All of the following conditions should be considered in the differential diagnosis EXCEPT

(A) autism

(B) developmental delay

(C) hearing impairment

(D) severe parental neglect

(E) childhood schizophrenia

5. All of the following conditions may cause sensorineural hearing loss EXCEPT

(A) rubella

(B) meningitis

(C) perinatal asphyxia

(D) otitis media

(E) aminoglycoside administration

6. All of the following statements regarding the use of stimulant medication in attention deficit-hyperactivity disorder (ADHD) are correct EXCEPT

(A) Tourette syndrome is a possible complication of stimulant usage

(B) stimulant drugs are the initial treatment for ADHD

(C) stimulants usually are administered only on school mornings

(D) methylphenidate, dextroamphetamine, and pemoline are the major stimulants in use at this time

### Questions 7–9

A fourth-year medical student is asked to evaluate a mildly obese 6-year-old boy. The boy is tall for his age, has a normal physical examination, and is described as an average student. His parents, who also are obese, believe he has a "glandular problem."

7. All of the following would be helpful in the initial evaluation and management of this child EXCEPT

(A) history of the child's dietary intake

(B) family history

(C) chromosomal analysis

(D) blood pressure measurement

(E) serum cholesterol and triglyceride studies

8. The most likely diagnosis for this boy is

(A) Laurence-Moon syndrome

(B) Prader-Willi syndrome

(C) hypothyroidism

(D) exogenous obesity

| | | |
|---|---|---|
| 1-C | 4-E | 7-C |
| 2-C | 5-D | 8-D |
| 3-B | 6-B | |

9. Which of the following would be the most appropriate initial treatment of this child?

(A) Psychotherapy
(B) Jaw wiring
(C) Positive reinforcement for dietary alterations
(D) Highly restrictive, low-calorie diet
(E) Rigorous daily exercise

**Directions:** Each item below contains four suggested answers of which **one or more** is correct. Choose the answer

A    if **1, 2, and 3** are correct
B    if **1 and 3** are correct
C    if **2 and 4** are correct
D    if **4** is correct
E    if **1, 2, 3, and 4** are correct

10. School phobia can result from

(1) a learning disability

(2) overprotective parents

(3) a death in the family

(4) a frightening teacher

11. A 16-year-old girl presents with signs of depression, including social withdrawal, anorexia, sadness, and inability to concentrate. Initial evaluation of this teenager should include

(1) measurement of serum ceruloplasmin levels to rule out Wilson's disease

(2) a toxic screen for evidence of drug abuse

(3) a CT scan

(4) a thorough examination for evidence of thyroid disease

**Directions:** The group of items in this section consists of lettered options followed by a set of numbered items. For each item, select the **one** lettered option that is most closely associated with it. Each lettered option may be selected once, more than once, or not at all.

**Questions 12–15**

For each characteristic, select the continence disorder with which it is associated.

(A) Encopresis
(B) Enuresis
(C) Both
(D) Neither

12. A familial tendency

13. Possible confusion with Hirschsprung's disease

14. Psychological origin in most cases

15. Involuntary in nature

---

 9-C        12-B        15-C
10-E        13-A
11-C        14-D

## ANSWERS AND EXPLANATIONS

**1. The answer is C** *[I A 4 b].*
In the treatment of failure to thrive, provision of a high-calorie diet is the first step in treatment. Further laboratory testing is rarely fruitful without indication from the patient's history and from the physical examination of its necessity. Hospitalization or referral to a dietitian may be necessary if there is no weight gain after a trial on a high-calorie diet. Referral to a subspecialist is indicated only if specific pathology is identified.

**2. The answer is C** *[VI D].*
Recurrent abdominal pain typically is periumbilical and diffuse. Well-localized pain, radiating pain, pain associated with other symptoms, and pain so severe as to awaken a child from sleep is less likely to be recurrent abdominal pain and more likely to be organic.

**3. The answer is B** *[III A 1].*
Implicit in the definition of learning disability is normal intellectual potential. Therefore, a diagnosis of mental retardation technically excludes an individual from being classified as learning disabled. Reading difficulties (termed dyslexia by some authorities) are extremely common among learning-disabled children. While math problems are less common, they certainly do occur. Various developmental deficits, including visual motor integration problems and sequential memory problems, are frequently found among learning-disabled children.

**4. The answer is E** *[VII B 1 b].*
Childhood schizophrenia usually does not present until after the age of 7 years. Autism develops by age 30 months and is associated with gross defects in language. Children with developmental delay also can present with limited language. Extreme parental neglect has been reported to cause delays in language acquisition and to cause depression, which can lead to elective mutism.

**5. The answer is D** *[V A 2 b].*
Otitis media is associated with conductive hearing loss, not sensorineural hearing loss. Rubella and other prenatal infections can cause sensorineural hearing loss, as can meningitis and other postnatal infections. Perinatal asphyxia has also been implicated. Aminoglycosides are ototoxic in high doses and should be carefully monitored.

**6. The answer is B** *[III B 4 c].*
Treatment of attention deficit-hyperactivity disorder (ADHD) with stimulant drugs should be initiated only after academic and behavioral approaches to the disorder have been attempted. A number of side effects, such as sleep and eating problems, headaches, growth retardation, and, rarely, Tourette syndrome, have been associated with stimulant use. Using medication only on school days and at lower doses helps to prevent some of these side effects.

**7–9. The answers are: 7-C** *[I B 2]*, **8-D** *[I B 3 a (1)]*, **9-C** *[I B 4].*
A chromosomal defect is an extremely rare explanation for obesity in a child with a normal physical examination, normal stature, and normal learning abilities. A review of the child's dietary history may reveal excessive caloric intake and suggest treatment recommendations. Family history is important, since the likelihood of a child being obese is greatly increased if family members also are obese. Blood pressure should be determined since it may be elevated in obese children. Obese individuals are more likely to have hyperlipidemia; therefore, serum triglycerides and cholesterol should be determined.

With obese parents, a normal physical examination, and normal mental status, this child most likely has exogenous obesity. Prader-Willi syndrome and Laurence-Moon syndrome are associated with short stature, mental retardation, and hypogonadism. Hypothyroidism would be unlikely in a child with normal stature and normal learning abilities.

Positive reinforcement through behavior modification is the most appropriate approach for a young, mildly obese child. Rigorous exercise, severe calorie restriction, and mechanical approaches such as jaw wiring are inappropriate in a growing child. Psychotherapy may be helpful in a morbidly obese child but is of little benefit at such a young age.

**10. The answer is E (all)** *[III C 2].*
School phobia can result from any situation at home or at school that can cause a vulnerable child to develop undue fears of leaving home and going to school. Often the phobia is due to the child's fear of

being separated from his mother under any circumstances. Often the child is fearful of someone at school or on the way to school.

**11. The answer is C (2, 4)** *[VII A 3 c, B 3 b].*
Symptoms of drug abuse and hypothyroidism both can mimic those of depression. Wilson's disease is more likely to mimic schizophrenia and, for diagnosis, an associated family history should exist. A CT scan should be ordered only if there is evidence of increased intracranial pressure.

**12–15. The answers are: 12-B** *[II A 2],* **13-A** *[II B 2],* **14-D** *[II A 2, B 2],* **15-C** *[II A 1, B 1].*
Both enuresis and encopresis are involuntary by definition. In general, enuresis is due to organic causes in only about 5% of children with this problem, but developmental delays and environmental factors are relatively common. Neither enuresis nor encopresis typically is solely of psychological origin. Enuresis is primarily inherited and maturational, while encopresis results from loss of bowel continence because of chronic constipation and is not familial. The differential diagnosis of encopresis should include Hirsch-sprung's disease, or aganglionic megacolon, because it frequently presents with severe constipation.

# 4
# Adolescent Medicine
Aric Schichor

## I. SCOPE AND GENERAL CONCEPTS OF ADOLESCENT MEDICINE

**A. Objectives.** Adolescence begins at puberty, a time of physical growth and personality development. The transition from childhood to adulthood is a confusing and ambiguous period for adolescents, parents, and health care providers. The time of onset of puberty and the manner of coping with the many physical, social, and emotional changes associated with adolescence vary widely from one adolescent to another. Adolescent medicine should focus on more than strictly medical issues—it also should consider the issues that affect a teenager's day-to-day well-being. Pediatric health care providers are required to:

1. Deal with acute health needs

2. Provide comprehensive health care, including:
   a. General medical care
   b. Care in high-risk health areas (e.g., sexual activity, substance abuse, depression, suicide, accidents)
   c. Guidance in general issues (e.g., peer relationships, school progress, home environment, relationship with parents)

3. Produce educated consumers of health services by providing health education

4. Encourage independence in health-seeking behavior

5. Support and counsel parents in providing supervision and guidance to their adolescents

6. Educate, assist, and work with other adults in the community who deal with adolescents

**B. General concepts**

1. **Common terms** are used to define the rights of adolescents.
   a. **Mature minors** are individuals 15 years of age or older who understand the risks and benefits of the services being provided.
   b. **Emancipated minors** are individuals 16 years of age or older who are married, have joined the armed forces, or have proven in a court of law that they are living on their own and managing their own financial affairs.

2. **State laws** vary regarding the right of adolescents to receive care without parental consent. In many states, mature minors may be treated for drug abuse and sexually transmitted diseases and may be given family planning, pregnancy, and abortion counseling without parental consent. Emancipated minors are eligible for comprehensive health care without parental consent, but emancipated minor status must be confirmed by a court in certain states.

3. **Confidentiality** is a central concept for adolescent health care. It permits the patient to form a relationship with the health care provider in which the patient can share information that is not given to anyone else without the formal consent of the patient. Confidentiality may be breached when life is at risk.

4. **The physician's office** should reflect the needs of adolescents and enhance the adolescent's attitude toward seeking health care. The decor of the waiting area and examination room should attract the adolescent. If possible, infants and children should not be seen in the same space at the same time.

**5. Family involvement** provides information about and support for adolescents and a way to increase their health care compliance.

## II. HEALTH MAINTENANCE ISSUES

### A. History

1. **Goals** of the patient history include:
   a. Obtaining information about high-risk areas in the adolescent's life from both the patient and the parents
   b. Determining specific concerns of the adolescent

2. **Methods**
   a. Information can be obtained through **interviews, discussion,** and **written questionnaires**. While questionnaires cannot replace verbal questioning, they can provide a focus for discussion, help for adolescents who are less verbal, and a way to use waiting time effectively.
   b. A **variety of approaches** to asking questions should be used, so that the patient has several opportunities to speak openly on the topics discussed. Three approaches to asking questions are:
      (1) **Direct approach** (e.g., Have you ever been in a hospital overnight?)
      (2) **Indirect approach** (e.g., Some people who get down or depressed sometimes think of ending it all or killing themselves. . . . Have you ever had such thoughts?)
      (3) **Open-ended approach** (e.g., What do you do for fun? What three things would you change to make your life better? On a scale of 1 to 5, with 1 being poor, 3 being average, and 5 being great, how would you rate your general health?). Follow-up to such questions should focus on what changes could be made to improve the situation and which changes the adolescent would like to pursue.

3. Discussing **key topics** can help address complex issues in the adolescent's life.
   a. **Sexual activity** (e.g., What are your plans for starting your own family? What would you use for protection against pregnancy?)
   b. **Substance abuse** (e.g., Do you ever get high? Do you have friends who use drugs and alcohol? What do you do when they ask you to try drugs and alcohol with them?)
   c. **Mental health** (e.g., Do you ever get down or depressed? What gets you down and depressed? Who do you talk to when you get down and depressed?)
   d. **Home situation** (e.g., What are your responsibilities at home? What would you change about your parents to make them better?)
   e. **Self-image** (e.g., How do you feel when you look at yourself in the mirror in the morning? What would you change to make yourself feel better when you look in the mirror?)

### B. Anticipatory guidance provides an opportunity to deal with the developmental issues of adolescence with both the adolescent and the parents (see Ch 1 II A 2).

1. **Early adolescence** includes the onset of puberty and continues through age 14 years.
   a. Most of the **pubertal physical changes** occur during this stage. Adolescents need reassurance that their bodies are developing normally.
   b. Issues of **independence** arise. Adolescents need to have the chance to make decisions for themselves and to be responsible for their actions. Parents need to be less protective and more comfortable in fostering responsible independence.
   c. A new **support group** is developed. Friends who were playmates now are peers and confidants. Adults outside the home are chosen as role models and counselors.
   d. Various changes occurring in the life of the adolescent may be accompanied by periods of rapid **mood swings**.
   e. Significant **school transition** from grammar school to middle school or junior high school results in increased school size, work load, and independence in school structure.

2. **Mid-adolescence** includes the ages 15 and 16 years.
   a. The **peer structure** becomes the support link in the transition from childhood, which has been left behind, to adulthood, which is yet to be reached. Parents can provide stability during this time by involving the adolescent in decision-making in the home and contracting with the adolescent on expected behavior.
   b. The adolescent undergoes a **cognitive transition** from **concrete operations** to **formal operations**. Living in the "here and now" becomes less important, while planning for the future and deferring gratification begin to take precedence.

   c. Adolescents need **privacy**.
   d. Adolescents develop an **adult identity** and their own opinions on sexuality, religion, and politics. They need to be informed of their right to health care. Parents may need assistance to recognize and deal with what they may feel is risk-taking behavior by their children.

3. **Late adolescence** begins at the age of 17 years.
   a. **Separation** from the home leads to physical independence. Parents need to realize that they are not losing their child; they are gaining an adult family member.
   b. The **decision-making process** relating to the future and to career goals is increasingly important.

C. **Physical examination** provides the physician with an opportunity to teach health maintenance, especially about routine breast and testicular examination. The adolescent's increasing need for privacy should be addressed by the use of appropriate drapes and gowns during the examination.

1. **Areas requiring special focus**
   a. **Skin.** The degree of acne and the patient's level of concern about acne should be evaluated. Facial and axillary hair development are markers used for the assessment of pubertal development.
   b. **Eyes.** Myopia may occur during pubertal development. The adolescent may ignore eye problems because of reluctance to wear glasses.
   c. **Dentition.** Evaluating the level of hygiene, discussion of the frequency of dental care, and a review of the development of the third set of **molar teeth** should be undertaken.
   d. **Neck.** The size of the thyroid gland should be noted.
   e. **Breast** examination should include determination of the stage of development as shown in Table 4-1. Tenderness, erythema, dimpling, asymmetric masses or size, discharge, and axillary adenopathy should be noted. Routine breast self-examination should be encouraged.
   f. **Heart sounds** may be accentuated because of a thin chest wall, and functional murmurs may become more apparent.
   g. **Male genitourinary tract** examination includes determination of the stage of development (Tables 4-2 and 4-3) and evaluation for urethral discharge, scrotal masses, testicular size, inguinal adenopathy, and evidence of inguinal hernia. In a boy with an uncircumcised penis, hygienic practices should be reviewed and particular attention given to possible lesions below the foreskin. Routine testicular self-examination should be encouraged.
   h. **Female genitourinary tract** examination includes determination of the stage of development (see Table 4-2) as well as an assessment of delayed puberty or abnormal pubertal development. A pelvic examination is indicated in evaluating vulvar lesions, vaginal symptoms (e.g., itching, unusual discharge, burning), lower abdominal pain, dysmenorrhea of greater than a 3-day duration, menstrual dysfunction, and exposure to a sexually transmitted disease (see IV A). Examination is also warranted in cases of maternal exposure to diethylstilbestrol (DES), desire for contraception, premarital assessment, and history of sexual intercourse.

**Table 4-1.** Stages of Female Breast Development

| | |
|---|---|
| Stage 1 | Preadolescent—The juvenile breast has an elevated papilla (nipple-shaped projection) and small flat areola. |
| Stage 2 | The breast bud forms under the influence of hormonal stimulation. The papilla and areola elevate as a small mound, and the areolar diameter increases. |
| Stage 3 | Continued enlargement of the breast bud further elevates the papilla. The areola continues to enlarge; no separation of breast contours is noted. |
| Stage 4 | The areola and papilla separate from the contour of the breast to form a secondary mound. |
| Stage 5 | Mature—The areolar mound recedes into the general contour of the breast. The papilla continues to project. |

Reprinted from Hoffmann A: *Adolescent Medicine*. Reading, MA, Addison-Wesley, 1983, p 18. Adapted from Tanner JM: *Growth at Adolescence*. Oxford, Blackwell, 1962.

**Table 4-2.** Stages of Pubic Hair Development

| | Male | Female |
|---|---|---|
| Stage 1 | Preadolescent—No pubic hair is present; a fine vellus hair covers the genital area | Preadolescent—No pubic hair is present; a fine vellus hair covers the genital area. |
| Stage 2 | A sparse distribution of long, slightly pigmented hair appears at the base of the penis. | A sparse distribution of long, slightly pigmented straight hair appears bilaterally along the medial border of the labia majora. |
| Stage 3 | The pubic hair pigmentation increases; it begins to curl and spread laterally in a scanty distribution. | The pubic hair pigmentation increases; it begins to curl and spread sparsely over the mons pubis. |
| Stage 4 | The pubic hair continues to curl and becomes coarse in texture. An adult type of distribution is attained, but the number of hairs remains fewer. | The pubic hair continues to curl and becomes coarse in texture. The number of hairs continue to increase. |
| Stage 5 | Mature—The pubic hair attains an adult distribution, with spread to the surface of the medial thigh. Pubic hair grows along the linea alba in 80% of males. | Mature—The pubic hair attains an adult feminine triangular pattern, with spread to the surface of the medial thigh. |

Reprinted from Hoffman A: *Adolescent Medicine.* Reading, MA, Addison-Wesley, 1983, p 16. Adapted from Tanner JM: *Growth at Adolescence.* Oxford, Blackwell, 1962.

   **2. Pubertal development** (for disorders of pubertal development see Ch 16 VI B)
      **a. The pubertal growth spurt** (Figure 4-1) is the third and last rapid growth stage during childhood. The first and second rapid growth stages occur in utero and shortly after birth.
         **(1)** Adolescents gain up to 25% of adult height and 50% of adult weight during this period.
         **(2)** Individuals vary widely in the onset and rate of pubertal development. It is important to talk about this variability with adolescents and, where appropriate, reassure them about the normal nature of their pubertal development.
         **(3)** This growth spurt is associated with muscle development in males and fat deposition in females.
      **b. Female pubertal changes** (Figure 4-2) start between ages 8 and 13 years and changes take place for 3–4 years. Breast development commonly precedes pubic hair development. Most girls reach adult height midway through puberty.
      **c. Male pubertal changes** (Figure 4-3) start between ages 9½ and 13½ years and changes take place for about 3 years. Testicular enlargement is usually the first sign of male pubertal development. Most boys reach adult height during the latter half of puberty.

   **D. Procedures**

      **1. Routine evaluations**
         **a. Height, weight, and blood pressure** should be measured and the data plotted in the appropriate charts. An adult blood pressure cuff should be used.

**Table 4-3.** Stages of Male Genital Development

| Stage 1 | Preadolescent—The testes, scrotum, and penis are the same as in childhood. |
|---|---|
| Stage 2 | As a result of canalization of seminiferous tubules, the testes enlarge. The scrotum enlarges, developing a reddish hue and altering in skin texture. The penis enlarges slightly. |
| Stage 3 | The testes and scrotum continue to grow. The length of the penis increases. |
| Stage 4 | The testes and scrotum continue to grow; the scrotal skin darkens. The penis grows in width, and the glans penis develops. |
| Stage 5 | Mature—The testes, scrotum, and penis are adult in size and shape. |

Reprinted from Hoffman A: *Adolescent Medicine.* Reading, MA, Addison-Wesley, 1983, p 17. Adapted from Tanner JM: *Growth at Adolescence.* Oxford, Blackwell, 1962.

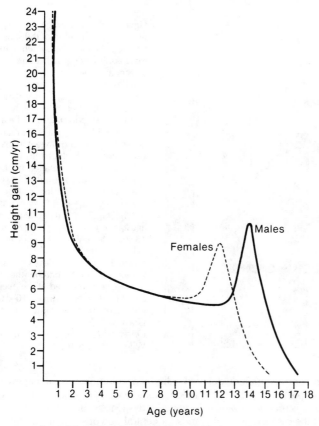

**Figure 4-1.** Graph showing the height gain (postnatal and pubertal growth spurts) in males and females between birth and age 18 years. The *curves* representing annual height gain are virtually identical for males and females until about age 9 years. At that point, the rate of height gain per year for females increases sharply until about age 12 years and then decreases sharply until it ends at about age 15½ years. The rate of height gain per year for males continues to decrease slightly from age 9 years to about age 12½ years. At that point, the rate of height gain per year for males increases sharply until about age 14 years and then decreases sharply until it ends at about age 17½ years. (Reprinted from Tanner JM, et al: Standards from birth to maturity for height, weight, height velocity, and weight velocity in British children, 1965. *Arch Dis Child* 41:454, 1965.)

   **b. Vision, hearing, and immunizations** should be checked. A tetanus booster should have been given within the past 10 years. Measles reimmunization should be performed if not administered by age 11–12 years (see Ch 1 II A 5 e).

**2. Laboratory studies**
   **a. Routine screening**
     **(1)** A complete blood count is helpful, especially to monitor changes in hematocrit levels due to increased erythropoietin activity subsequent to changes in the level of circulating androgens.
     **(2)** Sickle cell testing should be done in all black and Hispanic patients if it has not been done previously.
     **(3)** Other screening studies include urinalysis, tuberculin skin test, rubella titers in females, and mumps titers in males.
   **b. Special tests**
     **(1)** A Papanicolaou (Pap) test should be done annually on all sexually active adolescent females.
     **(2)** Pregnancy testing with a rapid urine immunoenzymatic assay for human chorionic gonadotropin (HCG) should be performed in sexually active females who are not using any form of contraception or who experience a delayed or abnormal menstrual period.
     **(3)** Cholesterol (non-fasting) level should be measured in adolescents who have a strong family history of cardiovascular disease or who are obese. If elevated, fasting cholesterol level and triglyceride level should be measured.

## III. GENITOURINARY AND GYNECOLOGIC DISORDERS

   **A. Disorders of menarche.** Normal menarche occurs at an average age of 12½ years, with bleeding lasting an average of 4–5 days. Menses may be irregular in the first 2 years. Twenty percent of young women are anovulatory into their late teens.

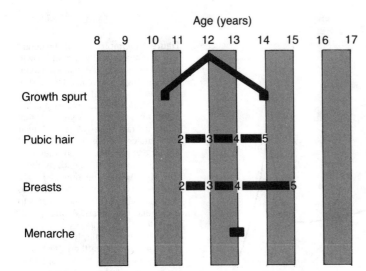

Age (years)

8    9    10   11    12   13    14   15    16   17

Growth spurt

Pubic hair     2▬3▬4▬5

Breasts     2▬3▬4▬5

Menarche

**Figure 4-2.** The average age in years of onset and duration of the stages of female pubertal development. The female adolescent growth spurt begins at the average age of 10½ years, reaches its peak at age 12 years (range, 9½–14½), and ends at the average age of 14 years. Pubic hair begins to develop in stage 2 at the average age of 11 years. Stage 3 is reached at age 12 years and stage 4 at age 13 years. Stage 5, in which the pubic hair achieves adult development, is reached at an average age of 14 years. Breasts begin to develop in stage 2 at the average age of 11 years (range, 8–13). Stage 3 is reached at the average age of 12 years and stage 4 at age 13 years. Stage 5, in which the breasts achieve adult development, is reached at an average age of 15 years (range, 13–18). Menarche (the onset of menses) is reached at the average age of 13 years (range, 10–16½). (Adapted from Grumbach MM, Grave GD, Mayer FE: *Control of the Onset of Puberty.* New York, John Wiley, 1974, p 460.)

1. **Amenorrhea**
    a. **Etiology.** Causes for amenorrhea include delayed pubertal development, significant weight gain or loss, stress or depression, pregnancy, medications (e.g., oral contraceptives, phenothiazines), structural obstruction or agenesis, gonadal dysgenesis, polycystic ovary syndrome, and tumors [of the ovaries, adrenal glands, or central nervous system (CNS)].
    b. **Primary amenorrhea** is the failure of menstruation and any other signs of pubertal development by age 14, or the failure of menstruation in spite of pubertal development by age 16.
    c. **Secondary amenorrhea** is the cessation of menstruation after it has been established at puberty (i.e., 6 months since the last menstrual period or a period of time equal to three or four previous cycles).
    d. **Oligomenorrhea** is marked by diminished menstruation, with each cycle occurring 2–3 months apart.

2. **Dysfunctional uterine bleeding** is characterized by regular menstrual cycles with heavy bleeding lasting more than 10 days, menstrual periods occurring more frequently than every 21 days, and irregular menstrual periods aside from those that commonly occur in the first 2 years after menarche.
    a. **Etiology**
        (1) Causes associated with the vagina and cervix include foreign bodies (tampons), adenosis subsequent to maternal DES exposure, and trauma or contact irritation (rape, rupture of hymen, or repeated intercourse).
        (2) Causes associated with the uterus, ovaries, and adnexa include intrauterine devices (IUDs), oral contraceptives, endometriosis, and polycystic ovary syndrome.
        (3) Other factors to consider include infections (vaginitis or salpingitis), masses (polyps or tumors), ectopic pregnancy, miscarriage, systemic disease, and bleeding disorders.
    b. **Evaluation**
        (1) **History.** The patient history should focus on the possible etiologies. The level of dysfunctional uterine bleeding should be determined.
            (a) **Mild dysfunctional bleeding** is characterized by an increase in duration of menses, a decrease in length of menstrual cycle, and a moderate increase in bleeding during menses.
            (b) **Moderate dysfunctional bleeding** is characterized by repeated episodes of prolonged menses, decreased length of menstrual cycle to the extent that menses occur every 2–3 weeks, and moderate to severe bleeding during menses.

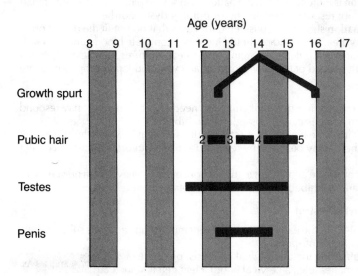

**Figure 4-3.** The average age in years of onset and duration of the stages of male pubertal development. The male adolescent growth spurt begins at the average age of 12½ years (range, 10½–16), reaches its peak rate at age 14, and ends at age 16 years (range, 13½–17½). Pubic hair begins to develop in stage 2 at the average age of 12 years. Stage 3 is reached at age 13 years and stage 4 at age 14 years. Stage 5, in which the pubic hair achieves adult development, is reached between the ages of 15 and 16 years. The testes begin to develop at the average age of 11½ years (range, 9½–13½). Maturation continues until adult development is reached at age 15 years (range, 13½–17). The penis begins to develop at the age of 12½ years (range, 10½–14½). Maturation continues until adult development is reached at an average age of 14½ years (range, 12½–16½). (Adapted from Grumbach MM, Grave GD, Mayer FE: *Control of the Onset of Puberty.* New York, John Wiley, 1974, p 460.)

 **(c) Severe dysfunctional bleeding** is characterized by menses that are so prolonged that the timing of the menstrual cycle is no longer clear and by very heavy bleeding during the menstrual cycle.
 **(2) Physical examination** should review the skin for signs of bleeding disorders and the organs (e.g., thyroid gland, liver) for indications of systemic disease. A pelvic examination should include a rectovaginal examination.
 **(3) Laboratory studies** should initially include a complete blood count, a pregnancy test, and wet preps and cultures for vaginitis or cervicitis. Thyroid and liver function tests as well as clotting studies should be done if indicated or as a secondary consideration. Gonadotropin and prolactin levels also should be evaluated.

**c. Therapy**
 **(1)** For **mild dysfunction** and normal hematocrit, the nature of the menstrual cycle should be reviewed and the adolescent reassured. The case is monitored for changes over time.
 **(2)** For **moderate dysfunction** and mild anemia, therapy may include a trial of oral contraceptives or medroxyprogesterone acetate. Iron and folic acid supplements are useful with repeated blood loss or associated anemia.
 **(3) Severe dysfunction** and moderate anemia may require hospitalization for initial stabilization and blood transfusion.
 **(4) Gynecologic consultation** is recommended in cases in which the above guidelines do not result in menstrual regulation.

**3. Dysmenorrhea** is menstrual pain (usually in the lower abdomen).
 **a. Primary dysmenorrhea,** which accounts for 75% of all cases of dysmenorrhea, is not associated with any other pelvic abnormality and lasts from a few hours to 2–3 days.
  **(1)** Symptoms include nausea, vomiting, headaches, back pain, and dizziness.
  **(2)** The exact etiology of the pain is unclear but it may be related to increased myometrial activity (contractions of the smooth muscle coat) of the uterus associated with increased production of prostaglandin.
 **b. Secondary dysmenorrhea** is caused by a definable pelvic abnormality such as inflammation, structural anomalies, adhesions, endometriosis, tumors, polyps, ovarian cysts, and IUDs.

### c. Evaluation

**(1) History.** The patient history should focus on the relation of pain to the menstrual cycle, the duration of pain, associated symptoms and degree of dysfunction, and familial history of similar pain. Knowledge about the level of sexual activity and exposure to a sexually transmitted disease (see IV A) is helpful. Systemic disease (e.g., gastroenteritis, urinary tract infection) should be ruled out.

**(2) Pelvic examination** is indicated when the patient is in severe pain that lasts longer than 3 days and does not respond to treatment for primary dysmenorrhea.

**(3) Laboratory evaluation** should be considered for cases that do not fit the definition of primary dysmenorrhea. Such studies should include a complete blood count and sedimentation rate for pelvic infection, vaginal wet smear, cultures for a sexually transmitted disease, ultrasound of the pelvis for ovarian cysts, and laparoscopy for severe unresolved cases.

### d. Therapy

**(1) Mild pain** with no limitation of activity may not need any treatment or may respond well to aspirin (an analgesic and prostaglandin inhibitor).

**(2) Moderate pain,** with some limitation of activity but a situation in which the adolescent does not miss school, may be eased by regular use of aspirin or an over-the-counter prostaglandin inhibitor.

**(3) Severe pain** that causes the adolescent to miss school may be relieved by a prescription-strength prostaglandin inhibitor or a trial of oral contraceptives.

## B. Maternal exposure to diethylstilbestrol

**1. DES** was used from the 1940s to the early 1970s to prevent miscarriage and was subsequently associated with disorders in the offspring.

**a.** Disorders in **female offspring** include vaginal adenosis, presence of columnar cells in the vagina, structural anomalies (e.g., a cervical hood), clear cell adenocarcinoma of the cervix and vagina, and structural changes in the endometrial cavity.

**b.** Disorders in **male offspring** have not been definitively identified. Cases have been reported in which male offspring have had microphallus, urethral stenosis, hypospadias, cryptorchidism, testicular hypoplasia, changes in semen (decreased mobility and density), and epididymal cysts.

**2. Evaluation** should document exposure to DES. Pelvic examination should include colposcopy, and histologic samples from the vagina, cervical opening, and endocervix should be obtained.

**3. Therapy** consists of tracking any structural changes, which may cause future problems with pregnancy, and repeated checks for cellular changes in the vagina and cervix. Any patient with cellular changes, such as those consistent with clear cell adenocarcinoma of the cervix, should be referred to a gynecologist for therapy.

## C. Pelvic masses

### 1. Sites

**a.** The **vagina** may contain foreign bodies or hematocolpos from an imperforate hymen.

**b.** The **uterus** may contain a fetus or a fibrous lesion.

**c.** **Adnexal sites** may hide an ectopic pregnancy, endometriosis, ovarian cysts, teratomas (tumors), or hydrosalpinx subsequent to inflammation.

**d.** Masses also may be located in the bowel, kidneys, or liver.

### 2. Evaluation

**a. History.** A history regarding menses, nature and frequency of symptoms, and level of sexual activity should be taken.

**b. Examination** can be augmented by pelvic ultrasound or laparoscopy if indicated.

**c. Laboratory studies** include complete blood count and sedimentation rate, analysis of any vaginal discharge, culture for a sexually transmitted disease (see IV A), a pregnancy test, and appropriate cytologic studies of any unidentified mass.

### 3. Therapy includes the following:

**a.** Perforation of the hymen to drain hematocolpos

**b.** Referral of cases involving ectopic pregnancy or tumors to a gynecologist

**c.** Hormonal or surgical therapeutic approach to endometriosis

**d.** Treatment of the cause of pelvic inflammation to resolve hydrosalpinx

**e.** Drainage of follicular cysts with guidance via laparoscopy if they do not resolve spontaneously

**D. Disorders of the breast and breast development**

1. **Abnormal development.** Initial breast development may be asymmetric. Congenital lack of glandular tissue and hypertrophy of the breasts both can be surgically corrected.

2. **Gynecomastia** is excessive development of the male mammary glands. Such development is often asymptomatic and unilateral. Gynecomastia occurs in up to 60% of all males and usually lasts 6 months to 2 years.

3. **Galactorrhea** is a discharge from the female breasts when lactation is not occurring. Evaluation for a pituitary tumor and hypothyroidism should be considered.

4. **Masses.** It is important to reassure the patient that most masses found during adolescence are benign.
   a. **Fibroadenoma** is the most common mass found in breasts of adolescents. These masses are rubbery, well-defined, movable, and usually unilateral. Fibroadenomas are benign and can be surgically removed if desired.
   b. **Fibrocystic disease** is characterized by typically bilateral changes in breast tissue (thickening, small cyst formation). The cysts usually require routine follow-up. Occasionally, surgical removal of large or malignant cysts is needed.
   c. **Malignancy** occurs very rarely in adolescents; however, any persistent breast lesion of unclear etiology should be biopsied.

**E. Testicular and scrotal disorders** (see also Ch 13 XI and Ch 15 XI)

1. **Varicocele** is dilatation of the veins of the spermatic cord. This disorder occurs in 15% of adolescents, more commonly on the left side of the scrotum, and, if extensive, may result in decreased fertility in adulthood.

2. **Priapism** is a sustained, painful erection. This disorder may be associated with sickle cell anemia, leukemia, or urethral inflammation.

3. **Inguinal hernias** occur up to five times more often in males than in females and occur more often on the right but are frequently bilateral.
   a. **Common terms** used to describe hernias include:
      (1) **Reducible.** The physician can displace hernia contents back into the abdomen.
      (2) **Incarcerated.** The hernia is not reducible.
      (3) **Strangulated.** An incarcerated hernia is likely to become gangrenous (i.e., the blood supply is cut off from the contents of the hernia).
      (4) **Sliding.** The wall of the hernia sac is composed of another organ (e.g., the colon).
   b. **Types.** Inguinal hernias are direct or indirect.
      (1) **Indirect** inguinal hernias are most common and protrude through the internal inguinal ring.
      (2) **Direct** inguinal hernias result from a weakness in the medial inguinal canal floor.

4. **Hydrocele** is a fluid-filled structure in the tunica vaginalis or the processus vaginalis located in the scrotum.

5. **Spermatocele** is cystic swelling of the epididymis or the rete testis containing spermatozoa.

## IV. GENITOURINARY AND GYNECOLOGIC INFECTIONS

**A. Sexually transmitted diseases (STDs)** are acquired by sexual contact and intercourse (including genital, rectal, and oral penetration). These diseases are most common in the adolescent and young adult population (age 15–24 years).

1. **Agents of specific STDs**
   a. *Chlamydia trachomatis* is the cause of the most common nonviral STD in the United States. It is an intracellular organism found in columnar lining cells of the cervix, uterus, fallopian tubes, liver capsule, urethra, rectum, pharynx, and skin. *C. trachomatis* is the most common cause of **nongonococcal urethritis (NGU)** in males. It also causes **lymphogranuloma venereum (LGV)** and **inclusion conjunctivitis**.

**(1) Clinical features**
  **(a)** Commonly associated findings include cervical ectopy and friability, mucoid cervical discharge with an increased number of white cells, and dysuria. In the male, dysuria is not always accompanied by a discharge.
  **(b)** Other related findings include pelvic tenderness with or without associated right upper quadrant pain in women, a painless vesicle (blister) with regional lymphadenopathy caused by LGV, pharyngitis, and rectal irritation and tenderness.
**(2) Diagnosis** is made by identification of chlamydia inclusion bodies either through cell culture or a rapid test using fluorescent antibody staining or spectrometric evaluation.

**b.** *Neisseria gonorrhoeae* is an intracellular, gram-negative diplococcus found in a distribution similar to that of *C. trachomatis;* in addition, joint involvement can cause arthritis. More than 1 million cases of **gonorrhea** are reported each year.
  **(1) Clinical features** are similar to those seen with *C. trachomatis* infection. Infection in males is more likely to be accompanied by purulent urethral discharge.
  **(2) Diagnosis** is based on finding gram-negative diplococci in male urethral discharge or a positive gonorrhea culture in females.

**c. Human immunodeficiency virus (HIV)** is acquired through sexual transmission or intravenous spread from blood products or illicit drug use.
  **(1)** Compared to adult HIV infection, HIV infection in adolescents has a lower male to female ratio, is more prevalent in black and Hispanic urban youths, and has a higher percentage of heterosexual transmission.
  **(2)** HIV infection causes acquired immune deficiency syndrome (AIDS) after a variable latency period (see Ch 8 II E).

**d.** *Ureaplasma urealyticum* is the second-most common cause of NGU in males. It is a T-strain mycoplasma with genital and pelvic distribution similar to that of *C. trachomatis*.

**e.** *Gardnerella vaginalis* is a gram-negative rod confined to the vagina.
  **(1) Clinical features** include a vaginal discharge with a "fishy" odor.
  **(2) Diagnosis** is made by identifying clue cells (vaginal epithelial cells covered with fragments of gram-negative rods) in the vaginal discharge.

**f.** *Treponema pallidum,* the cause of **syphilis,** had become a less common cause of infection up to the mid-1980s. It is now seen more regularly, partly as a result of changing patterns of illicit drug use. *T. pallidum* is a motile spiral microorganism that is 5–20 mm long. The infection generally starts in the genital area but can affect other parts of the body.
  **(1) Clinical features** are related to the stage of disease.
    **(a) Primary syphilis.** Patients present with chancres and regional lymphadenopathy 10–40 days after infection.
    **(b) Secondary syphilis.** Patients present with generalized malaise, lymphadenopathy, skin changes, and alopecia 2–6 months after infection.
    **(c) Late syphilis.** Patients present with CNS, cardiovascular, and musculoskeletal involvement 2–10 years after exposure.
  **(2) Diagnosis** is based on a serologic test for syphilis.

**g.** *Hemophilus ducreyi,* which causes **chancroid,** has become more common in the past 5 years. It should be considered in the differential diagnosis of a painful genital ulcer often accompanied by tender inguinal lymphadenopathy.

**h. Herpes simplex virus (HSV)** infection has increased in incidence, to more than 1 million cases per year in the United States. HSV is a DNA virus. The most common form causing genital involvement is HSV type 2.
  **(1) Clinical features.** Patients present with vesicles and ulcers on the external genitalia, in the vagina, on the cervix, around the rectal area, and on the lips and mouth. HSV infection also is associated with tender inguinal lymphadenopathy, dysuria, and dyspareunia.
  **(2) Diagnosis.** Clinical findings can be confirmed by a Tzanck test or a viral culture. Serum titers can be obtained from patients with possible past exposure but no active lesions.

**i. Condylomata acuminata** (venereal warts) are a form of DNA papillomavirus infection.
  **(1) Clinical features.** Patients present with single or groups of painless warts.
  **(2) Diagnosis** can be made by clinical appearance. Biopsy can be performed in cases of atypical presentation or of persistent warts. Follow-up colposcopic examination of the cervix is recommended in view of an increased association between the human papillomavirus and invasive cervical carcinoma. Males should also have a careful examination of the penis for identification of microscopic warts.

    **j. Molluscum contagiosum** is a poxvirus infection found in any part of the body, but it is usually present in greater concentration in the genital area when it is sexually transmitted.

        **(1) Clinical features.** Patients present with small papules with umbilical centers.

        **(2) Diagnosis** is made by clinical appearance. A potassium hydroxide smear of the contents of a papule shows molluscum bodies (cytoplasmic inclusions). Biopsy is performed in questionable cases.

    **k.** *Trichomonas vaginalis* is a flagellate protozoon present most commonly in the vagina in females but also found near the urethra of both sexes.

        **(1) Clinical features.** Female patients present with vaginal discharge that is bubbly, green, creamy, and malodorous. Dysuria, vaginal tenderness on examination, and a history of dyspareunia also are characteristic.

        **(2) Diagnosis** is made by microscopic identification of flagellate organisms. Sometimes the protozoa can be detected in urinary sediment.

    **l.** *Phthirus pubis* (pediculosis pubis, crab lice) is a parasite that is less than 4 mm long.

        **(1) Clinical features.** Patients present with a history of pruritus in the pubic or other hair associated with lice, tan egg cases, or both.

        **(2) Diagnosis.** Crab lice or egg cases are large enough to be visible clinging to pubic hair.

  **2. Therapy** for STDs should include all exposed individuals, whenever possible. The specific treatment depends on accurate identification of the causative organism; the choice of antibiotic must take into consideration the organism sensitivity and the patient's age and history of allergies. Examples of antibiotic choices include:

    **a.** Penicillin G benzathine for *T. pallidum*

    **b.** Ceftriaxone for *N. gonorrhea*

    **c.** Metronidazole for *T. vaginalis* and *G. vaginalis*

  **3. Prevention.** Proper use of condoms can reduce the risk of transmitting most of these STDs.

**B. Vaginitis**

  **1.** *Candida albicans,* the most common cause of vaginitis, is a form of fungus (yeast) that normally inhabits the vagina. Vaginitis occurs when the growth of *C. albicans* is not limited by the vaginal environment (i.e., the vaginal flora is more alkaline than it normally is).

    **a. Clinical features.** Patients present with a cheesy white discharge associated with vulvar pruritus. The infection occurs after systemic antibiotic therapy, with diabetes, and during pregnancy and is also associated with the use of birth control pills.

    **b. Diagnosis** is based on the presence of budding yeast and hyphae in a sample of vaginal discharge mixed with potassium hydroxide. The diagnosis is confirmed by culture.

    **c. Therapy.** Candidiasis is treated by the topical application of an antifungal preparation (e.g., miconazole nitrate) in the vagina at bedtime for 1 week.

  **2. Other causes** of vaginitis are *G. vaginalis, T. vaginalis,* and foreign bodies. Vaginal discharge can also be attributed to leukorrhea.

**C. Toxic shock syndrome (TSS)** was initially associated with menstruating women who used tampons. It has also been seen in women who use a diaphragm or contraceptive sponge for an extended period of time. TSS is caused by the release of endotoxin from a *Staphylococcus aureus* infection and may be potentially fatal.

  **1. Clinical features.** The patient presents with a fever higher than 102° F, a macular rash followed by desquamation especially on the palms and soles, hypotension, and three or more of the following symptoms and systemic changes:

    **a.** Vomiting and diarrhea

    **b.** Muscle cramps accompanied by elevation of creatine phosphokinase (CPK) levels

    **c.** Disorientation

    **d.** Hyperemia of the mucous membranes

    **e.** Hepatic changes [elevation of serum aspartate aminotransferase (AST), serum alanine aminotransferase (ALT), and bilirubin levels]

    **f.** Renal changes [elevation of blood urea nitrogen (BUN), creatinine levels, or both]

    **g.** Hematologic changes (decreased platelet count)

  **2. Therapy** includes controlling the symptoms of shock, removing any device from the vagina, and administering intravenous antibiotics. It may be useful to irrigate the vagina with normal saline or povidone-iodine. Counseling against the use of tampons and for appropriate use of barrier contraceptives is important, since there is a potential 30% recurrence of the problem.

**D. Pelvic inflammatory disease (PID)** is the spread of an infection from the vagina to the cervix, uterus, fallopian tubes, and peritoneum, potentially resulting in endometritis, salpingitis, parametritis, perihepatitis, and peritonitis. Such infections are most commonly seen in women age 15–24 years and may cause subsequent infertility, especially where significant fallopian tube damage occurs. PID is strongly associated with the use of an IUD.

1. **Clinical features.** The patient presents with significant abdominal pain and tenderness upon lateral motion of the cervix. The infection commonly starts during the menstrual period, and the patient may have a history of recent or past exposure to an STD. The erythrocyte sedimentation rate is elevated. An ultrasound of the pelvic area may show increased fluid outside these organs or formation of an abcess.

2. **Etiology.** The most common causes of PID are *N. gonorrhoeae* and *C. trachomatis*. Other causative organisms include *Mycoplasma hominis, S. aureus, Streptococcus, Escherichia coli,* and anaerobic bacteria such as *Bacteroides*. PID often is caused by multiple organisms.

3. **Therapy** for PID follows the **Centers for Disease Control guidelines**. Antibiotic coverage is determined by the causative organism.

**E. Perihepatitis** is perihepatic inflammation caused by such organisms as gonococcus (Fitz-Hugh Curtis syndrome) or by *C. trachomatis* subsequent to pelvic infection.

1. **Clinical features.** The patient may present with right upper quadrant pain, pleuritic irritation, and pain radiating to the right shoulder.

2. **Therapy** involves inpatient intravenous antibiotic treatment for the pelvic infection followed by outpatient oral antibiotic therapy depending on the causative organism.

**F. Epididymo-orchitis** occurs subsequent to an STD (usually gonorrhea or chlamydial infection) or after a urinary tract infection.

1. **Clinical features.** The patient presents with dysuria and urethral discharge. The involved area may be swollen and tender.

2. **Therapy** involves the administration of an appropriate antibiotic agent for the STD or the urinary tract infection.

**V. REPRODUCTIVE HEALTH ISSUES** have become increasingly more important to adolescents. Half of all adolescents are sexually active by age 17 years. Fewer than one-third of sexually active adolescents use any effective form of birth control. The most common reasons adolescents give for not using birth control are a denial of the ability to get pregnant and the unexpected nature of the intercourse.

**A. Contraception**

1. **Oral contraceptive pill.** The pill is the form of contraception most commonly used by adolescents. The **failure rate** of this method is 2%–4%.
   a. **Mechanism of action.** The pill suppresses ovulation, decreases the likelihood of implantation of the fertilized egg, and makes the cervical mucus more hostile to sperm.
   b. **Contraindications**
      (1) Absolute contraindications include pregnancy or a history of breast cancer, estrogen-stimulated reproductive tract neoplasm, thromboembolic disease, cerebrovascular accident, sustained hypertension, systemic disease involving the liver or coronary arteries, hyperlipidemia, or undiagnosed abnormal genital bleeding.
      (2) Relative contraindications include a history of labile or borderline hypertension, migraine headaches, diabetes, seizure disorder, oligomenorrhea, amenorrhea, sickle cell disease, or heavy cigarette smoking (over age 35).
   c. **Types of pills**
      (1) The **combination pill** contains both estrogen and progesterone and may have fixed doses of each or may vary the dose of these hormones through the cycle (**phasic pills**).
      (2) The **progesterone-only pill** works in a manner similar to the combination pill except that it may not regularly prevent ovulation. The failure rate is higher partly because the pill causes irregular menstrual periods. The progesterone-only pill is reserved for women who cannot tolerate estrogen.

(3) The **"morning after" pill** (diethylstilbestrol) is an intermediate- or high-dose estrogen preparation used 24–72 hours after intercourse to prevent pregnancy.

d. **Common side effects** of the pill include uterine bleeding between periods, nausea, weight gain, headaches, mood changes, and a period of anovulatory cycles after the pill is stopped.

e. **Advantages** of the pill include decreased menstrual bleeding; decreased dysmenorrhea; no interference with intercourse; improvement of acne; and potential help in decreasing or preventing problems with ovarian cysts, fibrocystic and fibroadenoma breast changes, and ovarian and endometrial cancer.

f. **Evaluation** prior to starting the pill should include a patient history for risk factors, a complete physical examination including a pelvic examination, and documentation of weight and blood pressure. **Clinical studies** should include a Pap smear; screening for gonorrhea, chlamydial infection, and syphilis; a blood count and urinalysis; and pregnancy test if indicated.

g. **Choosing the right pill** for an adolescent is important for consistent compliance. Most adolescents can be started on a low-dose combination pill. An obese adolescent needs a combination pill with the lowest dose of estrogen that can be tolerated. An adolescent with severe acne may be helped by a combination pill with a slightly higher dose of estrogen for a few months and then a switch to a lower-dose pill. A 28-pill package can increase compliance because of the necessity of taking a pill every day.

2. **Barrier methods of contraception** are used by less than one-fifth of the adolescent population who use any form of contraception. These methods tend to be more popular with older adolescents and young adults. The **failure rate** varies from 10%–20%, depending on the form of barrier contraceptive being used.

a. **Mechanisms of action.** Barrier contraceptives prevent sperm from entering the uterus, kill sperm while they are in the vagina, and absorb sperm.

b. **No contraindications** exist for the use of a barrier method of contraception.

c. **Types of barrier contraceptives** include:
   (1) The **diaphragm**—a circular rubber dome that, when properly placed, is an effective barrier between the vagina and cervix
   (2) The **cervical cap**—a firm plastic cap held in place by suction at the cervical opening
   (3) The contraceptive **sponge**
   (4) **Spermicides**—foams, jellies, or suppositories
   (5) The **condom,** which seems to be the most effective single barrier method of contraception. The combination of a condom and a spermicide approximates the effectiveness of the pill as a contraceptive method but with significantly fewer side effects. This method also serves as the most effective known deterrent to the spread of AIDS (barring celibacy.)

d. **Side effects** from barrier contraceptives are generally minor and consist of irritation or an allergic reaction. Vaginal infection and TSS can occur when the diaphragm or sponge is left in the vagina for extended periods of time (see IV C).

e. **Evaluation** for the use of these methods may not always occur since all of the methods except the diaphragm are available without a prescription. Sexually active adolescents should have a complete health evaluation (see V A 1 f). Women wishing to use a diaphragm must be measured for the appropriate size.

f. **Advantages** of barrier contraceptives include: They cause few, if any, systemic effects; they are used only at the time of intercourse; and they are inexpensive, easy to obtain, and may help prevent passage of sexually transmitted disease, including AIDS.

g. **Disadvantages** of barrier contraceptives include: They are considered messy, and they interrupt lovemaking.

3. **IUD.** This method should not be prescribed for use in sexually active teens.

a. **Mechanism of action.** The IUD blocks the implantation of a fertilized egg in the lining of the uterus, either by causing a mild endometritis or by affecting endometrial enzymes.

b. **Side effects** include pelvic infection, uterine perforation, ectopic pregnancy, and subsequent infertility.

4. **Injectable progesterone** is a frequently used form of contraceptive outside the United States.

a. **Mechanism of action.** Injectable progesterone is similar to the progesterone-only pill [see V A 1 c (2)] but is more effective in the suppression of ovulation.

    **b. Indications** include:
      **(1)** A patient who cannot tolerate estrogen
      **(2)** A patient who is unwilling to use a barrier contraceptive or progesterone-only pill
      **(3)** Failure of all other forms of contraception in a patient who does not wish to become pregnant
      **(4)** An adolescent who is mentally unable to understand the meaning of pregnancy and is unable to use other forms of contraception
    **c. Side effects** are similar to those seen with the progesterone-only pill. **Injectable progesterone** is not presently approved by the United States Food and Drug Administration (FDA) as a contraceptive. Studies show that it causes breast and uterine cancer in animals, it results in a delayed return to ovulation after injections are stopped, and it may cause infertility. It may be associated with teratogenic effects in the fetus. A patient who uses this contraceptive signs a statement indicating her awareness of the possible side effects. This is not a contraceptive choice for minors without parental consent.

## B. Pregnancy

  **1. General considerations.** Pregnancy occurs in more than 1 million teenagers in the United States each year, a frequency that is two to six times greater than that seen in other developed countries. More than half the women who become pregnant while in high school drop out of school. Nearly half the women who depend on state or federal support for their families had children before the age of 20 years. Teenage mothers have a 20%–40% chance of becoming pregnant again 1–2 years after the initial delivery.

  **2. Medical complications** of teenage pregnancy include toxemia and anemia. Infants born to mothers who are younger than 15 years have a high mortality rate and a high incidence of low birth weight. All of the developmental consequences for teenage mothers and their infants have not yet been clearly identified. Greater consequences for the younger adolescent are partially explained by the incomplete development of the pelvis.

  **3. Causes of teenage pregnancy**
    **a. During the concrete operational stage** (see II B 2 b) many teenagers deny their ability to get pregnant, are unable to think of events 9 months in the future, and exhibit poor compliance with contraception.
    **b. Family influence.** Often the mother or a sibling became a parent as a teen. Lack of an extended family decreases family support. In single-parent families or in families where both parents work, teenagers are not supervised much of the time.
    **c. Gradually decreasing age of menarche** has made pregnancy possible at an early age.
    **d. Situational stress** (e.g., school performance, family relations, pressure from a sexual partner or peer group) can also contribute to the problem.
    **e. Societal influences** may also play a role through lack of positive role models, lack of opportunities in the job market, increased emphasis on sex in the media, and relaxation of moral codes.
    **f. Desire to become pregnant** also has to be considered, as teenagers often feel that becoming a parent will give them someone to take care of, provide them with unconditional love, and will offer them a way to become independent.
    **g. Often the males involved are older** (in their late teens or early twenties). In these men, physical feelings and self-image interfere with their understanding of the consequences and responsibilities of their actions.

  **4. Evaluation for possible pregnancy**
    **a. History.** A patient history should correlate the frequency of sexual activity and the menstrual cycle with the understanding that often some menstrual bleeding can occur even in the presence of a pregnancy. Associated symptoms of pregnancy should be noted, including swelling of the breasts, nausea and vomiting, fatigue, and urinary frequency.
    **b. Physical examination** should check the size and color of the cervix as well as the size and consistency of the uterus.
    **c. Clinical studies** including a urine evaluation for HCG can determine the presence of a pregnancy within 10 days of conception. A subsequent blood analysis for the same gonadotropin can quantitate the duration of the pregnancy.

  **5. Decision-making for a pregnant teenager.** Allowing a teenager time to consider her options and having her talk to other teens who have been through the experience may be helpful. Involvement of the parents and the father of the child in discussions should be encouraged when possible.

  **a. Options.** Alternatives include keeping the baby, putting the baby up for adoption, placing the baby in foster care (thus allowing for a later decision), and abortion.

  **b. Factors influencing the decision.** Issues that may influence a pregnant adolescent's decision include decreased freedom when the child is born, financial and physical responsibility for the infant, need to develop a support system, and the effects of a pregnancy on her life-style and career goals.

**6. Care and support for a pregnant teenager.** When the pregnancy is to be carried to term, it is important to assist the teenager with early prenatal care, to facilitate continuation of school, and to help develop a support system, especially for future parenting.

**C. Abortion.** Teenagers undergo 500,000 abortions each year, nearly one-third of the total number of abortions performed. Nearly half (47%) of the pregnant teenagers from middle- and upper-income families choose abortion as compared to one-quarter (26%) of the pregnant teenagers from low-income families.

**1. Types of abortions**

  **a. First trimester** abortions, which account for the majority of abortions, are performed by vacuum curettage and are done as an outpatient procedure.

  **b. Second trimester** abortions are high-risk procedures, are more expensive than those performed in the first trimester, and often require overnight hospitalization. Few centers perform abortions in the second trimester. Methods include intra-amniotic cavity administration of hypertonic saline, urea, or dilation and curettage; and placement of prostaglandin as a suppository in the vagina.

**2. Mortality.** The mortality rate ranges from 1 in 400,000 when the abortion is done prior to 9 weeks gestation to 1 in 10,000 when it is done after 16 weeks gestation.

**3. Evaluation** should include a discussion of the meaning of abortion and related fears. The likely procedure should be reviewed, and the adolescent should be encouraged to have a support person with her. Examination and laboratory studies should confirm pregnancy, and ultrasound can be used to estimate gestational size.

**4. Follow-up.** A contraceptive method should be encouraged and made available immediately after the abortion. Follow-up pelvic exam is done 2 weeks after the abortion. This is a good time to assess the psychological consequences of the abortion and to plan future counseling visits to deal with unresolved feelings about the abortion and to help prevent another pregnancy.

## VI. MENTAL HEALTH ISSUES

**A. Depression** (see also Ch 3 VII A). More than half (60%) of teenagers surveyed while receiving routine health care indicated that they feel down or depressed as frequently as once a month to daily. Females experience depression more commonly than males.

**1. Etiology.** A number of factors may lead to depression, including:

  **a. Changes in peer relationships** (e.g., loss of a boyfriend or girlfriend, exclusion from the peer group, lack of peer group support, inability to be with peers)

  **b. Family influences** (e.g., lack of independence, poor communication, decreased availability of parents, problems between the parents)

  **c. School experiences** (e.g., poor performance, conflict with teachers, peer conflict or pressure, unrealistically high expectations from parents)

  **d. Poor self-image** (e.g., dissatisfaction with one's physical appearance, lack of self-confidence, a hopeless vision of the future)

**2. Clinical features.** Associated signs and symptoms include:

  **a. Recurrent somatic complaints** (e.g., headaches; chest, abdominal or back pains; changes in eating habits, sleep patterns, and levels of activity)

  **b. Mood swings** (manifested as restlessness; withdrawal from peers and family; decreased ability to function on a day-to-day basis; and "acting out" behavior such as violence, substance abuse, risk-taking, and little or no recognition of authority)

  **c. A decline in the level of school performance**

  **d. Apathy** (a loss of interest in sports, hobbies, and community-related activities)

3. **Therapy.** Attempts to prevent or treat depression include counseling programs associated with health services, school-based support services, and intervention in parent-adolescent conflict. The 24-hour phone availability of a health network can provide reassurance.

B. **Suicide** is the third most common cause of death in adolescents and young adults; suicide attempts outnumber successful suicides by as much as 200 to 1. Females make more attempts than males, but successful suicide is four times more common in males. More than half (60%) of teenagers who commit suicide have attempted suicide previously.

1. **Methods.** The most frequent methods by which adolescent suicide is committed in the United States are (in order) firearms, hanging, and drug overdose. (Females most commonly commit suicide by drug overdose.)

2. **Attempts to prevent suicide** should include the following steps.
   a. **Questioning.** All adolescent patients should be asked about suicidal thoughts, not just those who seem depressed. No clearly documented correlation exists between asking about suicidal thoughts and an increased incidence of suicide.
   b. **Assessment of risk.** If the adolescent has suicidal thoughts, the level of risk should be evaluated by a review of a history of suicide, by the level of familial support and recognition of the problems, and by a discussion of the methods of suicide that have been considered.
      (1) The **degree of depression** should be assessed. A severely depressed teenager may be unable to mobilize to commit suicide, but a teenager who is recovering from depression is more likely to commit suicide.
      (2) **Danger signs** should always be ascertained in depressed teenagers (e.g., getting affairs in order, giving away favorite possessions, withdrawing from friends and from social and school activities, a history of suicide or alcohol abuse in the family).
      (3) A **precipitating event** should be noted (e.g., a breakup with a girlfriend or boyfriend, a conflict with peers, pregnancy, and, most frequently, a conflict with parents).
   c. **Therapy** for a suicidal adolescent works well in a team approach including the services of a physician, a social worker, and a consulting psychiatrist. Appropriate information should be obtained to determine whether the patient can be treated on an ambulatory basis or requires inpatient evaluation.
      (1) An **ambulatory approach** should be considered in the following situations.
         (a) The patient has no significant history of depression or suicide.
         (b) The method used was less lethal and required no medical treatment.
         (c) The suicide attempt occurred at a time when help was available, or a suicide note was left in an accessible place prior to the attempt.
         (d) The family is supportive and recognizes the problem.
         (e) The teen and the family are willing to follow up on an ambulatory basis.
         (f) A mental health care provider is available.
      (2) **Hospitalization** is necessary in the following instances.
         (a) A safe environment is needed.
         (b) The family is not supportive or does not recognize the problem.
         (c) The patient has previously attempted suicide.
         (d) The patient has a history of depression.
         (e) A lethal method was used, or further medical care is needed.
         (f) The suicide attempt occurred without warning, and an ambulatory care arrangement cannot be found.

C. **Delinquency.** More than 50% of all arrests for major crimes in the United States involve individuals under the age of 21 years, and more than one-third of these arrests involve individuals under the age of 18 years. Males account for more then 75% of these arrests and for more than 90% of the arrests for violent crimes. A high level of delinquency is reported in the poorer population.

1. **Definitions**
   a. A **juvenile delinquent** is a minor age 7–17 years who commits a criminal act. Such a case usually is processed through juvenile or family court with emphasis on rehabilitation rather than punishment. Some cities have juvenile advisory teams who try to resolve such cases before they come to court. The youth usually is given a chance to clear his record.
   b. A **youthful offender** is an individual age 16–21 years who commits a criminal act. Such a case usually is processed through criminal court for punishment, but the youthful offender may be tried in family or juvenile court if the act committed is minor and if the youth will benefit from rehabilitation.

**c.** A **minor in need of supervision** is an individual age 7–17 years who commits an act that would not be illegal if he were an adult (e.g., running away or skipping school). These cases may be processed through juvenile or family court, but an attempt usually is made to resolve them outside the court system.

**2. Factors relating to delinquency** include medical, behavioral, and school problems; conflict with authority; disorder at home; and inappropriate peer structure.

**3. Prevention** may be aided by:

**a.** Development of more **early identification programs** that foster positive youth development, such as those run by boys clubs

**b.** Greater emphasis on **positive adult role models** (e.g., Big Brother or Big Sister programs)

**c.** A **change in national social priorities**

**(1)** The emphasis on material possessions, living for the moment, and sexual preoccupation should be decreased.

**(2)** It would also help to increase emphasis on education, family support, and self-achievement as well as to facilitate career development for the youth at risk.

**D. Eating disorders**

**1. Anorexia nervosa**

**a. Definition.** Anorexia nervosa is an eating disorder that typically occurs in early to late adolescence, predominantly (95% of cases) in girls. Anorexia is characterized by weight loss of at least 15% of original or anticipated body weight, disturbance of body image, absence of at least two consecutive menstrual cycles in post-menarchal females, and bulimia (see VI D 2).

**b. Etiology**

**(1)** Psychological causes appear to be extremely important. Often, the affected individual feels helpless and not in control of her life.

**(2)** Disordered family relationships may contribute to the etiology.

**(3)** Associated endocrine abnormalities exist but probably are secondary to the starvation.

**c. Evaluation**

**(1) History**

**(a)** The patient's chief complaint typically is, "I'm too fat," or, "My parents think I don't eat enough."

**(b)** Attempts should be made to document the chronology of the weight loss, and an extensive dietary history should be obtained.

**(c)** Queries should be made about vomiting, excessive exercise, and laxative abuse.

**(d)** Review of systems should be obtained to identify symptoms of systemic illness (e.g., inflammatory bowel disease, pituitary tumor, malignancy, depression, schizophrenia).

**(2) Physical examination.** Findings often include a wasted appearance, low blood pressure, low body temperature, and mottled skin. Physical examination should include funduscopy for papilledema and optic atrophy as well as examination of visual fields to identify possible intracranial pathology.

**(3) Laboratory studies**

**(a)** Routine laboratory tests should include complete blood count and erythrocyte sedimentation rate, urinalysis, BUN, electrolyte levels, thyroid studies, and liver function tests. An electrocardiogram (ECG) also is helpful.

**(b)** A computed tomography (CT) scan should be obtained in boys who present with weight loss, since the incidence of brain tumor is higher in boys.

**d. Therapy**

**(1) Medical management** of the anorectic patient involves nutritional support to prevent mortality and morbidity. Intervention may range from the mere presentation of a high-calorie diet to the placement of a nasogastric tube and, in some extremely resistant children, hyperalimentation.

**(2) Psychological management**

**(a) Behavior modification.** Strategies include positive reinforcement for eating and negative contingencies for refusing to eat. A system of privileges often is established, depending on the child's intake.

**(b) Psychotherapy,** both individual and family, is essential.

**(3) Psychopharmacology.** Antidepressant agents may be helpful.

**e. Prognosis.** Anorexia nervosa has a variable course. Many children who are hospitalized for anorexia nervosa require repeated hospitalizations. A 5%–10% mortality rate still is associated with this illness.

2. **Bulimia**
   a. **Definition**
      (1) Bulimia is repetitive binge eating associated with purging by vomiting and use of laxatives or diuretics. Affected adolescents have a disturbed self-image; they desire to lose weight but fear not being able to stop eating. Bulimia is considered a disorder distinct from anorexia nervosa; however, teenagers with anorexia nervosa may exhibit binging and purging behavior.
      (2) Bulimia is seen mainly in **older teenagers** (average age is 18 years); however, one study showed that binging and purging occurred in 13% of a group of 15-year-old teenagers. Prevalence varies between 5% and 19% in the general population. Bulimia is more common in females.
   b. **Clinical features.** The patient commonly presents with a poor self-image associated with depression (especially after a binge episode), thoughts about suicide, substance abuse (see VII), antisocial behavior (e.g., stealing), and self-mutilation.
   c. **Medical complications** may include esophagitis, gastric dilatation and possible rupture, aspiration, cardiac arrhythmia, pancreatitis, metabolic alkalosis associated with hypochloremia and hypokalemia, swelling of the parotid and submandibular glands, and dental problems such as erosion of dental enamel and dentin and loss of teeth.
   d. **Evaluation**
      (1) **History.** A patient history should consider eating patterns and food intake history, purging behavior, past weight fluctuations, body image, level of depression, risk-taking behavior, and family dynamics.
      (2) **Physical examination** includes assessment of vital signs for possible hypovolemia, assessment of dentition, examination for lymphadenopathy, and evaluation of cardiac function. The abdomen should be palpated for tenderness or distention. The skin should be evaluated (the hands should be checked for scars from repeated induced vomiting).
      (3) **Laboratory studies** should evaluate electrolyte level, hydration, and cardiovascular status.
   e. **Therapy** should initially stabilize the patient's medical condition. The focus of treatment is to normalize the metabolic state and encourage the adolescent to become involved in counseling. Antidepressant medication may be helpful in specific cases.

E. **Sexual abuse**

1. **Rape**
   a. **Definition.** Rape is sexual intercourse without the victim's consent. Penetration need not involve rupture of the hymen or entrance into the vagina; only contact of male genitalia with labia majora is necessary. Similarly, ejaculation need not occur for rape to be alleged. Women generally are the victims (in more than 90% of cases), with teenagers making up half of all rape victims. A significant number of rape cases go unreported.
   b. **Evaluation** should be done in a supportive setting by an experienced physician. The teenager needs to have a sense of control as well as a guarantee of confidentiality and privacy during the evaluation. All procedures should be explained before they are done.
      (1) **History.** A patient history should establish date, time, and nature of the rape as well as any acute symptoms. It is important to determine if the vaginal environment has changed since the rape. (Has the victim douched or bathed?) Menstrual, sexual, and contraceptive histories are helpful.
      (2) **Physical examination** aims to document the event as much as possible, with pictures when appropriate. Before the examination is begun, local legal requirements should be determined.
      (3) **Clinical studies** include checking for sperm, STDs, and pregnancy. Follow-up testing for AIDS should be performed if the perpetrator is unavailable or unwilling to undergo tests or if the perpetrator tests positive.
   c. **Therapy** focuses not only on possible pregnancy and STD but also on the mental health needs of the victim.

    **d. Sequelae of rape** initially include fear and shock, fatigue, and systemic responses (e.g., inability to eat, keep food down, or sleep). Later findings include impaired functioning at school, work, and home; sexual fear and dysfunction; poor self-image and depression; and decreased contact with peers.

  **2. Incest**

    **a. Definition.** Incest is sexual intercourse or molestation with a relative or guardian. Incest is most commonly reported between father (usually stepfather) and daughter and may also occur between siblings.

    **b. Associated behavioral changes** include somatic complaints, low self-esteem, substance abuse, running away, prostitution, depression, and thoughts about suicide.

    **c. Family dynamics** include a father figure with poor impulse control and associated alcohol abuse and a passive mother who has a poor relationship with the father and a tendency to neglect and eventually reject the daughter.

  **3. Molestation** is sexual contact short of intercourse without the victim's consent. It is most often committed by men through either exhibitionism, genital contact, or forced oral or anal sex. The evaluation, treatment, and sequelae are similar to those of rape.

## VII. SUBSTANCE ABUSE

  **A. Definition.** Substance abuse is consumption of cigarettes, alcohol, or drugs to the point of compromising health or causing dysfunctional behavior. Cigarette, marijuana, and alcohol use has decreased during the first half of the 1980s as compared to the high use levels reached in the latter half of the 1970s. Cocaine use has gradually increased, especially in the latter half of the 1980s, with the arrival of the "free base" form of this drug known as "crack." Chronic substance abuse causes the arrest of psychosocial development.

    **1. Stages of substance abuse**

      **a. Stage 1 is experimentation.** Experimentation usually starts with peers and under some peer pressure. Few if any behavioral changes take place. The user struggles between the euphoria achieved and associated guilt.

      **b. Stage 2 is abuse to relieve stress.** Use is more than just occasional and occurs in nonsocial situations. A supply of the substance is maintained, and the peer group develops around substance abuse. The user exhibits mood swings, and school performance declines.

      **c. Stage 3 is regular abuse.** The user becomes involved with the drug-oriented culture and most if not all peers use drugs. Behavioral problems now become chronic and may include trouble with the law. The user is depressed when not using drugs. The user needs to raise money to support the substance habit.

      **d. Stage 4 is dependence.** The drug is used not to produce euphoria but to prevent depression. The adolescent may drop out of school and become involved in destructive family dynamics. Physical changes may include weight loss, fatigue, blackouts, and chronic cough.

    **2. Evaluation** includes determining the pattern of substance abuse, level of dysfunction, and degree of depression.

      **a. Physical examination.** Signs of chronic drug abuse are ascertained (e.g., weight loss, skin and mucous membrane changes, compromise in lung function, depression).

      **b. Laboratory studies** can confirm drug abuse through urine or blood tests and can check for systemic changes in liver and pulmonary function.

    **3. Therapy** for adolescents in the first and second stages of involvement can usually be accomplished on an ambulatory basis, while those in the third and fourth stages may require hospitalization or placement in a residential rehabilitation facility. Difficulties arise because many substance abusers do not realize or do not admit that they have a problem.

  **B. Tobacco** abuse by teenagers strongly correlates with use by parents and peers. The rate of smoking in female adolescents now has equaled or surpassed that in males. Smoking is initiated about 2 years before the habit is established.

    **1. Hazards** of smoking in teenagers include altered lung function, resulting in chronic symptoms such as a productive cough; significant decrease in performance endurance, especially in sports; increased risk of lung cancer and coronary heart disease; and lifetime addiction.

2. **Using smokeless tobacco** (snuff) is a male-oriented activity (up to 25% of American male adolescents report some involvement). Snuff use is associated with development of oral squamous carcinoma. In one study, almost 63% of adolescent snuff users developed oral lesions.

C. **Marijuana** is derived from leaves of the hemp plant and is smoked in cigarettes (joints) or pipes or cooked in food. The active ingredient is tetrahydrocannabinol (THC). Hashish (hash), the resin from the hemp plant, is a purer form of THC. THC is metabolized in the liver but is also stored in body fat, resulting in a long half-life.

1. **Hazards** of marijuana use include impairment of lungs (to a greater extent than occurs in cigarette smoking), short-term memory and learning, immune function, reaction time, coordination and visual perception, and reproduction.

2. **Therapeutic effects** of marijuana include reduction of nausea in patients undergoing cancer chemotherapy and reduction of intraocular pressure in patients with glaucoma.

D. **Alcohol** is the most commonly abused substance.

1. Males more frequently use and abuse alcohol, and beer is the most common form of alcohol consumed. Adolescents are more likely to abuse alcohol if their parents and peers have a history of use.

2. **Hazards** of alcohol abuse include impairment of reaction time, coordination, and visual perception; acute illness (hangover) involving nausea, abdominal pain, and headaches; fatty liver changes and cirrhosis; a withdrawal syndrome after chronic use; chronic depression; and fetal damage when it is used to excess during pregnancy.

E. **Hallucinogens**

1. The most common hallucinogens are **lysergic acid diethylamide (LSD)**, which is derived from rye fungus; **mescaline**, which is derived from cactus; **psilocybin**, which is derived from *Psilocybe mexicana;* and **phencyclidine (PCP)**, a drug initially developed as a general anesthetic.

2. **Hazards** of hallucinogen abuse include self-inflicted physical harm during a hallucination, a "bad trip," "flashbacks," possible chronic CNS changes that can lead to "amotivation syndrome" (a condition in which individuals become passive and have little interest in achievement), and **overdose** (most frequently occurring with PCP and leading to psychosis or coma).

F. **Stimulants**

1. The most frequently used stimulants are **amphetamines** and **cocaine**. Cocaine is derived from leaves of *Erythroxylon coca* and other species of *Erythroxylon*.

2. **Hazards** of stimulant abuse include depression, cardiovascular impairment (e.g., arrhythmias, hypertension), irritation of nasal mucosa from inhaling cocaine, psychosis from amphetamine abuse, overdose (leading to convulsions, cardiovascular collapse, coma, and death), and rapid addiction from the use of crack.

G. **Depressants**

1. The most commonly abused depressants are **barbiturates** and **tranquilizers**.

2. **Hazards** of depressant abuse include slurred speech, ataxia, impulsive behavior, respiratory depression (from barbiturates), addiction, severe withdrawal reaction, and overdose leading to coma and death. The combining of these substances with alcohol dramatically increases their toxicity.

H. **Narcotics**

1. The most common narcotics are **heroin, methadone, meperidine,** and **propoxyphene**.

2. **Hazards** of narcotic abuse include complications from using injectable drugs (e.g., hepatitis, transmission of HIV and other forms of infection, abscesses, cellulitis), addiction, and possible overdose.

3. **Naloxone** is effective in counteracting the effects of narcotics and is used in treating overdose.

**I. Inhalants** usually have depressant and sedative effects.

    **1.** The most common in abuse are toluene (found in glue), trichloroethylene, gasoline, and fluorinated hydrocarbons and nitrous oxide (found in aerosol sprays).

    **2. Hazards** of inhalant abuse include nasal and bronchial irritation and systemic effects such as liver toxicity, renal toxicity, cardiac arrhythmias, and CNS damage. Lead toxicity from gasoline may cause further health problems.

## VIII. SKIN PROBLEMS

  **A. Acne** is the major skin problem in adolescents.

    **1. Pathophysiology.** Acne starts with increased sebum production stimulated by androgens during puberty. Sebum consists of a mixture of follicular keratin and secretions of the sebaceous glands. Bacteria (*Propionibacterium acnes*) in the follicles use substrate from the sebum to attract a white blood cell response. The white blood cell activity releases a variety of hydrolytic enzymes, which cause a local inflammatory reaction. Gradual resolution of the inflammation may lead to scarring.

    **2. Definition of terms**
      **a.** A **comedo** is hyperkeratosis of follicular epithelium, and its presence is the initial observable change in acne.
        **(1) Whiteheads** are closed comedones, resulting in slightly elevated papules in the skin.
        **(2) Blackheads** are a later stage of enlarged comedones that contain melanin and eventually open, leading to inflammatory responses.
      **b. Cystic acne** is not actually composed of cysts but of **nodules** formed during the inflammatory reaction, resulting in **erythematous papules (pimples)** or **pus-filled papules (pustules)**.

    **3. Therapy.** Acne is treated by reducing sebum production and decreasing bacterial activity with various agents.
      **a. Comedolytic and antikeratolytic agents** include topical retinoic acid and benzoyl peroxide (also noted to have an antibacterial effect) and systemic isotretinoin.
      **b. Antibacterial agents** generally consist of topical or systemic antibiotics.
      **c. Sebaceous gland inhibitor agents** include systemic isotretinoin and agents that decrease or counteract androgen production (e.g., birth control pills, dexamethasone).
      **d.** Other methods include **surgical removal** of comedones, use of **exfoliating agents** (e.g., ultraviolet light, cryotherapy), and use of **anti-inflammatory agents** such as steroids.
      **e.** The use of water-based instead of oil-based cosmetics is helpful.
      **f.** Diet manipulation has not proved effective.

  **B. Fungal infections** are the second most common skin infection in an adolescent population.

    **1. Agents.** The most common organisms causing fungal infection are dermatophytid fungi such as *Microsporum, Trichophyton, Epidermophyton,* and *Pityrosporum.*
      **a. Tinea corporis** (ringworm) develops on the trunk, extremities, and face and is marked by circular lesions of varying size with raised borders and flat, erythematous centers.
      **b. Tinea cruris** (jock itch) is common in the groin and thigh area of males (the scrotum is spared) and is demarcated by a raised border. This infection often follows from the prolonged use of an athletic supporter.
      **c. Tinea pedis** (athlete's foot) is marked by scaling between the toes and may result from poor foot care and infrequent change of socks.
      **d. Tinea versicolor** is marked by flat patches of hypopigmented or hyperpigmented areas with a distribution similar to that of tinea corporis. It is easily confused with **vitiligo,** an autoimmune condition.
      **e. Tinea capitis** is marked by scaly patches on the scalp and hair loss and frequently is caused by such organisms as *Microsporum* and *Trichophyton.* This infection often is associated with the use of hair products that contain significant amounts of grease or oil that remain on the scalp for extended periods of time. Superinfection with staphylococcal species is common in severe cases.

2. **Diagnosis** is made by the examination of a scraped specimen placed in potassium hydroxide and viewed under a microscope to reveal hyphae forms. A Wood's lamp is helpful in examining tinea capitis and tinea versicolor. Diagnosis may also be made by obtaining fungal cultures.

3. **Therapy.** Fungal infections are treated with topical antifungal preparations. Tinea versicolor responds to selenium sulfide therapy. Tinea capitis usually requires the use of systemic griseofulvin as well as treatment of any bacterial superinfection with the appropriate antibiotic. Tinea pedis is helped by improved foot hygiene. Tinea infections require several weeks of therapy before results are noticeable.

## IX. DISORDERS OF THE MUSCULOSKELETAL SYSTEM

A. **Scoliosis** is lateral curvature of the spine involving the thoracic and lumbar vertebrae. Incidence of scoliosis varies but generally is in the range of 3%–5% of the pediatric population. Seventy-five percent or more of the cases in adolescents have no known etiology. Scoliosis occurs more frequently in women when onset is in adolescence.

1. **Causes** of scoliosis other than idiopathic include congenital failure of spinal development, musculoskeletal disease (e.g., cerebral palsy), neurofibromatosis, Marfan syndrome, juvenile rheumatoid arthritis, trauma (e.g., fracture and destruction of vertebrae, severe burns), and structural defects (e.g., different leg lengths).

2. **Evaluation** includes determining an identifiable cause for the scoliosis. Physical examination of the back with the patient in an erect and a bent-at-the-hips position ascertains vertebral, scapular, and muscular asymmetry. Leg lengths should be checked as well as symmetry at the hips and shoulders. An x-ray of the spine can quantitate any curvature greater than 10°.

3. **Therapy** depends on the degree of back curvature.
   a. If curvature is less than 15° but greater than 10°, the adolescent should be seen by a physician every 6 months. Back exercises may be recommended.
   b. Scoliosis progresses more quickly during the pubertal growth spurt and should be checked every 3 months if the curvature is 15°–20°.
   c. If curvature is 20° or more, the patient should be referred to an orthopedic surgeon for additional therapy, which may include bracing and exercise or surgical stabilization for more advanced curvature.
   d. Change in scoliosis is not as rapid after the pubertal growth spurt but still occurs; thus, continued follow-up into adulthood is recommended.

4. **Sequelae** of uncontrolled scoliosis include deformity of the chest, limitation of lung function leading to polycythemia and pulmonary hypertension, and compromise in cardiac function from pressure on the chest cavity.

B. **Kyphosis** is excessive roundback of the thoracic spine, most often (in 95% of cases) caused by postural problems.

1. **Evaluation** consists of obtaining a history of postural difficulties and back pain. Physical examination should check for thoracic curvature, rounded shoulders, winging of the scapulae, excessive lumbar lordosis, and forward displacement of the head and neck. An x-ray of the back differentiates between a postural and a structural cause.

2. **Therapy** for mild curvature includes a review of posture in standing and sitting positions, back exercises, and appropriate supportive furniture (e.g., firm beds and chairs). Moderate to severe cases require referral to an orthopedic specialist for additional structural support.

C. **Slipped capital femoral epiphysis** is a displacement of the femoral head, usually posteriorly and medially off the femoral metaphysis. It occurs most often in males and is associated with obesity during the pubertal growth spurt.

1. **Evaluation** initially should include a history of any pain in the hip or the knee, antalgic gait, and obesity. Physical examination may reveal few positive findings except a limitation in the range of motion of the hip. An x-ray of the hip shows femoral head changes.

2. **Therapy** consists of referral of the patient to an orthopedic specialist for surgical correction.

D. **Osgood-Schlatter disease** causes stress changes in the tibial tuberosity at the site of attachment of the patellar tendon. The disease usually occurs during the pubertal growth spurt and is more common in males who are active in sports.

1. **Evaluation** includes a history of tenderness around the tibial tuberosity and a review of the patient's physical activities. Physical examination may identify some swelling of the tibial tuberosity with associated point tenderness. An x-ray helps to rule out any other knee pathology.

2. **Therapy** is mainly supportive and includes reduced physical activity when pain is severe. Bracing may become necessary if supportive care is not sufficient.

E. **Osteochondritis dissecans** is the separation of bone from cartilage in the medial or lateral femoral condyle. Most cases (90%) are unilateral. This condition occurs more often in males. In addition to the femur, it may be located in the elbow, hip, and ankle.

1. **Evaluation** includes obtaining a history of recurrent diffuse knee pain and a limp from holding the knee rigid. Physical examination may identify pain and swelling over the site of the lesion, which inhibits full flexion of the knee, and may reveal the absence of other physical deformities of the knee. An x-ray of the knee reveals bone separation.

2. **Therapy** with a long-leg cast is possible in cases identified early. Patients with more advanced disease may need to undergo surgery.

F. **Chondromalacia patellae** is instability of the patella leading to gradual destruction of the patellar cartilage. This is a common cause of knee pain, especially in women. The disease develops over a period of time and becomes worse with increased activity, especially when full knee flexion is required. This problem is generally unilateral but can be bilateral.

1. **Evaluation** includes a history of knee pain associated with the patella, episodes during which the knee gives out, trauma to the patella, and difficulty maintaining the knee in a flexed position for any length of time. Physical examination shows displacement of the patella with knee extension, and tenderness and crepitation with manipulation of the patella. The disease is limited to the patella and usually is not associated with limitation of the range of motion of the knee. An x-ray is not often diagnostic but is helpful in identifying other causes of pain.

2. **Therapy** includes limitation of activities requiring deep flexion of the knees (e.g., bicycling), pain control with aspirin or nonsteroidal anti-inflammatory agents, and improvement of muscle tone with isometric exercises. A rehabilitation program includes a gradual return to more complete physical activities under the direction of an orthopedist. Patients with severe damage and pain may require casting of the knee.

## BIBLIOGRAPHY

Emans SJH, Goldstein DP: *Pediatric and Adolescent Gynecology,* 3rd edition. Boston, Little, Brown, 1990.

Hofmann AD, Greydanus DE: *Adolescent Medicine,* 2nd edition. Norwalk, CT, Appleton & Lange, 1989.

Neinstein LS: *Adolescent Health Care: A Practical Guide,* 2nd edition. Baltimore, Urban and Schwarzenberg, 1990.

1989 STD Treatment Guidelines: *MMWR* 38(S–8): 1–43, 1989.

## STUDY QUESTIONS

**Directions:** Each of the numbered items or incomplete statements in this section is followed by answers or by completions of the statement. Select the **one** lettered answer or completion that is **best** in each case.

1. The first sign of puberty in males is

(A) development of pubic hair
(B) development of the glans penis
(C) pigmentation of the scrotum
(D) increased volume of the testes
(E) increased length of the penis

2. During mid-adolescence, the central issue for anticipatory guidance is

(A) peer support
(B) pubertal development
(C) adult role models
(D) separation
(E) school transition

3. Which of the following is the most effective birth control method with the fewest side effects?

(A) Diaphragm
(B) Oral contraceptive pill
(C) Rhythm
(D) Foam and condoms
(E) Injectable progesterone

4. Which of the following STDs is most prevalent in the United States?

(A) Gonorrhea
(B) Genital herpes
(C) Chlamydial infection
(D) Syphilis
(E) Trichomoniasis

5. Which of the following organisms is one of the most common causes of PID?

(A) *Mycoplasma hominis*
(B) *Chlamydia trachomatis*
(C) *Staphylococcus aureus*
(D) *Escherichia coli*
(E) *Ureaplasma urealyticum*

6. Which of the following complications is more likely to occur in a pregnant teenager who is age 15 or younger than in an older pregnant teenager?

(A) Anemia
(B) Pelvic complications
(C) Toxemia
(D) Low-birth-weight infant
(E) Infant mortality

7. The most common side effect in women using oral contraceptives is

(A) hair loss
(B) break-through bleeding
(C) depression
(D) dysmenorrhea
(E) longer menstrual periods

8. A 17-year-old female is evaluated for a menstrual period that has lasted twice as long as usual. Which of the following laboratory studies should be included in the initial evaluation of this patient?

(A) Liver function studies
(B) Clotting studies
(C) Pregnancy test
(D) Thyroid studies
(E) LH, FSH, and prolactin levels

9. All of the following statements about suicide are true EXCEPT

(A) it is the third leading cause of death for teenagers
(B) death by suicide is more frequently seen in males
(C) suicide is most commonly committed by overdose
(D) a history of a previous attempt is common
(E) attempts are more common in females

| | | |
|---|---|---|
| 1-D | 4-C | 7-B |
| 2-A | 5-B | 8-C |
| 3-D | 6-B | 9-C |

10. Acne therapy addresses all of the following factors EXCEPT

(A) diet
(B) local hygiene
(C) sebum production
(D) inflammatory response
(E) bacterial activity

11. All of the following statements about pubertal growth spurt are true EXCEPT

(A) it is early in males and late in females
(B) it is associated with muscle development in males
(C) it is the last of three growth spurts during childhood
(D) it is associated with fat deposition in females
(E) its average duration is about 3 years

12. A chlamydial genital infection can result in all of the following EXCEPT

(A) lower abdominal pain
(B) infertility
(C) epididymitis
(D) right shoulder pain
(E) arthritis

13. Oral contraceptives prevent pregnancy by all of the following mechanisms EXCEPT

(A) blocking sperm
(B) changing the cervical mucus
(C) decreasing implantation
(D) suppressing ovulation

14. Toxic shock syndrome is associated with all of the following findings EXCEPT

(A) vomiting and diarrhea
(B) disorientation
(C) increased platelet count
(D) elevated liver function tests
(E) elevated BUN

15. All of the following statements regarding substance abuse in adolescents are true EXCEPT

(A) substance abuse may retard psychosocial development
(B) cocaine is the most commonly abused substance
(C) tobacco use is associated with use by parents
(D) most forms of substance abuse are decreasing in adolescents

16. Absolute contraindications to the use of oral contraceptives include all of the following conditions EXCEPT

(A) hypertension
(B) diabetes
(C) hyperlipidemia
(D) cerebral vascular disease
(E) coronary artery disease

**Directions:** The group of items in this section consists of lettered options followed by a set of numbered items. For each item, select the **one** lettered option that is most closely associated with it. Each lettered option may be selected once, more than once, or not at all.

**Questions 17–20**

The diagnosis of genital infections is made from a smear of vaginal, cervical, or urethral discharge or by culture from the appropriate site of infection. For each microscopic finding listed below, select the causative organism with which it is most likely associated.

(A) *Neisseria gonorrhoeae*
(B) *Trichomonas vaginalis*
(C) *Candida albicans*
(D) *Chlamydia trachomatis*
(E) *Gardnerella vaginalis*

17. Budding hyphae

18. Flagellate protozoa

19. Inclusion bodies

20. Gram-negative diplococci

---

17-C        20-A
18-B
19-D

## ANSWERS AND EXPLANATIONS

**1. The answer is D** *[II C 2 c; Tables 4-2, 4-3]*.
Frequently, the start of puberty is missed because the physician is looking for the development of pubic hair. Testes that have enlarged to greater than 1.5 cc in volume indicate the onset of puberty. There may be a time interval between the onset of testicular enlargement and the development of pubic hair. The pigmentation of the scrotum, the increased length of the penis, and the development of the glans penis all follow the increase in the size of the testes.

**2. The answer is A** *[II B 2]*.
By mid-adolescence the availability of peer support and the right to privacy are integral issues in the transition to adulthood. Most pubertal development has occurred by this point, although an adolescent may still have concerns about his or her body. Separation does not become an issue until late adolescence. Adult role models are needed throughout adolescence. Middle and high school transitions occur during early adolescence.

**3. The answer is D** *[V A 2 c (5)]*.
The oral contraceptive pill and the combination of foam and condoms have almost identical success rates when used appropriately, but the latter has many fewer side effects. The diaphragm also has few side effects but has a failure rate of up to 15%–20%. The rhythm method (having sex at the time of the month when the woman is least likely to get pregnant) is only 70% effective, at best. Injectable progesterone is more effective than the progesterone-only pill in suppressing ovulation; however, it is linked to many side effects.

**4. The answer is C** *[IV A 1 a]*.
Chlamydial infection is the most common nonviral sexually transmitted disease in the United States today. Unfortunately, since *Chlamydia trachomatis* is hard to isolate and since the infection has only recently become a reportable disease, exact figures about its prevalence are not available. Chlamydial infection also is the leading cause of infertility in women.

**5. The answer is B** *[IV D 2]*.
Pelvic inflammatory disease (PID) can often be caused by more than one organism at a time. *Chlamydia trachomatis* and *Neisseria gonorrhoeae* are the most frequently isolated organisms from such infections. *Mycoplasma hominis, Escherichia coli* and *Staphylococcus aureus* may also cause this type of infection, but less commonly.

**6. The answer is B** *[V B 2]*.
Pelvic complications resulting from incomplete pelvic development are likely to occur in women who are younger than age 15 years. By age 16 or 17, most women have completed their pubertal development. Anemia, infant mortality, and low-birth-weight infants are complications associated with all ages of teen pregnancy and are usually due to poor nutrition and poor health habits during the pregnancy.

**7. The answer is B** *[V A 1 d]*.
Bleeding between menstrual periods is the most common reason many teenagers stop using oral contraceptives. This problem usually resolves after the first two to three cycles. Hair loss and depression are less common problems. Dysmenorrhea is decreased, and menstrual periods shorten with the use of birth control pills.

**8. The answer is C** *[III A 2 b (3)]*.
Mild dysfunctional vaginal bleeding is not uncommon in adolescents. Anemia, pregnancy, and vaginal infection need to be ruled out. After this is done, the patient can be reassured and followed for a period of 4–6 months. If the dysfunctional bleeding continues, further studies should be considered, including thyroid and liver function tests, clotting studies, and appropriate hormonal studies.

**9. The answer is C** *[VI B]*.
In the United States, many suicides are committed by drug overdose and poisoning, but they are not as common as those caused by firearms and hanging. Over two-thirds of those who commit suicide have tried it before, and many of those people have a history of depression or other mental health problems. Males are three to four times more likely to commit suicide than females, although females make more attempts. The ratio of suicides between males and females is influenced by the local culture. For example, the suicide rate is equal in men and women in Israel, but more women than men commit suicide in India.

**10. The answer is A** *[VIII A 3].*
Successful acne therapy involves counteracting the increased sebum production stimulated by elevated androgens and counteracting bacterial activity and the resulting local inflammatory response. Keeping the skin free from excessive oils has also proved to be helpful. Dietary restrictions, such as eliminating chocolate, have not proved very effective.

**11. The answer is A** *[II C 2; Figure 4-1].*
The pubertal growth spurt occurs during the first half of pubertal development in females and is associated with the deposition of fat. This early increase in physical stature may lead the female adolescent to link herself to an older peer group, the members of which are similar to her in physical development (rather than developing a link with peers her own age). In the male, the pubertal growth spurt occurs in the latter half of puberty and is associated with muscle development. These changes in the male need to be taken into account when he is given a sports physical examination. For example, the early pubertal male who is going out for football may not only be at a disadvantage because of the lack of muscle development but may also be at greater risk for physical injury. Pubertal development may last longer in females than in males, although the average duration is about 3 years.

**12. The answer is E** *[IV A 1 a, E, F].*
Since chlamydial infection is such a common sexually transmitted disease and may be asymptomatic (especially in women), it may spread to cause lower abdominal pain, infertility, epididymitis, and right shoulder pain. Lower abdominal pain is the result of a pelvic infection; infertility is caused by scarring of the fallopian tubes from infection; epididymitis may result from an untreated chlamydial urethritis; and right shoulder pain is caused by irritation of the phrenic nerve from perihepatitis as a result of infection. Joint involvement is not a characteristic of chlamydial infection, although it is a possible outcome of gonorrhea.

**13. The answer is A** *[V A 1 a].*
The hormones of oral contraceptives essentially turn off the ovulatory function of the ovaries. The uterine lining is not vascularized as extensively and, hence, is not as able to receive a fertilized egg. The cervical mucus becomes more hostile to sperm and makes it less likely that sperm enters the uterus.

**14. The answer is C** *[IV C 1].*
Toxic shock syndrome (TSS) is a total body response to the release of endotoxin from a *Staphylococcus aureus* infection. The platelet count decreases to less than 100,000/mm$^3$. Treatment requires the removal of the causative agent, such as a tampon or a diaphragm, and treatment with systemic antibiotics. Prevention requires the limited and careful use of diaphragms and tampons and the recognition of the symptoms associated with TSS.

**15. The answer is B** *[VII D].*
Alcohol is the most commonly abused substance among adolescents, although cocaine abuse is an increasing problem. Most forms of substance abuse in the adolescent population have gradually decreased in the 1980s from the levels seen in the late 1970s, with the exception of cocaine abuse, which has increased. In the past, it was thought that cocaine may not be addictive, but the new free-base cocaine is not only highly addictive but extremely dangerous because of its life-threatening side effects. Chronic substance abuse results in dissociation from normal socialization activities and leads to delay of psychosocial development.

**16. The answer is B** *[V A 1 b (1)].*
Since oral contraceptives can cause elevation in blood pressure as well as thromboembolic disease, they should not be used by a patient whose blood pressure is already elevated or by a patient in whom thromboembolic problems already exist, such as in cerebral vascular disease and coronary artery disease. Insulin requirements may change with the use of oral contraceptives by diabetics, but this can easily be adjusted.

**17–20. The answers are: 17-C** *[IV B 1 b],* **18-B** *[IV A 1 k (2)],* **19-D** *[IV A 1 a (2)],* **20-A** *[IV A 1 b (2)].*
Candidal vaginal infections are diagnosed by the presence of hyphae. This infection often is accompanied by a cheesy white discharge and vulvar pruritus. Such an infection often occurs after a course of systemic antibiotics taken for an unrelated infection. The antibiotics tend to decrease the normal vaginal flora and allow the yeast to proliferate.

*Trichomonas vaginalis* is a flagellate protozoa that causes vaginitis usually associated with a foul-smelling greenish discharge and vulvar tenderness. The organism tends to die quickly in a normal saline preparation. Such a preparation should be reviewed without delay.

Chlamydial infections are identified by inclusion bodies located in columnar lining cells in the endocervix of the female and about an inch into the urethra in the male. Unless samples of these cells are taken for culture or for a rapid analysis, a diagnosis of chlamydial infection is impossible to confirm. Samples of the cervical or urethral discharge may not contain the organism.

Gram-negative intracellular diplococci present in a smear from a male urethra are diagnostic for gonorrhea. In females, a culture is needed to confirm the presence of gonorrhea, since other gram-negative diplococci may be part of the normal vaginal flora.

**I. GENERAL PRINCIPLES.** Many problems that arise in the newborn are discussed in detail in other chapters. This chapter emphasizes those problems that are unique to the perinatal period. In this section, some general concepts are introduced, which are amplified in subsequent sections.

**A. Definition of terms**

**1.** The normal human **gestational period** is 280 days, or 40 weeks, calculated from the first day of the mother's last menstrual cycle.
   **a. Preterm gestation** refers to delivery at less than 38 weeks gestation.
   **b. Term gestation** refers to delivery at 38 to less than 42 weeks gestation.
   **c. Post-term gestation** refers to delivery at or after 42 weeks gestation.

**2.** The **neonatal period** is defined as the first 28 days (4 weeks) of life for term infants, although, from a practical standpoint, it is extended in the case of a prematurely delivered infant.

**B. Major concepts and concerns inherent to the neonatal period**

**1. Transition from fetal to neonatal life.** Changes in body and organ function occur as the fetus adapts to extrauterine life and begins to function independently. Organs mature at different rates and times during gestation. A preterm or complicated delivery may alter the normal sequence of these events (see I C 2). Some major changes occur in the following organ systems during the transition from fetal to neonatal life.
   **a. Cardiovascular system** (see also Ch 11 II A)
      **(1) Prenatal circulation** (Figure 5-1)
         **(a)** Oxygenation of the blood occurs in the **placenta**—an organ of low vascular resistance—and the oxygenated blood returns to the fetus via the **umbilical vein,** which enters the liver at the porta hepatis.
         **(b)** Blood passes via the **ductus venosus** to the inferior vena cava. Preferential shunting allows oxygenated blood to be shunted through the **foramen ovale** to the left atrium and left ventricle and on to the coronary, carotid, and cerebral arteries, while the desaturated blood of the inferior and superior venae cavae travels to the right atrium and right ventricle and on to the pulmonary artery.
         **(c)** Due to the high vascular resistance in the lung, 90% of the pulmonary artery blood bypasses the lung and is shunted through the **ductus arteriosus,** which enters the aorta below the takeoff of the brachiocephalic artery and left common carotid artery. In this way, the most highly oxygenated blood is supplied to the heart and brain.
         **(d)** Blood in the descending aorta, which is intermediately deoxygenated, is returned to the placenta via the **umbilical arteries**.
      **(2) Postnatal circulation**
         **(a)** At birth, there is a rise in systemic vascular resistance as a result of the cessation of blood flow through the placenta.
         **(b)** With the first few breaths, pulmonary vascular resistance falls, the foramen ovale closes, and the ductus arteriosus begins to constrict. These processes allow all deoxygenated blood returning to the right ventricle to go on to the lung and become oxygenated.
         **(c)** The oxygenated blood returns to the left ventricle and then is pumped throughout the body.

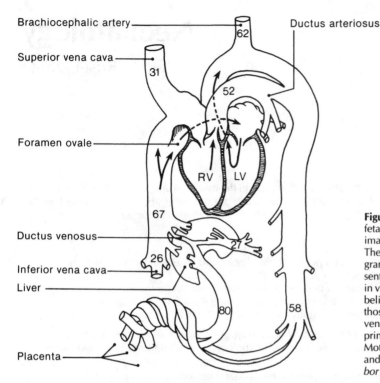

Brachiocephalic artery

Ductus arteriosus

Superior vena cava

Foramen ovale

RV   LV

Ductus venosus

Inferior vena cava

Liver

Placenta

**Figure 5-1.** Knowledge of the human fetal circulation is based on fetal animal studies, such as the fetal lamb. The fetal lamb circulation is diagramed here, with *numbers* representing the percent oxygen saturation in various segments. These values are believed to correspond closely to those in the human fetus. *RV* = right ventricle; *LV* = left ventricle. (Reprinted from Born GVR, Dawes GS, Mott JC, et al: Changes in the heart and lungs at birth. *Cold Spring Harbor Symp Quant Biol* 19:102, 1954.)

   **b. Pulmonary system** (see also Ch 11 II B)
     **(1)** By the end of gestation, the major airways and alveoli are filled with fluid that contains large amounts of **surfactant**.
     **(2)** At birth, the negative pressure created by the first breaths draws air into the lungs, and an air-fluid interface is formed. The surfactant spreads along the epithelial lining of the alveoli and decreases surface tension at the end of expiration.
   **c. Hepatobiliary system.** Prenatally, bilirubin conjugation in the liver is suppressed. In the first days of life, increased **glucuronyl transferase** activity results in conjugation and elimination of bilirubin, via reduction products, in the stool.
   **d. Renal system** (see Ch 13 II). Glomerular function, which is relatively low in fetal life as reflected by the glomerular filtration rate, increases with gestational age as well as with postnatal age. Tubular function also improves with age, which has important consequences for the elimination of many drugs from the body.

  **2. Growth.** The growth rate of the fetus is greater than that of the infant or older child. Growth slows just prior to birth, limited by placental substrate transport, and a loss of body weight occurs in the first few days after birth owing to loss of extracellular water and to inadequate nutritional intake. As the newborn acclimates to the extrauterine environment and improves her behavioral organization, feeding improves and growth accelerates again. Adequate nutrition along with control of possible hyperbilirubinemia or infection are crucial to normal growth and development in the newborn. (See IV B 2–3 for further discussion of growth and the nutritional needs of the newborn.)

  **3. Initial examination of the newborn.** It is the pediatrician's responsibility to perform a thorough physical examination and a series of screening tests so that common, preventable illnesses and congenital anomalies may be identified and rapidly treated, as a poor outcome often is related to a delay in detection and therapy. (See Ch 1 IV C–E for details of the newborn examination.)

**C. Somatic growth, organ maturation, and gestational age**

  **1. Somatic growth** refers to the process by which the body and its constituent parts increase in size. Somatic growth occurs by two processes: hyperplasia and hypertrophy.
   **a. Hyperplasia** is an increase in the size of a tissue or organ due to an **increase in cell number**. Growth during the first half of pregnancy is achieved by hyperplasia.

(1) Problems that interfere with somatic growth early in pregnancy inhibit cell division, causing a decrease in total body cell number. As a result, the fetus may be **symmetrically growth retarded** or small for weight, length, and head circumference.

(2) Factors that adversely affect hyperplastic growth of the fetus include:

(a) Congenital infection

(b) Chromosomal defects

(c) Nonchromosomal congenital syndromes

(d) Cell toxins (e.g., alcohol, narcotics)

b. **Hypertrophy** is an increase in the size of a tissue or organ due to an **increase in cell size**. Growth during the last trimester of pregnancy and postnatally is achieved primarily by hypertrophy.

(1) Aberrations in fetal nutrition in the last stage of pregnancy inhibit normal cell growth and may result in **asymmetric growth retardation**. Body weight is primarily affected, with preservation of brain growth.

(2) Factors that adversely affect fetal nutrition include:

(a) Maternal malnutrition

(b) Placental abnormalities or abnormal cord insertion

(c) Preeclampsia

(d) Multiple gestation

(e) Maternal use of cigarettes

2. **Organ maturation** refers to the structural and functional development of an organ system. Maturational growth is measured by comparison to the adult level of organ function.

a. The various **organ systems mature at different rates and at different times** during gestation. Premature birth may alter the normal sequence of organ maturation.

(1) The term infant has sufficient function of most organs to allow it to be independent at birth. Some organs (e.g., the liver, kidney) accelerate in function during the immediate perinatal period, whereas a few organs (e.g., the brain, lung) continue to mature for many years after birth.

(2) The preterm infant has inadequate function of some vital organs (e.g., the lung) at birth, but within a short period of time many of these organs will have accelerated development and function compared with a fetus of similar conceptional age. This allows for independent function of the preterm infant at a gestationally young age.

b. Usually, there is a **close correlation between the somatic growth and maturation of vital organs** (e.g., the lung) although various factors may accelerate or retard either or both of these processes. In the case of lung development, both fetal malnutrition and administration of betamethasone to the mother are factors that will accelerate biochemical maturation, whereas maternal diabetes and the associated fetal hyperglycemia and hyperinsulinemia will lead to delayed biochemical maturation of the lung.

3. **Gestational age.** Norms have been established for somatic growth at each week of gestation and are based on weight, length, and head circumference. However, size, per se, should not be used to infer gestational age or maturation.

a. If an infant's growth parameters are between the tenth and ninetieth percentiles for a specific time of gestation, the infant's growth is said to be **appropriate for gestational age**.

b. If an infant's weight is less than the tenth percentile for a specific time of gestation, the infant is said to be **small for gestational age** [see I C 1 a (2), b (2) for causative factors].

c. If an infant's weight is greater than the ninetieth percentile for a specific time of gestation, the infant is said to be **large for gestational age**. Causes include:

(1) Maternal diabetes

(2) Beckwith-Wiedemann syndrome

(3) Genetic predisposition (i.e., maternal history of large infants)

(4) Hydrops fetalis

d. If an infant's head circumference is greater than the ninetieth percentile for a specific time of gestation, regardless of other parameters, specific cerebral pathology should be investigated (see V G 4 and Ch 17 III C 3).

## II. PERINATAL ASPHYXIA

A. **Pathophysiology.** The ability of the fetus or infant to survive episodes of asphyxia is related to the mechanisms that regulate blood flow to the organs of the body. These mechanisms are designed to maintain oxygen delivery to the vital organs (i.e., the brain, heart, adrenal gland) during periods of hypoxia.

1. **During periods of hypoxia or hypercapnia,** blood flow to the brain is increased. The result is a stable delivery of oxygen to the brain to meet metabolic demands and maintenance of a normal intracellular pH. These flow changes are operational unless the infant is extremely hypotensive.

2. **During periods of mild asphyxia,** adaptive changes in blood flow allow adequate oxygen delivery to the brain, heart, and adrenal gland. This is accomplished via an increase and a redistribution of the cardiac output. Blood flow to the skin, muscle, kidney, and gastrointestinal tract is sacrificed to maintain perfusion of the vital organs.

3. **During periods of severe or prolonged asphyxia,** the underperfused (sacrificed) tissues and organs gradually become acidotic due to anaerobic metabolism and lactic acid production. This leads to myocardial depression and a gradual decrease in blood pressure so that blood fails to perfuse the vital organs, with resultant permanent tissue damage in such organs. The extent of the tissue damage depends on the amount of time that has elapsed between the failure of blood flow (i.e., tissue hypoxia) and the institution of resuscitation (i.e., reoxygenation of the tissues).

B. **Clinical features.** The ability to recognize the clinical signs and symptoms of perinatal asphyxia requires knowledge of the predisposing risk factors for asphyxia as well as the prenatal and postnatal symptoms of asphyxia.

1. **Prenatal risk factors for asphyxia** include:
   a. Extremes in maternal age (i.e., < 20 years or > 35 years)
   b. Placental abruption
   c. Placenta previa
   d. Preeclampsia
   e. Preterm gestation
   f. Post-term gestation
   g. Meconium-stained amniotic fluid
   h. Fetal bradycardia
   i. Malpresentation
   j. Multiple gestation
   k. Prolonged rupture of the fetal membranes
   l. Maternal diabetes
   m. Maternal use of illicit drugs

2. **Events that occur with the onset of asphyxia**
   a. **Sequence.** A clear understanding of the sequence of events that occur with the onset of asphyxia is of utmost importance in determining the condition of the asphyxiated infant and in initiating therapy (see III E).
      (1) Respiratory effort ceases abruptly, and the fetus (infant) experiences primary apnea. This is followed by a phase of gasping and, if resuscitation is not initiated, progression to terminal apnea.
      (2) A rapid decrease in the oxygenation of blood occurs, with resultant respiratory acidosis followed by a combined respiratory and metabolic acidosis.
      (3) The onset of hypoxia results in a rapid decrease in heart rate.
      (4) Blood pressure rises initially but, with progression to terminal apnea, falls to hypotensive levels.
      (5) The fall in blood pressure causes a decrease in the flow of blood to the organs and consequent tissue damage.
   b. **Recovery.** These events can be reversed with appropriate resuscitative measures [i.e., reoxygenation of the central nervous system (CNS); see III E].
      (1) As a result of such intervention, heart rate and blood pressure improve; gasping then occurs followed by regular breathing. Last to recover are body functions that are controlled by the higher regions of the brain.
      (2) The longer the episode of asphyxia, the longer it takes for heart rate, breathing, and other body functions to recover.

3. **Postnatal symptoms of asphyxia** vary with the degree of asphyxia. It is not clear why some infants exhibit multi-organ involvement, whereas others have only one or two organ systems involved. Some specific effects of asphyxia are listed below by organ system.

a. **Brain**

(1) **Mild asphyxia.** The infant who experiences mild asphyxia initially will be depressed. This is followed by a period of hyperalertness, which resolves within 1 or 2 days. There are no focal signs, and the prognosis is excellent for a normal outcome.

(2) **Moderate asphyxia.** The infant who experiences moderate asphyxia will be very depressed. This is followed by a prolonged period of hyperalertness and hyperreflexia. Generalized seizures often occur 12–24 hours after the episode of asphyxia but are controlled easily, resolving in a few days regardless of therapy. The prognosis is variable; normal results on electroencephalogram (EEG) are predictive of a normal outcome.

(3) **Severe asphyxia** is associated with coma, intractable seizure activity, cerebral edema, and intracranial hemorrhage. The infant often becomes progressively more depressed over the first 1–3 days, as the cerebral edema develops, and death may occur during this period. Survival generally is associated with a poor long-term outcome.

b. **Heart.** Severe or prolonged episodes of asphyxia may result in **hypoxic cardiomyopathy**. Signs and symptoms include hypotension, poor myocardial contractility, cardiomegaly, and congestive heart failure.

c. **Lung.** Respiratory distress and a need for oxygen can occur due to a delayed fall in pulmonary vascular resistance (see V A 2 h).

d. **Kidney.** Decreased renal blood flow during the asphyxial event causes **acute tubular necrosis**. This usually is self-limited.

e. **Gastrointestinal tract.** Asphyxia often is associated with poor gastrointestinal motility or ileus. The hypoxia also predisposes to secondary bacterial invasion and to the development of **necrotizing enterocolitis** (see V B).

f. **Blood.** Hypoxia depresses bone marrow function and initiates an intravascular coagulopathy, which results in thrombocytopenia, prolonged prothrombin time (PT) and partial thromboplastin time (PTT), and clinical evidence of bleeding.

C. **Therapy**

1. **General principles.** The primary objective in treating perinatal asphyxia is to restore an oxygen supply to the body tissues, especially the brain. This requires ventilation with oxygen and ensuring an adequate cardiac output. The secondary objective is to evaluate the degree of hypoxic injury and to plan treatment.

2. **Specific therapy.** Specific delivery room resuscitation procedures are discussed in III E. In addition, the following common problems should be anticipated or considered and treated if present:

a. Hypotension

b. Hypoxic encephalopathy and seizures

c. Persistent pulmonary hypertension

d. Hypoxic cardiomyopathy

e. Ileus and necrotizing enterocolitis

f. Acute tubular necrosis

g. Adrenal hemorrhage and necrosis

h. Hypoglycemia

i. Polycythemia

j. Hypocalcemia

k. Disseminated intravascular coagulation (DIC)

D. **Prognosis.** Outcome is related to the severity and duration of the asphyxial insult and to the adequacy of compensatory mechanisms, resuscitation procedures, and specific treatment of multiorgan system involvement. Neurologic outcome is the most difficult to predict but is best related to the degree of hypoxic encephalopathy and electroencephalographic activity in the neonatal period and to findings on physical examination of the infant at 9–12 months of age.

## III. DELIVERY ROOM MANAGEMENT OF THE NEWBORN

A. **Goals.** The goals of delivery room management are to assess and promptly attend to the immediate needs (e.g., oxygenation, ventilation) and potential problems (e.g., serious anomalies) of the newborn.

**B. Physical layout and equipment.** The newborn resuscitation area should have the following general characteristics:

1. Immediate proximity to the delivery room

2. Constant room temperature of 80° F (27° C)

3. Adequate light for thorough examination

4. Adequate space for necessary personnel (see III C 2)

5. Open bed with radiant heat source

6. Specific resuscitation equipment (see III C 3)

**C. Preparation for delivery**

1. **Obtaining information.** The pediatrician must have specific information concerning the mother and fetus to prepare for routine care of the mother and newborn as well as treatment of specific problems related to a particular delivery.
   a. **Obstetric history** should include all information that may be pertinent to the immediate fetal (newborn) condition. The information is best obtained from the obstetrician and the medical chart and by direct communication with the parents. Important items include:
      (1) Maternal age and medical and previous obstetric history
      (2) Length of gestation
      (3) Blood group incompatibilities
      (4) Maternal infection [e.g., syphilis, gonorrhea, rubella, herpes, human immunodeficiency virus (HIV), hepatitis]
      (5) Maternal drug usage
      (6) Ultrasound evaluation of fetal growth and amniotic fluid volume as well as for the possibility of congenital anomalies
      (7) Signs of chorioamnionitis, including prolonged rupture of the fetal membranes, maternal fever, and leukocytosis on complete blood count
      (8) Results of other fetal evaluations, including lecithin/sphingomyelin (L/S) ratio [see V A 1 b (1) (b)], non-stress test, and biophysical profile
   b. **Labor history** also should be obtained and should include:
      (1) Fetal heart tracing
      (2) Duration of fetal membrane rupture
      (3) Evaluation of amniotic fluid (color and quantity)
      (4) Progress of labor
      (5) Fetal scalp blood pH

2. **Forming the resuscitation team.** Personnel and their tasks vary with the type of delivery that is anticipated. High-risk deliveries or pregnancies include those with such complications as listed in Table 5-1.
   a. **Low-risk delivery team** includes:
      (1) **Team leader** (i.e., pediatrician, anesthesiologist, obstetrician, or nurse specialist trained in newborn resuscitation) to assess the newborn and institute any necessary resuscitation

**Table 5-1.** Factors Associated with High-Risk Pregnancies or Deliveries

| |
|---|
| Maternal diabetes |
| Maternal antibody sensitization (Rh, ABO) |
| Preterm gestation (delivery at < 38 weeks) |
| Post-term gestation (delivery at > 42 weeks) |
| Multiple gestation |
| Maternal bleeding (placental abruption, placenta previa) |
| Severe preeclampsia |
| Intrauterine growth retardation |
| Maternal narcotic addiction |
| Known fetal anomalies |
| Breech presentation |
| Cesarean delivery |
| Fetal distress |

        **(2) One assistant** (i.e., nursery or delivery room nurse) to assist in basic newborn resuscitation, including drying and warming the infant and assessing heart rate

  **b. High-risk delivery team** includes:

        **(1) Team leader** to direct resuscitation and, possibly, to direct and institute airway management

        **(2) Three assistants**

           **(a)** One to assess heart rate and to initiate cardiac compression if needed

           **(b)** One to assist with drying, suctioning, ventilating, and preparing drugs for injection

           **(c)** One to gain intravenous access and to administer drugs

**3. Readying equipment.** The equipment needed is directly related to the basic principles of newborn resuscitation.

  **a. Equipment needed for airway management** includes:

      **(1)** Wall-unit suction pump with regulator (a pressure of 80 cm of $H_2O$ is appropriate for most suctioning) and connector tubing

      **(2)** De Lee suction catheter with trap

      **(3)** Oral airway (various sizes)

      **(4)** Endotracheal tubes of appropriate sizes

      **(5)** Laryngoscope

      **(6)** Suction catheters

  **b. Equipment needed for ventilation and oxygenation** includes:

      **(1)** Oxygen source, which preferably should be warmed and humidified

      **(2)** Masks of appropriate sizes

      **(3)** Bag with oxygen reservoir, mechanism to deliver positive end-expiratory pressure (PEEP), and manometer to measure airway pressure

  **c. Drugs that may be needed** include:

      **(1)** Epinephrine

      **(2)** Plasma volume expanding agent (i.e., 5% albumin or 5% purified protein fraction solution)

      **(3)** Sodium bicarbonate

      **(4)** Naloxone

  **d. Equipment needed for intravenous access** includes:

      **(1)** Umbilical catheters (3.5 F and 5.0 F)

      **(2)** Instruments for umbilical cutdown

      **(3)** Saline solution (0.9%)

**D. Assessment of the newborn and the Apgar score.** The goal of the initial assessment is to determine the newborn's state of oxygenation and ventilation. This usually is done by performing an abbreviated **Apgar evaluation**.

**1.** The Apgar score was devised as a means of assessing the oxygenation, ventilation, and degree of asphyxia in a uniform manner that quickly communicates information to all persons involved in the resuscitation of the newborn. The Apgar evaluation is performed at 1 and 5 minutes after birth. Five signs—heart rate, respiratory effort, muscle tone, reflex irritability, and skin color—are examined and assigned a score of 0, 1, or 2 (Table 5-2). The Apgar score is obtained by adding all individual scores.

  **a.** A **score of 8–10** reflects good oxygenation and ventilation and indicates no need for vigorous resuscitation.

  **b.** A **score of 5–7** indicates a need for stimulation and supplemental oxygen.

**Table 5-2.** Apgar Evaluation of the Newborn

| Sign | Score | | |
|---|---|---|---|
| | **0** | **1** | **2** |
| Heart rate | Absent | < 100 beats/min | > 100 beats/min |
| Respiratory effort | Absent | Weak, irregular | Strong, regular |
| Muscle tone | Flaccid | Some flexion | Well flexed |
| Reflex irritability (response to catheter in nostril) | No response | Grimace | Cough or sneeze |
| Skin color | Blue, pale | Body pink, extremities blue | Entire body pink |

    **c.** A **score of less than 5** indicates a need for assisted ventilation and possible cardiac support (see III E 1 c, d).

  **2.** The Apgar score is a useful method of communicating the well-being of the newborn. However, urgently needed resuscitation should not be delayed while a full examination is performed. Bradycardia or a poor respiratory effort alone indicates a need for immediate resuscitation.

  **3.** The Apgar score at 5 minutes reflects the adequacy of resuscitation and the degree of perinatal asphyxia.

**E. Resuscitation.** The purpose of resuscitation is to reoxygenate the CNS of the newborn by providing oxygen, establishing ventilation, and ensuring an adequate cardiac output. Although it may be difficult to differentiate primary apnea from secondary apnea, a quick assessment of the newborn's skin color, respiratory activity, and heart rate should allow prompt institution of appropriate resuscitation.

  **1. Routine procedures.** The evaluations and procedures that constitute the resuscitation of the newborn are listed below in the order in which they should be initiated.

    **a. Maintenance of body heat.** The infant should be dried and provided with radiant heat to maintain body temperature. It is important to avoid hypothermia, which will increase the newborn's oxygen consumption.

    **b. Establishment of an airway.** Immediately after delivery, the infant's head should be placed in a neutral or slightly extended position and an airway established by clearing the mouth, nose, and pharynx of thick secretions or meconium (see III E 2 a). Deep and frequent oropharyngeal suctioning should be avoided, as it will increase vagal output, causing apnea and bradycardia.

    **c. Ventilation.** The adequacy of air exchange in the newborn must be assessed. In most cases, drying off, suctioning, and tactile stimulation (e.g., gentle flicking of the feet or rubbing of the back) are adequate to induce effective spontaneous ventilation.

      **(1)** If ventilation is adequate, **supplemental oxygen** may be given to improve heart rate or skin color.

      **(2)** If supplemental oxygen does not improve heart rate or skin color or if ventilation is inadequate, **mechanical ventilation** should be initiated, using mask and bag ventilation.

        **(a)** If spontaneous ventilation improves, mechanical ventilation should be stopped and supplemental oxygen resumed.

        **(b)** If the response is poor or if airway obstruction occurs, an endotracheal tube should be inserted and mechanical ventilation continued.

    **d. Circulation.** If mechanical ventilation does not improve the heart rate or skin color, one of the following steps is taken.

      **(1)** If **heart rate is less than 60 beats/min,** or between 60 and 80 beats/min and not improving, cardiac compression is initiated; if heart rate does not improve, epinephrine is administered via an umbilical venous catheter or endotracheal tube.

      **(2)** If **heart rate is 80 beats/min or greater** but there is poor perfusion or weak pulse, a plasma volume expanding agent is administered at a dose of 15 ml/kg.

    **e. Drug support.** The following medications may be useful during resuscitation.

      **(1) Sodium bicarbonate** should be reserved until it is clear that a metabolic acidosis exists.

      **(2) Naloxone** may be helpful for poor spontaneous respiratory effort secondary to maternal narcotic usage during labor. Naloxone is contraindicated in an infant born to a mother who is addicted to narcotics.

  **2. Special problems requiring resuscitation** are discussed in further detail in section V (see specific cross-references noted below).

    **a. Meconium aspiration syndrome** (see V A 3 c). Meconium-stained amniotic fluid may be a sign of perinatal asphyxia. Thin meconium rarely is a significant problem. Thick meconium, however, is a serious concern as it may be aspirated and result in aspiration pneumonia. Although an affected infant may be depressed due to asphyxia, **it is imperative that the meconium be removed from the airway before any attempt is made to ventilate the infant** [see V A 3 c (3)].

    **b. Choanal atresia** (see V A 2 b) is a membranous or bony obstruction of the posterior nasal passages. It is a life-threatening anomaly, and failure to recognize it may result in respiratory arrest.

c. **Progressive respiratory distress or cyanosis** that occurs in an infant despite appropriate resuscitation usually suggests an underlying disorder of the cardiopulmonary system, which requires immediate investigation and intervention. Such disorders include:
   (1) Cyanotic heart disease (i.e., pulmonary stenosis, transposition of the great vessels)
   (2) Congenital or acquired disorders of lung formation or function [i.e., diaphragmatic hernia (see V A 2 d), pneumothorax (see V A 3 b)]
   (3) Sepsis (see V F 2)

# IV. CARE OF THE NEWBORN. In this section, some specific aspects of newborn physiology, pathophysiology, and therapy are reviewed.

A. **Fluid and electrolyte requirements** (see also Ch 13 VII A). Water represents 94% of the fetal weight at 3 months gestation. At term, water content has declined to 80% of the birth weight of the newborn.

1. **Fluid loss and replacement**
   a. **Fluid loss**
      (1) During the first week of life, the extracellular fluid space contracts, resulting in a large reduction in body water. This water loss is responsible for the 5% weight loss observed in term infants. The preterm infant may lose up to 10%–15% of his birth weight.
      (2) Water loss through evaporation from the skin and from expired air is referred to as **insensible water loss**. Water loss through the urine and stool is referred to as **sensible water loss**. Stool accounts for a very small amount of sensible water loss.
   b. **Fluid replacement** is based on fluid loss and is calculated as the sum of insensible and sensible water losses. Initial parenteral fluid replacement should be accomplished with a 10% dextrose solution.
      (1) Insensible water loss varies with gestational age and factors related to the nursing environment, such as the heat source, humidity, and use of phototherapy (for treatment of hyperbilirubinemia).
      (2) In addition to water lost in the urine, other sensible losses such as gastric secretions (i.e., vomitus) should be included in the calculation of total water loss.
   c. **Fluid balance** is monitored by examining:
      (1) Urine output
      (2) Change in body weight
      (3) Serum sodium concentration
      (4) Urine specific gravity

2. **Electrolyte loss and replacement**
   a. **Sodium, potassium, and chloride** are the principal salts that are lost through the urine and should be replaced accordingly. Assuming an adequate urine output, replacement is begun 24 hours after birth at the following rates:
      (1) **Sodium:** 1–3 mEq/kg/day
      (2) **Potassium:** 1–2 mEq/kg/day
      (3) **Chloride:** 1–3 mEq/kg/day
   b. **Calcium.** A decrease in serum calcium concentration frequently occurs during the first week of life. Serum calcium concentrations below 7 mg/dl (total) or below 3–3.5 mg/dl (ionized) are considered **hypocalcemic**.
      (1) **Early neonatal (physiologic) hypocalcemia.** Nearly all infants experience a small decline in total serum calcium during the first few days of life due to intrauterine parathyroid hormone (PTH) suppression. Early neonatal hypocalcemia rarely requires treatment except in preterm infants, infants of diabetic mothers, and asphyxiated infants.
      (2) **Late neonatal (nonphysiologic) hypocalcemia** is seen at the end of the first week of life. Etiologies include:
         (a) Increased phosphate ingestion, as occurs in infants who are fed cow's milk or high-phosphate rice cereal
         (b) Hypomagnesemia
         (c) Hypoparathyroidism
      (3) **Therapy** generally consists of calcium replacement with calcium gluconate and treatment of any underlying cause of the hypocalcemia.

    **c. Other required minerals** include:
      **(1)** Phosphorus
      **(2)** Magnesium
      **(3)** Iron
      **(4)** Trace metals

**B. Nutritional requirements.** Adequate caloric intake with the correct balance of carbohydrate, protein, and fat is needed for homeostasis and growth. The specific nutritional requirements of the newborn are reviewed here, after a brief overview of prenatal gastrointestinal system development and fetal and neonatal growth.

  **1. Prenatal development of the gastrointestinal tract**
    **a. Anatomic development** proceeds in a series of orderly steps. By 4 weeks gestation, the primitive foregut is identified; by 6 weeks, foregut, midgut, and hindgut divisions are present. Malformations of the gastrointestinal tract occur due to failure in division or normal rotation or to vascular accidents.
      **(1) Esophagus**
        **(a) Normal development.** The esophagus begins as a common tubular structure that invaginates to form the esophagus, the pharynx, and the respiratory tree.
        **(b) Developmental anomalies** include **esophageal atresia** and **tracheoesophageal fistula,** which result from failure in division. (The latter disorder rarely occurs in the absence of the former; see also V A 2 a.)
      **(2) Stomach**
        **(a) Normal development.** The stomach is formed by dilation of the caudal end of the foregut. Development is complete by 5 weeks gestation.
        **(b) Developmental anomalies** of the stomach are rare.
      **(3) Intestines**
        **(a) Normal development.** The **duodenum** is formed as the terminal foregut and proximal midgut grow and form a loop. The remainder of the midgut forms the **jejunum** and **ileum**. Between 5 and 10 weeks gestation, the growing midgut is forced out of the abdominal cavity and into the umbilical cord. The **mesentery** grows within the loop. By the end of this period, the intestines reenter the abdominal cavity, proceeding cranially to caudally and making a 270° rotation.
        **(b) Developmental anomalies**
          **(i) Small bowel atresia** is thought to result from a vascular accident, probably during rotation and reentry of the bowel into the abdominal cavity.
          **(ii) Malrotation** results from failure of normal rotation and fixation, which predisposes to the development of a **volvulus** (i.e., twisting of the bowel about the superior mesenteric artery with resulting obstruction).
          **(iii) Omphalocele** is a herniation of intra-abdominal viscera into the umbilical cord. A membranous sac containing bowel, liver, or both arises from failure of reentry of the bowel from the yolk sac. The sac has a common insertion with the umbilical cord into the abdominal wall.
          **(iv) Gastroschisis** results from a defect in the closure of the abdominal wall, through which a variable portion of intestine protrudes.
      **(4) Colon**
        **(a) Normal development.** The colon develops from the hindgut and cloaca, which divides into the urogenital sinus and rectum by 6 weeks gestation.
        **(b) Developmental anomalies** include:
          **(i) Imperforate anus,** which results from failure of the cloacal membrane to rupture
          **(ii) Hirschsprung's disease** (congenital megacolon), which is failure of the normal innervation of the distal colon (see Ch 10 VIII E)
    **b. Biochemical development**
      **(1) Gastric functional development** begins during the second trimester. Gastric acid activity does not begin until after 32 weeks gestation and increases rapidly in the first 24 hours of life.
      **(2) Small intestine functional development** also extends into postnatal life.
        **(a) Disaccharidase activity.** Sucrase, maltase, and isomaltase activity begins by 12 weeks gestation and is at 70% by 34 weeks. Lactase activity remains low until term.

**(b) Disaccharidase deficiency.** The most common congenital enzyme deficiency is a combined deficiency of sucrase and isomaltase. Congenital lactase deficiency is much less common, but a transient lactase deficiency frequently follows an episode of infectious gastroenteritis.

**2. Fetal and neonatal growth**

**a. Fetal growth.** The fetal growth rate is 5 g/day at 14–15 weeks gestation, 10 g/day at 20 weeks, and 30 g/day at 32–34 weeks. The growth rate slows after 36 weeks gestation.

**(1)** During the first trimester, growth parameters (i.e., weight, length, head circumference) are fairly uniform in all fetuses.

**(2)** Variability in fetal growth during the last trimester is due to several factors, including genetic endowment, fetal nutrition, and multiple gestation (fetal growth rate declines at 31 weeks gestation in twins and at 29 weeks gestation in triplets).

**(3)** Abnormalities of fetal growth and their etiologies are discussed in I C 1.

**b. Neonatal growth**

**(1)** After birth, there is a loss of weight due to a loss of extracellular water and suboptimal caloric intake. Term infants lose 5% of their birth weight; preterm infants lose up to 15% of their birth weight.

**(2)** Term infants regain their birth weight by the end of the first week of life and, thereafter, gain 20–30 g/day.

**3. Nutritional considerations.** The composition of the nutritional solution and the route of delivery depend on the gestational age, general medical condition, and possible special nutritional needs of the newborn.

**a. Enteric nutrition**

**(1) Route of feeding**

**(a)** The **term infant** can be bottle-fed or breast-fed on demand, as long as attention is paid to intake and fluid balance.

**(b)** The otherwise healthy **preterm infant who is between 34 and 38 weeks gestational age** should be fed every 3 hours by bottle, breast, or gavage, depending on the infant's strength and alertness.

**(c)** The **preterm infant who is less than 34 weeks gestational age** does not have a well-coordinated suck and swallow reflex and, therefore, should be fed via a feeding tube. The feedings may be gastric bolus every 2–3 hours, except in infants weighing less than 1000 g.

**(d)** Continuous gastric or transpyloric feeding is employed in the **infant who weighs less than 1000 g,** as this infant has a limited gastric volume and may experience intermittent hypoglycemia and hypoxia when given bolus feedings.

**(e)** The **infant who requires an endotracheal tube and mechanical ventilation** should be fed continuously via a transpyloric tube to prevent gastric reflux and aspiration.

**(2) Feeding solution.** The composition of the feeding solution depends on the presence or absence of special protein, carbohydrate, or fat requirements or intolerances, which, in turn, depends on gestational age, gastrointestinal motility status, and the possibility of intestinal enzyme deficiencies or other metabolic disorders [e.g., phenyiketonuria (PKU)].

**(a) Term infants who do not have complicating metabolic problems.** All of the water, calorie, protein, and vitamin requirements of the normal term infant are met by human milk or 20 kcal/oz cow's milk–based formula. The specific nutritional needs of these infants for normal growth are as follows.

**(i)** The normal term infant needs 100–120 kcal/kg/day to meet basal and growth requirements.

**(ii)** The infant also needs 2–3 g/kg/day of protein for cellular growth, which represents approximately 10% of the total daily calorie intake.

**(iii)** In addition, 40% of the daily calorie requirements should be derived from carbohydrates, with the remainder provided by dietary fats.

**(b) Preterm infants** have decreased gastric motility and intestinal lactase activity as well as increased calcium and phosphorus requirements, among other nutritional problems. The initial feeding solution should be a dilute, whey-based formula or human milk. As positive nitrogen balance is achieved, the infant may be advanced to a formula that is high in calcium, phosphorus, and protein or to supplemented human milk. A 24 kcal/oz formula is reserved for infants whose water intake must be restricted and infants who cannot tolerate adequate feeding volumes.

(c) **Infants with special metabolic needs.** Special formula solutions are available for infants with selected intestinal enzyme deficiencies (e.g., sucrase-isomaltase deficiency) or metabolic diseases (e.g., PKU).

(3) **Vitamins and minerals.** Commercially available formulas now are fortified with vitamins, minerals, and trace elements. Therefore, formula-fed term infants do not routinely require vitamin or mineral supplementation.

(a) **Special vitamin needs**

(i) Infants who are fed human milk should receive a multiple vitamin supplement containing vitamins A, D, and C.

(ii) Due to small body stores and inadequate feeding volumes, preterm infants should routinely receive a multiple vitamin supplement containing the fat-soluble vitamins (A and D) and the water-soluble vitamins (B and C). In addition, the preterm infant who is less than 36 weeks gestational age should receive vitamin E to prevent hemolytic anemia.

(b) **Special mineral and trace element needs**

(i) **Iron.** All infants require iron supplementation, which may be obtained via iron-fortified formula or via a separate supplement. Iron supplementation may be delayed in the preterm infant until enteric feedings are tolerated. Due to the increased bioavailability of iron in human milk, iron supplementation in term breast-fed infants may await the introduction of iron-fortified cereal at 4–6 months of age.

(ii) **Fluoride** supplements should be given to infants living in areas where the water is not fluoridated and to infants who are fed human milk.

(iii) **Calcium and phosphorus.** The needs of the growing term infant are met by either commercial formula or human milk. Due to rapid bone growth, the calcium and phosphorus requirements of the preterm infant are greater and necessitate special fortified formulas or supplementation if fed human milk.

b. **Total parenteral nutrition.** Preterm and other sick infants may require total parenteral nutrition due to gastrointestinal disorders (e.g., neonatal necrotizing enterocolitis) as well as nongastrointestinal disorders (e.g., respiratory disease, sepsis). An intravenous solution of dextrose, amino acids, fat, vitamins, and minerals can be administered by either peripheral or central venous access. Appropriately used, total parenteral nutrition can provide adequate calories and protein to support the basal needs and growth of the sick infant.

C. **Principles of drug therapy.** The administration and dosing of drugs are different in neonates. Disregarding this fact may result in toxicity or nontherapeutic usage of drugs. After administration of a drug, the effect and disposition will depend on a number of the factors discussed below. A neonatology or pharmacology text should always be consulted regarding dosages of drugs for preterm and term infants.

1. **Route of administration** determines the peak drug level, how quickly the peak level is reached, and how long the peak drug level is sustained.

2. **Solubility and pH** determine the compatibility of drugs, tissue penetration, and excretion rate.

3. **Protein binding.** The plasma total protein and albumin levels of the newborn are lower than the adult levels.

a. When similar total drug concentrations are considered, in the newborn there will be a larger unbound drug fraction for drugs with strong protein binding compared to the adult. Since the unbound fraction is the active fraction in the blood, lower total drug concentrations are needed to achieve a therapeutic effect in newborns.

b. Drug competition for albumin-binding sites in the infant with hyperbilirubinemia (see V C) also poses a problem. If all the albumin binding sites are occupied with bilirubin, there will be a larger free fraction of drug in the blood. Conversely, if the drug displaces bilirubin or is already occupying the binding site, the increase in free bilirubin may increase the risk of kernicterus.

4. **Metabolism of drugs by the liver** often is suboptimal due to low levels of glucuronyl transferase. This often results in an increase in plasma drug levels and excretion of unchanged drug compared to the adult.

5. **Excretion of drugs by the kidney** often is impaired due to low renal blood flow, low glomerular filtration rate, and immature tubular function.

**V. SPECIAL MANAGEMENT PROBLEMS IN THE NEWBORN.** Many of the disorders mentioned in this section are covered more extensively in other chapters of this book. However, their clinical presentation and management warrant special consideration in the newborn.

**A. Disorders of the respiratory system.** The newborn may present with a variety of respiratory disturbances, which may be developmental in origin or may occur at birth or soon after. Specific respiratory disorders of the newborn are reviewed here, after a brief overview of prenatal respiratory system development.

    **1. Prenatal development of the respiratory system**

        **a. Anatomic development** begins at 3 weeks gestation, with the division of the foregut into the esophagus and trachea. Major bronchial branching occurs by 4 weeks gestation.

            **(1)** The **pseudoglandular stage of lung development** (5–16 weeks) is characterized by further branching of the conducting airways, the development of tracheal cartilage, and the appearance of bronchial arteries. At 10 weeks, goblet cells appear within the bronchioles. By 15 weeks, capillaries have developed and undifferentiated cuboidal cells have appeared.

            **(2)** The **canalicular stage of lung development** (16–25 weeks) is characterized by formation of terminal alveolar sacs, capillary approximation with the alveolar sacs, and differentiation of types I and II alveolar cells.

            **(3)** The **alveolar,** or **terminal sac, stage** (26–40 weeks) is characterized by a progressive increase in the number of alveolar sacs, which creates a greater surface for gas exchange. Surfactant also appears during this stage of development.

        **b. Biochemical development.** The most important prenatal event is the production of **surfactant** by type II alveolar cells.

            **(1) Function and composition of surfactant**

                **(a)** The major function of surfactant is to decrease alveolar surface tension and increase lung compliance. Surfactant prevents alveolar collapse at the end of expiration and allows for opening of the alveoli at a low intrathoracic pressure.

                **(b)** The group of phospholipids comprising surfactant also is referred to as lecithin. The ratio of **lecithin (L)** to **sphingomyelin (S)** in the amniotic fluid is a reflection of the amount of intrapulmonary surfactant and lung maturity. An **L/S ratio** of 2:1 or greater usually indicates biochemical lung maturity.

                **(c)** The most abundant component of surfactant is **phosphatidylcholine**. Less abundant but essential for optimal reduction in surface tension is **phosphatidylglycerol**.

            **(2) Pathways for surfactant production.** There are two major pathways.

                **(a)** The **methylation pathway** is functional by 22–24 weeks gestation but is easily inhibited by acidosis and hypoxia.

                **(b)** The **choline incorporation pathway** matures at 35 weeks gestation and is resistant to hypoxia and acidosis.

             **(3) Rate of surfactant production**

                **(a)** The production of surfactant is accelerated by several factors, including:

                    **(i)** Maternal steroid administration in the presence of a female fetus

                    **(ii)** Prolonged rupture of the fetal membranes

                      **(iii)** Maternal narcotic addiction

                      **(iv)** Preeclampsia

                      **(v)** Chronic fetal stress (i.e., placental insufficiency)

                      **(vi)** Thyroid hormone [i.e., long-acting thyroid stimulator (LATS)-associated maternal hyperthyroidism or hypothyroidism with secondary fetal hyperthyroidism]

                    **(vii)** Theophylline

                  **(b)** The production of surfactant is delayed by combined fetal hyperglycemia and hyperinsulinemia, as occurs in maternal diabetes.

    **2. Developmental disorders**

        **a. Esophageal atresia with tracheoesophageal fistula** (see also Ch 10 II C 1 and Ch 12 VII C). Esophageal atresia is a lack of continuity of the esophagus. Although it may occur alone, it most often is accompanied by a fistula between the trachea and the distal esophagus (tracheoesophageal fistula). These developmental disorders are the result of defective differentiation.

(1) **Clinical features.** These infants have difficulty with copious oral and pharyngeal secretions. If the secretions obstruct the airway or if aspiration occurs, respiratory distress can result.

(2) **Diagnosis** is suggested by failure to pass a nasogastric tube into the stomach and is confirmed by a chest x-ray that reveals the tube coiled up in the blind pouch of the esophagus.

(3) **Therapy.** Emergency management involves constant suction of the esophagus, 30° elevation of the head to prevent reflux of gastric contents into the lungs, and preparation for definitive therapy (i.e., surgical repair).

b. **Choanal atresia** is a unilateral or bilateral obstruction of the posterior nasal airway by a membranous or bony septum. This anomaly results from failure of the bucconasal mucosa to rupture.

(1) **Clinical features.** Due to the fact that most newborns are obligate nose breathers, bilateral atresia usually presents in the delivery room as airway obstruction, apnea, and cyanosis. Unilateral obstruction may be asymptomatic.

(2) **Diagnosis** is confirmed either by inability to pass a suction catheter through the nostrils into the oropharynx or by x-ray using radiopaque dye to show the area of nasal obstruction.

(3) **Therapy.** Emergency management consists of establishing an airway either with an oral airway or by endotracheal intubation. Definitive therapy is surgical reconstruction, performed in the neonatal period.

c. **Pulmonary hypoplasia** histologically is seen as a decrease in the number of alveoli and capillary beds. The level of bronchial branching that is affected depends on the time during gestation when the insult occurs.

(1) **Etiology.** Major causes of pulmonary hypoplasia include:
  (a) Diminution of amniotic fluid volume due to:
    (i) Rupture of the fetal membranes
    (ii) Lack of fetal urine secondary to nonfunctioning (e.g., dysplastic, polycystic) kidneys or to urinary tract obstruction
  (b) Intrathoracic space-occupying lesion, such as:
    (i) Diaphragmatic hernia
    (ii) Pulmonary tumor

(2) **Clinical features.** The clinical presentation is one of severe respiratory distress and cyanosis.
  (a) The chest x-ray may show a small thoracic cavity and small lungs. Pneumothorax, pleural effusion, or both are frequently seen bilaterally.
  (b) When oligohydramnios is present, the characteristic facies of **Potter syndrome** are present.
  (c) On palpation, kidneys may be normal, absent, or large, if there is a renal etiology.

(3) **Diagnosis.** With severe hypoplasia, chest x-ray is helpful for establishing the diagnosis.

(4) **Therapy** consists of vigorous ventilatory support and treatment of coexistent persistent pulmonary hypertension. Almost all infants with associated renal anomalies die shortly after birth, and treatment should be tailored accordingly.

d. **Diaphragmatic hernia** is a displacement of abdominal contents into the thoracic cavity through a defect in the diaphragm.

(1) **Types**
  (a) **Hernias through the foramen of Bochdalek** are by far the most commonly seen diaphragmatic hernias. The defect, which almost always is on the left, occurs in the posterolateral portion of the diaphragm. It results from failure of the pleuroperitoneal canal to close, which normally occurs between 6 and 8 weeks gestation. This is the most urgent of all neonatal thoracoabdominal emergencies.
  (b) **Hernias through the foramen of Morgagni** are somewhat rare. The hernia, which usually is on the right, occurs in the anterior portion of the diaphragm through defects that are secondary to a developmental failure of the retrosternal segment of the septum transversum. Frequently, the hernia contains only omentum, and the affected newborn is asymptomatic.

(2) **Pathophysiology.** Ipsilateral pulmonary hypoplasia results from compression of the affected lung by the displaced gastrointestinal organs. A shift of the mediastinal structures, resulting in compression of the contralateral lung, may cause hypoplasia of that lung to a lesser degree.

**(3) Clinical features.** Severe respiratory distress, with cyanosis and dyspnea, usually is apparent shortly after birth. Breath sounds are diminished on the affected side, and heart sounds are shifted to the right. The abdomen may be scaphoid in cases of extensive displacement.

**(4) Diagnosis** is confirmed by a chest x-ray demonstrating air-filled bowel in the left hemithorax.

**(5) Therapy** includes intubation, vigorous oxygenation and mechanical ventilation, decompression of the intestinal tract with a nasogastric tube, correction of metabolic acidosis, and surgical removal of the abdominal contents from the thorax with repair of the hernia.

    **(a)** Mask and bag ventilation should be avoided or minimized, as it results in distension of the bowel and further compromises the pulmonary function of the affected newborn.

    **(b)** Pulmonary hypertension frequently complicates the pre- and postoperative course.

    **(c)** Extracorporeal membrane oxygenation may be helpful in selected infants.

**(6) Prognosis.** Survival rates depend on the degree of lung hypoplasia and the presence of other anomalies. With conventional therapy, survival rates are approximately 50%; however, the use of extracorporeal membrane oxygenation may improve survival.

**e. Congenital lobar emphysema** is due to developmental abnormalities in either the conducting airways or the alveoli that result in the trapping of air in the affected lobe of the lung.

**(1) Clinical features.** Infants generally present at birth or soon after with mild to severe respiratory distress, including tachypnea and cyanosis.

**(2) Diagnosis** is established by chest x-ray, which initially reveals a dense, opaque, overinflated area of lung. Later, with further air trapping, the area may display hyperlucency.

**(3) Therapy** varies with the particular clinical presentation. The asymptomatic infant needs little immediate treatment. The severely affected infant may be helped by bronchoscopy but, in most cases, eventually requires removal of the involved lobe.

**f. Hyaline membrane disease (respiratory distress syndrome of the newborn)** is a respiratory disorder that primarily affects preterm infants who are born prior to the biochemical maturation of their lungs.

**(1) Pathophysiology.** The lungs are poorly compliant due to a deficiency of surfactant, resulting in the classic complex of progressive atelectasis, intrapulmonary shunting, hypoxemia, and cyanosis. The hyaline membrane that forms and lines the alveoli is composed of protein and sloughed epithelium—the result of oxygen exposure, alveolar capillary leakage, and the forces generated by the mechanical ventilation of these infants.

**(2) Clinical features.** Affected infants characteristically present with tachypnea, grunting, nasal flaring, chest retraction, and cyanosis in the first 3 hours of life. There is decreased air entry on auscultation.

**(3) Clinical course.** The natural course is a progressive worsening over the first 48–72 hours of life.

    **(a)** After the initial insult to the airway lining, the epithelium is repopulated with type II alveolar cells.

    **(b)** Subsequently, there is increased production and release of surfactant, so that there are sufficient quantities in the air spaces by 72 hours of life. This results in improvement in lung compliance and resolution of the respiratory distress.

**(4) Diagnosis** is confirmed by a chest x-ray that reveals a uniform ground-glass pattern and an air bronchogram that is consistent with diffuse atelectasis.

**(5) Therapy and prognosis**

    **(a)** Conventional therapy for the affected premature infant includes supportive care as well as the administration of oxygen. It also may be necessary to increase the mean airway pressure by use of continuous positive airway pressure or intermittent assisted ventilation. Outcome with conventional therapy is good.

    **(b)** Therapy with artificial or bovine surfactant has been shown to improve this condition dramatically in clinical trials and is likely to be the primary mode of therapy in the future.

**(6) Prevention.** When amniotic fluid assessment reveals fetal lung immaturity and preterm delivery cannot be prevented, administration of corticosteroids to the mother 48 hours before delivery can induce or accelerate the production of fetal lung surfactant.

**(7) Complications** associated with hyaline membrane disease are a result of organ immaturity, associated with asphyxia, and mechanical ventilation. Common complications and associated findings include pneumothorax, patent ductus arteriosus, intraventricular hemorrhage, necrotizing enterocolitis, bronchopulmonary dysplasia, and retinopathy of prematurity (retrolental fibroplasia).

**g. Transient tachypnea of the newborn** is thought to result from decreased lymphatic absorption of fetal lung fluid. It most commonly occurs in infants born near term by cesarean section, without preceding labor. (The catecholamine surge associated with labor and delivery, which is thought to enhance pulmonary lymphatic drainage, does not occur in this setting.)

**(1) Clinical features.** The tachypnea is quiet or mild and usually not associated with retractions. The infant appears comfortable and rarely is cyanotic.

**(2) Diagnosis** is based on the delivery history and a chest x-ray, which characteristically reveals fluid in the major fissure, prominent vascular markings, increased interstitial markings, and hyperinflation. Auscultation may reveal rales.

**(3) Therapy** is supportive. The tachypnea resolves in a few days. Low concentrations of supplemental oxygen may be required.

**h. Persistence of the fetal circulation,** or **persistent pulmonary hypertension of the newborn,** generally is a disease of term infants who have experienced acute or chronic in utero hypoxia. It is seen frequently in infants with meconium aspiration syndrome (see V A 3 c).

**(1) Pathophysiology.** The primary abnormality is a failure of the pulmonary vascular resistance to fall with postnatal lung expansion and oxygenation.

**(a)** Normally, at birth, the systemic vascular resistance rises as a result of cessation of blood flow through the placenta, and pulmonary vascular resistance falls with the first breaths.

**(b)** With persistence of the fetal circulation, the pulmonary vascular resistance continues to be high and may, in fact, be higher than the systemic resistance. This results in shunting of the deoxygenated blood, which is returning to the right side of the heart, away from the lungs. The right-to-left shunt can occur at both the atrial level (foramen ovale) and through the ductus arteriosus. Since the lungs are bypassed, the blood is not oxygenated and hypoxemia ensues.

**(2) Clinical features.** These infants have rapidly progressive cyanosis associated with mild to severe respiratory distress. There is a varied response to oxygen administration, depending on the size of the shunt.

**(3) Diagnosis**

**(a)** The diagnosis is suggested by a history of perinatal hypoxia and clinical cyanosis at birth combined with a normal cardiovascular examination and normal chest x-ray, although parenchymal disease may coexist (e.g., group B streptococcal pneumonia, hyaline membrane disease, meconium aspiration syndrome).

**(b)** Echocardiography should be used to establish the diagnosis and should demonstrate:

**(i)** The absence of cyanotic heart disease

**(ii)** An increased pulmonary vascular resistance

**(iii)** The presence of right-to-left shunt at the foramen ovale, ductus arteriosus, or both

**(4) Therapy** includes supplemental oxygen, mechanical ventilation, hyperventilation, support of systemic blood pressure, and administration of sodium bicarbonate and pulmonary vasodilators.

**(5) Prognosis.** The overall mortality rate associated with this disease is high. Extracorporeal membrane oxygenation may improve the outcome in certain patients.

**3. Acquired disorders**

**a. Pneumonia**

**(1) Etiology.** Pneumonia often is associated with chorioamnionitis and may be caused by aspiration of infected amniotic fluid. The infectious agent also may cross the placenta, enter the fetal circulation, and spread to the lungs. Sepsis often is present (see V F 2).

**(2) Clinical features.** The infant presents with signs of respiratory distress, including tachypnea, cyanosis, and retractions. Auscultation may reveal rales, rhonchi, or diminished breath sounds. Other signs of systemic infection may be noted, including poor perfusion, hypotension, acidosis, and leukopenia or leukocytosis.

**(3) Diagnosis** is confirmed by a chest x-ray that reveals any one of a variety of patterns, including diffuse or patchy infiltrates or consolidation. The process may be unilobar or multilobar. A tracheal aspirate also may reveal bacteria and an increased number of neutrophils.

**(4) Therapy and prognosis.** Treatment includes administration of appropriate antibiotics (see V F 2 f), supplemental oxygen, and mechanical ventilation (if needed). The outcome usually is good.

**b. Pneumothorax** is the presence of free air in the pleural space. The air often is under tension (i.e., at greater than atmospheric pressure) and in this setting is referred to as **tension pneumothorax**.

**(1) Incidence and etiology.** Asymptomatic, spontaneous pneumothorax occurs in 1%–2% of otherwise healthy newborns at birth. Symptomatic pneumothorax more commonly occurs in the infant who is receiving mechanical ventilation or who has underlying lung disease (e.g., hyaline membrane disease, pulmonary interstitial emphysema, meconium aspiration pneumonia).

**(2) Clinical features.** Symptoms and signs include cyanosis, tachypnea, and elevation of the affected hemithorax. Auscultation reveals diminished breath sounds on the affected side.

**(3) Diagnosis**

  **(a)** The diagnosis is made by a chest x-ray that demonstrates a dense, partially collapsed lung surrounded by a large area of radiolucent air within the hemithorax. Depending on the degree of tension and lung compliance, the mediastinal structures are shifted toward the opposite side of the chest.

  **(b)** Transillumination of the thorax may aid in the diagnosis of pneumothorax in emergencies; positive evidence is the transmission of light through the affected side.

**(4) Therapy** varies with the severity of the symptoms.

  **(a)** If no other lung disease exists and there is minimal respiratory distress, supplemental 100% oxygen (nitrogen washout technique) for several hours usually is sufficient.

  **(b)** If a significant degree of tension, respiratory distress, or some other lung disease exists, the air should be evacuated by aspiration with a syringe and needle or by a chest tube. Constant suction should be applied to the chest tube if a continuous air leak exists.

**c. Meconium aspiration syndrome** is a multiorgan disorder with perinatal asphyxia as the underlying cause. It most commonly occurs in post-term infants and infants who are small for gestational age due to intrauterine growth retardation. Both have placental insufficiency as a common pathway for fetal hypoxia.

**(1) Pathophysiology.** The fetal hypoxia triggers, via a vagal reflex, the passage of thick meconium into the amniotic fluid. The contaminated amniotic fluid is swallowed into the oropharynx and aspirated at birth with the initiation of breathing. With severe fetal asphyxia and acidosis, the meconium may be aspirated prenatally due to fetal gasping. Other organs affected by the perinatal hypoxia include the brain, heart, gastrointestinal tract, and kidneys.

**(2) Diagnosis** is established by the presence of meconium in the tracheal or amniotic fluid combined with symptoms of respiratory stress and a chest x-ray that reveals a pattern of diffuse infiltrates with hyperinflation.

**(3) Therapy.** Since most episodes of aspiration occur with the initiation of respiration, the most effective therapy is prevention. This consists of removal of the meconium prior to the initiation of ventilation. The meconium is removed from the infant's airway as follows.

  **(a)** The oropharynx is suctioned prior to both delivery of the thorax and initiation of breathing and again when the infant is on the warmer bed.

  **(b)** The vocal cords are visualized using a laryngoscope, and a large endotracheal tube or De Lee catheter is inserted.

  **(c)** Direct wall-unit suction (at a pressure of 80 mm of $H_2O$) is applied to the tube or catheter as it is removed. The procedure is repeated if significant meconium is recovered. **Only after the trachea is cleared of any meconium should spontaneous or artificial ventilation be initiated.**

  **(d)** If aspiration has occurred and the infant is in distress, therapy consists of administration of oxygen and mechanical ventilation.

        **(e)** Persistent pulmonary hypertension also may coexist and should be vigorously treated.

   **d. Bronchopulmonary dysplasia** (see Ch 12 V) is a chronic pulmonary disease of infants that can result from oxygen and mechanical ventilation therapy for hyaline membrane disease in a preterm infant. It is characterized by the need for oxygen therapy beyond 28 days of life. A characteristic series of changes is seen on x-ray.

**4. Breathing disorders**
  **a. Regulation of breathing**
    **(1) Initiation of breathing.** Although the fetus has periodic breathing movements in utero, it is not until after birth that breathing becomes regular and sustained. It is still not clear what mechanism initiates the infant's first breath.
      **(a)** With the first breath, the pulmonary stretch receptors do not cause complete exhalation, and, instead, a second inhalation follows. This is called **Head's paradoxical reflex**. It never occurs again throughout life.
      **(b)** Prior to birth, the alveoli are only minimally distended with lung fluid, and surface tension is high. The first few breaths must create a large negative intrathoracic pressure to open and distend the alveoli.
      **(c)** The first few breaths also allow dispersion of surfactant, which prevents alveolar collapse at the end of expiration by lowering the surface tension. Therefore, minimal negative pressure must be created by subsequent breaths to reexpand the alveoli.
    **(2) Maintenance of breathing.** Normal function of the respiratory center in the brain results in rhythmic inhalation and exhalation. The respiratory rate and depth of each breath are modulated by the Hering-Breuer reflex, carotid bodies, diaphragmatic strength, and cerebrospinal fluid (CSF) pH.
  **b. Apnea** (see also Ch 12 VI) is the cessation of breathing for longer than 20 seconds. Apnea often occurs in preterm infants (**apnea of prematurity**) and reflects immaturity of the respiratory control mechanisms in the brain stem.
    **(1) Clinical features.** Bradycardia (i.e., heart rate < 80 beats/min) often is associated with apnea. Apnea of prematurity is characterized by periodic breathing and intermittent hypoxia, which further diminish respiratory drive.
    **(2) Diagnosis** of apnea of prematurity is made after excluding other reasons for the apnea, including:
      **(a)** Infection
      **(b)** Intracranial hemorrhage
      **(c)** Airway obstruction
      **(d)** Gastroesophageal reflux
      **(e)** Seizures
      **(f)** Hypoxia
      **(g)** Pulmonary edema
      **(h)** Metabolic disturbances (e.g., hypoglycemia, hypocalcemia, hyponatremia)
      **(i)** Inappropriate environmental temperature (hot or cold)
    **(3) Therapy**
      **(a) Apnea of prematurity.** Treatment measures include tactile stimulation, maintenance of the neutral thermal zone and core body temperature, supplemental oxygen, use of an oscillating water bed, and administration of respiratory stimulants (e.g., theophylline, caffeine). It also may be necessary to increase the mean airway pressure by use of continuous positive airway pressure or intermittent assisted ventilation.
      **(b) Other causes of apnea.** Treatment of the underlying disorder usually leads to cessation of the apneic episodes.

**B. Neonatal necrotizing enterocolitis** refers to a spectrum of varying degrees of acute intestinal necrosis usually following ischemic injury of the bowel with secondary invasion and devitalization of the bowel wall.

  **1. Incidence.** This is a serious and common problem, affecting 1%–5% of all newborns admitted to intensive care units. Affected infants most commonly are premature, asphyxiated, and suffering from other medical problems. Necrotizing enterocolitis rarely is observed in healthy term infants.

2. **Etiology and pathogenesis**
   a. **Bowel ischemia** secondary to preceding perinatal asphyxia generally is regarded as the cause of bowel wall injury. The introduction of formula or human milk then provides the substrate for bacterial overgrowth. Bacterial invasion of the bowel wall, often with gas production (**pneumatosis intestinalis**), leads to tissue necrosis and perforation.
   b. **Other predisposing factors** include:
      (1) Systemic hypotension
      (2) Patent ductus arteriosus
      (3) Placement of an umbilical artery catheter
      (4) Exchange transfusion
      (5) Previous treatment with systemic antibiotics
      (6) Use of hyperosmolar formula
      (7) Rapid advancement of the feeding volume

3. **Clinical features and diagnosis**
   a. **Signs and symptoms** generally are noted during the first 2 weeks of life, shortly after enteric feeding has begun, and include:
      (1) Gastric residuum, which often is bile-stained
      (2) Abdominal distension
      (3) Blood in stool (occult or gross)
      (4) Apnea
      (5) Lethargy
      (6) Poor perfusion, with hypotension or shock
      (7) Abdominal wall discoloration
      (8) Unstable temperature
      (9) Hyperglycemia
      (10) Metabolic acidosis
   b. **Laboratory findings**
      (1) Suggestive blood findings include:
         (a) Leukocytosis, with neutropenia
         (b) Thrombocytopenia
      (2) Suggestive findings on abdominal x-ray include:
         (a) Dilated, thickened bowel loops
         (b) Pneumatosis intestinalis, which generally starts in the right lower quadrant
         (c) Perforation, with free abdominal air and portal vein air

4. **Clinical course.** Two distinct clinical patterns are noted.
   a. Most infants follow a course characterized by feeding intolerance, abdominal distension, occult blood in the stool, and dilated bowel loops on x-ray. These infants improve rapidly with therapy.
   b. The other group of infants has severe, progressive symptoms, including gross blood in the stool, extreme abdominal tenderness, hypotension, DIC, and sepsis. Pneumatosis intestinalis and perforation frequently occur in this setting.

5. **Therapy**
   a. Treatment should begin with discontinuation of enteric feeding, gastric drainage, and administration of intravenous fluids.
   b. Once cultures have been taken, systemic antibiotics (e.g, ampicillin, gentamicin) should be given. Also, any accompanying disorders (e.g., DIC) should be treated.
   c. Surgical resection of the necrotic bowel segment is indicated for infants who have had a progressive downhill course and for those in whom intestinal perforation has occurred.

6. **Prognosis.** The mortality rate associated with necrotizing enterocolitis, which is highest in the most premature infants, is approximately 30%.

C. **Neonatal hyperbilirubinemia** is a condition characterized by an excessive concentration of bilirubin in the blood. There are two types of hyperbilirubinemia: **unconjugated,** which can be physiologic or pathologic in origin, and **conjugated,** which always stems from pathologic causes. Both types may lead to **jaundice**. Neurotoxic concentrations of unconjugated bilirubin can cause **kernicterus**.

1. **Normal bilirubin metabolism** (Figure 5-2). Bilirubin is a bile pigment formed from the degradation of heme that is mainly derived from red blood cell destruction (75%) but also from ineffective red blood cell production (25%).
   a. The intermediary product of hemoglobin degradation—**biliverdin**—is converted to bilirubin via a reduction reaction.
   b. Fat-soluble bilirubin normally circulates in plasma bound to albumin, from which it is transported into hepatocytes.
   c. Conjugation with glucuronide converts bilirubin to a water-soluble product, which is excreted into the bile.

2. **Unconjugated or indirect hyperbilirubinemia** may occur due to excessive bilirubin production (hemolysis), defective bilirubin clearance from the blood, or defective bilirubin conjugation by the liver. The most common cause in the neonatal period is a physiologic delay in the ability of the liver to clear, metabolize, and excrete the relatively large bilirubin burden at birth. At extremely high levels, fat-soluble unconjugated bilirubin enters the brain and causes neuronal dysfunction and death.
   a. **Clinical manifestations**
      (1) **Jaundice** occurs in 50% of all newborns and reflects an accumulation of unconjugated bilirubin in the blood and other tissues. Jaundice can be clinically observed at blood concentrations of 5 mg/dl or greater. Unconjugated hyperbilirubinemia or jaundice may be due to physiologic or nonphysiologic causes.
         (a) **Physiologic jaundice** refers to the increased serum concentration of unconjugated bilirubin that is observed during the first few days of life.
            (i) **Causative factors** include delayed activity of glucuronyl transferase, increased bilirubin load on hepatocytes, and decreased bilirubin clearance from the plasma.
            (ii) **Clinical features.** Physiologic jaundice is associated with an umbilical cord serum bilirubin concentration of less than 2 mg/dl, a peak serum bilirubin level of less than 12–15 mg/dl on the third day of life, and a return to normal

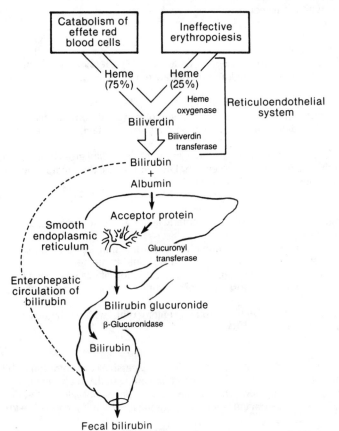

**Figure 5-2.** Bilirubin metabolism in the neonate. (Reprinted from Avery GB: *Neonatology: Pathophysiology and Management of the Newborn.* Philadelphia, JB Lippincott, 1981, p 476.)

levels by the end of the first week of life. In preterm infants, bilirubin levels usually are higher and the physiologic jaundice lasts longer. Breast-fed infants also may have higher bilirubin levels.

(b) **Nonphysiologic jaundice** refers to hyperbilirubinemia that is secondary to a pathologic process. Specific **causes** of nonphysiologic indirect hyperbilirubinemia include:

- (i) Hemolytic diseases of immune etiology (e.g., fetomaternal blood group incompatibilities) as well as nonimmune etiology (e.g., spherocytosis, hemoglobinopathy, red blood cell enzyme deficiency) [see also V D 1 a (1) and Ch 14 III D]
- (ii) Extravascular blood loss and accumulation (e.g., due to cephalhematoma)
- (iii) Increased enterohepatic circulation (e.g., due to intestinal obstruction)
- (iv) Breast-feeding associated with poor intake
- (v) Disorders of bilirubin metabolism (e.g., Lucey-Driscoll syndrome, Crigler-Najjar syndrome, Gilbert syndrome)
- (vi) Metabolic disorders (e.g., hypothyroidism, panhypopituitarism, galactosemia)
- (vii) Bacterial sepsis

(2) **Kernicterus** is a severe neurologic condition associated with very high levels of unconjugated bilirubin in the blood. Kernicterus is characterized by yellow staining of the basal ganglia and hippocampus, which is accompanied by widespread cerebral dysfunction.

(a) **Causative factors.** Kernicterus occurs when free bilirubin crosses the blood-brain barrier and enters the brain cells.

- (i) Normally, unconjugated bilirubin is bound tightly to albumin, which prevents bilirubin from crossing the blood-brain barrier. Free bilirubin exists when the **amount of unconjugated bilirubin exceeds the binding capacity of albumin**.
- (ii) **Bilirubin also may enter the brain at low concentrations** due to displacement from the albumin-binding site by another compound (e.g., sulfa drug), which leads to an increased free bilirubin concentration, or due to disruption of the blood-brain barrier by sepsis, asphyxia, acidosis, or infusion of hyperosmolar solutions.

(b) **Clinical features** of kernicterus include the following neurologic manifestations:

- (i) Lethargy or irritability
- (ii) Hypotonia
- (iii) Opisthotonus
- (iv) Seizures
- (v) Mental retardation
- (vi) Hearing loss

b. **Diagnosis**

(1) **Physiologic jaundice** should be suspected if underlying pathologic causes of the hyperbilirubinemia can be excluded. Because the most common causes of unconjugated hyperbilirubinemia are physiologic and hemolytic, the initial evaluation should include:

- (a) Complete blood count with peripheral smear and reticulocyte count
- (b) Determination of maternal and infant blood types
- (c) Coombs' test (indirect and direct)
- (d) Determination of direct and indirect concentrations of bilirubin

(2) **Nonphysiologic jaundice** should always be suspected when the umbilical cord serum bilirubin concentration is elevated, when the clinical appearance of jaundice is within the first 24 hours of life, or when the conjugated fraction of the serum bilirubin concentration exceeds 2 mg/dl.

c. **Therapy** consists of treatment of any underlying causes of hyperbilirubinemia and the prevention of kernicterus.

(1) **Treatment modalities**

(a) **Phototherapy** converts unconjugated bilirubin into several water-soluble photoisomers that can be excreted without conjugation. **Lumirubin,** a structural isomer, is the major excretory product; **4Z, 15E-bilirubin,** a geometric isomer, is a minor photoconversion product.

**(b) Exchange transfusion** is used principally in hemolytic disease or when the bilirubin concentration is very high. This procedure directly removes the bilirubin from the intravascular space. Unbound antibodies that initiate the hemolytic process also are removed.

**(2) Specific indications for the use of phototherapy and exchange transfusion** are discussed in detail in most neonatology texts. In the term infant, phototherapy may be initiated when the serum bilirubin concentration reaches 12–15 mg/dl before the third day of life. Exchange transfusion is generally performed when the serum bilirubin concentration is 20 mg/dl or greater. The specific bilirubin concentration that requires treatment varies with gestational age, the cause of the jaundice, and the presence of medical complications (e.g., sepsis, acidosis).

3. **Conjugated or direct hyperbilirubinemia**
   a. **Clinical manifestations.** Jaundice associated with conjugated hyperbilirubinemia always is pathologic in origin. Specific **causes** of direct hyperbilirubinemia include:
      **(1)** TORCH infection (see Ch 7 II B)
      **(2)** Metabolic disorders (e.g., galactosemia)
      **(3)** Bacterial sepsis
      **(4)** Obstructive jaundice (e.g., due to biliary atresia)
      **(5)** Prolonged administration of intravenous protein solutions
      **(6)** Neonatal hepatitis
   b. **Diagnosis** is based on a conjugated fraction of the serum bilirubin concentration that exceeds 2 mg/dl. Further evaluation should be directed to possible underlying causes of the direct hyperbilirubinemia.
   c. **Therapy** is directed to the underlying causes of the hyperbilirubinemia.

D. **Hematologic disorders**

1. **Anemia** (see also Ch 14 III). In the newborn, anemia is defined as a hematocrit less than 40%. Normally, the hematocrit at term gestation is 50%–55%.
   a. **Etiology.** The principal causes of anemia in the newborn can be divided into those associated with acute blood loss, those associated with chronic blood loss, and those associated with impaired red blood cell production. The most frequent cause—**hemolytic disease of the newborn**—is discussed first in somewhat more detail than the other causes.
      **(1) Hemolytic disease of the newborn** (erythroblastosis fetalis) usually is the result of blood group incompatibility between the mother and the fetus. Hemolysis occurs when maternal antibodies to a particular blood group antigen cross the placenta and bind to fetal red blood cells, which are then destroyed in the spleen.
         **(a)** The most commonly involved antigen is $Rh_0(D)$—from the Rh blood group system. Rh incompatibility is associated with **extravascular hemolysis**.
         **(b)** Less commonly involved are ABO blood group antigens.
         **(c)** Rarely, hemolytic disease of the newborn is caused by other blood group incompatibilities (e.g., c, E, Kell), a congenital defect or deficiency in red blood cell enzymes [e.g., glucose-6-phosphate dehydrogenase (G6PD)], a red blood cell membrane defect, infection, or vitamin deficiency (e.g., vitamin E).
         **(d)** In utero, if the anemia is severe (usually involving Rh incompatibility), the fetus (infant) will exhibit the signs and symptoms of **hydrops fetalis** (see V E 3).
      **(2) Anemia caused by acute blood loss** can be due to:
         **(a)** Placenta previa
         **(b)** Placental abruption
         **(c)** Fetomaternal transfusion
         **(d)** Fetoplacental transfusion
         **(e)** Cord rupture
         **(f)** Internal hemorrhage
      **(3) Anemia caused by chronic blood loss** can be due to:
         **(a)** Hemolytic disease
         **(b)** Twin-to-twin transfusion in monochorionic twin pregnancy
         **(c)** Fetomaternal transfusion
         **(d)** Chronic phlebotomy
      **(4) Anemia caused by impaired red blood cell production** can be due to a congenital disorder (i.e., Diamond-Blackfan syndrome; see Ch 14 III D 2 a).

**b. Clinical features.** The clinical differentiation of acute from chronic blood loss is based on the following physical findings.

  **(1) Acute blood loss** is associated with:
  - **(a)** Acute distress
  - **(b)** Shallow, rapid respirations
  - **(c)** Tachycardia
  - **(d)** Weak to absent pulse
  - **(e)** Hypotension
  - **(f)** Absence of hepatosplenomegaly
  - **(g)** Low blood volume

  **(2) Chronic blood loss** is associated with:
  - **(a)** Pallor disproportionate to the degree of distress
  - **(b)** Weak to normal pulse
  - **(c)** Normal blood pressure
  - **(d)** Signs of congestive heart failure
  - **(e)** Hepatosplenomegaly
  - **(f)** Normal blood volume

**c. Diagnosis.** The specific cause of the anemia is established on the basis of information collected from the following sources:

  **(1)** History
  **(2)** Complete blood count with peripheral smear and reticulocyte count
  **(3)** Evaluation of maternal and infant blood for Rh or ABO incompatibility
  **(4)** Coombs' test
  **(5)** Other tests [e.g., Kleihauer test (to identify and quantify fetal red blood cells), hemoglobin electrophoresis, G6PD evaluation]

**d. Therapy**

  **(1) Hemolytic disease of the newborn.** Therapy is indicated when the hemoglobin and hematocrit are low enough to compromise the oxygen-carrying capacity of the blood, which can cause congestive heart failure, respiratory distress, acidosis, poor perfusion, and hypotension. The blood volume usually is normal. Therefore, the anemia is corrected by performing a partial exchange transfusion with packed red blood cells.

  **(2) Acute blood loss** should be treated rapidly. Therapy includes restoration of blood volume and red blood cell mass and elimination of the cause of blood loss, if it is still present.

  **(3) Chronic blood loss.** Therapy varies depending on the clinical condition and cause of blood loss and may consist of transfusion of packed red blood cells, partial exchange transfusion with packed red blood cells, iron therapy, or no intervention.

**2. Polycythemia** occurs in 2%–5% of all newborns and is defined as a hematocrit of 65% or greater when a freely flowing blood sample is taken from a large vein. **Hyperviscosity** of the blood almost always exists in association with polycythemia.

**a. Etiology.** Polycythemia has been associated with the following conditions:

  **(1)** Fetoplacental transfusion associated with birth asphyxia or delayed cord clamping
  **(2)** Twin-to-twin transfusion
  **(3)** Chronic intrauterine hypoxia secondary to placental insufficiency (e.g., pregnancy-induced hypertension with fetal growth retardation) or increased fetal metabolism (e.g., with maternal diabetes)
  **(4)** Endocrine disorders (e.g., hyperthyroidism)
  **(5)** Genetic disorders (e.g., Down syndrome, Beckwith-Wiedemann syndrome)

**b. Pathophysiology**

  **(1)** Many of the problems associated with polycythemia were originally thought to be due to organ ischemia and hypoxia secondary to an increase in blood viscosity. It is now known that most of the blood flow reduction is due to an increased oxygen content in the arterial blood. This reciprocal relationship of decreased blood flow and increased arterial oxygen content results in a normal or increased delivery of oxygen to most organs.

  **(2)** Therefore, most of the problems associated with polycythemia are more likely the result of the perinatal events (i.e., acute or chronic hypoxia) that also are responsible for the development of the polycythemia rather than any flow disturbances attributable to the polycythemia itself.

    **c. Clinical features**
      **(1) Symptoms and signs** associated with polycythemia include:
        **(a)** Tachypnea and cyanosis
        **(b)** Jitteriness and seizures
        **(c)** Hypoglycemia
        **(d)** Renal dysfunction
        **(e)** Necrotizing enterocolitis
      **(2) Complications.** Polycythemia is associated with an abnormal long-term neurologic outcome.
    **d. Therapy** generally is supportive. Reduction of the hematocrit by partial exchange transfusion may be helpful in alleviating renal dysfunction and hypoglycemia but may increase the risk of necrotizing enterocolitis. No study has shown a beneficial effect of partial exchange transfusion on long-term neurologic outcome.

**E. Hydrops fetalis** is a condition that develops in utero, usually as a result of chronic anemia due to hemolytic disease, although many etiologies exist. Its chief features include anemia and hypoproteinemia.

    **1. Etiology.** The causes of hydrops fetalis are varied and include:
      **a.** Severe chronic anemia due to:
        **(1)** Isoimmunization ( i.e., Rh incompatibility)
        **(2)** Homozygous α thalassemia
        **(3)** Twin-to-twin or fetomaternal transfusion
      **b.** Cardiac disease, such as:
        **(1)** Structural defects
        **(2)** In utero closure of the foramen ovale
        **(3)** Paroxysmal atrial tachycardia
      **c.** Hypoproteinemia
      **d.** Intrauterine infection, including:
        **(1)** Syphilis
        **(2)** Toxoplasmosis
        **(3)** Cytomegalovirus infection
      **e.** Chromosomal disorders (e.g., Turner syndrome, 45 XO)
      **f.** Idiopathic causes

    **2. Pathophysiology.** The exact pathophysiology is unknown, but the central factor in the development of hydrops fetalis appears to be severe chronic anemia with loss of oxygen-carrying capacity, leading to hypoxia and acidosis. A contributing factor is hypoproteinemia, which together with anemia causes the development of congestive heart failure, edema, pleural effusions, and ascites. All of these problems contribute to the respiratory distress seen at birth.

    **3. Clinical features**
      **a. Signs and symptoms** include:
        **(1)** Congestive heart failure
        **(2)** Pallor
        **(3)** Ascites
        **(4)** Pleural effusions
        **(5)** Peripheral edema
        **(6)** Hepatosplenomegaly
      **b. Laboratory findings** include:
        **(1)** Anemia
        **(2)** Hypoproteinemia
        **(3)** Hypoxia
        **(4)** Acidosis

    **4. Diagnosis** is based on the maternal medical and obstetric history (e.g., Rh sensitization of the mother) and the clinical and laboratory findings.

    **5. Therapy** is aimed at correcting the anemia and treating the congestive heart failure and respiratory distress. In addition, appropriate treatment should be provided for associated etiologies and conditions (e.g., infections).

    **6. Clinical course and prognosis** vary depending on the etiology, how severely affected the infant is at birth, the presence of perinatal asphyxia or congenital anomalies, and the response to therapy. Idiopathic causes of hydrops fetalis are associated with a high mortality rate.

**F. Infection** continues to be a major cause of neonatal morbidity and mortality despite advances in therapy. Although perinatally acquired bacterial infections are the most common, infections that are acquired in utero remain an important source of long-term disability.

1. **General considerations**
   a. **Predisposing factors.** The newborn is particularly susceptible to infection due to immaturity of immune system mechanisms, including:
      (1) Neutrophil chemotaxis
      (2) Neutrophil phagocytosis
      (3) Bactericidal activity
      (4) Humoral components
   b. **Timing and route of infection.** The causative organism and abnormalities associated with neonatal infections vary with the time and route of infection.
      (1) **Transplacental infections prior to birth**
         (a) **Common causative organisms** include:
            (i) Cytomegalovirus
            (ii) *Treponema pallidum* (the agent of syphilis)
            (iii) HIV, the agent of acquired immune deficiency syndrome (AIDS)
            (iv) Rubella virus
            (v) *Toxoplasma gondii*
            (vi) Echovirus
            (vii) *Listeria monocytogenes*
         (b) **Abnormalities associated with infection acquired in the first trimester** include:
            (i) Congenital malformation
            (ii) Intrauterine growth retardation
            (iii) Microcephaly
            (iv) Hydrocephalus
            (v) Stillbirth
         (c) **Abnormalities associated with infection acquired later in pregnancy** include:
            (i) Microcephaly
            (ii) Hydrops fetalis
            (iii) DIC
            (iv) Anemia
            (v) Intracranial hemorrhage
            (vi) Hepatosplenomegaly
            (vii) Jaundice
            (viii) Skin and eye lesions
            (ix) Stillbirth
      (2) **Perinatal infections** include infections acquired through the fetal membranes, ascending infections acquired after rupture of the fetal membranes, and infections acquired via the birth canal.
         (a) **Common causative organisms** include:
            (i) Group B β-hemolytic streptococcus
            (ii) *Escherichia coli*
            (iii) *Klebsiella* species
            (iv) *Streptococcus pneumoniae*
            (v) Herpes simplex virus
            (vi) *Chlamydia trachomatis*
            (vii) *Neisseria gonorrhoeae*
            (viii) *Neisseria meningitidis*
         (b) **Abnormalities associated with perinatal infections** include:
            (i) Respiratory distress
            (ii) Temperature instability
            (iii) Septic shock
            (iv) Neutropenia
            (v) Thrombocytopenia
            (vi) Meningitis
            (vii) Death
      (3) **Postnatal infections** most often are acquired as a result of nosocomial or community exposures. Hospitalized newborns who are premature or require instrumentation are particularly susceptible.

    (a) **Common causative organisms** include:
        (i) *Staphylococcus aureus*
        (ii) *Staphylococcus epidermidis*
        (iii) *Pseudomonas aeruginosa*
        (iv) *Candida albicans*
        (v) *E. coli*
        (vi) *Klebsiella pneumoniae*
        (vii) *Clostridia* species
        (viii) *Bacteroides* species
        (ix) Enterococcus
    (b) **Abnormalities associated with postnatal infections** include:
        (i) Respiratory distress
        (ii) Feeding intolerance
        (iii) Apnea
        (iv) Anemia
        (v) Shock
        (vi) DIC
        (vii) Hypoglycemia or hyperglycemia
        (viii) Temperature instability

2. **Bacterial infection and neonatal sepsis.** Bacterial infections most frequently are acquired via the birth canal or nosocomially. The infection almost always is bacteremic (often with seeding of the meninges via the blood) and associated with systemic symptoms—a condition referred to as **neonatal sepsis**.
  a. **Incidence.** Neonatal sepsis is common in premature infants. About 1%–4% of these infants develop at least one episode of sepsis during their hospitalization. Sepsis in term infants is rare, occurring in less than 1%.
  b. **Risk factors** for early neonatal sepsis include:
    (1) Premature labor
    (2) Prolonged rupture of the fetal membranes
    (3) Low birth weight
    (4) Chorioamnionitis
    (5) Maternal fever
  c. **Etiology.** The most common causative organisms include:
    (1) Gram-positive cocci, especially group B β-hemolytic streptococci but also *S. aureus* and *S. epidermidis*
    (2) Gram-negative rods, especially *E. coli* and *K. pneumoniae*
    (3) Gram-positive rods (e.g., *L. monocytogenes)*
  d. **Clinical features**
    (1) **Signs and symptoms** of bacterial infection include:
      (a) Unexplained respiratory distress
      (b) Unexplained feeding intolerance
      (c) Temperature instability
      (d) Hypoglycemia or hyperglycemia
      (e) Apnea
      (f) Lethargy
      (g) Irritability
    (2) **Laboratory findings** include:
      (a) Abnormal white blood cell count, including neutropenia or neutrophilia
      (b) Prolonged PT and PTT
      (c) Tracheal aspirate containing bacteria and neutrophils
  e. **Diagnosis.** In addition to the physical examination, the laboratory evaluation for neonatal sepsis should include:
    (1) Complete blood count [neutropenia (< 1800/mm³) or an elevated ratio of immature to total neutrophils suggests sepsis]
    (2) Blood cultures
    (3) A lumbar puncture
    (4) Culture and counterimmunoelectrophoresis (CIE) or latex agglutination testing of the urine
    (5) Gram stain and culture of a tracheal aspirate, if the infant is intubated
    (6) Chest x-ray
    (7) Gastric aspirate (at the time of delivery) for neutrophil count, Gram stain, and culture

**f. Therapy**
- **(1)** Empiric antibiotic therapy should begin after the diagnostic workup and consist of a broad-spectrum penicillin (usually ampicillin) and an aminoglycoside (usually kanamycin or gentamicin). Once culture data are available, therapy should be tailored to the specific organism.
- **(2)** The initial choice of antibiotics for nosocomial infection depends on nursery, community, and individual patient exposure information.
- **(3)** The duration of therapy usually is 7–10 days except for invasive infections (e.g., meningitis, osteomyelitis), which require longer courses of antibiotic therapy.
- **(4)** Other complications (e.g., DIC) always should be investigated and treated.

**3. Viral infection** is uncommon in the newborn but can be devastating. Viral infections can be divided into those acquired prenatally and those acquired perinatally or postnatally.
- **a. Prenatal viral infections**
  - **(1) Etiology.** Common causes include:
    - **(a)** Rubella virus
    - **(b)** Cytomegalovirus
    - **(c)** Echovirus
    - **(d)** Herpes zoster virus
    - **(e)** HIV (see Ch 8 II E)
  - **(2) Clinical features** include:
    - **(a)** Intrauterine growth retardation
    - **(b)** Congenital anomalies
    - **(c)** Skin lesions
    - **(d)** CNS defects
    - **(e)** Hepatosplenomegaly
    - **(f)** Ocular lesions
    - **(g)** Hearing loss
- **b. Perinatal and postnatal viral infections**
  - **(1) Common causes** include:
    - **(a)** Herpes simplex virus
    - **(b)** Herpes zoster virus
    - **(c)** Hepatitis A and B viruses
    - **(d)** Respiratory syncytial virus
    - **(e)** Echovirus
    - **(f)** Coxsackievirus
    - **(g)** Cytomegalovirus (via blood transfusion)
  - **(2) Clinical features**
    - **(a) Herpes virus infections.** Symptoms do not appear until at least 3–7 days and up to 4 weeks after birth. These infections manifest as vesicular skin eruptions, DIC, shock, pneumonia, and encephalitis.
    - **(b) Respiratory syncytial virus infections** manifest as temperature instability, respiratory distress, apnea, clear nasal discharge, and poor feeding.
- **c. Diagnosis** begins with a high index of suspicion and is based primarily on infant culture data, cord immunoglobulin M (IgM) level, changing infant serum antibody titers, results of rapid antigen or antibody tests, maternal medical history and culture data, and time of the year.
- **d. Therapy** is available for herpes virus and respiratory syncytial virus infections.
  - **(1)** Herpes virus infections are treated systemically with vidarabine or acyclovir and ophthalmologically with vidarabine ointment.
  - **(2)** Respiratory syncytial virus infections are treated with aerosolized ribavirin.

**G. Neurologic disorders** generally result in abnormalities of tone, strength, and state of consciousness. The most common neurologic problems occurring in newborns are reviewed here.

**1. Asphyxial brain injury** (see also II) is the most common neurologic abnormality in the neonatal period.
- **a. Risk factors for perinatal asphyxia** (see II B 1)
- **b. Pathophysiology** (see also II A and II B 2)
  - **(1)** During mild to moderate perinatal asphyxia, blood flow to the brain is preserved due to redistribution of the cardiac output.
  - **(2)** During severe perinatal asphyxia, cerebral hypoxia and ischemia occur, initially in the cerebral cortex and eventually in the cerebellum and brain stem.

    **c. Clinical features** (see II B 3 a)

    **d. Therapy** (see also II C)

      **(1)** Treatment primarily is supportive (i.e., ventilation with oxygen and maintenance of cardiac output) while awaiting spontaneous recovery, especially with a mild insult.

      **(2)** Severely asphyxiated infants may require more extensive support of neurologic function as well as respiratory, cardiac, and renal function.

      **(3)** Anticonvulsants are helpful in controlling seizures, although the seizure activity generally is self-limited.

      **(4)** Therapy to reduce cerebral edema or to lower the cerebral metabolic rate has not been shown to improve outcome.

    **e. Prognosis** is variable and sometimes difficult to predict. Mild asphyxia almost always is associated with a good outcome, whereas severe asphyxia frequently is associated with significant morbidity and mortality. The EEG in the neonatal period is somewhat predictive of long-term outcome.

**2. Seizures** (see also Ch 17 V A) are not uncommon in the neonatal period. Subtle seizures—which manifest as rhythmic eye deviation or blinking, lip smacking, "bicycling," or apnea—are the most common form, followed by generalized tonic, multifocal clonic, focal clonic, and myoclonic seizures.

    **a. Etiology.** Underlying causes of seizure activity include:

      **(1)** Asphyxia

      **(2)** Brain anomalies (e.g., holoprosencephaly)

      **(3)** Intracranial hemorrhage, particularly within the brain parenchyma

      **(4)** Systemic metabolic disorders (e.g., hypoglycemia, hyponatremia, hypocalcemia, hypernatremia, hyperammonemia) and inborn errors of amino acid and organic acid metabolism

      **(5)** Meningitis and encephalitis

      **(6)** Pyridoxine dependency

    **b. Diagnosis.** The following evaluations should be made in an effort to pinpoint the cause of the seizure activity:

      **(1)** Neurologic examination

      **(2)** EEG

      **(3)** Ultrasound and computed tomography (CT) scanning, especially in the presence of lateralization of the seizure or EEG

      **(4)** Screening for metabolic disorders (e.g., involving glucose, calcium, or sodium), for inborn errors of metabolism (e.g., involving amino acids or organic acids), and for pyridoxine dependency

      **(5)** Lumbar puncture (in the absence of increased intracranial pressure) and evaluation of the CSF for sepsis

    **c. Therapy** should be initiated with phenobarbital, diphenylhydantoin, or both. Alternative or additional treatment agents include lorazepam, paraldehyde, and valproate. Pyridoxine dependency should be considered in term infants who show no clear cause for the seizure activity and who do not respond to routine therapy. Resolution of the seizure activity after pyridoxine administration is diagnostic of dependency.

    **d. Prognosis** varies with the underlying etiology.

**3. Pericranial and intracranial hemorrhage** (see also Ch 17 VI A) can be classified according to the location of the bleeding within the brain.

    **a. Subaponeurotic, or subgaleal, hemorrhage** is a collection of blood beneath the thin, tendinous sheet covering the skull and above the periosteum of the bones of the skull; it is a large potential space that crosses cranial suture lines. Subaponeurotic hemorrhage generally follows head trauma at birth. On examination, the scalp and head feel firm and boggy over a large area, and there may be scalp discoloration and a large amount of blood loss. Failure to recognize subaponeurotic hemorrhage may yield disastrous results due to shock.

    **b. Cephalhematoma** is a subperiosteal collection of blood; hence, it does not cross cranial suture lines. It is seen following birth trauma and is self-limited, almost always disappearing without residual effects. Therapy to evacuate the collection of blood is contraindicated, as it is associated with a significant risk of infection.

    **c. Subarachnoid hemorrhage** may occur after a normal or traumatic delivery. Bleeding is self-limited, and symptoms (e.g., irritability, seizure activity) resolve in a few days. The infant may be asymptomatic in some cases.

d. **Subdural hemorrhage** also is seen with birth trauma. A significant amount of blood can accumulate and cause focal neurologic deficits due to pressure exerted on the brain. However, drainage is necessary only if symptoms are severe or do not resolve.

e. **Intraventricular hemorrhage** is seen almost exclusively in preterm infants and is the result of bleeding of the germinal matrix frequently following an asphyxial insult.

   (1) Small intraventricular hemorrhages that are confined to a germinal matrix (grade I) or that are associated with a small amount of blood in the ventricle (grade II) often resolve without sequelae.

   (2) Large intraventricular hemorrhages that are associated with ventricular dilatation (grade III) or with extension into the brain parenchyma (grade IV) are associated with permanent functional impairment and hydrocephalus.

4. **Hydrocephalus** (see also Ch 17 III D) refers to an excessive collection of CSF within the ventricular system due to imbalanced production and absorption of CSF.

   a. **High-pressure, or obstructive, hydrocephalus** results when normal drainage and reabsorption of CSF do not occur. It is seen in congenital aqueductal stenosis, Dandy-Walker malformation, and myelomeningocele with Arnold-Chiari malformation and following intraventricular hemorrhage and meningitis.

   b. **Low-pressure, or communicating, hydrocephalus** (also called **hydrocephalus ex vacuo**) is seen after intracranial hemorrhage and in some malformations. This is to be distinguished from the fluid seen in the large intracerebral space in some malformations, such as holoprosencephaly. Communicating hydrocephalus does not require therapeutic intervention.

5. **Hypotonia**, a condition characterized by diminished tone of the skeletal muscles, is the most common neurologic motor disorder of the neonatal period. An evaluation must be performed to determine at which level in the progression of nerve impulse to muscular contraction the defect exists. Common etiologies include:

   a. Asphyxia (brain defect)

   b. Werdnig-Hoffmann disease (spinal cord defect)

   c. Congenital myasthenia gravis (neuromuscular junction defect)

   d. Muscular dystrophy (muscle defect)

   e. Myotonic dystrophy (muscle defect)

   f. Hypothyroidism (metabolic defect)

6. **Myelomeningocele** (see also Ch 17 III B 1 a, b) is the most common congenital anomaly of the nervous system. It results from failure of the neural tube to close.

   a. **Clinical features** depend on the location of the myelomeningocele. Not uncommonly, there is an associated Arnold-Chiari malformation, hydrocephalus, or both.

   b. **Diagnosis.** Prenatal screening (see Ch 7 I F) of maternal serum and amniotic fluid for alpha-fetoprotein and fetal ultrasonography allow for early diagnosis of myelomeningocele and potential intervention.

   c. **Therapy.** Primary surgical closure of the sac is the treatment of choice to prevent infection. Hydrocephalus often develops after closure of the sac. A shunting procedure may be necessary to relieve the hydrocephalus and prevent intracranial hypertension.

   d. **Prognosis** depends on the location of the myelomeningocele, the presence or absence of associated brain lesions, the occurrence of shunt infections, and the effectiveness of physical therapy and other supportive care.

H. **Ophthalmologic disorders** are unusual in the newborn, which is fortunate, as the pediatrician's ability to detect specific abnormalities is limited. However, a careful examination of the newborn's eyes usually allows for gross detection of all ophthalmologic problems, which can then be delineated further by a pediatric ophthalmologist.

1. **Ophthalmia neonatorum** is an acute conjunctivitis of the newborn, which has a limited number of common etiologies. Since the routine eye examination does not allow for a specific diagnosis, a Gram stain and culture should be obtained. (See Ch 1 IV F 2 for further discussion of ophthalmia neonatorum.)

2. **Cataract** refers to any clouding of the lens. Early intervention is important if future blindness and amblyopia are to be prevented.

   a. **Etiology.** Cataracts result from numerous causes, including hereditary disorders, intrauterine infections (e.g., rubella), and metabolic diseases (e.g., galactosemia). The cause in some cases is unknown.

  **b. Therapy** includes removal of the lens combined with either corrective glasses or intraocular artificial lens implantation.

 **3. Glaucoma** is characterized by increased intraocular pressure resulting in ocular damage and vision impairment. Glaucoma may be inherited or may be acquired as a component of some other disorder (e.g., retinopathy of prematurity, chorioretinitis, rubella).

  **a. Clinical features** include conjunctival injection, excessive lacrimation, light sensitivity, blepharospasm, and corneal clouding.

  **b. Therapy** is surgical and should be instituted as soon as possible.

  **c. Prognosis** is related to the duration of the glaucoma. Early intervention most frequently is associated with good vision.

 **4. Retinopathy of prematurity** (retrolental fibroplasia) was first seen during the 1940s and 1950s, after oxygen therapy became commonly used in the nursery to sustain life in very small premature infants. Incidences of 10%–70% have been reported in infants with a birth weight less than 1500 g.

  **a. Etiology and pathogenesis.** The development of retinopathy of prematurity appears to be related to **immaturity of the retinal vessels** of preterm infants. Contributing factors include **hyperoxia,** hypercarbia, and intermittent hypoxia.

   **(1)** The hyperoxia induces vasospasm and endothelial damage in the retinal vessels, with resultant tissue edema and injury.

   **(2)** Over the following weeks, reactive proliferative neovascularization occurs, causing traction (i.e., pulling up) of the retina, which may result in retinal detachment. This sequence occurs without further insult but may regress at any time prior to detachment.

  **b. Therapy.** The retinopathy generally resolves spontaneously. In infants with active, rapidly progressive disease, **cryotherapy** is indicated to prevent traction and retinal detachment.

  **c. Prognosis** is related to the severity of the vascularity and subsequent spontaneous regression. Myopia is common. Blindness follows retinal detachment.

 **5. Neuroblastoma** should be suspected when an abnormal red reflex (**leukokoria**) is observed in a newborn.

 **6. Intrauterine infection associated with ophthalmologic abnormalities**

  **a. Toxoplasmosis** is associated with a chorioretinitis. Focal or multifocal lesions are seen. Prognosis is poor.

  **b. Cytomegalovirus infection** is associated with chorioretinitis. No therapy is available.

  **c. Rubella** is associated with glaucoma, cataract, microphthalmus, and uveitis. Therapy is symptomatic.

 **7. Aniridia** is a rare developmental disorder characterized by a lack of development of the iris. It is associated with other congenital abnormalities, especially Wilms' tumor (see Ch 15 VI), which must always be suspected when aniridia is detected.

**I. Multiple gestation** always should be seen as a high-risk event due to its increased association with intrauterine accidents, growth abnormalities, prematurity, and problems at the time of delivery (e.g., abnormal fetal position, asphyxia).

 **1. Incidence.** Approximately 1%–1.3% of all live births are the result of twin gestation. The true incidence of twin gestation probably is slightly higher. The monozygotic twinning rate is 3.5—4.0 in 1000 live births, or 35%–40% of all twins who are born.

 **2. Etiology**

  **a. Monozygotic twinning** may be viewed as a teratogenic event, as it occurs more frequently with increasing maternal age, is associated with more congenital malformations, and can be caused by teratogens. A problem of symmetry in the developing embryo may result in conjoined twins.

  **b. Dizygotic twinning** is due to double ovulation, which may be related to elevated gonadotropin levels.

 **3. Placentation**

  **a. Monochorionic placentation** always is associated with monozygotic twins; 1% of monozygotic twins are monoamniotic.

  **b. Dichorionic placentation** almost always is associated with dizygotic, diamniotic twins.

  **c. Twin placentas** are associated with a sixfold to ninefold increase in the incidence of velamentous cord insertion and with a high incidence of vasa previa.

4. **Prenatal problems**
   a. **Death.** Monoamniotic twins have only a 40% chance of both surviving. Death may occur due to cord accidents and to twin-to-twin transfusions, which may lead to the death of one fetus, with thromboplastin release and subsequent DIC in the second twin.
   b. **Growth disturbances** are the rule.
      (1) **Intrauterine growth retardation.** There is decreased potential for growth in twin fetuses as compared to a single fetus, probably due to the limitations of placental surface area for nutrient transfer.
      (2) **Twin-to-twin transfusion,** resulting in a large, polycythemic twin and a small, anemic twin, is a significant risk in monochorionic placentation.
   c. The incidence of **congenital malformations** is doubled in twin pregnancy.
   d. The incidence of **spontaneous abortion** also is increased.
   e. **Preterm delivery** occurs in up to 50% of twin pregnancies; the incidence is even higher in triplet and quadruplet pregnancy.
      (1) Preterm delivery is a significant factor in the increased morbidity and mortality associated with multiple gestation.
      (2) The incidence of preterm delivery and growth retardation can be decreased by early identification of multiple gestation and by placing the mother on strict bed rest. Maternal compliance is higher in the hospital setting.
   f. **Maternal complications** include:
      (1) Pregnancy-induced hypertension
      (2) Polyhydramnios
      (3) Hyperemesis and nausea
      (4) Anemia

5. **Postnatal problems**
   a. **Prematurity,** with all of its sequelae, is the most common management problem. Complications of prematurity include:
      (1) Low birth weight
      (2) Hyaline membrane disease, which occurs more often and is more severe in the second-born twin
      (3) Intracranial hemorrhage
      (4) Infection
   b. **Growth retardation,** both symmetrical and asymmetrical, occurs more frequently in multiple gestation. This may be associated with developmental abnormalities as well as long-term growth disturbances.
   c. **Perinatal asphyxia,** especially of the second-born twin and in instances of malpresentation or vasa previa, may result in long-term morbidity or mortality.

6. **Management** is aimed at:
   a. Identifying multiple gestation as early as possible
   b. Managing other medical problems
   c. Controlling preterm labor
   d. Identifying the ideal route of delivery
   e. Avoiding asphyxia in the second twin (in twin pregnancy) or in subsequent infants (in other multiple pregnancies)

J. **Hypoglycemia** is defined as a plasma glucose concentration less than 30 mg/dl during the first 24 hours of life and less than 45 mg/dl thereafter. Hypoglycemia is very common in infants of diabetic mothers as well as in infants who are born following various perinatal complications, including prematurity, intrauterine growth retardation, and asphyxia.

1. **Pathogenesis.** The pathogenesis varies depending on the clinical setting and the associated conditions affecting the infant.
   a. **Maternal diabetes.** The hypoglycemia in infants of diabetic mothers is the result of a hyperinsulinemic state that persists after the umbilical cord is cut and the maternal supply of glucose is interrupted.
   b. **Prematurity.** Preterm infants become hypoglycemic due to diminished glycogen stores and to immaturity of gluconeogenic enzymes.
   c. **Growth retardation.** Growth-retarded infants frequently are depleted of hepatic glycogen and quickly become hypoglycemic.
   d. **Perinatal asphyxia** forces the fetus (infant) to use anaerobic metabolism, which quickly depletes stored glycogen and results in hypoglycemia.

    **e. Cold stress** increases oxygen consumption as well as glucose consumption. It also may increase free acids and result in hypoglycemia.

    **f. Sepsis** may cause hypoglycemia, although hyperglycemia also is observed, which presumably is due to insulin insensitivity.

    **g. Beckwith-Wiedemann syndrome** is characterized by hypoglycemia, visceromegaly, macroglossia, and omphalocele. Hyperinsulinism secondary to pancreatic islet cell hyperplasia is responsible for the hypoglycemia.

    **h. Nesidioblastosis** and **pancreatic islet cell adenoma** are associated with hyperinsulinemia and hypoglycemia.

    **i. Metabolic disorders,** such as galactosemia and panhypopituitarism, also are associated with hypoglycemia.

**2. Clinical features.** Infants with hypoglycemia are not always symptomatic. However, the following symptoms may occur:

    **a.** Hypotonia or jitteriness

    **b.** Apnea or tachypnea

    **c.** Seizures

**3. Diagnosis.** Screening for hypoglycemia may be done using any of a number of bedside reagent strips. The diagnosis is confirmed by the actual measurement of the plasma glucose concentration by the clinical laboratory.

**4. Therapy**

    **a.** Primary therapy is intravenous glucose. The glucose infusion may be required for several days until the basal insulin secretion rate decreases, glycogen stores are replenished, or gluconeogenesis improves. Bolus infusions of hypertonic glucose should be avoided, as they may result in a rebound hypoglycemia.

        **(1)** Intravenous glucose should be administered as a constant infusion begun at a rate of 6–8 mg/kg/min. This may be increased to a rate of up to 20 mg/kg/min. (A central venous access should be employed for infusions given at a rate above 12–15 mg/kg/min.)

        **(2)** A small (0.5–1.0 g/kg) bolus of glucose may be used for extreme hypoglycemia or if severe symptoms related to hypoglycemia occur. This should always be followed by a constant infusion.

    **b.** Hypoglycemia that is secondary to hyperinsulinemia and resistant to intravenous glucose should be treated with corticosteroids or diazoxide. If drug treatment fails, pancreatectomy should be performed. These more aggressive forms of therapy rarely are necessary except for hypoglycemia that is associated with Beckwith-Wiedemann syndrome, nesidioblastosis, or islet cell adenoma.

**K. Disorders associated with maternal diabetes.** The pregnancy of a diabetic woman is one that is associated with multiple complications affecting both mother and fetus. The key to an optimal outcome is consistent euglycemia in the mother.

**1. Diabetic embryopathy**

    **a. Caudal regression** is a congenital anomaly that is specifically associated with **infants of diabetic mothers**. It clearly is related to maternal hyperglycemia during organogenesis.

    **b. Other anomalies** also occur at an increased rate. The specific genetically related anomalies vary depending on geographic location and race. In the United States, congenital anomalies of the heart and CNS are common.

**2. Prenatal growth abnormalities.** Glucose easily crosses the placenta, whereas insulin does not; therefore, maternal hyperglycemia causes fetal hyperglycemia and a reactive fetal hyperinsulinemia. This combination results in increased somatic growth of the fetus due to cellular hyperplasia and hypertrophy. The large size of the fetus often results in dystocia. The brain is the only organ whose growth is not affected by the fetal hyperglycemia and hyperinsulinemia.

**3. Late fetal death** occurs more frequently in the poorly controlled diabetic pregnancy than in the normal pregnancy or euglycemic diabetic pregnancy. Animal studies show that fetal hyperglycemia and hyperinsulinemia are associated with an increase in fetal metabolism and respiration. As the fetus approaches term, oxygen transport becomes limited, and the hypermetabolic state may lead to fetal hypoxia and death.

**4. Preterm delivery** is common and the result of fetal distress or a planned early delivery. Complications largely depend on the gestational age and lung maturity of the infant at the time of

delivery. Effective production of surfactant is delayed in these infants; therefore, an L/S ratio always should be determined prior to an elective delivery to indicate the level of lung maturity.
   **a.** An L/S ratio of 3:1 or greater indicates lung maturity in an infant of a diabetic mother.
   **b.** A lower ratio reflects lung maturity only if significant amounts of phosphatidylglycerol are present.

5. **Hypoglycemia** is very common in infants of diabetic mothers and is related to the mother's overall glycemic control as well as the intrapartum glucose levels (see V J for more information).

6. **Other metabolic disturbances** seen in infants of diabetic mothers include:
   **a.** Hypocalcemia
   **b.** Hyperbilirubinemia (see V C)

7. **Polycythemia** associated with elevated erythropoietin levels is observed and probably reflects chronic fetal hypoxia.

8. **Alterations in normal neonatal behavior** commonly are observed in infants of diabetic mothers. Abnormalities include lethargy, hypotonia, and poor feeding. An etiology is not clear.

9. **Large body size.** Those infants who are large for gestational age are more likely to continue to be large for age beyond infancy.

L. **Intrauterine drug exposure.** Recent studies have documented fetal exposure to numerous drugs, including antibiotics, caffeine, nicotine, alcohol, aspirin, and antihistamines. Over the past decade, the use of illicit drugs (e.g., heroin, cocaine, marijuana) by pregnant women also has grown. The intravenous use of illicit drugs is associated with a high risk for preterm birth as well as a significant risk of hepatitis and AIDS in both the mother and infant. The drug-seeking behavior of these mothers often makes it difficult for them to care for their infants. The following are some commonly used drugs that may have major effects on the developing fetus and newborn.

1. **Nicotine** is absorbed through the lungs from cigarette smoke and is accompanied by the diffusion of carbon monoxide across the alveoli into the mother's blood. Nicotine is a vasoconstrictor that may limit uterine blood flow, and carbon monoxide decreases the arterial oxygen content. Together the two substances reduce the transfer of oxygen and nutrients from mother to fetus. The result is decreased intrauterine growth and chronic hypoxia.

2. **Alcohol** is a well-established teratogen. Fetal exposure may result in a spectrum of effects ranging from mild reduction in cerebral function to classic **fetal alcohol syndrome** (see also Ch 7 II G 1). Features of this syndrome include microcephaly with cerebral dysfunction, characteristic facies (short palpebral fissures, diminished philtrum, small upper lip), and intrauterine and extrauterine growth failure. The amount of alcohol consumed by the mother appears to correlate with the degree to which the fetus is affected.

3. **Heroin and methadone**
   **a.** Narcotic use by the mother is associated with intrauterine growth retardation, increased risk of sudden infant death, and infant narcotic withdrawal syndrome. There is accelerated maturation of several fetal organs, including the liver and lung (surfactant production).
   **b.** It is not clear whether the abnormalities of fetal growth and maturation are due directly to the effects of the drugs or to other environmental factors (e.g., poor maternal nutrition) often associated with maternal narcotic use.
   **c.** Many of these infants will experience **narcotic withdrawal syndrome,** which is characterized by irritability, poor sleeping, high-pitched cry, diarrhea, sweating, sneezing, seizures, poor feeding, and poor weight gain. Naloxone should never be given to such infants in the delivery room, as it will precipitate acute withdrawal.
   **d.** The long-term neurologic consequences of fetal narcotic exposure have not been investigated completely.

4. **Cocaine** use by pregnant women has increased dramatically over the past decade. Such use is associated with congenital anomalies, intrauterine growth retardation, intracranial hemorrhage, placental abruption, and preterm birth. Infants may undergo withdrawal (irritability, poor feeding). Recent studies have demonstrated abnormalities in control of respiration and an increased risk for sudden infant death.

**VI. CARE OF THE PARENTS AND ETHICAL DECISION MAKING.** Whether the parents have the happy experience of bonding to a healthy newborn or the tragic experience of mourning a dying infant, it is the pediatrician's role to provide the parents with support and information and to answer their questions.

**A. Parent-infant bonding**

1. **Bonding between the healthy term infant and her parents**
   a. Bonding, or the process of psychological attachment of the parents to the newborn, appears to begin during pregnancy and to intensify as the fetus begins to move inside the uterus and react to external stimuli. During this period, the parents often form a mental image of what the infant will look like at birth.
   b. At the time of delivery, it is thought that the mother experiences a unique psychological state or "window." This close contact with the infant in the delivery room will foster ideal bonding and promote optimal future mother-infant interactions.
      (1) The **maternal behavior pattern** is typical. It begins with touching of the infant's fingers and palms followed by central caressing. Eye contact is also made.
      (2) **Paternal behavior** is quite similar.
      (3) While every effort should be made to ensure parent-infant bonding in the delivery area, medical problems (e.g., hypothermia, respiratory distress) must take precedence.
   c. The process of bonding continues for hours and days after birth. Even if the delivery room bonding experience does not occur, it has been shown that strong mother-infant ties will be established if the mother and infant are given long periods of contact together over the next few days.

2. **Problems in bonding between the sick infant and his parents**
   a. The establishment of neonatal intensive care units, the advancement of technology, and the honing of clinical skills have allowed the survival of an increasing number of small and sick infants. The size and fragility of the newborn, the equipment used to care for the infant, and the long periods of hospitalization may make the normal bonding process more difficult for parents.
   b. At the turn of the century, it was recognized that institutional care improved the outcome of the feeble infant, yet the separation of the infant from the mother often led to abandonment. The ideal solution to this problem has not been found, as evidenced by the high rate of child abuse among infants who have been cared for in neonatal intensive care units. The following procedures are recommended to minimize the physical separation of the infant from the parents and to encourage the formation of a strong bond.
      (1) Whenever possible, the mother should be transported to a tertiary care center prior to delivery.
      (2) When the infant is transported to another hospital, the father should travel immediately to the referral center so that he may keep close contact with the infant and bring photographs and information back to the mother.
      (3) Visitation should be available 24 hours a day.
      (4) A strong line of communication should be established between the medical staff (i.e., physicians, nurses, social workers) and the parents.
      (5) The parents should be encouraged to keep in contact by telephone when visitation is difficult.
      (6) The parents should be prepared regarding what to expect during their first visit to the nursery, and they should be made aware of any sudden change in the infant's condition.
      (7) Information should be conveyed in a positive and truthful manner.
      (8) Psychological evaluation and support should be made available to parents who are having a particularly difficult time coping with their sick infant or the intensive care unit setting. Parents' groups often are helpful.
      (9) Plans for discharge should be made in advance and should include the parents. Having the parents stay overnight in the hospital prior to discharge can significantly help them adapt to new roles that they will perform after they leave the hospital. Any current or future medical problems and follow-up plans should be explained to the parents.

**B. Support of the parents of a malformed infant.** The birth of a malformed infant is a tragedy that creates a complex challenge for the pediatrician who must care for the child and help the parents through the disappointment and period of adjustment.

1. **Stages of parental reaction.** Parents go through four stages in reacting to their malformed infant, starting with mourning the loss of the expected healthy infant and ending with acceptance of the actual infant. These stages are:
   a. Shock
   b. Denial
   c. Sadness and anger
   d. Reorganization and acceptance

2. **Supportive actions** that will help the parents through this tragic period include the following.
   a. The parents should be encouraged to spend as much time as possible with the infant.
   b. The infant should be shown to the parents as soon as possible, because a mental image of the anomaly is often worse than the actual malformation.
   c. Good lines of communication should be maintained, and information should be conveyed in a truthful manner.
   d. The parents need support through each stage of adjustment and should not be rushed through the various stages.
   e. Plans for adequate support of the infant and parents should be made prior to discharge.

C. **Support of the parents of a dying infant during the illness and after the death**

1. **Parental reactions**
   a. **Grief** experienced after the loss of a newborn is unique in that the attachment one has for a parent, sibling, spouse, or older child has not been formed. Rather, the newborn is perceived as a part of the parent, especially the mother. As such, the grieving behavior of the parents includes both the classic grieving behaviors plus behaviors reflecting detachment, similar to the feelings experienced when a limb has been amputated. The feelings include anger, guilt, fury, helplessness, and horror. As opposed to the feelings when a spouse or sibling dies, the feelings following the loss of an infant are not relieved by identification.
   b. Loss of a newborn often results in a **breakdown in communication** between the parents due to their difficulty in expressing emotions and their feelings of guilt, blame, or both.

2. **Supportive actions.** The parents can best be supported through the following actions.
   a. The parents should be prepared if death is anticipated.
   b. The parents should be together when they are told of the death.
   c. Every effort should be made to allow the parents to hold the infant before and after death if they desire to.
   d. Time for the immediate grieving should be allowed to pass prior to discussion of autopsy and burial arrangements.
   e. Support should be offered to the parents 3–4 months after the death. This may be in the form of an office visit or contact with a parents' group.
   f. Autopsy reports should be made available and discussed with the parents in a timely fashion.

D. **Ethical decision making.** Over the past 25 years, advances in knowledge of fetal and neonatal physiology and improvements in clinical skills and technology have allowed the survival of many immature and congenitally malformed infants. Ethical problems arise when this "high tech" care is given to potentially nonviable infants. Some guidelines for ethical decision making are as follows.

1. The parents always should be involved, with the physician, in the decision-making process. It is the role of the physician to provide knowledge so that the parents can participate in life-or-death decisions regarding their infant.

2. When viability is in doubt due to inadequate knowledge concerning the nature and severity of the infant's condition or prognosis, life support always should be provided until adequate data can be gathered.

3. All hospitals should have an ethics committee to assist the pediatrician when issues of life support or proper treatment are not clear, when the parents' wishes conflict with the physician's, or when the parents are not competent and cannot participate in the decision-making process.

4. The decision to terminate life support should be made only when it is clear that therapy is prolonging the dying process or when the burden of therapy outweighs any potential benefit to the infant.

## BIBLIOGRAPHY

Avery GB: *Neonatology: Pathophysiology and Management of the Newborn,* 3rd edition. Philadelphia, JB Lippincott, 1987.

Avery ME, Taeusch HW: *Schaffer's Diseases of the Newborn,* 5th edition. Philadelphia, WB Saunders, 1984.

Creasy RK, Resnik R: *Maternal-Fetal Medicine,* 2nd edition. Philadelphia, WB Saunders, 1989.

Klaus MH, Fanaroff AA: *Care of the High-Risk Neonate,* 3rd edition. Philadelphia, WB Saunders, 1986.

Volpe JJ: *Neurology of the Newborn,* 2nd edition. Philadelphia, WB Saunders, 1987.

# STUDY QUESTIONS

**Directions:** Each of the numbered items or incomplete statements in this section is followed by answers or by completions of the statement. Select the **one** lettered answer or completion that is **best** in each case.

1. Which of the following events occurs during the canalicular stage of lung development?

(A) Development of bronchiolar arteries and goblet cells
(B) Development of terminal alveolar sacs and differentiation of alveolar cells
(C) Development of tracheal cartilage
(D) Appearance of phosphatidylglycerol
(E) Appearance of undifferentiated cuboidal cells

2. Which of the following conditions is a cause of asymmetric growth retardation?

(A) Twin pregnancy
(B) Trisomy 18
(C) Cytomegalovirus infection
(D) Fetal alcohol syndrome

3. The primary goal of resuscitation of the newborn is to

(A) establish spontaneous breathing
(B) improve the heart rate
(C) reoxygenate the CNS
(D) improve the infant's color
(E) make the infant cry spontaneously

4. The most common complication of a multiple-gestation pregnancy is

(A) premature birth
(B) maternal hypertension
(C) maternal anemia
(D) hyperemesis

5. Hyperbilirubinemia is diagnosed in a 2-day-old infant whose serum bilirubin concentrations are 17.5 mg/dl (indirect fraction) and 0.2 mg/dl (direct fraction). All of the following statements concerning the evaluation and management of this infant are true EXCEPT

(A) the indirect and direct bilirubin concentrations are consistent with a physiologic jaundice
(B) the initial evaluation should include a complete blood count with reticulocyte count, maternal infant blood types, and Coombs' test
(C) breast-feeding may have contributed to the elevated bilirubin concentration
(D) phototherapy should be administered

6. All of the following are components of the Apgar score EXCEPT

(A) heart rate
(B) muscle tone
(C) blood pressure
(D) reflex irritability
(E) skin color

7. All of the following statements about tracheoesophageal fistula are true EXCEPT

(A) the fistula most commonly is found between the distal esophagus and trachea
(B) the proximal esophagus usually ends in a blind pouch
(C) the goal of initial management is to keep the airway clear of secretions
(D) the diagnosis is established by a radiologic study using contrast to outline the defect
(E) definitive therapy consists of surgical repair of the fistula and reanastomosis of the proximal and distal portions of the esophagus

---

| | | |
|---|---|---|
| 1-B | 4-A | 7-D |
| 2-A | 5-A | |
| 3-C | 6-C | |

8. Newborn infants often require lower doses of drugs compared to adults (adjusted for body mass and weight) for all of the following reasons EXCEPT

(A) newborns have lower blood protein and albumin concentrations
(B) newborns have a lower glomerular filtration rate
(C) glucuronyl transferase activity is reduced in newborns
(D) renal tubular secretion is lower in newborns
(E) newborns have a lower normal blood pH

9. Infants may develop hypoglycemia due to hyperinsulinemia under all of the following conditions EXCEPT

(A) Beckwith-Wiedemann syndrome
(B) nesidioblastosis
(C) maternal diabetes
(D) asymmetric growth retardation
(E) pancreatic islet cell adenoma

10. Signs and symptoms of neonatal necrotizing enterocolitis include all of the following EXCEPT

(A) bile-stained gastric fluid
(B) pneumatosis intestinalis
(C) guaiac-positive stools
(D) apnea
(E) jaundice

11. Immediate preparation for a high-risk delivery involves all of the following steps and procedures EXCEPT

(A) obtaining the obstetric history
(B) gathering the appropriate personnel
(C) requesting a neonatology consultation
(D) obtaining the labor history
(E) readying the resuscitation equipment

12. All of the following complications of pregnancy are risk factors for perinatal asphyxia EXCEPT

(A) placental abruption
(B) hyperemesis gravidarum
(C) prematurity
(D) preeclampsia
(E) meconium-stained amniotic fluid

13. Which of the following statements regarding retinopathy of prematurity is FALSE?

(A) Its development is related to retinal vessel immaturity and hyperoxia
(B) The retinopathy resolves spontaneously in most infants
(C) Cryotherapy is the treatment of choice for all stages of disease
(D) Myopia is a common sequela

14. Which of the following is NOT a cause of symmetrical growth retardation?

(A) Congenital infection
(B) Chromosomal defects
(C) Cell toxins
(D) Preeclampsia
(E) Fetal alcohol syndrome

8-E    11-C    14-D
9-D    12-B
10-E   13-C

**Directions:** Each item below contains four suggested answers of which **one or more** is correct. Choose the answer

- A   if **1, 2, and 3** are correct
- B   if **1 and 3** are correct
- C   if **2 and 4** are correct
- D   if **4** is correct
- E   if **1, 2, 3, and 4** are correct

15. During fetal life, oxygen saturation is highest in which of the following fetal arteries?

(1) Carotid

(2) Renal

(3) Coronary

(4) Pulmonary

16. True statements concerning fluid balance in the newborn include

(1) sensible water loss includes urine, stool, and pulmonary and gastric fluid losses

(2) insensible water loss is increased by the use of radiant warmers, phototherapy, and an elevated environmental temperature

(3) replacement of sodium, potassium, and chloride in physiologic amounts is begun at birth

(4) water loss in the first week of life is greater in the preterm infant

17. An infant born at 30 weeks gestation begins to experience apnea on the second day of life. Included in the initial management of this infant should be

(1) therapy with theophylline

(2) evaluation for evidence of hypoxia, infection, or intracranial hemorrhage

(3) placement of an oscillating bed

(4) complete blood count, arterial blood gas studies, and plasma glucose and electrolyte measurement

18. A nurse believes that a 12-hour-old infant has experienced a seizure lasting 2 minutes. Labor history includes the rupture of the fetal membranes 24 hours prior to delivery and a difficult delivery with forceps. The Apgar score was 7 at 1 minute and 8 at 5 minutes. The nurse reports that the infant had been feeding poorly and was lethargic prior to the seizure. The differential diagnosis includes

(1) asphyxia

(2) meningitis

(3) kernicterus

(4) intracranial hemorrhage

15-B       18-C
16-C
17-C

## ANSWERS AND EXPLANATIONS

**1. The answer is B** *[V A 1 a (2)]*.
During the pseudoglandular stage of lung development, there is the ingrowth of major airways and blood vessels into the undifferentiated intrathoracic mesenchyme. The tracheal cartilage develops, bronchial arteries appear, and goblet cells line the airways. During the canalicular stage, there is further branching of airways down to the terminal alveolar sacs. The lining cells differentiate into types I and II alveolar cells. During the alveolar, or terminal, sac stage, there is production of surfactant by the type II alveolar cells. Phosphatidylglycerol, a component of surfactant, appears at 35 weeks gestation. It is present in small quantities, but it is very important in lowering lung surface tension and preventing hyaline membrane disease.

**2. The answer is A** *[I C 1 b]*.
Asymmetric growth retardation occurs as a result of an insult late in gestation; cell number is normal, but cell size is decreased. Asymmetric growth retardation is associated with factors that decrease uterine, placental, or umbilical blood flow and transfer of nutrients to the fetus. In the case of multiple pregnancy, the collective fetal nutritional requirements are greater than the ability of the placenta to transfer such nutrients from the maternal circulation. Chromosomal defects (e.g., trisomy 18), congenital infection (e.g., with cytomegalovirus), and maternal use of drugs (e.g., alcohol) are factors that adversely affect fetal growth early in gestation, causing symmetrical growth retardation.

**3. The answer is C** *[III E]*.
The primary goal of resuscitation of anyone—infant, child, or adult—is to reoxygenate the central nervous system. This is achieved by providing adequate oxygen and ventilation and by establishing adequate cardiac output. Improvement in heart rate and color and spontaneous respiration are signs that the goal is being achieved.

**4. The answer is A** *[V I 4 e]*.
Multiple-gestation pregnancies are fraught with problems for both the mother and the fetuses (infants). The most common problem is premature birth.Other problems include maternal hypertension, anemia, hyperemesis, and growth disturbances in the fetuses.

**5. The answer is A** *[V C]*.
In physiologic jaundice, the maximum bilirubin concentration should not exceed 12–15 mg/dl. The initial investigation should include tests that will evaluate for the presence of hemoloytic disease, the most common cause of hyperbilirubinemia aside from decreased glucuronyl transferase activity (physiologic jaundice). Appropriate tests include a complete blood count with reticulocyte count, determination of maternal and infant blood types, Coombs' tests, and indirect and direct bilirubin concentrations. Initiation of phototherapy is appropriate in this infant. As long as the infant is well hydrated, breast-feeding should be encouraged.

**6. The answer is C.** *[III D 1]*.
Blood pressure is not a component of the Apgar score. The Apgar score determines the state of oxygenation and ventilation as reflected by heart rate, respiratory effort, muscle tone, reflex irritability, and skin color.

**7. The answer is D** *[V A 2 a]*.
The diagnosis of esophageal atresia with tracheoesophageal fistula is established by the inability to pass a nasogastric tube into the stomach and the observation on chest x-ray that the tube is coiled up in the esophageal pouch. While the fistula between the trachea and distal esophagus may be seen on a lateral chest x-ray as a column of air between the stomach and trachea, special studies generally are not necessary since the fistula almost always starts at the level of the carina and connects to the superior aspect of the distal esophagus. Contrast studies of the esophageal pouch may result in aspiration and should not be undertaken.

**8. The answer is E** *[IV C]*.
Several factors must be considered when administering drugs to newborn infants, but blood pH is not one of them; normal pH is similar in infants and adults. The lower blood protein concentration in newborns compared to adults results in higher unbound fractions of drugs at given total drug concentrations. Lower drug metabolism in the newborn liver and lower renal clearance result in longer drug half-lives in newborns compared to adults. These factors require appropriate adjustments in drug dosing and monitoring of drug concentrations in neonates.

**9. The answer is D** *[V J 1].*
Infants with asymmetric growth retardation usually are the result of a pregnancy complicated by placental insufficiency; these infants have been "starved" in utero. They have virtually no glycogen stores and become hypoglycemic soon after birth. Conditions that cause hypoglycemia due to hyperinsulinemia include Beckwith-Wiedemann syndrome (a condition associated with pancreatic islet cell hyperplasia), nesidioblastosis, and pancreatic islet cell adenoma. Infants of diabetic mothers are both hyperglycemic and hyperinsulinemic in utero. The hyperinsulinism continues after birth and results in hypoglycemia if proper therapy is not provided.

**10. The answer is E** *[V B 3, 4, C 2 a (1) (b)].*
Jaundice is not a feature of necrotizing enterocolitis, although it may occur if sepsis develops. Neonatal necrotizing enterocolitis is accompanied by an ileus as evidenced by abdominal distention, loss of bowel sounds, and bile-stained gastric fluid. The bacterial invasion of the intestinal wall leads to inflammation and tissue breakdown, which result in blood in the stool. Gas formation by the bacteria in the intestinal wall can be seen on x-ray and is referred to as pneumatosis intestinalis. Apnea, a nonspecific sign of infection, often is seen in association with necrotizing enterocolitis and other infections in the newborn.

**11. The answer is C** *[III C].*
To prepare for a high-risk delivery, the pediatrician must gather information about problems in the present and past pregnancies, such as Rh sensitization, herpetic infections, and malformations. The length of gestation and the results of fetal evaluation must also be ascertained. Additionally, the labor history yields information concerning the risk for asphyxia. An optimal resuscitation requires an appropriate number of trained personnel and properly functioning equipment. While a neonatology consultation may be needed for some high-risk deliveries, it is not part of the immediate preparation.

**12. The answer is B** *[II B 1].*
Hyperemesis gravidarum is not a risk factor for perinatal asphyxia. Placental abruption, prematurity, preeclampsia, and meconium-stained amniotic fluid do predispose to perinatal asphyxia. Placental abruption is the separation of the placenta from the uterine wall. With progressive separation, there is decreasing surface area for oxygen transfer from mother to fetus, and an increasing degree of fetal hypoxia results. Premature infants frequently suffer perinatal asphyxia due to their inability to tolerate labor and to respiratory problems at birth. The incidence of perinatal asphyxia increases with decreasing gestational age at birth. Preeclampsia predisposes newborns to hypoxia and perinatal asphyxia due to chronic placental insufficiency and superimposed intermittent uteroplacental hypoperfusion during labor. Meconium-stained amniotic fluid is the result of fetal passage of meconium, which is triggered by hypoxia-stimulated vagal reflexes.

**13. The answer is C** *[V H 4].*
Retinopathy of prematurity generally resolves spontaneously. In the few infants with active, rapidly progressive disease, cryotherapy has been shown to be effective in many, but not all, cases. Retinopathy of prematurity appears to be related to immaturity of retinal vessels in preterm infants and to hyperoxia. The degree of insult to the retina varies with the severity of the vascularity and subsequent spontaneous regression. Myopia is a common outcome.

**14. The answer is D** *[I C 1].*
Early fetal growth is due to cellular hyperplasia. Congenital infection, chromosomal defects, cell toxins, and maternal alcohol use all affect the fetus during early gestation and result in a decrease in both the total cell number and the growth of all organs. This is termed symmetrical growth retardation. Preeclampsia, a complication that occurs in the last trimester, results in fetal malnutrition, which primarily reduces birth weight but does not affect the brain (head circumference) or linear growth. This is termed asymmetric growth retardation.

**15. The answer is B (1, 3)** *[I B 1 a (1)].*
Highly saturated blood returns to the fetus via the umbilical vein, ductus venosus, and inferior vena cava. This blood is preferentially shunted across the foramen ovale to the left side of the heart to supply the coronary and cerebral circulation. Desaturated blood from the head and rest of the body returns to the right ventricle, is pumped out to the pulmonary artery, and is shunted across the ductus arteriosus to the descending aorta. Therefore, aside from umbilical vein blood, the most highly saturated blood is preductal, and the postductal blood is relatively desaturated.

**16. The answer is C (2, 4)** *[IV A 1].*
Total body water and extracellular water and fluid loss are greater in the preterm infant than in the term

infant; these parameters increase in an exponential manner with decreasing gestational age. Electrolyte replacement begins at 24 hours of age, after the establishment of an adequate urine output. An overload of total body sodium, potassium, and chloride may result if electrolytes are replaced prior to 24 hours of age or before an adequate urine output is established. Insensible water loss is increased by the use of radiant warmers, phototherapy, and an elevated environmental temperature, because these factors all increase evaporative water loss through the relatively thin and poorly keratinized skin of the infant. Pulmonary water losses are not directly measured and are not sensible water losses.

**17. The answer is C (2, 4)** *[V A 4 b (2)].*
Although apnea of prematurity is the most common cause of apnea in a 2-day-old preterm infant, other etiologies must be evaluated before initiating therapy. Failure to perform the appropriate evaluations may result in a delay in the diagnosis and, thus, appropriate treatment of correctable and potentially life-threatening causes of the apnea (e.g., infection, hypoxia, airway obstruction, metabolic disturbances).

**18. The answer is C (2, 4)** *[V F 1 b (2), G 3].*
The two important points in the history described in the question are the length of time between the rupture of the fetal membranes and delivery, which increases the risk for infection, and the use of forceps, which is associated with intracranial trauma and hemorrhage. Although asphyxia is a major cause of seizures during the first day of life, there is nothing in the history to suggest its occurrence (i.e., there has been no history of abnormal fetal heart tracing or meconium-stained fluid, and the Apgar score was normal). Clinical signs of kernicterus are not seen at 12 hours of age.

# 6
# Critical Care
Betty S. Spivack

**I. GOAL AND SCOPE OF CRITICAL CARE MEDICINE.** Critical care is a new and evolving medical specialty concerned with the management of patients whose homeostatic mechanisms have failed. The goals of the specialty are to maintain physiologic balance while treating the underlying derangement. Intensive care physicians have special expertise in ventilatory support, promotion of cardiac output, treatment of acute electrolyte disorders and acute coma, and nutritional support for the critically ill patient. The boundaries of critical care medicine intersect with those of many other specialties, most notably pulmonology, cardiology, neurology, and surgery.

## II. RESUSCITATION

### A. Primary concerns

1. **Basic life support.** Appropriate measures to provide basic life support should preclude all advanced life support measures.

2. **Prompt intervention.** All emergency interventions must be performed immediately and not after time-consuming laboratory tests.

3. **Reassessment** is required after any intervention.

### B. Basic life support

1. **Ventilation** is the most important intervention in the apneic child. The correct amount of ventilation will provide moderate, but not excessive, chest rise.
   a. The airway is assessed for patency. If breathing is not apparent, help is summoned and the head is repositioned in the sniffing position.
   b. Breathing is reassessed and, if not apparent, two slow breaths are administered.
   c. If air entry is impeded, the head is repositioned and the procedure is repeated. If the airway remains impeded, obstructed airway intervention should follow (see II B 3).

2. **Circulation**
   a. The pulse is assessed by palpating the **femoral or brachial pulse** of infants under 12 months and the **carotid pulse** of children older than 1 year.
   b. If no pulse is present, **chest compression** should be initiated and should be coordinated with ventilation (Table 6-1).

3. **Obstructed airway intervention.** Foreign body aspiration should be suspected in children with sudden onset of respiratory distress associated with coughing, gagging, and stridor.
   a. **Infant.** Back blows and chest thrusts are given alternately in sequences of four each, until spontaneous breathing is reestablished or until a manual breath can be delivered.
      (1) **Back blows.** The infant should be straddled over the rescuer's arm, with the head supported, and the blows delivered by the heel of the hand between the infant's shoulder blades.
      (2) **Chest thrusts.** The infant should be turned over, with head and neck supported, and the thrusts performed like slow chest compressions.
   b. **Child.** Subdiaphragmatic thrusts (the **Heimlich maneuver**) are performed until the object is expelled or 10 thrusts have been given. The patient is then reassessed.
      (1) **Unconscious child.** The maneuver is performed with the child on the ground and the

**Table 6-1.** Basic Life Support Maneuvers in Infants and Children

| Resuscitative Maneuver | Infants | Children |
|---|---|---|
| Maintenance breathing | 20 breaths/min | 15 breaths/min |
| Pulse check | Brachial/femoral | Carotid |
| Compression site | Lower third of sternum | Lower third of sternum |
| Compression depth | 0.5–1.0 inch | 1.0–1.5 inch |
| Compression rate | 100/min | 80–100/min |
| Compression:breath ratio | 5:1 with pause for ventilation | 5:1 with pause for ventilation |

rescuer straddling the child. The heel of a fisted hand is placed in the subxiphoid region of the abdomen, with the fist covered by the other hand, and the thrust is given upward, taking care to stay in the midline.

    **(2) Conscious child.** The rescuer stands or sits behind the child, holding the thumb side of the fist against the subxiphoid region of the abdomen. The thrust is given as a quick upward movement, avoiding the xiphoid and internal organs.

  **c. Contraindications**

    **(1)** Airway clearing maneuvers should not be attempted if there is gradual **onset of respiratory symptoms** over hours or days, particularly if the symptoms are associated with fever or other signs of infectious disease.

    **(2)** The Heimlich maneuver should never be performed on **infants younger than 1 year**.

**C. Advanced life support** involves quick cardiopulmonary assessment, therapeutic intervention, and reevaluation.

  **1. Quick cardiopulmonary assessment.** This assessment of the physiologic status of the patient will determine the treatment priorities. The procedure is performed in rapid sequence, taking approximately 30 seconds to 1 minute.

    **a. Assessment areas**

      **(1) Airway.** The airway is assessed for patency and is described as either patent, maintainable by positioning, or unmaintainable (i.e., requiring assisted ventilation, intubation, or other intervention).

      **(2) Breathing** is assessed on the basis of the rate and work of breathing, quality of air entry, and skin color.

      **(3) Circulation** is assessed on the basis of the heart rate, blood pressure, peripheral and central arterial pulses, and skin and central nervous system (CNS) perfusion.

    **b. Sequence of assessment** is as follows:

      **(1) Inspection** of the patient's rate and work of breathing, skin color, and alertness

      **(2) Palpation** of the peripheral and central arterial pulses, skin temperature, capillary refill, response to painful stimulation, and liver edge

      **(3) Auscultation** of the quality of air entry and cardiac sounds

    **c. Physiologic classifications** are defined as follows:

      **(1) Stable:** adequate airway, breathing, and circulation

      **(2) Respiratory distress:** impaired airway and/or breathing but adequate ventilation and maintained alertness

      **(3) Respiratory failure:** impaired ventilation but adequate circulation (see Ch 12 II)

      **(4) Early shock:** decreased perfusion but maintained blood pressure

      **(5) Late shock:** marked hypoperfusion with frank hypotension

      **(6) Cardiopulmonary failure:** bradycardia, agonal respirations, and absence of pulses (it is impossible to know whether cardiopulmonary failure is the result of respiratory or circulatory embarrassment)

      **(7) Cardiopulmonary arrest:** absence of breathing or effective cardiac output

  **2. Therapeutic intervention**

    **a. Stable condition.** Care of the stable child includes evaluation of factors suggested by a more detailed history and physical examination and periodic reassessment of physiologic status.

**b. Respiratory distress.** Children with respiratory distress should be kept in a position of comfort with a parent, with professional staff nearby. Cardiac monitoring and oximetry are appropriate, and oxygen should be applied as tolerated. The diagnostic and therapeutic course should be determined by more complete history and physical examination, and reassessment should be frequent.

**c. Respiratory failure** (see also Ch 12 II). The child in respiratory failure should be separated from parents and monitored with a cardiac monitor and oximetry. The patient should receive high-concentration oxygen via bag-mask or intubation. The patient should be reassessed immediately after any intervention and at frequent intervals thereafter.

**d. Shock.** The child in shock should be separated from parents, monitored with a cardiac monitor, and reassessed frequently. Vascular access should be established with a peripheral intravenous or central venous catheter or by intraosseous technique. Shock due to dysrhythmia or congestive heart failure should be distinguished from that due to other physiologic causes (e.g., dehydration, sepsis). The patient should be reassessed immediately after any intervention and at frequent intervals thereafter.

    **(1)** In the absence of dysrhythmia or congestive heart failure, a fluid bolus of crystalloid or colloid should be given and the child reassessed. Repeat boluses may be required.

    **(2)** In the presence of congestive heart failure, inotropic support via continuous infusion may be necessary (this is relatively uncommon in children). For treatment of dysrhythmia, see II C 2 g.

**e. Cardiopulmonary failure.** The child in cardiopulmonary failure should be monitored with a cardiac monitor, given 100% oxygen ($O_2$) via bag-mask or intubation, and reassessed.

    **(1)** If circulatory status improves, the event most likely is respiratory in origin and should be treated appropriately after further evaluation.

    **(2)** If the patient appears to be in shock, circulatory embarrassment is the apparent triggering event (see II C 2 d for treatment of shock).

**f. Cardiopulmonary arrest.** Ventricular tachycardia and fibrillation are rare causes of cardiac arrest in childhood and should be treated as described in II C 2 g.

    **(1)** The first step in treating cardiac arrest is to initiate basic life support and to begin cardiac monitoring and ventilation with bag-mask or intubation. If possible, vascular access should be established but should not delay therapy. If circulation is not restored with assisted ventilation and cardiac compression, epinephrine should be administered vascularly or endotracheally.

    **(2)** The patient should be reassessed and, if there is persistent asystole or bradycardia, atropine should be given vascularly or endotracheally.

    **(3)** The second reassessment should include blood gas analysis. If marked metabolic acidosis exists in the presence of adequate ventilation, sodium bicarbonate ($NaHCO_3$) may be given but only via the vascular route. **Do not administer bicarbonate via an endotracheal tube.**

**g. Dysrhythmia.** Only unstable dysrhythmias require immediate treatment. Those without cardiac or circulatory instability may await consultation with a pediatric cardiologist prior to treatment.

    **(1) Treatment of bradycardia (slow rhythm).** Most bradycardia in childhood is respiratory in origin. With decreased heart rate, there is low cardiac output.

        **(a)** The initial steps are to oxygenate and ventilate and then reassess.

        **(b)** If bradycardia persists despite adequate oxygenation and ventilation—and hypoperfusion is present—atropine or isoproterenol should be administered. Patients refractory to drug therapy require electrical pacing.

    **(2) Treatment of tachycardia (fast rhythm).** A small stroke volume produces a low cardiac output.

        **(a)** The first step is to determine whether there is a **narrow or wide complex tachycardia**. If narrow complex, the dysrhythmia must be classified as **sinus tachycardia** or **supraventricular tachycardia** (Table 6-2).

            **(i)** Sinus tachycardia in an unstable patient suggests a primary problem with ventilation or perfusion, which should be addressed with appropriate measures.

            **(ii)** Sinus tachycardia in a stable patient may be due to fever, dehydration, anxiety, or pain. The source of the tachycardia should be treated, not the symptom.

            **(iii)** Unstable supraventricular tachycardia and wide complex tachycardia both are treated by prompt synchronized cardioversion.

**Table 6-2.** Distinguishing Sinus from Supraventricular Tachycardia

| Feature | Sinus Tachycardia | Supraventricular Tachycardia |
|---------|-------------------|------------------------------|
| Heart rate | Usually < 200 but may exceed 200 | Usually > 230 |
| ECG | Usually P waves; variable | No P waves; very regular |
| History | Cause for increased rate found (e.g., fever, dehydration, respiratory distress) | Nonspecific symptoms |
| Physical examination | Consistent with history | Instability greater than suggested by history; congestive heart failure usually present in infants |

        **(iv)** Supraventricular tachycardia without instability should not be treated with emergency intervention. A pediatric cardiologist should be consulted promptly.

    **(b)** A pediatric cardiologist should be contacted as soon as possible to coordinate further therapy, but **treatment of unstable patients should not be delayed to get a consult**.

  **(3) Treatment of absent pulse.** Absent pulse (i.e., no effective cardiac output) may result from asystole (most commonly), ventricular tachycardia, ventricular fibrillation, or electromechanical dissociation (which may be due to cardiac failure but more commonly is due to treatable causes such as hypoxia, hypovolemia, electrolyte disturbances, tension pneumothorax, or cardiac tamponade).

    **(a)** The first steps are to ventilate with 100% $O_2$ and initiate basic life support.

    **(b)** If there is asystole, the child should be treated for cardiopulmonary arrest (see II C 2 f).

    **(c)** If there is ventricular fibrillation or pulseless ventricular tachycardia, defibrillation should be performed using an unsynchronized discharge.

    **(d)** If three consecutive shocks are ineffective, epinephrine, lidocaine, bretylium, or procainamide may assist defibrillation. **Note: Ingestion of sympathomimetic or anticholinergic drugs is the most common cause of ventricular tachycardia in childhood.**

**III. RESPIRATORY INTENSIVE CARE.** The purpose of respiratory support is to maintain oxygenation and ventilation at levels consistent with baseline physiologic needs while avoiding complications due to $O_2$ toxicity and barotrauma. The proper level of support is the lowest level required to achieve these goals.

  **A. Derangements of oxygenation and ventilation**

    **1. Oxygenation defects**

      **a. Arterial hypoxemia** may occur with or without an increased alveolar-arterial (A-a) $PO_2$ gradient (Table 6-3). Conditions that do not increase the A-a $PO_2$ gradient cause a decrease in alveolar $PO_2$. Arterial hypoxemia is caused by some combination of the following factors:

        **(1) Shunt ($\dot{V}/\dot{Q}$ = 0).** Blood flow does not come into contact with alveolar gas.

**Table 6-3.** Alveolar-Arterial (A-a) $PO_2$ Gradient and Arterial Hypoxemia

| Cause of Hypoxemia | A-a $PO_2$ Gradient | Effect of Added $O_2$ |
|--------------------|---------------------|------------------------|
| Shunt | Increased | Little or no effect |
| Low $\dot{V}/\dot{Q}$ ratio | Increased | Small effect |
| Hypoventilation | Normal | Increase in $PO_2$ |
| Diffusion defect | Increased | Little or no effect |
| Altitude | Normal | Increase in $PO_2$ |

(2) **$\dot{V}/\dot{Q}$ mismatch ($0 < \dot{V}/\dot{Q} < 1$).** Blood flow to a region exceeds the amount of alveolar gas in that region.

(3) **Hypoventilation ($\dot{V}/\dot{Q} > 1$).** Diminished blood flow in the region of ventilation (equivalent to an increase in dead space ventilation).

(4) **Diffusion deficit.** Ventilation and perfusion are matched, but diffusion is impaired due to an intrinsic membrane defect (rare) or because the time available for gas diffusion is limited (common in patients with decreased compliance or other causes of extreme tachypnea).

(5) **Altitude.** Barometric pressure is decreased, causing a decrease in atmospheric $P_{O_2}$.

  b. **Tissue hypoxia** may be caused by:
  (1) Arterial hypoxemia
  (2) Diminished cardiac output or hypoperfusion
  (3) Shift to the left in the oxyhemoglobin dissociation curve
  (4) Hypoglycemia
  (5) Enzyme deficiency or block in Krebs cycle or electron-transport chain
  (6) Uncoupling of the electron-transport chain from oxidative phosphorylation

2. **Ventilation defects.** Two factors can cause an increase in $P_{CO_2}$.
  a. **Decreased alveolar minute ventilation** may be due to:
  (1) Decreased respiratory drive
  (2) Increased dead space
  (3) Increased work of breathing, exceeding the capacity of the child
  (4) Decreased capacity to perform the work of breathing
  b. **Increased $CO_2$ production** (i.e., in excess of ability to increase alveolar ventilation) may be due to:
  (1) Increased metabolic rate
  (2) Increased metabolic ratio (i.e., ratio of $CO_2$ produced to $O_2$ consumed)

## B. Respiratory support techniques

1. **Supplemental $O_2$** may be provided by nasal cannula, mask, or tent or in association with other techniques of assisted ventilation.
  a. **Purpose.** Supplemental $O_2$ is used to provide sufficiently high $P_{O_2}$ (and $O_2$ content) to maintain the body's physiologic activities. It has no major role in treatment of hypoventilation or hypercarbia.
  b. **Limitations**
  (1) The utility of $O_2$ is limited by its toxicity. In high concentrations (80%–100%) used for long periods (more than 24 hours), $O_2$ is damaging to biologic membranes, including the alveolar capillary membrane.
  (2) Supplemental $O_2$ is not useful for all causes of hypoxemia. It is moderately useful for treating low $\dot{V}/\dot{Q}$ processes but of little or no use in treating processes involving a shunt or diffusion deficit. In general, if adequate oxygenation ($P_{O_2} > 60$) is not obtained using 60% $O_2$ and the need for therapy extends beyond 24 hours, another mode of therapy is needed.

2. **Aids to spontaneous ventilation and oxygenation**
  a. **Continuous positive airway pressure (CPAP),** or the related use of **positive end-expiratory pressure (PEEP),** improves end-expiratory lung volumes in poor compliance–low volume disease states. CPAP (PEEP) may be used in combination with supplemental $O_2$, pressure-supported ventilation, or mechanical ventilation.
  (1) CPAP (PEEP) provides an end-expiratory pressure exceeding ambient barometric pressure (Figure 6-1). This causes an increase in end-expiratory volumes (functional residual capacity), which yields improved $\dot{V}/\dot{Q}$ ratios, decreased shunting, and improved oxygenation.
  (2) Higher lung volumes also mean improved lung compliance, which decreases the work of breathing. This encourages the patient to breathe in a slower, deeper pattern that is more consistent with good gas distribution and diffusion. This effect may improve both oxygenation and ventilation.
  b. **Pressure-supported ventilation** may decrease the work of breathing and increase spontaneous ventilation in a patient in respiratory failure. This technique may be used in association with supplemental $O_2$, PEEP, or mechanical ventilation.

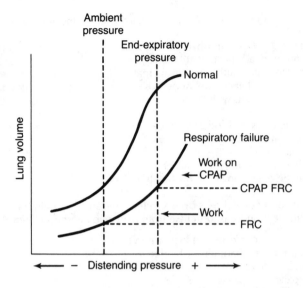

**Figure 6-1.** Effect of the use of continuous positive airway pressure (*CPAP*) on end-expiratory lung volumes in respiratory failure. *FRC* = functional residual capacity.

(1) The technique consists of a machine that increases air flow through a tube as the patient begins to breathe. The machine senses the initiation of a breath, but the patient controls the rate, tidal volume, and inspiratory time.

(2) Resistance to inspiration is substantially decreased by the increase in air flow through the tube, resulting in a larger tidal volume for a given amount of work performed by the patient. This improves the patient's respiratory mechanics, thereby improving gas distribution and diffusion and, subsequently, enhancing ventilation and oxygenation.

c. **Helium-oxygen (He-O$_2$) mixtures** provide less airway resistance, because He is a lighter and less viscous gas than nitrogen. He-O$_2$ mixtures may be used in conjunction with some, but not all mechanical ventilators.

(1) Mixtures containing more than 50% He may improve spontaneous ventilation, breathing pattern, gas distribution, and oxygenation.

(2) This technique may not be tolerated by patients requiring a high fraction of inspired O$_2$ (Fio$_2$).

**3. Mechanical ventilation**

a. **Positive-pressure ventilation** supplies gas directly to the trachea via an endotracheal tube or a tracheostomy. The delivery of gas may be controlled by setting the flow rate and inspiratory time, the volume, or the pressure. All modes may be used with supplementary O$_2$ and PEEP.

(1) With **time-cycled, pressure-limited ventilation,** gas is delivered by setting flow rate, inspiratory time, and a pressure limit. Pressure is determined by the volume and compliance of the patient.

(a) Flow rate will be constant unless the pressure limit is reached.

(b) If the pressure limit is not reached, volumes increase linearly during inspiration. This tends to worsen gas distribution.

(2) With **volume-cycled, pressure-limited ventilation,** gas is delivered by setting tidal volume, inspiratory time, and a pressure limit. Pressure is determined by the preset volume and compliance of the patient.

(a) Flow rate may be constant—essentially the same as a time-cycled ventilator—or decelerating, depending on the ventilator model. A decelerating flow provides most of the volume early in inspiration, resulting in better gas distribution and diffusion.

(b) If the pressure limit is reached, the remaining volume is dumped. Thus, in a patient with worsening compliance, preset volumes may not be reached, causing unsuspected hypoventilation.

(3) With **pressure-cycled ventilation,** gas is delivered by setting inspiratory pressure and inspiratory time. Volume is determined by the preset pressure level and compliance of the patient. This mode of ventilation requires continuous monitoring of expired volumes.

**(a)** Pressure-cycled ventilation is the most effective way to distribute gas in a patient with poor compliance and impaired diffusion. It is most effective combined with a relatively long inspiratory time.

  **(i)** Inspiratory pressure levels are reached almost instantly and continue throughout inspiration.

  **(ii)** This pattern generates high flow rates initially, which diminish over the remainder of the inspiratory period.

**(b)** In a patient with worsening compliance, tidal volumes may decrease at a constant inspiratory pressure level.

  **b. Negative-pressure ventilators** are appropriate only for patients with neuromuscular problems.

  **(1)** With this technique, a vacuum is established around the patient's chest, and the applied negative pressure yields a tidal volume dependent on the compliance of the chest and lung.

  **(2)** Limitations on the negative pressure will unduly limit the tidal volumes and minute ventilation of the patient with poor chest or lung compliance.

## IV. CARDIOVASCULAR INTENSIVE CARE

**A. Invasive monitoring techniques.** In a critically ill patient, any parameter that may indicate a life-threatening change prior to severe deterioration should be monitored frequently or continuously. Such parameters may include cardiac rate and rhythm, arterial pressure, central venous pressure, pulmonary arterial pressure, and cardiac output.

  **1. Arterial pressure.** To monitor, a vascular catheter is placed percutaneously or by cutdown in a peripheral or central artery.

  **a. Indications** include shock, hypertensive crisis, and intravenous (IV) infusion of sympathomimetic antidysrhythmic medications.

  **b. Complications** primarily relate to thrombosis within the artery.

  **2. Central venous pressure.** To monitor, a vascular catheter is placed percutaneously or by cutdown, with the tip in the central veins of the chest or in the right atrium (the latter is more dangerous).

  **a. Indications** include all conditions in which volume status is key to critical management, such as severe congestive heart failure and renal failure.

  **b. Complications** include hemorrhage, air embolus, pneumothorax, and arrhythmias from improper placement in the ventricle or adjacent to the coronary sinus.

  **3. Pulmonary arterial catheterization.** To monitor, a vascular catheter is introduced percutaneously or by cutdown into one of the central veins, and the catheter is advanced through the right atrium and right ventricle and into one of the pulmonary arteries, aided by balloon flotation.

  **a. Data supplied**

  **(1)** With the balloon deflated, a **pulmonary arterial pressure wave** is displayed. With the balloon inflated and properly positioned, a **pulmonary capillary wedge tracing** is displayed, reflecting left atrial filling pressures.

  **(2)** The catheter may be used to determine **cardiac output** by thermodilution technique.

  **(3)** After the pressure and output data have been obtained, **other variables** may be calculated, including pulmonary and systemic vascular resistance and right and left myocardial work.

  **b. Indications** include any condition in which central venous pressure may not accurately reflect left atrial filling pressure or in which repeated, accurate measurement of cardiac output may be required. Such conditions include septic shock, cardiogenic shock, acquired respiratory distress syndrome (ARDS), and post-operative management of patients with impaired cardiovascular function.

  **c. Complications** include those caused by central venous catheterization (see IV A 2 b) as well as pulmonary infarction, ventricular arrhythmias, perforation of the pulmonary artery or cardiac chambers, and rupture of cardiac valves.

**B. Shock** is a complex metabolic state characterized by impaired delivery of $O_2$ and other substrates to the tissues.

1. **General principles**
   a. **Causes**
      (1) **Noncardiovascular causes** include hypoxemia, hypoglycemia, and toxins (e.g., cyanide) that impair delivery and utilization of $O_2$ by the tissues.
      (2) **Cardiovascular causes** include disorders of preload, contractility, or afterload.
   b. **Phases.** All forms of untreated shock go through three phases, which vary in duration depending on the cause. These are:
      (1) **Compensated shock** (normal blood pressure)
      (2) **Uncompensated shock** (low blood pressure)
      (3) **Irreversible shock** (multiple organ system damage)

2. **Types of cardiovascular shock**
   a. **Hypovolemic shock** is due to decreased preload.
      (1) **Compensatory mechanisms** include:
         (a) Antidiuretic hormone (ADH) secretion
         (b) Aldosterone-renin-angiotensin secretion
         (c) Endogenous catecholamine secretion
      (2) **Physiologic responses** include:
         (a) Decreased urine output
         (b) Vasoconstriction
         (c) Tachycardia
         (d) Increased contractility
      (3) **Clinical features** include:
         (a) Tachycardia
         (b) Cool, pale extremities
         (c) Prolonged capillary refill time (> 2 seconds)
         (d) Impaired mental status (late)
         (e) Hypotension (very late)
      (4) **Therapy**
         (a) Circulating volume should be reestablished with crystalloid or colloid solution (see also Ch 13 VII B 5 a).
         (b) Inotropic support is used only in very late hypovolemic shock, when myocardial damage has occurred due to prolonged hypoperfusion. It should be started only after normal circulating volume has been restored.
   b. **Cardiogenic shock** is due to decreased contractility.
      (1) **Compensatory mechanisms** include:
         (a) ADH secretion
         (b) Aldosterone-renin-angiotensin secretion
         (c) Endogenous catecholamine secretion
      (2) **Physiologic responses** include:
         (a) Decreased urine output, leading to hypervolemia
         (b) Vasoconstriction, leading to increased afterload
         (c) Tachycardia
         (d) Further decrease in contractility and cardiac output (due to increased demands from three changes noted above)
      (3) **Clinical features** include:
         (a) Tachycardia
         (b) Cool pale extremities
         (c) Delayed capillary refill
         (d) Impaired mental status
         (e) Hypotension (early)
      (4) **Therapy** consists of:
         (a) Inotropic support with dopamine, dobutamine, or epinephrine
         (b) Vasodilation with nitroprusside (acute) or captopril (chronic)
         (c) Diuresis
   c. **Distributive shock** is due to poor perfusion of tissue beds (afterload).
      (1) **Compensatory mechanisms** are limited to endogenous catecholamine secretion.
      (2) **Physiologic responses** include:
         (a) Tachycardia
         (b) Increased contractility

(3) **Clinical features**
   (a) **Early signs** include fever, extreme tachycardia, low diastolic pressure, normal or slightly increased systolic pressure, bounding pulses, prolonged capillary refill, and impaired level of consciousness.
   (b) **Late signs** are those features seen in cardiogenic shock [see IV B 2 b (3)].
(4) **Therapy** consists of:
   (a) Maintaining circulating volume
   (b) Prolonging the hyperdynamic phase, using inotropic support
   (c) Vasoconstriction, if needed, using an α-agonist
   (d) Correcting the triggering derangements

## C. Postoperative cardiovascular patient

1. **Acute management.** Patients who have been placed on cardiopulmonary bypass for "open heart" procedures exhibit decreased myocardial contractility for the first 24–48 hours postoperatively. This is exaggerated in patients who have undergone vagotomy.
   a. In such patients, there is continuous monitoring of arterial pressure, central venous pressure, left atrial or pulmonary arterial pressure, and ECG tracing.
   b. Cardiac output may be supported by infusion of inotropic agents (e.g., dopamine, dobutamine, epinephrine).
   c. Perfusion may be enhanced by a vasodilator (e.g., nitroprusside).
   d. Monitoring devices and drainage tubes are removed as the patient continues to stabilize.

2. **Complications**
   a. **Pleural or pericardial effusions** may appear in the first week postoperatively or later, as part of the postpericardiotomy syndrome. These usually disappear without treatment but should be monitored until they do. The effusion may require intervention if cardiac output or ventilation is impaired.
   b. Patients with intracardiac repairs may have conduction defects that predispose to **dysrhythmias**. Such patients may require medication to suppress the arrhythmia or may need an implantable pacemaker or, rarely, a defibrillator.
   c. Patients with indwelling grafts or valve devices are at increased risk for **thrombogenesis** and bacterial colonization. Such complications may lead to **stroke** or **endocarditis**.

# V. NEUROLOGIC INTENSIVE CARE

## A. Increased intracranial pressure

1. **Normal physiology**
   a. Intracranial pressure (ICP) is generated as a function of the **compliance of the cranial vault** and the **volume of the intracranial contents,** which include brain parenchyma, cerebrospinal fluid (CSF), intravascular blood, and interstitial fluid. Compliance of the system may vary depending on the degree of ossification of the skull, splitting of the sutures, or the presence or absence of fontanelles.
   b. In the normal situation, cerebral blood flow remains stable over a wide range of states of hydration and blood pressures due to **autoregulation**.

2. **Causes of increased ICP** include:
   a. Increased intracerebral mass (brain tumor)
   b. Increased CSF volume (hydrocephalus)
   c. Increased intravascular blood volume (arteriovenous malformation)
   d. Increased interstitial fluid (cerebral edema)
   e. Extravascular fluid collections (epidural, subdural, subarachnoid, or intracerebral hemorrhage)

3. **Pathophysiology**
   a. ICP may remain constant for a variable period of time after intracranial volume begins to rise through:
      (1) Shunting of blood out of the venous sinuses to the central veins of the chest
      (2) Shunting of CSF out of the ventricles into the spinal cord

    **b.** Whenever intracranial volume exceeds the capacity of the cranial vault to expand, and when shunting of CSF and venous blood have been maximally accomplished, ICP begins to rise dramatically.

    **(1)** The capacity for autoregulation may be lost (i.e., cerebral blood flow may become directly proportional to mean arterial blood pressure).

    **(2)** Pressure exerted on the brain stem may cause the **Cushing reflex** (i.e., bradycardia, hypertension).

    **(3)** Continued increase in ICP may cause herniation and death by compression of brain stem structures (more likely with a mass or with severe cerebral edema).

**4. Therapy**

  **a. Monitoring**

    **(1) ICP** may be measured directly by several devices.

    **(2) Arterial pressure** should be assessed continuously in any patient requiring ICP monitoring.

    **(3) Central venous pressure** monitoring may be required.

    **(4) Cardiac rate and rhythm** should be monitored continuously.

  **b. Reduction of intracranial volume**

    **(1) Brain mass.** Partial or total resection of a tumor may normalize ICP. Other interventions may be required first in a quickly progressive, unstable patient.

    **(2) CSF** may be removed directly from the ventricles via ventriculostomy (useful only in the setting of hydrocephalus).

    **(3) Intravascular blood volume** may be reduced.

      **(a)** Cerebral blood flow is directly proportional to $P_{CO_2}$ within the physiologic range (20–60 mm Hg). Thus, hyperventilation ($P_{CO_2}$ = 25–30 mm Hg) reduces blood volume and ICP.

      **(b)** Cerebral vasoconstriction also may be achieved by using continuous infusion of short-acting barbiturates (e.g., pentobarbital).

      **(c)** Elevation of the head may promote drainage of venous blood into the internal jugular veins.

    **(4) Interstitial fluid** may be reduced with:

      **(a)** Osmotic diuresis with mannitol

      **(b)** Mild dehydration

      **(c)** Barbiturates

      **(d)** Steroids

    **(5) Extravascular fluid collections** should be removed if they demonstrate a significant mass effect. Other, quicker techniques (e.g., hyperventilation) should be used initially in the acute situation.

  **c. Increased cranial compliance** may be accomplished by:

    **(1) Craniotomy** (burr holes)

    **(2) Hemicraniectomy** is a deforming, palliative technique, not often used anymore.

    **(3)** Opening of the sutures may temporarily decrease pressure and symptoms, even in the presence of an expanding mass.

**B. Brain death** is a state characterized by **complete and irreversible brain and brain stem failure**. Physical examination or other testing reveals no brain or brain stem function at any level.

**1. General principles**

  **a. Somatic death.** Brain death is invariably followed by somatic death, even if the body is maintained by mechanical ventilation and inotropic support.

    **(1)** The usual mechanism of somatic death is progressive hypotension that becomes increasingly unresponsive to catecholamines.

    **(2)** This process may take anywhere from several days to several weeks.

  **b. Legality of brain death.** All states now accept brain death as actual death.

    **(1)** Some states have appellate rulings that declare brain death to be equivalent to somatic death, thus negating the need for treatment.

    **(2)** The remaining states have legislation dictating that brain death is equivalent to actual death.

  **c. Pediatric brain death**

    **(1)** Brain death is difficult to assess in young children due to developmental issues. States of apparent brain death have been followed by prolonged survival and some degree of recovery in very young children and frequently in premature infants.

    **(2)** Standards for diagnosis of brain death in various age-groups are summarized in Table 6-4.

**2. Physical examination** must be performed when the body temperature is greater than 35° C and when no medications or toxins are present in concentrations that may cause coma. This will require artificial warming of the patient, as the brain-dead patient is unable to control temperature and is hypothermic. Function in any of the following areas is incompatible with the diagnosis of brain death.

  **a. Cortical functions**
    **(1)** Any pain response other than simple withdrawal, which may be a spinal cord response
    **(2)** Presence of deep tendon reflexes and nonflaccid limbs
    **(3)** Voluntary movement, localization, decorticate or decerebrate posturing
  **b. Midbrain functions**
    **(1)** Temperature control
    **(2)** Oculovestibular responses ("doll's eyes," "caloric" responses)
  **c. Cranial nerve functions**
    **(1)** Pupillary, corneal, and gag reflexes
    **(2)** Sucking movements
  **d. Respiratory drive** is assessed via **apnea test**.
    **(1)** The patient is preoxygenated with 100% $O_2$ for 5 minutes but must have a normal $P_{CO_2}$ (> 35 mm Hg) at the beginning of the test.
    **(2)** Mechanical ventilation is stopped, and heart rate and respiration are observed continuously for 5 minutes or until heart rate begins to fall.
    **(3)** A greater than 20 mm Hg increase in arterial $P_{CO_2}$, without spontaneous ventilation, is required.

**3. Neurophysiologic testing** is used to rule out continued activity or perfusion of the brain. Absence of the expected finding is compatible with brain death.

  **a. EEG** is the oldest technique available for this assessment, but it is time-consuming and prone to produce artifacts. To be reliable, the EEG requires:
    **(1)** A body temperature above 35° C
    **(2)** Absence of coma-producing levels of drugs (e.g., barbiturates), which may reversibly suppress cortical function
    **(3)** Careful attention to eliminate electrical artifact caused by life-support equipment
    **(4)** Recording of response to painful stimulation
    **(5)** ECG and muscle tracings as well as the standard cephalic leads
    **(6)** High sensitivity (3 mV) recording
  **b. Evoked brain stem potentials** assess brain stem transmission of external stimuli and may be helpful in assessing absence of brain stem function at certain levels. Both auditory and somatosensory evoked responses have been studied in this setting.
  **c. Four-vessel cerebral angiography** studies cerebral blood flow after injection of dye into the internal carotid and vertebral arteries. Brain death is associated with absence of cerebral blood flow for reasons that are not well understood. This test is very invasive and difficult to perform in a child who is on multiple forms of life support.
  **d. Isotope brain scanning** may be used in the pediatric intensive care setting, if a portable gamma counter is available. Otherwise, it too is difficult to perform in a critically ill child, although less so than angiography. Isotope brain scanning is somewhat less reliable than four-vessel angiography.

**Table 6-4.** Standards for Pediatric Brain Death Determination

| Age-Group* | Observation Period | EEG Testing |
|---|---|---|
| 7 days–2 months | Two examinations separated by 48 hours | Two examinations separated by 48 hours |
| 2 months–1 year | Two examinations separated by 24 hours | Two examinations separated by 24 hours |
| Older than 1 year | Two examinations separated by 12–24 hours | None required; observation period may be reduced if isoelectric EEG is obtained |

*No standards exist for premature infants or for term infants during the first week of life.

## VI. TRAUMA

### A. General principles

**1. Mortality**

    **a. Accidental trauma** is the leading cause of death in children older than 1 year of age (see Ch 2 I B).

    **b. Inflicted trauma** (child abuse) may be the leading cause of death in children between 1 month and 1 year of age (see Ch 3 VIII).

**2. Management.** Children with severe trauma are treated in a hospital with pediatric surgeons and a pediatric intensive care unit. They should be rapidly transferred to such a facility after initial stabilization and not delayed in an inappropriate facility for time-consuming diagnostic tests.

**3. Prevention.** While appropriate management of the traumatized child will improve survival and morbidity statistics, the largest improvement in these areas will come from injury prevention programs and recognition of abusive families.

### B. Initial assessment

**1.** Quick assessment of **airway stability, respirations, circulation,** and **organ function** is required. Large-bore intravenous access is established at this time.

**2.** A rapid **physical examination** is done, which assesses external evidence of trauma and neurologic status after the neck has been stabilized.

**3.** Initial **emergent interventions** (see VI C) are performed.

**4.** Appropriate **x-rays,** including cervical spine films, are done rapidly, preferably in an appropriately equipped trauma room rather than in a radiology suite.

**5. Blood tests** (e.g., arterial blood gas, hematocrit, coagulation studies, electrolytes, cardiac enzymes, hepatic enzymes, amylase, lipase) are performed.

**6.** The **bladder is cannulated,** and urine is evaluated for flow and presence of blood.

**7. Further radiologic tests,** such as a cystogram and head or abdominal CT scans, are done if indicated.

**8. Diagnostic peritoneal lavage** is done if emergent treatment of another site requires immediate surgery and precludes abdominal CT studies.

### C. Therapy. The patient should be observed and treated in a pediatric intensive care unit.

**1. Airway instability** is treated by endotracheal intubation, tracheotomy, or cricoidotomy.

**2. Respiratory distress** is treated by manual or mechanical ventilation and, depending on the examination or setting, placement of thoracostomy tubes to both diagnose and treat potential pneumothorax and hemothorax.

**3. Hypoperfusion** is treated by volume therapy with isotonic crystalloid, colloid, or blood. A pericardial tap may be indicated to rule out and treat potential cardiac tamponade from hemopericardium. Inotropic support is rarely indicated.

**4. Surgical intervention** is guided by the patient's status and the results of the diagnostic evaluation.

### D. Specific injuries

**1. Head injuries** may require neurosurgical procedures for relief of **intracranial hematomas.** Fewer than 20% of children with severe head injury have such lesions. Most have severe **cerebral edema** associated with increased ICP not susceptible to surgical intervention.

    **a. Patients with cerebral edema and evidence of increased ICP** should have an intracranial pressure monitoring device placed and be treated as described in V A 4. Appropriate rehabilitation should begin as early as possible, with passive range of motion (to prevent joint contractures) performed as soon as such stimulation does not cause a dangerous rise in ICP.

    **b. Infants with intracranial injuries suggestive of child abuse** must be evaluated completely for other occult injuries, particularly **occult fractures.**

**(1)** Intracranial injuries highly suggestive of abuse include interhemispheric subarachnoid/subdural bleeds, acute and chronic subdural hematomas, retinal hemorrhages, and cerebral edema.

**(2)** The likelihood of abuse increases dramatically if these injuries are found in a child with no history of severe impact or deceleration trauma. Falls from less than 3 feet are insufficient to explain such injuries.

**2. Hepatic and splenic lacerations** are best diagnosed by abdominal CT scan. Surgical repair or resection rarely is required; usually, such lesions tamponade, followed by hemostasis and healing.

  **a. Nonoperative management,** best performed in a pediatric intensive care unit, is predicated on close observation for evidence of:

  **(1)** Hypoperfusion

  **(2)** Hypotension

  **(3)** Falling hematocrit

  **(4)** Change in physical examination

  **b. Operative management** is indicated for:

  **(1)** Continued bleeding requiring large volume transfusions

  **(2)** Shock

  **(3)** Associated trauma or medical conditions that make appropriate observation impossible

**3. Seat belt injuries**

  **a. Types.** Inappropriate use of lap belts in small children may lead to a triad of **abdominal injuries,** including hepatic or splenic laceration, dislocation of the lumbosacral spine, and visceral contusion. The small bowel and pancreas are frequent sites of injury; vascular trauma also may occur.

  **b. Signs.** Seat belt injury may be indicated by external bruising of the abdomen where the lap belt applied pressure.

  **c. Therapy** is specific for the lesions that are identified.

**4. Spinal cord trauma**

  **a. Evaluation**

  **(1)** Evaluation of the spinal column should be done immediately in all cases of multiple or severe trauma. Cervical support should be continued until the entire cervical spine, including the odontoid process, has been adequately evaluated.

  **(2)** The comatose drowning victim must also be evaluated for cervical trauma secondary to vertex compression from a diving accident.

  **b. Complications.** Unrecognized fractures or dislocations of the spinal column may lead to paraplegia, quadriplegia, or death due to inappropriate handling.

  **c. Therapy**

  **(1)** Stabilization of the vertebral column by halo traction or operative spinal fusion is mandatory.

  **(2)** Glucocorticoid or $GM_1$ ganglioside administration in the initial post-trauma period may limit ultimate severity of sequelae.

  **(3)** Supportive care may include mechanical ventilation, bladder catheterization, and adaptive equipment.

  **(4)** Associated injuries must be treated appropriately.

**5. Orthopedic injuries.** Any fracture occurring in a child younger than 6–12 months of age is highly suggestive of abuse etiology and should be followed by a complete plain film and isotope skeletal survey to rule out other occult fractures. Metabolic bone diseases should be ruled out by appropriate x-ray and blood testing.

  **a.** Fractures especially indicative of abusive trauma include:

  **(1)** Metaphyseal corner fractures

  **(2)** Posterior rib fractures

  **(3)** Spiral or oblique fractures in a pre-ambulatory child

  **(4)** Stellate or widely diastatic skull fractures

  **b.** Abusive fractures in infancy are frequently associated with intracranial injury, and head CT should be done in all such cases.

  **c.** Damage to growth plates in young children may be difficult to assess by x-ray and may result in disparity of growth in those regions.

## VII. NUTRITIONAL SUPPORT DURING CRITICAL ILLNESS

### A. High stress states (sepsis and multiple trauma)

1. **Metabolic pathophysiology**
   a. Secretion of counter-regulatory hormones (e.g., endogenous catecholamines, glucocorticoids, glucagon) leads to **relative insulin resistance** and **hyperglycemia**.
   b. Hyperpyrexia, increased cardiac demands, and healing of wounds lead to a **marked increase in metabolic activity, oxygen** and **energy consumption,** and **carbon dioxide generation**.
   c. These increased metabolic demands lead to a requirement for **increased alveolar ventilation** and may predispose to early **respiratory failure**.
   d. In the absence of adequate caloric and protein sources, muscle proteins are broken down for gluconeogenesis and amino acids for protein synthesis.
   e. These processes may lead to severe **malnutrition** in a short period. This state is associated with anergy, infectious complications, and high mortality.

2. **Nutritional support**
   a. **General guidelines**
      (1) Multiple organ failure or abdominal trauma may prevent early enteral feeding. In this case, parenteral alimentation using the specific guidelines given in VII A 2 b should be established within the first 48 hours of treatment.
      (2) Enteral feeding during the hypermetabolic phase should also conform to the need for increased protein sources. This may be accomplished by using formulas designed for the severely stressed patient or by adding protein supplements to more standard enteral formulas.
   b. **Specific guidelines**
      (1) A **positive nitrogen balance** should be provided as soon as possible. This will require higher protein/calorie ratios than a normal diet, as carbohydrates are being handled inefficiently.
      (2) Provision of **fat** in the early period will prevent essential fatty acid deficiency and may decrease $CO_2$ production by lowering the metabolic ratio. This may help prevent or ameliorate respiratory failure.
      (3) The increased metabolic requirements in such patients imply that **calories** must be provided in substantially more than normal amounts to prevent muscle breakdown for energy generation.

### B. Renal failure (see also Ch 13 IX)

1. **Metabolic pathophysiology**
   a. Impaired excretion of nitrogen as urea leads to **uremia** with the potential for contributing to platelet dysfunction and hyperosmolar states. Limited caloric intake, causing muscle breakdown for gluconeogenesis as an energy source, may increase urea production and worsen uremia.
   b. Impaired ability to excrete water leads to **hypervolemia,** exacerbated by excess sodium ingestion.
   c. Impaired ability to synthesize vitamin $D_3$ leads to **hypocalcemia, hyperphosphatemia,** and **secondary hyperparathyroidism**.

2. **Nutritional support** may be provided parenterally using relatively low amounts of well-balanced essential amino acid preparations in conjunction with carbohydrates and lipids. Enteral nutrition should be done with a diet or enteral formula that conforms to the following guidelines.
   a. The nutritional source must be low in protein, sodium, and phosphate.
   b. The nutritional source must provide adequate calories to meet metabolic needs.

### C. Hepatic failure (see also Ch 10 IX D)

1. **Metabolic pathophysiology**
   a. Extreme hepatic insufficiency causes an inability to detoxify $NH_3$ to urea and, thus, may result in **hyperammonemia,** a state that is highly toxic to the brain.
   b. A relative inability to metabolize aromatic amino acids may lead to high concentrations of these substances. In association with hyperammonemia and the other derangements caused by fulminant hepatic failure, this may lead to **hepatic encephalopathy**.

    **c.** An inability to store glucose as glycogen and impaired hepatic gluconeogenesis create an intolerance of fasting and result in **hypoglycemia**.

    **d.** Impaired production and secretion of bile acids may cause **impaired absorption of long-chain fatty acids**.

  **2. Nutritional support**

    **a.** Protein sources must be limited to help prevent hyperammonemia. Some authorities recommend additionally limiting sources containing aromatic amino acids.

    **b.** High carbohydrate density sources should be used as continuous infusions (parenteral or enteral) to prevent hypoglycemia.

## BIBLIOGRAPHY

Chameides L: *Textbook of Pediatric Advanced Life Support.* Dallas, American Heart Association, 1988.

Plum F, Posner JB: *The Diagnosis of Stupor and Coma,* 3rd edition. Philadelphia, FA Davis, 1980.

Rogers MC: *Handbook of Pediatric Intensive Care,* Baltimore, Williams & Wilkins, 1989.

Touloukian RJ: *Pediatric Trauma,* 2nd edition. St. Louis, Mosby-Year Book, 1990.

West JB: *Pulmonary Pathophysiology,* 2nd edition. Baltimore, Williams & Wilkins, 1982.

## STUDY QUESTIONS

**Directions:** Each of the numbered items or incomplete statements in this section is followed by answers or by completions of the statement. Select the **one** lettered answer or completion that is **best** in each case.

1. Which of the following statements is true regarding the treatment of a child with an obstructed airway?

(A) Airway clearing maneuvers should be used in all situations where a child cannot spontaneously ventilate because of an obstructed airway

(B) Foreign body aspiration is suggested by the sudden onset of respiratory distress and stridor

(C) The Heimlich maneuver is used only in children older than 2 years

(D) When the Heimlich maneuver is inappropriate, back blows should be given until the airway is cleared

(E) Correct placement of the hands for the Heimlich maneuver is over the lower third of the sternum

2. Quick cardiopulmonary assessment includes evaluation of all of the following EXCEPT

(A) ECG tracing

(B) work of breathing

(C) skin perfusion

(D) airway patency

3. Increased intracranial pressure may be reduced by all of the following EXCEPT

(A) mannitol

(B) pentabarbital infusion

(C) ventriculostomy

(D) hypoventilation

(E) resection of a brain tumor

4. Which of the following statements regarding hepatic lacerations due to blunt abdominal trauma is true?

(A) The injury is best demonstrated by radionuclide liver and spleen scan

(B) The laceration typically requires surgical exploration and repair

(C) The injury may be prevented in young children by appropriate use of seat belts

(D) Hepatic lacerations usually are not associated with other significant injuries

**Directions:** Each item below contains four suggested answers of which **one or more** is correct. Choose the answer

**A**   if **1, 2, and 3** are correct
**B**   if **1 and 3** are correct
**C**   if **2 and 4** are correct
**D**   if **4** is correct
**E**   if **1, 2, 3, and 4** are correct

5. Results of pressure-supported ventilation in a patient with respiratory failure may include

(1) improved lung compliance due to increased functional residual capacity

(2) increased alveolar ventilation due to decreased work of breathing

(3) increased tidal volume due to improved lung compliance of the patient

(4) increased oxygenation due to improved gas distribution and diffusion

| | |
|---|---|
| 1-B | 4-C |
| 2-A | 5-C |
| 3-D | |

6. True statements regarding management of pediatric dysrhythmias include which of the following?

(1) Children with a heart rate greater than 200 require emergent antidysrhythmic therapy
(2) Atropine may be given for unstable bradycardia via endotracheal tube if vascular access has not been obtained
(3) Verapamil is the treatment of choice for infants with supraventricular tachycardia
(4) Defibrillation is performed using an unsynchronized discharge

7. All forms of shock are characterized by

(1) impaired delivery of $O_2$ and other metabolic substrates to the tissues
(2) decreased blood pressure
(3) impaired level of consciousness
(4) decreased cardiac output

8. Forms of mechanical ventilation include

(1) time-cycled, pressure-limited ventilation
(2) volume-cycled, pressure-limited ventilation
(3) pressure-cycled ventilation
(4) negative pressure ventilation

**Directions:** Each group of items in this section consists of lettered options followed by a set of numbered items. For each item, select the **one** lettered option that is most closely associated with it. Each lettered option may be selected once, more than once, or not at all.

**Questions 9–12**

For each case described below, select the therapeutic intervention most likely to be of benefit.

(A) Isotonic crystalloid infusion
(B) Dobutamine infusion
(C) Atropine administration
(D) Synchronized cardioversion

9. An infant presents with cardiac arrest. After intubation and ventilation, the patient is centrally pink and has a heart rate of 40 and systolic blood pressure of 50 mm Hg.

10. An infant presents with a 3-day history of profuse diarrhea. The patient has a heart rate of 200 and decreased perfusion with diminished peripheral pulses.

11. A child with known cardiomyopathy and congestive heart failure presents with decreased level of consciousness and hypotension after 1 day of symptoms of upper respiratory infection.

12. A child who has been involved in an automobile accident presents with impaired perfusion and a systolic blood pressure of 60 mm Hg.

**Questions 13–17**

Match each statement concerning respiratory support techniques with the technique it best describes.

(A) CPAP
(B) Pressure-supported ventilation
(C) Supplemental $O_2$
(D) Positive pressure ventilation
(E) He-$O_2$ mixtures

13. This technique decreases work of breathing by increasing the flow provided during spontaneous inspiration.

14. With this technique, breaths are mechanically generated.

15. This technique is ineffective if $O_2$ requirements exceed 50% $O_2$.

16. With this technique, arterial oxygenation may improve secondary to increased alveolar $P_{O_2}$.

17. This technique decreases work of breathing by improving compliance and increasing functional residual capacity.

| | | | |
|---|---|---|---|
| 6-C | 9-C | 12-A | 15-E |
| 7-B | 10-A | 13-B | 16-C |
| 8-E | 11-B | 14-D | 17-A |

## ANSWERS AND EXPLANATIONS

**1. The answer is B** *[II B 3]*.
Foreign body aspiration is suggested by the sudden onset of respiratory distress, stridor, coughing, and gagging. Airway clearing maneuvers should not be performed when fever, symptoms of upper respiratory infection, or slow onset of distress suggests an infectious etiology for the airway obstruction. The Heimlich maneuver (subdiaphragmatic thrusts) is the intervention of choice in children older than 1 year with airway obstruction secondary to suspected foreign body aspiration. The maneuver is performed by thrusting upward with a double fist placed midline below the diaphragm. In infants too young for the Heimlich maneuver, foreign body aspiration with obstruction should be treated with sequences of four back blows alternating with four chest thrusts.

**2. The answer is A** *[II C 1 a]*.
The quick cardiopulmonary assessment is an abbreviated physical examination designed to evaluate airway patency, breathing, and circulation rapidly. Breathing is assessed by rate, quality of air entry, work of breathing, and skin color. Circulation is assessed through heart rate, blood pressure, peripheral and central arterial pulses, and skin and central nervous system (CNS) perfusion. An ECG tracing is not included in the quick cardiopulmonary assessment.

**3. The answer is D** *[V A 4 b]*.
Cerebral blood flow is directly proportional to carbon dioxide tension ($PCO_2$). Therefore, hypoventilation tends to increase cerebral blood flow, increasing intracranial volume and intracranial pressure (ICP). Hyperventilation is a technique used to lower ICP. Other techniques include osmotic diuresis, barbiturate infusions, removal of intracranial masses, and removal of cerebrospinal fluid (CSF) via ventriculostomy.

**4. The answer is C** *[VI D 2–3]*.
Hepatic lacerations are best demonstrated by abdominal CT scan. Most typically, the lesion tamponades and does not require surgical repair. These injuries may occur in conjunction with other abdominal or extra-abdominal injuries and often are the result of inappropriate use of a lap belt by very young children. In this setting, the laceration often is accompanied by surface bruising, intestinal injury, and lumbar vertebral dislocation.

**5. The answer is C (2, 4)** *[III B 2 b]*.
Pressure-supported ventilation is a technique that aids spontaneous ventilation of a patient. The tidal volume, respiratory rate, and inspiratory time all are under the control of the patient. The increased flow rates provided by the machine during spontaneous inspiration decrease the work of breathing and may improve alveolar ventilation. This improvement in respiratory mechanics also may lead to improved gas distribution and diffusion, thus improving oxygenation. Functional residual capacity is not significantly affected by pressure-supported ventilation.

**6. The answer is C (2, 4)** *[II C 2 g; Table 6-2]*.
Sinus tachycardia may be in excess of 200 beats/min in young infants, whereas supraventricular tachycardia usually exceeds 230 beats/min in this age-group. Sinus tachycardia usually is caused by anxiety, respiratory distress, or shock and should not be treated by antidysrhythmic drugs or cardioversion. Unstable supraventricular tachycardia is best treated by prompt synchronized cardioversion. Defibrillation is performed in an unsynchronized fashion, since there is no regular QRS tracing with which to synchronize.

**7. The answer is B (1, 3)** *[IV B 1–2]*.
Shock is a state characterized by inadequate delivery of oxygen ($O_2$) and other substrates to the tissues. The CNS is highly sensitive to this; thus, level of consciousness will decrease regardless of the cause of shock. Low blood pressure is characteristic of uncompensated shock and is not a requirement for the diagnosis of shock. Children compensate for decreased circulating volume remarkably well. As a result, frank hypotension occurs very late in pediatric hypovolemic shock, long after lethargy, anuria, and metabolic acidosis have appeared. Distributive forms of shock (e.g., septic shock) are characterized by an increase in cardiac output in the early phase; this form of shock is due to vasodilation and shunting of blood away from the capillary beds.

**8. The answer is E (all)** *[III B 3]*.
There are two main types of mechanical ventilators: positive-pressure ventilators and negative-pressure

ventilators. In positive-pressure ventilation, machine cycling may be determined by flow rate and inspiratory time (time-cycled), volume (volume-cycled), or inspiratory pressure (pressure-cycled). Time-cycled and volume-cycled ventilators have a pressure limit setting, so that dangerously high pressures may be avoided.

**9–12. The answers are: 9-C** *[II C 2 g (1)],* **10-A** *[II C 2 d (1); IV B 2 a],* **11-B** *[II C 2 d (2); IV B 2 b],* **12-A** *[VI C 3].*
The child with bradycardia that is not relieved by oxygenation and ventilation requires pharmacologic support with an agent such as atropine. Children with hypovolemia require fluid support, whether the hypovolemia is due to dehydration (as in the child with a history of diarrhea) or trauma (as in the child who was involved in an automobile accident). A heart rate of 200 in an infant is more likely to be sinus tachycardia than supraventricular tachycardia, which typically involves a heart rate exceeding 230 and a nonspecific history. Children with cardiogenic shock (as in the child with congestive heart failure) need inotropic support with an agent such as dobutamine.

**13–17. The answers are: 13-B** *[III B 2 b],* **14-D** *[III B 3 a],* **15-E** *[III B 2 c],* **16-C** *[III B 1],* **17-A** *[III B 2 a].*
Aids to spontaneous ventilation include pressure-supported ventilation (which diminishes work of breathing by decreasing airway resistance), helium-oxygen ($He-O_2$) mixtures (which are ineffective with less than 50% He), and continuous positive airway pressure, or CPAP (which improves functional residual capacity and compliance). Positive-pressure ventilators generate gas flow mechanically and then push it into the patient's airway. Supplemental $O_2$ does not change respiratory mechanics but improves oxygenation by raising alveolar $Po_2$ levels.

# 7

# Birth Defects and Genetic Disorders

Suzanne B. Cassidy
David A. H. Whiteman

## I. OVERVIEW

**A. Definition.** Medically significant birth defects are congenital anomalies that require some form of medical intervention. Birth defects range in severity from relatively minor anomalies (e.g., polydactyly) to severe or systemic conditions (e.g., hydrocephalus, Down syndrome).

**B. Incidence.** The population risk for medically significant birth defects is approximately 3% of all live-born infants. However, not all birth defects are detected at birth; for example, some forms of kidney disorders, congenital heart disease, and mental retardation are diagnosed later in life. Congenital anomalies cause 10% of all neonatal deaths.

**C. Etiologic classification.** The entire spectrum of human development is guided by the interaction of genetic makeup and the environment. Most birth defects are caused by environmental factors, genetic alterations, or a combination of both. In some cases, birth defects are caused by unknown factors and are called sporadic disorders.

**1. Environmental factors** are known to cause at least 10% of all birth defects. **Teratogens** are environmental agents that cause congenital anomalies by interfering with embryonic or fetal organogenesis, growth, or cellular physiology or by disrupting previously normal tissue (see II).

**2. Genetic disorders.** Genetic factors are responsible for many **single birth defects** as well as many **syndromes** (see I D 2).
  **a. Major forms of genetic disorders** are:
    **(1)** Single gene disorders (see III)
    **(2)** Chromosome disorders (see IV)
    **(3)** Multifactorial disorders (see V)
  **b. Contiguous gene deletion syndromes** are a newly recognized class of human genetic disorders due to the absence of several neighboring genes. These defects cause recognizable but variable conditions, often with several diverse manifestations. In some cases, microdeletions are visible by high-resolution chromosome analysis; in others, they are not. The recognition of such syndromes can be aided by review of the rapidly accumulating information on the human gene pool.

**3. Sporadic disorders** present no risk to future offspring. These disorders often are due to accidents of embryonic development or gestation (e.g., blood vessel occlusion). Some birth defects probably are due to new autosomal dominant mutations that are lethal prior to reproductive age or that interfere with the reproductive potential of affected individuals. These defects are difficult to distinguish from sporadic disorders.

**D. Dysmorphism and syndromes**

**1. Dysmorphism** is an abnormality in form or structural development. The presence of abnormal physical features often suggests an underlying (often genetic) disorder and sometimes portends the presence of other (internal) abnormalities of form or function.
  **a. Dysmorphic features** are those that fall outside the range of normal.
    **(1) Causes of dysmorphic features** fall into three major categories.
      **(a) Malformations** result from poor tissue formation caused by single gene, multifactorial, or chromosomal disorders or to accidents or teratogens.

         **(b)** **Deformations** result from unusual forces on normal tissues, particularly abnormal mechanical forces in utero.

            **(i)** **Maternal causes** include a small or malformed uterus, crowding due to fibroids or multiple gestation, and oligohydramnios.

            **(ii)** **Fetal causes** include poor fetal movement (e.g., neuromuscular problems), malformation, and abnormal position.

         **(c)** **Disruptions** involve a breakdown of normal tissues due to infection, vascular occlusion, or mechanical forces (e.g., amniotic bands).

     **(2)** **Objectively measurable features.** For many features (e.g., height, weight, head circumference), there are objectively measurable norms.

         **(a)** An example is interpupillary distance: Patients whose distance is measurably smaller than normal have **hypotelorism,** and patients whose distance is greater than normal have **hypertelorism**.

         **(b)** Other measurable features include inner canthal and outer canthal distances, ear length, hand and foot length, penis and clitoral length, and upper-to-lower segment ratios.

     **(3)** **Subjectively observable features.** Some features must be judged subjectively by contrast with the normal population.

         **(a)** Examples of subjectively observable dysmorphic features include a flat facial profile, a small chin, a down-turned mouth, an abnormally curled ear, and abnormal palmar creases.

         **(b)** Subjectively observable dysmorphic features require careful observation. The features of a dysmorphic-appearing child should be compared with those of the parents in an attempt to distinguish between subjectively dysmorphic features and familial characteristics. One or more dysmorphic features may be present in otherwise completely normal individuals.

  **b.** **Minor anomalies** are unusual morphologic features that are of no serious medical or cosmetic consequence to the patient.

     **(1)** Examples include ear pits, toe syndactyly, curved fifth fingers, and unusual ear shape.

     **(2)** The significance of minor anomalies is that they serve as valuable clues to a possible underlying pattern of malformation or to isolated major internal malformations.

     **(3)** The presence of **two or more minor anomalies** should lead to a more extensive evaluation of the patient.

**2.** **Syndromes** are recognizable patterns of internal and/or external structural and functional abnormalities or malformations that are known or presumed to be due to a single cause. Recognizable patterns of dysmorphic features, with or without other abnormalities, often constitute syndromes; Down syndrome is a classic example of dysmorphic features in a recognizable pattern [see IV B 1 b (1)]. Some syndromes, however, have no associated dysmorphic features.

  **a.** Every feature that is part of a syndrome need not necessarily be present in a given individual with the syndrome. Individuals with the same syndrome share a number of features, but not necessarily any one feature or any specific combination of them. In most cases, no one feature is pathognomonic for a syndrome.

  **b.** It is not uncommon for the features characteristic of syndromes to develop over time, so that it may not always be possible to make a diagnosis in a very young child.

  **c.** Syndromes can be sporadic of unknown etiology, or caused by single gene abnormalities, chromosomal anomalies, teratogens, or deformations.

**3.** **Patient evaluation.** The presence of dysmorphic features in a patient should lead to the search for other abnormalities and for an underlying disorder. A careful evaluation of the dysmorphic child is important so that a diagnosis can be reached. Diagnosis currently is achieved in about 50% of dysmorphic children.

  **a.** A **prenatal history** should be taken, with particular attention to potential causes of abnormal features such as mechanical forces (e.g., oligohydramnios, abnormal uterine structure, abnormal fetal position, abnormal fetal activity, twinning, fibroids) or teratogens (e.g., medications, illicit drugs).

  **b.** A **family history,** including a **pedigree,** should be obtained, paying special attention to physical or mental abnormality, pregnancy loss, and consanguinity.

  **c.** A thorough **physical examination** should be performed, focusing on physical features and growth and development to seek a pattern of features that has been previously described.

    **d.** A complete **neurologic examination,** including an ophthalmologic examination, is important.

    **e.** **Laboratory studies** should be performed to determine whether there are internal organ abnormalities. Tests may include cardiac and renal ultrasound, cranial ultrasound, computed tomography (CT) scan or magnetic resonance imaging (MRI), a chromosome study, and a skeletal x-ray survey.

**E. Genetic counseling** is made available to individuals who have a positive history of genetic disorders or other birth defects and to those who are at increased risk for having a child with a birth defect.

    **1. Establishing a specific diagnosis.** Genetic diagnosis and counseling involve examination by trained individuals, leading to specific diagnosis. The ability to make a specific diagnosis allows better medical management of affected individuals, since the natural history of etiologically separate disorders with similar manifestations may be very different.

    **2. Evaluating recurrence risk.** Once a diagnosis has been made, it becomes possible to discuss recurrence risks for birth defects and **prenatal diagnosis** for future pregnancies.

        **a.** If a couple has a child with a specific genetic condition, that couple's risk for having another child with a birth defect equals their risk for having a child with this specific condition plus the background risk of 3% with each pregnancy.

        **b.** If a birth defect is caused by a known environmental agent (e.g., radiation, alcohol), the risk for recurrence of the specific birth defect in future pregnancies can sometimes be eliminated by avoidance of that (or a related) environmental agent during pregnancy, although there remains the background risk of 3% for all birth defects in each pregnancy.

    **3. Pedigree analysis** is the first step in most genetic counseling. A four-generation pedigree is constructed for each family, including all medical information.

        **a. Ethnic background** is ascertained for all family members, since some conditions (especially autosomal recessive disorders) occur with increased frequency in specific populations. Certain ethnic subgroups of individuals are at increased risk for having children with specific autosomal recessive disorders due to inbreeding.

            **(1)** Ashkenazi Jews and French Canadians are at increased risk for **Tay-Sachs disease**.

            **(2)** Individuals of Greek, Italian, and other Mediterranean descent are at increased risk for β **thalassemia**.

            **(3)** African blacks and African-Americans have an increased risk for **sickle-cell disease**.

            **(4)** Southeast Asians have an increased risk for α **thalassemia**.

            **(5)** Individuals of Northern European descent have an increased risk for **cystic fibrosis**.

        **b. Family history of birth defects and pregnancy loss** is noted, since they may give clues to genetic disorders.

        **c. Husband-wife consanguinity** is noted, since this leads to an increased risk for having a child with a birth defect, particularly an autosomal recessive disorder or multifactorial disorder, because people who are related are more likely to carry the same rare genes than are those who are not related.

**F. Prenatal diagnostic procedures** allow detection of birth defects and genetic disorders prior to delivery and usually prior to the third trimester. Detection of birth defects in pregnancy allows parents the option of pregnancy termination or additional time for emotional adjustment. Early detection also affects how the physician manages the remainder of the pregnancy, delivery, and neonatal period. Available prenatal diagnostic procedures include the following.

    **1. Maternal serum α-fetoprotein (AFP)** level can be used as a screening test at 16–18 weeks gestation. This test, which reflects fetal protein in maternal blood, can be offered to every pregnant woman since there are no risks involved.

        **a.** Elevated maternal serum AFP levels can be associated with neural tube defects, abdominal wall defects (e.g., omphalocele), and fetal bleeding.

        **b.** Low maternal serum AFP levels can be associated with an increased risk for Down syndrome or other trisomies.

    **2. Fetal ultrasound** is a safe test that can be offered in pregnancies where there is a risk for structural fetal anomalies. Currently there are no known associated risks for the fetus or mother from ultrasound testing.

        **a. Level I** ultrasound is performed in most obstetric office settings to evaluate fetal size, growth, number of fetuses, and viability. If abnormalities are suspected, most patients are referred to centers where level II ultrasound is available.

**b. Level II** ultrasound is offered at centers that specialize in the care of high-risk pregnancies and management of fetal abnormalities. Major structural abnormalities of most organ systems can be diagnosed and evaluated. Level II ultrasound is often performed in conjunction with amniocentesis and chorionic villus sampling (see I F 4).

**3. Amniocentesis**

**a. Technique**

**(1) Timing.** Amniocentesis usually is performed at 16 weeks gestation. The safety and success rate for earlier amniocentesis, at 13–15 weeks, is currently being evaluated.

**(2) Procedure.** A needle is inserted into the amniotic cavity and approximately 30 ml of amniotic fluid is removed for the following evaluations:

**(a)** Chromosome analysis

**(b)** Confirmation of elevated maternal serum AFP level

**(c)** Study of specific cell or fluid biochemical or DNA markers

**(d)** Fetal sexing (offered when no other studies are available for an X-linked disorder known to be carried by the mother, since termination of a male fetus would avoid birth of an affected child)

**b. Complications.** Amniocentesis is associated with a 0.25%–0.50% complication rate. Complications include:

**(1) Spontaneous labor,** leading to spontaneous abortion

**(2) Amniotic fluid leakage,** leading to spontaneous labor or oligohydramnios

**(3) Needle puncture of the fetus** (rare)

**(4) Infection** (rare, since the procedure is done aseptically)

**c. Indications.** Amniocentesis generally is offered primarily to women whose risk for having an affected fetus is greater than the underlying risk for complications from the procedure. This high-risk group includes:

**(1)** Women age 35 years and older, since beyond this age the risk for having a fetus with a chromosome trisomy rises significantly

**(2)** Pregnant women who have elevated maternal serum AFP levels

**(3)** Pregnant women who have low maternal serum AFP levels

**(4)** Women with a prior history of having a child with trisomy 21, since their risk for having another child with a trisomy is about 1%–2%

**(5)** Families in whom the mother or father carries a balanced reciprocal chromosome translocation and who, thereby, have a high risk of having a chromosomally unbalanced fetus

**(6)** Families in whom there is a positive family history of a known autosomal or X-linked disease and in whom it is possible to do carrier testing in the fetus either by enzyme studies or recombinant DNA marker studies on amniocytes (amniotic fluid cells)

**4. Chorionic villus sampling (CVS)**

**a. Technique**

**(1) Timing.** CVS is a relatively new prenatal diagnostic test that is performed between 8 and 11 weeks gestation.

**(2) Procedure.** A polyethylene catheter is placed through the cervix via the transvaginal route under ultrasound guidance, or a needle is inserted transabdominally into the developing placenta. Chorionic villus cells of the placenta are aspirated through the tube and can be used for:

**(a)** Chromosome analysis

**(b)** Enzyme studies (if the fetus is at risk for having a known enzyme deficiency)

**(c)** DNA marker studies (if the fetus is at risk for having a single gene disorder with no measurable gene product)

**(d)** Fetal sexing (if a male fetus is at risk for a known X-linked disorder)

**b. Complications.** CVS is not a widely offered prenatal diagnostic test due to the 1%–1.5% risk of complications. Compared to amniocentesis, CVS poses a greater risk for fetal loss and for maternal infection (chorioamnionitis).

**c. Advantages.** A major advantage of CVS is the early gestational age at which the test is offered. This allows lower anxiety for the family, compared to amniocentesis, since fetal movements have not been felt yet and the fetus is not yet completely formed. If an abnormality is detected and the parents opt to terminate the pregnancy, the procedure is less psychologically traumatic and of lower risk at 12 weeks (when CVS results are available) than at 18–20 weeks (when amniocentesis results are available).

   **d. Disadvantages**

      **(1)** It is not possible to perform amniotic fluid AFP testing with CVS, since this test is done so early in pregnancy and only fetal cells are obtained.

      **(2)** Due to the possibility of chromosomally differing cell lines in the chorionic villi (**mosaicism;** see IV A 1 c), CVS results occasionally are ambiguous, necessitating further evaluation with amniocentesis.

**5. Fetoscopy**

   **a. Technique.** Fetoscopy is a procedure whereby a small fiberoptic instrument is inserted under ultrasound guidance transabdominally into the uterine cavity where the fetus is visualized and can be examined.

      **(1)** This procedure can be used to **aspirate blood** from a cord vessel for prenatal diagnosis of hemoglobinopathies and bleeding disorders.

      **(2)** The technique can also be used to obtain **fetal skin biopsy specimens** for prenatal diagnosis of genetic skin disorders such as ichthyosis.

   **b. Complications.** The risk of this procedure is approximately 5%, with complications involving bleeding, pregnancy loss, infection, and amniotic fluid leakage.

**6. Fetal blood sampling** from the umbilical cord can also be performed with ultrasound guidance but without direct visualization. The test is used for chromosome analysis and biochemical study of fetal blood for conditions such as hemophilia. Since the instrument is smaller and the time taken is shorter, the risks are lower (approximately 2%–3%).

**7. Direct DNA analysis** has increased the ability to make diagnoses in single gene disorders, even in some conditions where the mutant gene product has not yet been identified. Through the use of restriction endonucleases from bacteria and recombinant DNA technology, it has been possible to find **restriction fragment length polymorphisms (RFLPs),** which permit detection of abnormal genes through linked gene markers.

   **a. Linkage analysis.** Many RFLPs are not located within the gene being sought but are located sufficiently close on the same chromosome that linkage analysis can be used, because the RFLP segregates with the gene.

      **(1)** For most disorders, the use of this technique requires that several family members—including one affected individual—undergo DNA analysis of their leukocytes or skin fibroblasts. In informative families,* this allows the possibility of prenatal diagnosis from amniocytes or CVS.

      **(2)** This technique can be used for some autosomal dominant disorders (e.g., Huntington's disease), some autosomal recessive disorders (e.g., cystic fibrosis), and some X-linked disorders (e.g., Duchenne muscular dystrophy).

   **b. Direct detection.** In a few disorders, genetic analysis allows direct detection of the abnormal gene itself (e.g., in sickle-cell disease) through the use of a DNA probe complementary to the gene. In these cases, other family members do not need to be tested, since linkage analysis is not needed.

## II. ENVIRONMENTAL FACTORS

   **A. General principles.** Proving the relationship between a substance to which a fetus is exposed and a birth defect involves the consideration of several important factors. Usually, not every exposed fetus shows the effect of a teratogen.

     **1. Teratogen specificity.** A teratogen increases the risk for a specific malformation or a specific pattern of malformations. A general increase in all malformations usually is due to a bias of ascertainment.

---

*Informative families** are those in which the RFLPs on the chromosome carrying the mutation are different than the RFLPs on the chromosome with the normal gene, or those in which the RFLPs in the parent with the gene are different than those of the parent not carrying the gene. When both chromosomes or both parents have the same RFLPs, they cannot be distinguished by linkage analysis and so are **noninformative**.

2. **Timing of exposure** is vital, since morphogenesis occurs for only the first 8–12 weeks, so that any structural abnormality in tissue development must occur prior to 12 weeks gestation. Growth and central nervous system (CNS) development are primarily affected thereafter. Exposure prior to implantation (day 7–10 postconception) results in loss of the embryo or produces no effect.

3. **Dosage** is important. In many cases, there is a threshold below which no effect is demonstrable.

4. **Genetic constitution** of the mother and, especially, the fetus determine whether a specific fetus will be affected. For example, only 11% of fetuses whose mothers take hydantoin during pregnancy will exhibit fetal hydantoin syndrome.

5. **Interaction** between a potential teratogen and other exposures also must be considered.

B. **Infectious agents,** especially the **"TORCH" organisms,** are known to be responsible for a significant proportion of birth defects.

1. **Toxoplasma (T)** interferes with fetal growth and CNS development.

2. **Syphilis (O** for others) interferes with fetal growth, brain development, and skeletal development.

3. **Rubella (R)** can cause cataracts, deafness, mental retardation, and congenital heart disease.

4. **Cytomegalovirus (C)** can cause fetal growth disturbance and CNS anomalies, although the only manifestation may be hearing loss.

5. **Herpes virus (H)** infections generally do not cause malformations, although perinatal exposure to herpes virus can cause neonatal encephalitis.

C. **Medication, drugs, and chemicals** can interfere with embryonic and fetal development.

1. **Alcohol.** Fetal exposure to alcohol can be associated with fetal growth disturbance, abnormal brain development, congenital heart disease, and skeletal abnormalities. A specific pattern of abnormalities called the **fetal alcohol syndrome** can be seen in some offspring of chronically alcoholic women (see II G).

2. **Hydantoin** exposure during pregnancy can cause fetal growth disturbance and skeletal and CNS abnormalities. A specific pattern of anomalies, the **fetal hydantoin syndrome,** is seen in some exposed infants.

3. **Thalidomide** exposure during pregnancy has been associated with limb malformations and cleft palate.

4. **Retinoic acid** exposure during pregnancy, especially exposure to isotretinoin, results in brain, ear, and heart malformations.

5. **Tetracycline** exposure causes dark staining of teeth.

6. **Other teratogenic chemicals** have been described, including anticonvulsants, anticoagulants, antithyroid medications, cancer chemotherapeutic agents, iodine-containing agents, lead, lithium, and mercury.

D. **High-dose radiation** is a teratogenic agent that causes fetal malformations by interfering with cell division and organogenesis. Usually, the dose received by the fetus from diagnostic x-ray studies falls below the threshold for teratogenic effect.

E. **Maternal metabolic disorders** also can adversely influence fetal development.

1. **Diabetes.** Infants of diabetic mothers have a 10%–15% risk for birth defects, particularly those involving the heart, skeleton, brain, and spinal cord. The causative factor is believed to be hyperglycemia. Careful control of diabetes before conception and throughout pregnancy decreases the risk for birth defects.

2. **Phenylketonuria (PKU).** Infants of mothers who have PKU are exposed during pregnancy to excess metabolites of the amino acid phenylalanine. Brain and congenital heart defects occur in nearly every exposed fetus [see III B 3 b (2)].

### F. Mechanical forces

1. **Intrauterine mechanical forces** result in **deformations**.
   a. Intrauterine tumors or fibroids or abnormal uterine anatomy may result in a fetus that is constrained, thereby causing breech presentation, facial distortions, dislocations of the hips, or club feet.
   b. Inadequate amniotic fluid (oligohydramnios) results in severe fetal constraint and may also be associated with hypoplasia of the lungs.

2. **External mechanical forces** can result in **disruptions of fetal blood supply**. These forces can include the formation of bands of tissue from the amniotic sac that can cause hypoplasia of limbs or transverse amputations.

### G. Maternal alcoholism.
Alcohol is the most common major teratogen to which the fetus may be exposed. The amount of alcohol consumed appears to correlate with the degree of adverse affect to the fetus. A genetic predisposition may play a significant role in determining which fetus will be severely or mildly affected by maternal alcohol use and which will be unaffected, although specific genetic factors have not been identified.

1. **Fetal alcohol syndrome** represents a frequent and striking example of a teratogenic disorder.
   a. **Incidence**
      (1) In most populations, fetal alcohol syndrome occurs in 1–2 in 1000 newborns. The syndrome affects 30%–45% of the offspring of women who drink more than 4–6 drinks per day while pregnant.
      (2) An estimated 10%–20% of cases of mild to moderate mental retardation are due to the effects of alcohol in utero.
   b. **Clinical features** of fetal alcohol syndrome include CNS dysfunction, growth deficiencies, facial dysmorphism, and other anomalies.
      (1) **CNS dysfunctions** include developmental delay and intellectual defects (an average IQ of 63), poor fine motor coordination, tremulousness and irritability in infancy, hyperactivity, brain disorganization (e.g., abnormal structure and aberrant nerve cell migration), and microcephaly due to micrencephaly.
      (2) **Growth deficiencies** include birth weight and length below the third percentile and subnormal linear growth and weight gain (decreased subcutaneous fat).
      (3) **Facial dysmorphism** (Figure 7-1) includes a small midface area; long, smooth philtrum; and smooth, thin upper lip with poor definition.
      (4) **Other anomalies** include decreased joint mobility, clinodactyly or camptodactyly of the fifth fingers, rib abnormalities, renal structural malformations, and Klippel-Feil anomaly (cervical vertebral fusions).

2. **Possible fetal alcohol effects.** In those offspring of alcoholic women who do not manifest the complete fetal alcohol syndrome, one or more of the anomalies seen in that syndrome can sometimes be found. This has been called possible fetal alcohol effects. It is important to rule out some other etiology for the abnormalities found in offspring of alcoholic women without the complete fetal alcohol syndrome before ascribing the effects to alcohol exposure. This is particularly important as it relates to possible associated findings and recurrence risk.

3. **Miscarriage.** There is an increase in the risk for miscarriage, which is proportional to the amount of alcohol consumed.

4. **Other effects.** Lesser amounts of alcohol have been shown to produce milder symptoms in a proportion of exposed offspring, particularly as regards size and behavior. While there is no demonstrated medically significant adverse effect from ingestion of small amounts of alcohol during pregnancy or from an occasional episode of greater intake (binge drinking), there are no data to support a "safe" amount of alcohol use during pregnancy. Thus, the most cautious approach is to avoid alcohol entirely during pregnancy.

### H. Environmental pollutants
of various types have been suggested as possible teratogens, although it has been very difficult to study such agents. Birth defects registries, which exist in many states, may be helpful in implicating or absolving specific environmental pollutants as causes of birth defects.

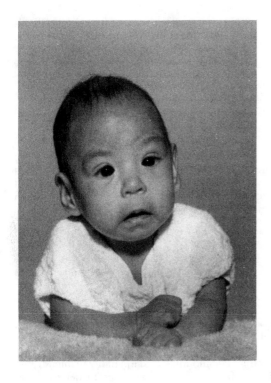

**Figure 7-1.** Characteristic dysmorphic facial features in an infant with fetal alcohol syndrome. Note mild ptosis, epicanthal folds, flat nasal bridge, short nose, long smooth philtrum, and thin upper vermillion border. (Photograph courtesy of T. Kellerman.)

**III. SINGLE GENE DISORDERS.** Each human normally has between 30,000 and 50,000 **genes** that are packaged in the 46 chromosomes (22 pairs of **autosomes** and 1 pair of **sex chromosomes**). All genes come in pairs except for the genes on the sex chromosomes of males. Over 3000 different single gene disorders have been described, which are classified by their mode of inheritance (i.e., autosomal dominant, autosomal recessive, or X-linked).

**A. Autosomal dominant disorders** occur when one gene of a gene pair is altered, or mutated.

    **1. General characteristics**
        **a. Defect.** Autosomal dominant disorders often are due to a **mutation in a gene coding for a structural protein**.
        **b. Recurrence risk.** Any individual with an autosomal dominant disorder has a 50% chance of passing on the mutant gene to offspring. Thus, each child of an affected individual has a 50% chance of being affected.
        **c. Inheritance.** A mutant gene usually is inherited from one parent who is affected with the same condition. Occasionally, an individual will be the first person in a family to display an autosomal dominant trait. This is caused by a **fresh mutation** of that gene in the ovum or spermatocyte that produces the affected individual. The recurrence risk for the parents of a child with a fresh mutation is very low (i.e., equivalent to the chance that another spontaneous mutation will occur). However, the risk for the offspring of the affected individual is 50%.
        **d. Clinical features**
            **(1)** It is common for autosomal dominant genes to cause conditions that manifest differently and vary in degree of severity among affected individuals. This is called **variable expressivity**. For example, in polycystic kidney disease, some people present with early renal failure, whereas others have only hypertension and normal renal function

at the same age. The severity or type of expression of an autosomal dominant disorder in an offspring is usually independent of the way the parent is affected.

(2) A mutant dominant gene often has an effect on more than one tissue or organ system, which is called **pleiotropy**.

2. **Marfan syndrome** is an example of an autosomal dominant disorder, which affects 1 in 20,000 newborns. Marfan syndrome demonstrates variable expressivity, pleiotropy, and a high rate of new mutation.

   a. **Defect.** Marfan syndrome is believed to be due to abnormal fibrillin (the major protein of myofibrils), which results in connective tissue abnormalities.

   b. **Clinical features**

     (1) **Skeletal manifestations** produce a characteristic body habitus (Figure 7-2) and may include:

       (a) Unusually long, thin digits (arachnodactyly) and limbs (dolichostenomelia), resulting in disproportionate tall stature

       (b) Scoliosis and chest deformity (pectus carinatum, excavatum, or both)

       (c) Hypermobile joints

       (d) Long, thin face with a high, narrow palate

     (2) **Ocular manifestations**

       (a) Myopia often is present and may be very severe.

       (b) Lens subluxation may occur.

     (3) **Cardiovascular manifestations** are the most severe medical complications of Marfan syndrome.

       (a) **Dilatation of the aortic root** due to abnormal connective tissue in the vessel wall can cause aortic insufficiency, and dissection and rupture of the aorta may occur at any time due to **cystic medial necrosis. Monitoring** of affected individuals for aortic root diameter and treatment with β-blockers to prevent additional enlargement or **preventive surgery** to replace the proximal aorta significantly diminishes the mortality rate.

       (b) **Mitral valve prolapse** is a very common cardiac finding.

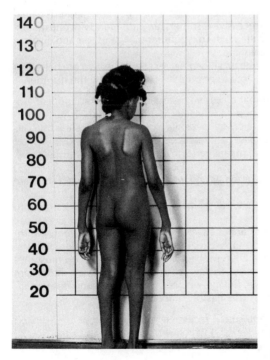

**Figure 7-2.** Characteristic body habitus in a 3½-year-old child with Marfan syndrome. Note tall stature; thin body habitus with long limbs, long hands, and long flat feet; and scoliosis. (Photograph courtesy of R. Pyeritz, M.D.)

(4) **Pulmonary manifestations,** less common in childhood, include a high incidence of spontaneous pneumothorax due to ruptured pulmonary blebs and emphysema due to abnormal connective tissue in the bronchial tree.
  c. **Diagnosis** of Marfan syndrome must be made on a purely clinical basis; as yet there is no specific biochemical or molecular marker.
   (1) **Diagnostic criteria**
     (a) To make the diagnosis, at least two of the following major manifestations must be present:
       (i) Typical skeletal findings
       (ii) Typical ocular findings
       (iii) Typical cardiovascular findings
       (iv) Positive family history
     (b) Once a diagnosis is made, the other manifestations should be sought by skeletal measurements, ophthalmologic evaluation, and echocardiography.
   (2) **Diagnostic challenges.** Only 70%–85% of affected individuals have an affected parent, due to the high incidence of new dominant mutations in Marfan syndrome. Variability in severity and in manifestations also can make it difficult to prove a positive family history. Usually it is necessary to examine the parents and siblings of a possibly affected individual and to obtain and review medical records of family members who died suddenly or of unknown causes.
  d. **Follow-up.** Individuals with or suspected of having Marfan syndrome should be followed with annual physical examinations, ophthalmologic evaluations, and echocardiography. Treatment with β-blockers should be considered, to reduce the progression of aortic root dilatation.

B. **Autosomal recessive disorders** occur when both genes of a gene pair have mutations.

  1. **General characteristics**
    a. **Defect.** Many autosomal recessive disorders are due to mutations in genes coding for **enzymes**. Since half of the normal enzyme activity is adequate under most circumstances, a person with only one mutant gene will not be affected.
    b. **Inheritance.** An individual in whom both members of a gene pair have mutations is called **homozygous** for that gene. In autosomal recessive disorders, an individual with one mutant and one normal gene for a gene pair is called **heterozygous** for that gene pair and displays no clinical effects from the single mutant gene.
    c. **Recurrence risk.** Both parents of a child with an autosomal recessive disorder are heterozygous for that gene; each child of such a couple has a 25% risk of having the disorder.
  2. **Cystic fibrosis** is the most common autosomal recessive disorder in whites of European descent. It affects 1 in 2000 newborns in this population (see Ch 10 X A 1 and Ch 12 IV).
    a. **Defect.** A defect in membrane transport of chloride results in an inability to clear mucous secretions in the lungs and causes decreased pancreatic exocrine function. Molecular genetic and linkage analysis has located the mutant gene on the long arm of chromosome 7.
    b. **Clinical features and course**
     (1) Affected children have recurrent pneumonias and intestinal malabsorption. Males are infertile. Growth is secondarily poor.
     (2) Cystic fibrosis usually causes death in early adulthood from pulmonary destruction.
    c. **Diagnosis**
     (1) Although the specific gene product cannot be measured directly at present, the increased concentration of chloride ion in sweat allows for early definitive diagnosis.
     (2) At present, direct DNA analysis using DNA probes can identify 70% of chromosomes carrying a specific cystic fibrosis mutation. In many of the remaining cases, the mutant gene can be detected through genetic linkage of DNA markers, starting from an affected family member. Prenatal diagnosis has been accomplished.
  3. **Inborn errors of metabolism** usually are autosomal recessive, although a few are X-linked [e.g., ornithine transcarbamylase deficiency (OTCD) which is discussed in III C 3].
    a. **General features**
     (1) **Incidence and epidemiology**
       (a) Although individual metabolic disorders are rare, the hundreds of such disorders together are responsible for a significant amount of mental retardation and mental illness.

**(b)** Certain ethnic groups are at increased risk for specific metabolic errors (e.g., Tay-Sachs disease is seen most frequently in Ashkenazi Jews and French Canadians).

**(2) Defect**

**(a)** Metabolic disorders generally are caused by specific **defects in enzyme structure or function** or by **abnormalities of proteins that transport metabolites** to cells or across cell membranes. The consequent metabolic alterations manifest as physiologic disturbances, mental deficiencies, or both.

**(b)** Inborn metabolic errors may be associated with accumulation of excess precursor, toxic metabolites of excess precursor, or deficiency of products needed for normal metabolism.

**(3) Categories** of common metabolic disorders are listed in Table 7-1.

**(4) Clinical features** that are helpful in detecting inborn errors of metabolism are listed below and summarized in Table 7-2.

**(a) Vomiting and acidosis** after initiation of feeding with breast milk or formula may herald a disorder of **amino acid** metabolism or **carbohydrate** metabolism.

**(b) Unusual odor of urine or sweat** may be seen in several conditions. For example, **maple syrup urine disease** is named for the odor given off by urine of affected children.

**(c) Hepatosplenomegaly** can be caused by metabolic disorders where there is an accumulation (storage) of metabolites within the cells of the liver and spleen.

**(d) Mental retardation,** especially if progressive, may be caused by inborn metabolic errors. **Brain atrophy** or other toxic effects can be caused by harmful effects of circulating metabolites, such as occurs in PKU. **Megalencephaly** (enlarged brain) with mental retardation can result from the inability to metabolize intracellular substances, such as occurs in **mucopolysaccharide** disorders.

**(e) Severe acidosis** with a high anion gap can be caused by the presence of abnormal metabolites, most commonly in **aminoacidurias**.

**(f) Hyperammonemia** usually is associated with **urea cycle** disorders and **organic acid** disorders.

**(g)** A family history of **early infant death** should suggest the possibility of an inborn error in metabolism.

**(h) Growth retardation** is frequently seen in infants with inborn errors of metabolism.

**(i) Seizures** commonly occur when a metabolic disturbance is present.

**(5) Diagnosis.** In most metabolic disorders, an enzyme activity can be measured as abnormal or a metabolite can be measured as abnormally high or low. Thus, in many such disorders, it is possible to detect heterozygous gene carriers and to make a prenatal diagnosis from amniocytes or chorionic villus tissue. A few inborn errors may be diagnosed using RFLPs or DNA probes.

**b. Disorders of amino acid and organic acid metabolism**

**(1) General features**

**(a) Defect.** These disorders usually involve a block in a synthetic pathway, causing buildup of either the precursor or catabolites of the precursor.

**(b) Clinical features**

**(i)** Symptoms, which usually begin in early infancy, are due to inadequate synthesis of necessary metabolic compounds. Excess precursors or their metabolites may interfere with normal metabolic function and regulation (e.g., by causing severe acidosis or alkalosis).

**(ii)** Symptoms may become evident after the initiation of protein-containing feedings, which increase the substrate for the deficient enzyme.

**Table 7-1.** Categories of Common Metabolic Disorders

| Category | Common Examples |
|---|---|
| Disorders of amino acid and organic acid metabolism | Phenylketonuria, homocystinuria, isovaleric acidemia |
| Disorders of ammonia metabolism | Ornithine transcarbamylase deficiency |
| Disorders of carbohydrate metabolism | Galactosemia, glycogen storage diseases |
| Mucopolysaccharidoses | Hurler syndrome |

**Table 7-2.** Clinical Clues to Inborn Errors of Metabolism

| | |
|---|---|
| Recurrent episodes of vomiting | Megalencephaly or brain atrophy |
| Acidosis with anion gap | Hyperammonemia |
| Unusual odor of urine or sweat | Unexplained seizures |
| Hepatosplenomegaly | Episodic illness with coma |
| Growth retardation | Family history of early infant death |
| Mental retardation | |

- (c) **Diagnosis.** Specific diagnosis requires evaluation of urine or plasma for the concentration of amino acids, organic acids, and their metabolites.
- (d) **Therapy.** Some of these disorders are untreatable and associated with early death or mental retardation. Others are treatable with dietary manipulation or replacement of deficient cofactors. Most organic acid disorders lead to decreased level of consciousness, mental and neurologic deficiency, and death in infancy or childhood.

- (2) **Phenylketonuria (PKU),** the best studied and most common of the amino acid disorders, occurs in 1 in 12,000 live births.
    - (a) **Defect.** A deficiency in the enzyme **phenylalanine hydroxylase** prevents conversion of phenylalanine to tyrosine, with subsequent buildup of the toxic metabolites phenylacetic acid and phenyllactic acid.
    - (b) **Clinical features.** Unlike most amino acid disorders, PKU is not symptomatic early in infancy. Symptoms are seen later in infancy and during childhood, if the disorder is untreated.
        - (i) The most significant manifestation is moderate to severe **mental retardation**.
        - (ii) **Neurologic manifestations,** including hypertonicity and tremors, and behavior disorders are common.
        - (iii) Since there is a block in the conversion of phenylalanine to tyrosine, **hypopigmentation** is a common sign (tyrosine is a necessary intermediate in production of the pigment melanin).
    - (c) **Prevention of mental retardation** in PKU can be achieved by **early identification** of the defect and restriction of dietary intake of phenylalanine.
        - (i) Most states have mandatory **newborn screening programs** to identify infants with PKU, to initiate the diet sufficiently early to prevent mental retardation.
        - (ii) **Dietary restriction** should start very early in infancy (by age 1 month) to be optimally effective, and life-long restriction is recommended to prevent loss of intellectual capability.
        - (iii) Individuals with PKU who **maintain careful dietary management** are able to live normal lives. However, women with PKU who have discontinued dietary restriction are at substantially increased risk for having children with birth defects, especially microcephaly, congenital heart disease, and mental retardation.
- (3) **Homocystinuria** occurs in several distinct biochemical forms. The incidence has been estimated from newborn screening for one biochemical form as 1 in 100,000 live births. If it were possible to screen for all biochemical forms, which can have very nonspecific symptoms, the incidence would be higher.
    - (a) **Defect.** Homocystinuria is due to deficiency of the enzyme **cystathionine synthetase,** leading to accumulation of homocystine, which is excreted in the urine and can be measured there. There is **genetic heterogeneity** in the cause of homocystinuria, and the disorder may also occur as a result of a **cofactor deficiency**. The cofactor involved is **5-methyl-tetrahydrofolate**.
    - (b) **Clinical features.** There are no symptoms in infancy. The major manifestations during childhood are skeletal, ocular, and intellectual.
        - (i) There is a typical **body habitus** similar to that seen in Marfan syndrome, with long thin limbs and digits. Scoliosis, sternal deformity, and osteoporosis are common.
        - (ii) **Dislocated lenses** are a frequent feature.
        - (iii) **Mental retardation,** generally mild to moderate, is seen in some affected individuals.
        - (iv) **Vascular thrombosis** occurs commonly, and childhood strokes and myocardial infarctions are reported.

(c) **Management**
- (i) When the cofactor deficiency is the cause, the disorder can be treated with pharmacologic doses of vitamin $B_6$.
- (ii) In non-$B_6$–responsive homocystinuria, dietary management is extremely difficult since the necessary restriction of sulfhydryl groups leads to a very low protein, foul-tasting diet.

**(4) Isovaleric acidemia**
(a) **Defect**
- (i) Isovaleric acidemia is a prototypic organic acid disorder due to deficiency of **isovaleryl CoA dehydrogenase,** the enzyme responsible for the oxidative decarboxylation of leucine.
- (ii) A secondary deficiency of **L-carnitine** may develop due to consumption of dietary and body stores of carnitine by conjugation to the water-soluble isovaleryl glycine and elimination in the urine.

(b) **Clinical features**
- (i) The presentation varies from severe neonatal ketoacidosis with encephalopathy (which, untreated, will progress to death) to a more indolent form with failure to thrive, developmental delay, and episodic metabolic acidosis.
- (ii) During ketoacidotic episodes, patients may demonstrate neutropenia and pancytopenia and have the odor of "sweaty feet."
- (iii) Myopathy, cardiomyopathy, or both may occur with L-carnitine deficiency.

(c) **Diagnosis** is by demonstration of isovaleric acid, isovaleryl glycine, and isovaleryl carnitine in the urine.

(d) **Therapy** includes moderate protein restriction and dietary supplementation with glycine and L-carnitine. If begun at an early age, treatment leads to resolution of the ketoacidotic episodes and normal development.

c. **Disorders of ammonia metabolism** occur in at least 1 in 50,000 newborns.
- **(1) General features**
  - (a) **Defect.** Disorders of the urea cycle are associated with hyperammonemia, since they are involved with the metabolism of ammonia for excretion from the body.
  - (b) **Clinical features**
    - (i) Ammonia levels generally rise after initiation of protein-containing feedings or breast feeding.
    - (ii) Affected children are well at birth but become progressively more lethargic and may develop seizures or decreased level of consciousness.
- **(2) Ornithine transcarbamylase deficiency (OTCD)** is a prototypic disorder of ammonia metabolism, but—unlike most metabolic disorders—it is inherited as an X-linked recessive trait (see III C 3).
- **(3) Other urea cycle disorders** (e.g., citrullinemia, argininosuccinic aciduria, carbamyl phosphate synthetase deficiency) have similar clinical courses to OTCD. A fifth disorder, arginase deficiency, tends to present with less severe hyperammonemia and with progressive spastic quadriplegia and mental retardation.

d. **Disorders of carbohydrate metabolism.**
- **(1) Galactosemia** is a severe example of an inborn error of carbohydrate metabolism.
  - (a) **Defect.** It is an autosomal recessive disorder caused by deficiency of the enzyme **galactose-1-phosphate uridyl transferase,** resulting in impaired conversion of galactose-1-phosphate to glucose-1-phosphate.
  - (b) **Clinical features** are noted within a few days to weeks after initiation of formula or breast milk feedings. Initial symptoms include hepatomegaly, vomiting, anorexia, aminoaciduria, and growth failure.
  - (c) **Diagnosis** is initially made by detection of non-glucose–reducing substances in the urine (galactose and galactose-1-phosphate) and is confirmed by demonstrating absence of galactose-1-uridyl transferase in erythrocytes. Many states have mandatory newborn screening for galactosemia, since it is treatable when diagnosed early.
  - (d) **Therapy** for galactosemia is the elimination of all formulas and foods containing galactose.
    - (i) **Treated individuals** often have normal intelligence if the diagnosis is made and treatment is initiated early. However, there is an increase in the incidence of learning disorders even in treated individuals. Affected females have a high incidence of **ovarian hypofunction** and premature ovarian failure.

      **(ii)** **Untreated infants** often die, either from inanition or ***Escherichia coli* sepsis**. Untreated survivors suffer from growth retardation, mental retardation, and cataracts.

   **(2)** **Glycogen storage diseases (GSDs)** are a group of conditions caused by a lack of enzymes involved in glycogen synthesis or breakdown, with a resultant buildup of glycogen in tissues (see also Ch 17 X D 3 a). Representative autosomal recessive types listed below illustrate the variable clinical picture.

      **(a)** **GSD type I (von Gierke's disease)** is caused by a deficiency of the enzyme **glycogen-6-phosphatase**. The disorder presents in infancy as hepatomegaly, nephromegaly, hypoglycemia, and acidosis. Therapy is geared toward prevention of hypoglycemia, either by continuous nasogastric feeding or by initiating a diet high in complex carbohydrates (e.g., corn starch) that are slowly absorbed from the gastrointestinal tract.

      **(b)** **GSD type II (Pompe's disease)** is caused by a deficiency of **acid maltase**. Symptoms are evident in infancy due to deposition of glycogen in the liver (causing hepatomegaly), heart (causing cardiomegaly), and skeletal muscle (causing hypotonia). All tissues are affected. No therapy is available, and most children die before age 1 year from cardiac failure or respiratory failure.

      **(c)** **GSD type V (McArdle's disease)** is caused by a deficiency of the skeletal muscle enzyme **phosphorylase**. Beginning in later childhood and adulthood, muscle exertion causes fatigability, cramps, and occasionally myoglobinuria. No specific therapy is available.

  **e.** **Mucopolysaccharidoses (MPSs)** are a group of disorders characterized by deficiency of lysosomal enzymes responsible for intracellular catabolism of mucopolysaccharides. All are autosomal recessive conditions except for **Hunter syndrome** (MPS type II; iduronate sulfatase deficiency), which is an X-linked recessive disorder (see III C). The incidence of this group of disorders is 1 in 25,000 newborns.

   **(1)** **Clinical features** are caused by intracellular accumulation (storage) of mucopolysaccharides and are not apparent at birth.

      **(a)** All tissues can be affected, but effects are most commonly seen in the liver and spleen (hepatosplenomegaly), skeleton (skeletal dysplasia, dwarfism, joint contracture), brain (megalencephaiy, mental retardation), heart (aortic and mitral valve incompetence), and respiratory system (tracheal stenosis).

      **(b)** Mucopolysaccharidoses usually are associated with deterioration of neurologic function and progressive mental retardation. In some MPSs, the brain is unaffected and intelligence is normal.

   **(2)** **Diagnosis** of the mucopolysaccharidoses is suggested by the presence of specific mucopolysaccharides in the urine. The diagnosis is confirmed by performing specific enzyme assays on leukocytes or fibroblasts.

**C.** **X-linked disorders** occur when a male inherits a mutant gene on the X chromosome, which always is maternal in origin. Common X-linked disorders include hemophilia A, color blindness, and Duchenne muscular dystrophy.

  **1.** **General characteristics**

    **a.** **Inheritance**

      **(1)** The affected male is termed **hemizygous** for the gene, since he has only a single X chromosome and a single set of X-linked genes.

      **(2)** The mother of the affected individual is **heterozygous** for the gene, since she has two X chromosomes, one normal and one with a mutant gene. She may demonstrate partial manifestations of the disorder, since only one of the two X's in any cell is transcriptionally active **(Lyon hypothesis)**.

    **b.** **Recurrence risks** for X-linked disorders differ depending on whether the mother or the father has the abnormal gene.

      **(1)** **If the mother has the gene** on one of her two X chromosomes and, thus, is a **carrier,** there is a 50% chance that the gene will pass to each offspring. If the offspring is a daughter, she, too, will be a carrier. If the offspring is a son, he will be affected since he will not have a second X chromosome to compensate for the effects of the abnormal gene. Thus, each daughter has a 50% chance of being a carrier, and each son has a 50% chance of being affected.

**(2) If the father has the gene** and, thus, is **affected,** he can only pass that abnormal gene to his daughters; all his daughters, therefore, will be carriers. Since the Y chromosome is normal, all his sons will be unaffected. **There is no male-to-male transmission.**

2. **Fragile X syndrome** is a common cause of mental retardation, which is associated with a chromosomal marker.
    a. **Incidence.** An X-linked form of mental retardation is found in 1 in 1000 males, and 40% of males with X-linked mental retardation have the fragile X syndrome. Some women with mental retardation also may display the fragile X chromosome.
    b. **Diagnosis** can be made by detecting a chromosomal marker called a **fragile site** on the distal end of the long arm of the X chromosome.
        (1) In order to demonstrate the fragile site on the X chromosome, it is necessary to culture the lymphocytes in a **folate-deficient medium** via a fragile X study.
        (2) The frequency of this syndrome calls for all children (male and female) with mental retardation of unspecified etiology to undergo a fragile X study.
    c. **Recurrence risk.** Because the fragile X syndrome is an X-linked disorder with a chromosomal marker, recurrence risks (for the mutation) are the same as for other X-linked disorders. Occasionally, a male will carry the fragile X gene without expressing it clinically or cytogenetically. This complicates genetic counseling.
    d. **Clinical features** may be quite variable.
        (1) **Physical features**
            (a) Infants are often **large** at birth. Head circumference often is greater than the ninety-fifth percentile for age.
            (b) **Macro-orchidism** is a commonly seen feature, although it is usually not detected until puberty.
            (c) **Dysmorphic facial features** may include a large jaw, large ears, and a prominent forehead.
        (2) **Mental retardation** usually is in the moderate range. Speech and language function are usually the most affected.
            (a) Some males with fragile X syndrome have no unusual clinical features other than mental retardation.
            (b) Some female carriers of the fragile X chromosome have a lower IQ than normal.
        (3) **Autistic features** are seen in greater than expected frequency in patients with the fragile X syndrome. A characteristic personality is described.
    e. **Therapy.** There is **no specific therapeutic modality** for the fragile X syndrome, although the value of folate supplementation is being investigated.

3. **OTCD**
    a. **Defect.** OTCD is a prototypic disorder of ammonia metabolism, which is inherited as an X-linked recessive trait.
        (1) Although males primarily are severely affected, up to one-third of female carriers may manifest symptoms due to lyonization [see III C 1 a (2)].
        (2) Genetic heterogeneity exists, so that some affected males have a less severe mutation and clinical course.
    b. **Clinical features**
        (1) Typically, overwhelming illness develops in affected males within 24–48 hours of birth (i.e., after initiation of protein-containing feedings). The newborn becomes progressively more lethargic and may develop seizures and a decreased level of consciousness as serum ammonia levels rise to > 500 μg/dl and, ultimately, to about 1000 μg/dl.
        (2) Female carriers may present with headache and vomiting after protein meals and, later, with learning disabilities or an altered response to protein loading.
    c. **Therapy and prognosis**
        (1) Treatment may be attempted with intravenous fluids, glucose, and agents that exploit alternative pathways for nitrogen excretion (e.g., benzoic acid, phenylacetate).
        (2) Early aggressive treatment can improve the prognosis for survival and function, but the outlook often remains poor unless the infant is managed prospectively from birth (based on a positive family history). Even then, the management is complex and demanding of the parents.

**IV. CHROMOSOME DISORDERS.** Each human normally has 22 pairs of autosomes and 1 pair of sex chromosomes, with females having two X chromosomes and males having one X and one Y chromosome. One member of each pair of chromosomes comes from each parent, with a carefully regulated amount of genetic material. An alteration in the amount or nature of chromosome material usually is associated with birth defects or other abnormalities. Chromosome disorders are seen in 5 in 1000 live births (0.6%).

**A. General characteristics**

1. **Defect.** Most chromosome defects arise de novo (i.e., no other family member has a defect). The defects usually are classified as abnormalities of **number** or of **structure and content**. They may involve either the autosomes or the sex chromosomes; birth defects due to autosomal abnormalities generally are more severe than those due to sex chromosome abnormalities.
   a. **Numerical defects** may be **aneuploid** (chromosome number is not an exact multiple of the diploid number) or **euploid** (chromosome number is an exact multiple of the diploid number). **Examples** of numerical chromosome abnormalities include trisomy 21 (Down syndrome), trisomy 18, trisomy 13, Klinefelter syndrome, and Turner syndrome.
   b. **Structural defects** result from chromosome breakage and include unbalanced translocation, deletion, duplication, inversion, isochromosome, and centric fragment. **Examples** of disorders due to structural chromosome abnormalities include Prader-Willi syndrome, cri du chat syndrome, and Wilms' tumor.
   c. **Mosaicism** is another type of chromosome defect characterized by two or more cell lines with different chromosome compositions. Mosaicism occurs as a result of mitotic nondysjunction after fertilization. Therefore, recurrence risk for parents of a child with mosaicism is negligible.

2. **Indications for chromosome analysis**
   a. Children who have **recognizable phenotypes** (clinical features) consistent with known chromosomal disorders should have confirmatory chromosome studies.
   b. Children with **multiple congenital abnormalities or dysmorphic features** and no clinically identifiable etiology require chromosome studies.
   c. Children with **mental retardation** and no identifiable etiology require chromosome studies, including a fragile X study.
   d. Parents who have had **recurrent** (two or more) **pregnancy losses** should have chromosome studies.
      (1) Of couples with two or more miscarriages, 5% will have one member with a balanced reciprocal chromosome translocation.
         (a) Miscarriage can result when an embryo or fetus has an inherited unbalanced chromosome translocation that is incompatible with life.
         (b) Such couples are at risk for having a live-born child with multiple congenital anomalies due to an unbalanced translocation and should be offered prenatal diagnosis.
      (2) Some women with recurrent pregnancy loss have been found to have **mosaicisms** involving the sex chromosomes; however, the etiologic significance of this, if any, is not clear.
   e. Since 40% of all spontaneous abortions are caused by chromosome abnormalities (usually extra or missing chromosomes), all **spontaneously aborted and stillborn fetuses** should have chromosome studies.
   f. Chromosome studies are valuable for aiding in the diagnosis and management of patients with **ambiguous genitalia**.
   g. Sex chromosome abnormalities are often found in **infertile men and women**.
   h. Chromosome studies should be obtained on bone marrow samples from all **leukemic patients** since leukemic cells often have chromosome abnormalities.
   i. **Solid tumors** often contain cytogenetic alterations, which may give clues to their gene origin.

3. **Methods of chromosome analysis.** Chromosome studies can be performed on any tissue in which cells are actively undergoing mitosis. A **karyotype** is an arrangement of the chromosomes that is made from micrographs; it allows the analysis of chromosome number and structure.
   a. **Peripheral blood studies** are the most common, since blood is the easiest tissue to obtain.
      (1) The T cells are stimulated with phytohemagglutinin (PHA), which causes the cells to undergo mitosis.

**(2)** Results from peripheral blood chromosome studies usually take a minimum of 3 days to obtain, since that is the time required for the cells to enter metaphase.
  **b. Bone marrow studies.** Bone marrow cells are constantly undergoing mitosis, making it possible to obtain results within 6 hours of obtaining a sample.
  **(1)** Bone marrow chromosomes may be studied when management decisions regarding newborn infants who have multiple birth defects may be altered by knowing whether there is a chromosome abnormality associated with a very poor prognosis [e.g., trisomy 18 (see IV B 3)].
  **(2)** The most common use of bone marrow chromosome studies is for evaluation of leukemias. The exact type of chromosomal anomaly in leukemic cells aids in diagnosis, management, and determination of prognosis (see Ch 15 II A 1).
  **c. Organ tissue studies.** Chromosome studies also can be performed on solid tissues and organs.
  **(1)** Occasionally it is not possible to obtain peripheral blood, as in the case of a **stillborn fetus,** and another tissue is evaluated.
  **(2)** In the case of **chromosome mosaicism,** tissue biopsies (usually taken from the skin) are grown in culture to diagnose or confirm the defect. Generally, it takes at least 3–4 weeks for solid tissue cells to grow in culture before chromosome analysis can be performed.

**B. Numerical autosomal abnormalities.** Characteristic phenotypes are associated with specific autosomal trisomies. **Trisomy** refers to the fact that three—rather than the normal two—copies of a specific chromosome are present in the cells of an individual. Such trisomies occur because of a meiotic division error called **nondisjunction** in either the oocyte of the mother or the spermatocyte of the father. Only a few trisomies are found in live-born infants; others are seen only in aborted fetuses.

**1. Down syndrome** is the most common autosomal trisomy.
  **a. Types of defects.** The characteristic finding and etiology of Down syndrome is trisomy 21, although some cases are due to translocation or, more rarely, mosaicism.
  **(1) Trisomy.** Ninety-five percent of children with Down syndrome have 47 chromosomes with three number 21 chromosomes. Trisomy 21 occurs in 1 in 700 live births.
  **(a)** The risk for having a child with an extra chromosome 21 increases with **advancing maternal age.** This risk rises dramatically after age 35 years. Most children with trisomy 21 are born to women younger than 35 years of age, however, since most women give birth prior to age 35 years. The mechanism for the increased incidence of trisomy 21 in fetuses of older mothers is not understood. The extra chromosome comes from the father in a small percentage of cases.
  **(b)** The **recurrence risk** for parents of children with trisomy 21 increases to 1%–2% (unless age-related risk is greater).
  **(2) Translocation.** Four percent of children with Down syndrome have 46 chromosomes, with a translocation of the third number 21 chromosome to another chromosome—usually a **D-group** (number 13, 14, or 15) or a **G-group** (number 21 or 22) chromosome.
  **(a)** Of all cases of translocation Down syndrome, three-fourths are **de novo** (i.e., not familial).
  **(b)** One-fourth of cases are **familial,** meaning that one of the parents has a balanced translocation involving one number 21 chromosome and another chromosome. In these cases, the **recurrence risk** may be as high as 15% in future pregnancies (depending on which other chromosome is involved and on the sex of the partner carrying the balanced translocation).
  **(3) Mosaicism.** One percent of children with Down syndrome have chromosome mosaicism, with some cells having 46 chromosomes and two number 21 chromosomes and some cells having 47 chromosomes and three number 21 chromosomes. The mosaicism results from a mitotic division error that occurred during early embryonic development.
  **b. Clinical features.** Children with Down syndrome have a characteristic appearance that can be defined in terms of their **dysmorphic features**. They also have a number of other characteristic **functional and structural abnormalities** that are part of the syndrome. Children with mosaic Down syndrome may have a milder clinical presentation than those with trisomy 21 in all of their cells.
  **(1) Dysmorphic features** (Figure 7-3)

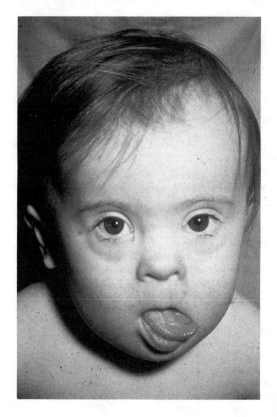

**Figure 7-3.** Characteristic dysmorphic features in an infant with Down syndrome. Note small palpebral fissures with epicanthal folds, flat nasal bridge, small nose and mouth, protruding tongue, and small chin. Brushfield spots can be seen on the iris. (Photograph courtesy of K. Jones, M.D.)

- **(a) Common dysmorphic facial features** are a flat facial profile; short, upslanting palpebral fissures; Brushfield spots; a flat nasal bridge with epicanthal folds; a small mouth with protruding tongue; a small, retroplaced chin; and short ears with abnormal ear lobes that are usually downfolded.
- **(b) Other dysmorphic features** include microcephaly, flat occiput (brachycephaly), excess posterior neck skin, short stature, short sternum, small genitalia, short hands and fingers marked by incurved fifth fingers with hypoplastic middle phalanx, single palmar creases (simian creases), and a gap between the first and second toes.
- **(2) Functional and structural abnormalities**
    - **(a) Hypotonia** is a frequent accompaniment to the dysmorphic features of Down syndrome and is most noticeable in the newborn.
    - **(b) Cardiac defects,** especially endocardial cushion defects and septal defects, are seen in 50% of people with Down syndrome; about half of these may be fatal.
    - **(c) Gastrointestinal abnormalities** (especially duodenal atresia and Hirshsprung's disease) are the next most common internal organ abnormalities in Down syndrome.
    - **(d) Developmental delay** is seen in young children, and **mental retardation** is diagnosed once the age of IQ testing is reached. The mean IQ is 50, with most individuals performing in the moderately retarded range.
    - **(e) Hypothyroidism** and **leukemia** occur at higher frequency than in the general population.

**(f)** With improved medical, educational, and vocational management, life expectancy for Down syndrome patients can be well into adulthood. A newly recognized problem of the third and fourth decade is a pattern of dementia much like **Alzheimer's disease**.

    **c. Prognosis.** With increased life expectancy in Down syndrome, issues relating to employment, financial security, health care, and living situation must be addressed by families and social service agencies. Supervised group home living has become a successful alternative for these and other mentally retarded adults.

**2. Trisomy 13.** From 1 in 4000 to 1 in 10,000 newborns are affected by trisomy 13.

    **a. Types of defects**

      **(1) Trisomy.** Seventy-five percent of cases of trisomy 13 are due to a free extra chromosome 13—a result of a parental meiotic nondisjunction. There is a relationship between the occurrence of trisomy 13 and advanced maternal age, although it is not as strong as that for trisomy 21.

      **(2) Translocation.** Twenty percent of the cases of trisomy 13 are the result of translocation involving chromosome 13.

        **(a)** Three-fourths of these cases are **de novo**.

        **(b)** One-fourth are due to a familial translocation involving the number 13 chromosome, and in these cases the **recurrence risk** can be as high as 14% in future pregnancies.

      **(3) Mosaicism.** Five percent of the cases of trisomy 13 are mosaics for normal 46 chromosome cell lines and cell lines with 47 chromosomes with an extra number 13 chromosome.

    **b. Clinical features.** Trisomy 13 is associated with **severe birth defects,** including:

      **(1) Microcephaly** with open skin lesions of the scalp (**aplasia cutis congenita**)

      **(2) Cleft lip with or without cleft palate** (often severe and bilateral)

      **(3) Severe CNS malformations,** including **holoprosencephaly** (absence of midline structures, often with a single ventricle)

      **(4) Eye malformations,** including microphthalmos and colobomata

      **(5) Polydactyly** of the hands and feet

      **(6) Omphalocele**

      **(7) Genital malformations,** including ambiguous genitalia in males

      **(8) Congenital heart disease**

      **(9) Severe mental retardation**

    **c. Prognosis** for patients with trisomy 13 is extremely poor: 50% percent of patients die before 1 month of age, 70% die before age 6 months, and 90% die before age 1 year.

**3. Trisomy 18** occurs in 1 in 8000 live births. There is a relationship between advanced maternal age and the occurrence of trisomy 18, but this is less marked than that seen in trisomy 21 and trisomy 13.

    **a. Types of defects.** Trisomy 18 rarely is caused by a chromosome translocation.

      **(1)** Ninety percent of the cases of trisomy 18 are a result of **meiotic nondisjunction**.

      **(2)** Ten percent of the cases of trisomy 18 are **mosaics**—caused by a postzygotic (postfertilization) mitotic nondisjunction.

    **b. Clinical features**

      **(1)** Trisomy 18 is associated with **multiple congenital anomalies,** including intrauterine growth retardation, microcephaly with prominent occiput, CNS malformations and severe mental retardation, hypertonia (spasticity) after initial hypotonia, and micrognathia (small mandible).

      **(2) Other congenital anomalies** include characteristic overlapping of the second and fifth fingers over the third and fourth fingers, with fixed finger contractures and absence of interphalangeal flexion creases, dislocated hips, rocker bottom feet, congenital heart disease, and occasional neural tube defects. The variability and subtlety of the dysmorphic features can sometimes make this condition difficult to recognize.

    **c. Prognosis** for patients with trisomy 18 is extremely poor: 30% of patients die within 1 month of birth and 90% die before 1 year of age.

**C. Sex chromosome disorders** involve abnormalities in the number or structure of the X or Y chromosome.

    **1. Turner syndrome** affects 1 in 2500 newborn girls.

      **a. Types of defects.** In Turner syndrome, only one X chromosome exists or is normal. Several different chromosomal anomalies can result in the Turner phenotype.

**(1)** In 55% of girls with Turner syndrome, there is a 45,X karyotype.

**(2)** In 25% of cases, the structure of one of the X chromosomes is altered. The structural anomaly usually is a **deletion** of a segment of the chromosome or a duplication of the long or short arm of the chromosome with a subsequent loss of the other arm (called an **isochromosome**).

**(3)** In 15% of cases, there is a **mosaic** for two or more cell lines, one of which usually is 45,X and the other is 46,XX or 46,XY. A third cell line may be present, most commonly leading to a karyotype of 45,X/46,XX/47,XXX. Mosaicism is caused by postzygotic mitotic nondisjunction.

**b. Recurrence risk** for Turner syndrome is the same as the general population risk (i.e., 1 in 5000 live births).

**c. Clinical features** of Turner syndrome may be noted at birth, although many girls are not diagnosed until puberty.

**(1) Dysmorphic features** include lymphedema of hands and feet at birth, a shield-shaped chest, webbing of the neck, cubitus valgus (increased carrying angle), short stature (average adult height is 135 cm), and multiple pigmented nevi.

**(2) Functional and structural abnormalities**

**(a) Gonadal dysgenesis** is present in 100% of patients and is associated with primary amenorrhea and lack of pubertal development due to absence of ovarian hormones. It is important to replace ovarian hormones at puberty as part of the management of Turner syndrome patients. With rare exception, women are unable to become pregnant.

**(b) Gonadoblastoma** (a tumor of abdominally located gonads with Y-containing cells) may develop in patients who have a cell line with a Y chromosome. It is essential to perform bilateral gonadectomy in girls with such a cell line.

**(c) Renal anomalies** occur in 40% of patients and include duplication of the collecting system and horseshoe kidney.

**(d) Congenital heart disease** occurs in 20% of patients. Defects include aortic stenosis, bicuspid aortic valve, and coarctation of the aorta.

**(e) Autoimmune thyroiditis** is common.

**(f) Learning disabilities** are common.

**d. Diagnosis.** Some girls suspected of having Turner syndrome have a 46,XX karyotype in peripheral blood.

**(1)** Most of these girls have mosaic Turner syndrome, and a skin biopsy is necessary to find the mosaicism in fibroblasts.

**(2)** Some of these patients have a phenotypically similar but genetically unrelated condition called **Noonan syndrome,** which, unlike Turner syndrome, can also affect males and has a number of additional clinical findings, including mental retardation in many cases.

**e. Prognosis** depends on the type and severity of malformations. Lifespan probably is normal in most cases.

**2. Klinefelter syndrome** affects 1 in 1000 newborn boys and is due to an extra X chromosome.

**a. Types of defects**

**(1)** In 80% of boys with Klinefelter syndrome, there is a **47,XXY karyotype.**

**(2)** In 20% of cases, there is a mosaic, with one cell line having a **47,XXY karyotype.**

**b. Recurrence risk** for Klinefelter syndrome is the same as the general population risk (i.e., 1 in 2000 live births).

**c. Clinical features** are variable and nonspecific.

**(1)** Males usually are taller than average in relation to their families, with an arm span generally greater than their height.

**(2)** At puberty, males are incompletely masculinized and usually have a female body habitus and female escutcheon with decreased body hair.

**(a)** Gynecomastia is a common feature.

**(b)** The testes remain small, and there is hyperplasia of Leydig cells and greatly diminished spermatozoa production, with infertility.

**(3)** The mean IQ is 90, and there is a slight increase in the incidence of mild mental retardation.

**(4)** Behavioral problems and immaturity are common.

3. **Other sex chromosome abnormalities**
   a. Men with **46,XX karyotype** have a phenotype similar to Klinefelter syndrome. The incidence of 46,XX males is 1 in 25,000 live births. This condition is caused by a translocation of genetic material from the short arm of the Y chromosome to another chromosome.
   b. A **47,XXX karyotype** is seen in 1 in 1000 live-born females. Most cases have a normal phenotype, although tall stature for the family is a frequent finding. The average IQ is 90, but there is no apparent increased incidence of mental retardation. There may be an increased tendency for schizophrenia.
   c. A **47,XYY karyotype** is seen in 1 in 1000 live-born males. The phenotype generally is normal, although most patients are taller than average for their families (the average height is 180 cm). Previous concerns about behavioral disorders in these individuals have been challenged by subsequent research.

D. **Structural chromosome abnormalities**

   1. **Partial deletions**
      a. **Types of defects**
         (1) Some syndromes can be caused by the loss of chromosome material from the ends of a chromosome (**terminal chromosome deletion**) or loss of material from the middle or inner portion of a chromosome (**interstitial deletion**).
         (2) Although most chromosome deletions arise de novo, terminal deletions may result from the child inheriting an **unbalanced chromosome translocation** (unequal exchange of chromosome material between two chromosomes) from a parent who has a balanced reciprocal translocation (equal exchange of chromosome material between two chromosomes).
      b. **Clinical features.** Children with terminal deletions usually have growth deficiency, mental retardation, dysmorphic features, and multiple malformations.
      c. **Detection**
         (1) It often is necessary to perform special chromosome studies to detect small or subtle deletions. These **high-resolution, or prometaphase, studies** capture cells in an early stage of the mitotic cycle, so the chromosomes are longer and have more regions (bands) visible for analysis.
         (2) In cases of terminal deletion, it is necessary to perform karyotypes of both parents.
         (3) A family history of recurrent pregnancy loss may be found when parents have balanced chromosome translocations, since other family members also may carry the translocation.
      d. **Disorders caused by partial deletions**
         (1) **Cri du chat syndrome** occurs in 1 in 50,000 newborns.
            (a) **Defect.** The syndrome is caused by a deletion of material from the terminal end of the short arm of chromosome 5 (**5p−**).
            (b) **Clinical features**
               (i) Affected children have a characteristic cat-like cry.
               (ii) Profound mental retardation and CNS abnormalities are consistent findings.
               (iii) Congenital heart disease is common, as are ocular malformations (e.g., cataracts, optic atrophy).
            (c) **Prognosis.** Many patients can survive into adulthood.
         (2) **Prader-Willi syndrome** occurs in 1 in 15,000 newborns.
            (a) **Defect.** The syndrome is associated with an interstitial deletion of the long arm of chromosome 15 (**deletion of 15q11–13**), detected by prometaphase analysis or molecular genetic analysis.
               (i) About 70% of patients with Prader-Willi syndrome have a chromosome deletion, always in the paternally derived chromosome 15.
               (ii) A small proportion (about 5%) have a rearrangement involving 15q.
               (iii) The remainder, who have a normal-appearing chromosome complement, recently have been found to be missing the paternal contribution of 15q on the basis of absence of the paternal chromosome 15 and presence of two number 15 chromosomes of maternal origin. This is called **maternal disomy**.
               (iv) The existence of maternal disomy as a cause of Prader-Willi syndrome is an example of **genetic imprinting,** a newly recognized phenomenon in which some genes are modified differently (and therefore expressed differently), depending on whether they were inherited from the mother or the father, even though the genetic code is the same.

        **(v)** The others lack visible microscopic chromosome mutations, but the extent of molecular abnormalities in this group of patients is still being characterized.

    **(b) Recurrence risk.** The empiric recurrence risk is less than 1 in 100, unless the chromosome 15 deletion is the result of parental translocation or some other rearrangement (very rare).

    **(c) Clinical features**

        **(i)** Children with Prader-Willi syndrome have severe infantile hypotonia associated with feeding difficulties and failure to thrive in infancy. Later (between age 1 and 4 years), these children develop central obesity due to an appetite disorder. They eat large amounts of food unless strict dietary control is enforced.

        **(ii)** Developmental delay is a major feature. Most patients are mildly mentally retarded, although some have a normal IQ. Behavior problems are common, and a characteristic personality type is seen.

        **(iii)** Dysmorphic features (Figure 7-4) include narrow bifrontal diameter, almond-shaped palpebral fissures, a down-turned mouth, and small hands and feet.

        **(iv)** There is hypogonadotrophic hypogonadism, which manifests as small genitalia and incomplete puberty.

        **(v)** Short stature in adulthood is the rule.

    **(d) Prognosis.** Lifespan is shortened only by the complications of obesity (e.g., diabetes mellitus, hypoventilation).

**(3) Retinoblastoma** (see also Ch 15 XIII)

    **(a) Defect.** Some children with retinoblastoma have an interstitial deletion of the long arm of chromosome 13 (**deletion of 13q14**), detected by prometaphase analysis.

    **(b) Clinical features**

        **(i)** The onset of retinoblastoma in these cases usually is in the first 2 years of life. The disease usually is bilateral.

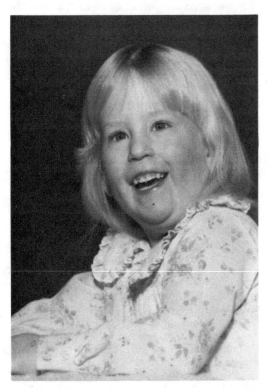

**Figure 7-4.** Characteristic dysmorphic features in a child with Prader-Willi syndrome. Note narrow bifrontal diameter, almond-shaped palpebral fissures, thin upper lip, and ropy saliva. (Photograph courtesy of T. Kellerman.)

    **(ii)** Mental retardation usually is seen.
    **(iii)** Patients often have some degree of facial dysmorphism.
  **(4) Wilms' tumor** (see also Ch 15 VI)
    **(a) Defect.** Children with Wilms' tumor and aniridia (absent irises) may have an interstitial deletion of the short arm of chromosome 11 (**deletion of 11p13**), detected by prometaphase analysis.
    **(b) Clinical features**
      **(i)** Mental retardation is a consistent feature.
      **(ii)** Males often have ambiguous genitalia.
      **(iii)** Children with 11p13 deletion are at high risk for developing abdominal tumors, especially Wilms' tumor and gonadoblastoma; therefore, they should be monitored frequently with abdominal ultrasound.

 **2. Partial trisomy**
  **a. Defect.** Partial trisomy results when extra chromosome material is found in the karyotype, but there is less than an entire extra chromosome present.
   **(1)** The extra chromosome material can occur at the end of the long or short arm of the chromosome, or it may be inserted into the normal chromosome at any point.
   **(2)** It also may occur as a separate piece of chromosome material (a chromosome **marker** or **minute**), with or without its own centromere.
  **b. Clinical features.** The origin of the extra chromosome material determines the phenotypic effects. When the extra material is autosomal, dysmorphic features, growth insufficiency, malformations, and developmental abnormalities are commonly seen.
  **c. Diagnosis**
   **(1) High-resolution banding or special staining techniques** sometimes can identify the origin of the extra chromosome material, especially if it is large. **DNA probe analysis** also may be helpful in identifying the origin of markers.
   **(2) Parental karyotypes** should be obtained, since the partial trisomy sometimes results from a balanced parental translocation. Such a translocation gives a parent an increased risk for future chromosomally unbalanced offspring, with clinical consequences of an increased risk for miscarriage, stillbirth, malformations, or mental retardation. It may also aid in the identification of the chromosome of origin of the extra material in the child.
   **(3)** In many cases, especially of **de novo partial trisomy,** the extra material cannot be identified. In that case, it is impossible to specifically predict the prognosis for the child, since the origin of the extra genetic material remains unknown.

**V. MULTIFACTORIAL DISORDERS** are conditions that are believed to be caused by a combination of genetic liability and environmental (nongenetic) factors. Many common birth defects and many common disorders of midlife are ascribed to multifactorial inheritance.

 **A. General characteristics**

  **1. Incidence.** The general population incidence of most multifactorial disorders is 1.0–1.5 per 1000 for each condition.

  **2. Recurrence risk.** Individuals who have a multifactorial disorder or who have a child with a multifactorial disorder have approximately a 2%–5% empiric risk for recurrence of the disorder with each subsequent pregnancy.
   **a.** The increased risk for recurrence implies that there must be some genetic factors, probably several genes, that play a role in the occurrence of these disorders.
   **b.** The fact that these conditions do not recur in 25% or 50% of offspring as do autosomal recessive, autosomal dominant, and X-linked disorders implies that environmental factors also must play a role in their occurrence.
   **c.** Unlike single gene disorders, the recurrence risk for multifactorial disorders increases with an increasing number of affected relatives and increasing severity of the disorder.
   **d.** There is a difference in male (M) to female (F) ratio of several multifactorial disorders [e.g., congenital hip dislocation (F > M) and pyloric stenosis (M > F)]. When this is the case, the recurrence risk for first-degree relatives is greater when the affected individual is of the less often affected sex.

    **e.** The recurrence risk is greater when the affected individual is more severely affected. For example, the recurrence risk is greater when a child has bilateral cleft lip and palate when compared to isolated cleft lip.

    **f.** The recurrence risk for multifactorial disorders decreases rapidly with decreasing degree of relatedness.

**3. Examples.** Common multifactorial disorders include:

    **a. Common birth defects** [e.g., club foot, cleft lip with or without cleft palate, neural tube defects (meningomyelocele, anencephaly), congenital heart defects, congenital hip dislocation, pyloric stenosis]

    **b. Mental retardation**

    **c. Affective disorders** (e.g., bipolar disorder, schizophrenia)

    **d. Common disorders of midlife** (e.g., hypertension, peptic ulcer disease, hyperlipidemia, diabetes mellitus, coronary artery disease)

**B. Neural tube defects** (see also Ch 17 III B 1) occur in 1–2 in 1000 newborns in the United States.

**1. Types of defects.** The two major types of neural tube defect—anencephaly and meningomyelocele—both are caused by failure of the neural groove to fuse completely into a tube by the twenty-eighth day of pregnancy.

    **a. Anencephaly** represents failure of closure of the caudal neural tube.

        **(1)** Children with anencephaly have no cranium and have only the most basal portions of the brain.

        **(2)** They are profoundly neurologically abnormal and generally die within the first few hours to days of life, surviving to that time on brain stem functions.

    **b. Meningomyelocele** represents failure of closure of the neural tube distal to the brain, leading to hernial protrusion through the vertebral column, as in **spina bifida**.

        **(1)** Lesions may be anywhere along the spine but most commonly occur in the lumbar area.

        **(2)** Failure of development of normal vertebral architecture allows the cord to bulge out of the protective confines of the spine, with resultant loss of neurologic function below the level of the lesion.

        **(3)** The dura and skin must be surgically closed over the lesion to prevent meningitis. Very often, the consequence is hydrocephalus due to the associated presence of an **Arnold-Chiari malformation** of the ventricular system (downward displacement of the hindbrain through the foramen magnum).

        **(4)** Additional neurologic and other associated findings in children with meningomyelocele depend on the level of the lesion.

            **(a)** Bladder control may be absent, with consequent recurrent urinary tract infections, reflux, and the need for urinary diversion.

            **(b)** Bowel function may be lost, with consequent severe chronic constipation.

            **(c)** Club foot and other orthopedic problems below the level of the lesion are common.

            **(d)** Mental retardation and seizures are frequent when hydrocephalus is or has been present.

**2. Risk factors.** Anencephaly and meningomyelocele are two expressions of the same disorder, and an individual at risk for this disorder may have a child with either manifestation. Neural tube defects show classic multifactorial inheritance, but the incidence varies with a number of factors.

    **a. Geographic location** is important, with the incidence being highest in Ireland and Wales.

    **b. Social class** is an important variable, with a higher incidence in poorer groups.

    **c. Maternal age** is a factor, and both teenage mothers and older mothers are at increased risk.

    **d. Prenatal exposure** to known contributory environmental factors, such as valproic acid and maternal diabetes, results in an increased risk.

**3. Recurrence risk** increases with each additional first-degree relative who is affected.

    **a.** If a couple has one child with a neural tube defect, the risk for each subsequent child to be affected is 3%–5%. It is 7%–10% after a second affected child.

    **b.** A person with a meningomyelocele has a 2%–4% risk of having an affected child with each pregnancy.

4. **Prenatal diagnosis** of neural tube defects almost always can be accomplished in the second trimester.
   a. Most neural tube defects, being open defects, are reflected by **elevated AFP levels** in amniotic fluid and in maternal serum (see I F 1).
   b. Elevated maternal serum AFP levels can be followed by a **level II ultrasound** (to examine the fetus for anencephaly or a spinal defect) and **amniocentesis** (to determine whether amniotic fluid AFP and acetylcholine esterase levels are elevated), since the presence of both of these is more specific for neural tube defect. The parents of an affected fetus then have options of terminating the pregnancy or continuing the pregnancy with knowledge of the condition, which allows improved perinatal management and allows the parents to prepare emotionally for having a child with a serious birth defect.

5. **Preventive therapy.** Current studies suggest that the recurrence risk for neural tube defects may be lowered significantly by taking 1 mg of **folic acid** daily from the time of conception through the time of formation of the neural tube (end of first trimester). As a result, many physicians recommend starting prenatal vitamin preparations that contain adequate folate from the time conception is attempted.

C. **Orofacial clefts** are common birth defects with multifactorial inheritance.

1. **Cleft lip with or without cleft palate** is seen in 1–2 per 1000 live births.
   a. **Risk factors**
      (1) Twice as many boys are born with cleft lip with or without cleft palate as girls.
      (2) The incidence of cleft lip is highest in Asian and American Indian populations and lowest in blacks.
   b. **Differential diagnosis.** There are over 50 syndromes that include cleft lip with or without cleft palate, and these must be excluded before making the diagnosis of isolated cleft lip with or without cleft palate. These syndromes may be autosomal dominant, autosomal recessive, X-linked, or sporadic.
      (1) An example is **Van der Woude syndrome,** an autosomal dominant condition where lip pits are seen in all gene carriers but only some individuals have cleft lip with or without cleft palate due to variable expressivity. The recurrence risk for gene carriers is 50% versus 3%–5% in the multifactorial isolated cleft lip.
      (2) Cleft lip may be associated with exposure to teratogenic agents, particularly alcohol.
   c. **Recurrence risk**
      (1) Recurrence risk if one child or one parent is affected is 3%–5%.
      (2) Recurrence risk if two children or one child and one parent are affected is 10%.
      (3) Recurrence risk is higher if affected individuals have bilateral cleft lip and palate or if females are affected.

2. **Isolated cleft palate** is a multifactorial condition distinct from cleft lip with or without cleft palate that is seen in 1 in 2000 live births.
   a. **Risk factors**
      (1) Girls are affected more frequently than boys.
      (2) The recurrence risks for cleft palate are similar to those for cleft lip with or without cleft palate; however, there is no increased risk for having a child with cleft lip.
   b. **Differential diagnosis.** There are over 150 syndromes that involve cleft palate; therefore, other abnormalities must be excluded before making a diagnosis of isolated cleft palate.
   c. **Subtypes**
      (1) Microforms of cleft palate are **bifid uvula** and **submucous cleft** of the palate. These conditions usually are not of functional significance. However, the **recurrence risk** is 3%–5%, which includes a risk for having a child with a complete cleft of the palate.
      (2) Another form of cleft palate is caused by **micrognathia (hypoplastic mandible)** and projection of the tongue posteriorly during development, preventing closure of the palate. This phenomenon is called **Pierre Robin (Robin) sequence.**
         (a) The cleft usually is U-shaped.
         (b) The **recurrence risk** generally is low, since the Pierre Robin sequence usually is sporadic; however, the Pierre Robin sequence can be associated with syndromes such as **Stickler syndrome** and **Treacher Collins syndrome**. When a syndrome is present, the recurrence risk depends on the inheritance of the syndrome. There are over 50 syndromes in which the Pierre Robin sequence may be seen.

## VI. WHEN TO CONSIDER A GENETIC OR MULTIFACTORIAL DISORDER

### A. Prenatally

1. **Fetal wastage** may be an indication of a balanced chromosome translocation, a lethal autosomal recessive disorder, or a new dominant disorder.

2. **Fetal growth deficiency** is seen in many chromosomally abnormal pregnancies, in some syndromes, and in many fetuses with malformations.

3. **Oligohydramnios** may reflect genetic urinary tract disorders, where there is decreased fetal urine production.

4. **Polyhydramnios** can be seen in neurologically impaired fetuses, including those with genetic neurologic disorders, and in fetuses with malformations of the gastrointestinal tract, where swallowing is impaired.

### B. In the newborn

1. **Congenital malformations** often are due to a genetic disorder or condition with a genetic component. A careful evaluation should consider other anomalies, dysmorphic features, and neurologic abnormalities that suggest syndromes, chromosome disorders, and multifactorial isolated birth defects.

2. **Infants who are small for gestational age** may have a genetic disorder.
   a. Examination should seek possible dysmorphic features, malformations, neurologic abnormalities, and a significant prenatal history.
   b. Chromosome disorders, syndromes, and dwarfing conditions should be considered in addition to teratogens, placental abnormalities, and in utero constraint.

3. **Large size at birth** also may be a reflection of an abnormality. One of the disorders of overgrowth is the **Beckwith-Wiedemann syndrome,** which is associated with macrosomia, omphalocele, macroglossia, and hypoglycemia. Infants of diabetic mothers often are large (macrosomic) at birth.

4. **Infants with short stature at birth** may have a dwarfing condition or may be small for gestational age.

5. **Dysmorphism** often is an indicator of a chromosomal abnormality, a single gene or sporadic syndrome, or deformation. An evaluation for other anomalies of function or structure should be undertaken. A careful prenatal history may indicate deformation as the cause.

6. **Hypotonia** may indicate a genetic disorder, such as a CNS malformation, neuromuscular disease, or one of a variety of syndromes associated with central hypotonia (e.g., chromosomal disorders, Prader-Willi syndrome, some dwarfing conditions).

7. **Seizures** resulting from a metabolic derangement or CNS malformation associated with a genetic disorder may present in the newborn. Chromosomal disorders and single gene disorders frequently are the cause.

8. **Ambiguous genitalia** imply a genetic disorder unless the fetus was exposed to hormones. The differential diagnosis of ambiguous genitalia includes metabolic disorders, multifactorial abnormalities, chromosome anomalies, single gene disorders, teratogenic exposures, and sporadic syndromes.

9. **Abnormal pH** (e.g., acidosis, alkalosis) occurs in a number of inborn metabolic errors, such as amino acidurias and organic acidurias.

### C. In the infant and toddler

1. **Failure to thrive,** or insufficient growth rate, has many causes, some of which are genetic (see also Ch 3 I A). It often is helpful diagnostically to distinguish between conditions with prenatal-onset growth deficiency (such as fetal alcohol syndrome and chromosomal disorders) and those with only postnatal-onset failure to thrive (such as metabolic disorders).
   a. **Inborn errors of metabolism** commonly have associated failure to thrive, as do **neurodegenerative disorders** and other severe neurologic conditions that may be genetic in origin.
   b. Many **chromosome abnormalities and syndromes** have associated growth deficiency.
   c. **Dwarfing conditions** may initially present as failure to thrive, although growth rate may eventually normalize.

**d.** Some **teratogens,** such as alcohol, may also produce postnatal as well as prenatal growth deficiency.

**2. Developmental delay** also has many causes, but it should raise suspicion of a genetic condition.

   **a. Delays in motor development** alone may reflect a neuromuscular disorder, either central or peripheral.

   **b. Delays in cognitive development** alone or cognitive plus motor delays may presage mental retardation, which should raise suspicion of a genetic cause.

   **c.** Many syndromes have associated **developmental delays and mental retardation,** and, thus, delays should trigger the search for associated anomalies or dysmorphism.

**3. Loss of developmental milestones,** or **regression,** suggests neurodegenerative disorders, most of which are genetic in origin (e.g., neuronal storage disorders).

**4. Microcephaly** (see also Ch 17 III C 2)

   **a.** Microcephaly usually is a sign of poor brain development **(micrencephaly),** as the skull generally grows in response to brain growth. There are many causes of micrencephaly, including single gene disorders, chromosomal abnormalities, syndromes, anoxic or vascular brain damage, and teratogen exposure.

   **b.** Occasionally, microcephaly can be a reflection of premature closure of the sutures **(craniosynostosis).** This can occur on the basis of a genetic disorder or syndrome or can occur sporadically.

**5. Macrocephaly** can be familial and isolated or can reflect an abnormality that may be genetic in origin.

   **a.** Macrocephaly may be caused by increased ventricular size (as in hydrocephalus), or it may be due to increased brain size **(macrencephaly).**

   **b.** Some disorders and syndromes are associated with macrocephaly without apparent consequence, such as **neurofibromatosis.** Associated signs and symptoms should be sought.

   **c. Fragile X syndrome** has associated macrocephaly, so patients with macrocephaly should be evaluated for mental retardation.

   **d.** Some inborn metabolic errors causing **storage of material in nerve cells** can produce macrocephaly. Mucopolysaccharidoses, for example, are associated with macrocephaly.

   **e. Intracranial malformations** may present as large head size, reflecting **hydrocephalus.** In most cases, it is appropriate to do a cranial CT or MRI scan if macrocephaly of unknown etiology is present.

**6. An unusual growth pattern** may be an indication of a genetic condition.

   **a.** Some disorders associated with **limb asymmetry or hypertrophy** include neurofibromatosis, **Klippel-Trenaunay-Weber syndrome,** and **Russell-Silver syndrome.** Such asymmetry should also raise suspicion of an intra-abdominal tumor, such as Wilms' tumor. Abdominal ultrasound is indicated when limb hypertrophy is present.

   **b. Generalized overgrowth** may suggest Beckwith-Wiedemann syndrome or Sotos' syndrome.

   **c. Disproportionate growth** often is indicative of a bony dysplasia or connective tissue abnormality.

      **(1)** Short limbs, often resulting in short stature, should trigger the search for radiologic abnormalities of bone growth.

      **(2)** Unusually long limbs for race might suggest Marfan syndrome, homocystinuria, or Stickler syndrome.

      **(3)** A short trunk usually indicates a bony abnormality of the spine, generally either a bony dysplasia, scoliosis, or structural vertebral anomalies.

**7. Abnormal pigmentation,** diffusely or focally, may reflect a genetic disorder (see also Ch 17 VIII A, B).

   **a. Neurocutaneous disorders** often present in this age-group with dermatologic findings. Such disorders include **neurofibromatosis** (café au lait spots), **tuberous sclerosis** (hypopigmented spots), **basal cell nevus syndrome** (multiple nevi), and **incontinentia pigmenti** (swirls of hyperpigmentation).

   **b.** Generalized hypopigmentation may be seen with **albinism** or **ectodermal dysplasias.**

**8. An unusual odor** of an infant or the infant's urine may be a manifestation of an inborn metabolic error, such as PKU (mousy odor) or maple syrup urine disease.

### D. In childhood

1. **Mental retardation** is the most common indication of a genetic problem that is recognized in the school-age child. Frequently, it is preceded by developmental delay.
   a. The causes of mental retardation are many. Identifying the specific etiology is important, as it allows the determination of prognosis, educational planning. possible associated problems, and the recurrence risk. Table 7-3 lists the major categories of causes of mental retardation and some examples (see also Ch 3 Table 3-1).
   b. The evaluation of the child with mental retardation is discussed in Chapter 3 IV B. When no cause for mental retardation can be found, multifactorial inheritance is the most likely etiology, with a 3%–5% recurrence risk.

2. Some **metabolic disorders, genetic neurologic conditions, and neurodegenerative disorders** may present in mid-childhood.

3. **Chronic anemia** may reflect hemoglobinopathy (e.g., thalassemia) or a disorder of red blood cell metabolism [e.g., glucose-6-phosphate dehydrogenase (G6PD) deficiency].

### E. In adolescence and adulthood

1. Failure of expected secondary sexual development and other **pubertal disorders** may indicate a genetic condition.
   a. Some single gene disorders, such as testicular feminization, are associated with primary amenorrhea.
   b. Sex chromosome abnormalities, such as Turner syndrome (45,X) or Klinefelter syndrome (47,XXY), lead to incomplete or inadequate sexual development.
   c. Several syndrome disorders have associated delayed, precocious, or abnormal pubertal development (e.g., Prader-Willi syndrome).

2. Several genetic **neurologic disorders** may present in adolescence, such as the hereditary and sensory motor neuropathies [e.g., Charcot-Marie-Tooth disease (see Ch 17 X B 1)], some spinocerebellar degenerations, and some ataxias [e.g., Friedreich's ataxia (see Ch 17 IX C 1)].

3. **Genetic kidney disorders** (see Ch 13 X) commonly present in adulthood, including autosomal dominant polycystic kidney disease and hereditary nephritis. The initial presenting symptom may be hypertension.

4. **Cancer** may occur at an earlier age than is commonly seen due to genetic predisposition (see Ch 15 I C 1).

**Table 7-3.** Causes of Mental Retardation

| Category | Examples |
| --- | --- |
| Autosomal dominant | Tuberous sclerosis<br>Myotonic dystrophy |
| Autosomal recessive | Phenylketonuria<br>Mucopolysaccharidoses |
| X-linked | Fragile X syndrome<br>Aqueductal stenosis |
| Multifactorial | Nonspecific mental retardation<br>Hydrocephalus |
| Chromosomal | Down syndrome<br>Prader-Willi syndrome |
| Teratogenic | Fetal alcohol syndrome<br>Congenital rubella syndrome |
| Accidental | Perinatal anoxia<br>Intracranial hemorrhage |
| Unknown etiology | Williams syndrome<br>Cornelia de Lange syndrome |

    **a.** Some single gene disorders cause a predisposition to cancer, including those causing multiple endocrine neoplasias, breast cancer, Peutz-Jeghers syndrome (colon cancer), familial polyposis, and Gardner syndrome.

    **b.** Some families have an increased risk for several different types of cancer. These so-called cancer families present as though they have an autosomal dominant disorder with variable expressivity.

    **c.** Some chromosomal deletions can predispose to cancer (e.g., deletion of band 11p13 with Wilms' tumor).

**5. Early onset of common disorders of midlife,** such as coronary artery disease and hypertension, are caused in some families by genetic predisposition, which may be due to a single gene disorder or may be multifactorial.

**6. Infertility** or **recurrent pregnancy loss** may be caused by a parental balanced translocation, a genetic lethal disorder in the fetus, or a structural uterine abnormality in the woman. Oligospermia associated with infertility in men can be seen in Klinefelter syndrome, cystic fibrosis, and immotile cilia syndrome.

**7.** Several autosomal dominant **seizure disorders** present during adolescence or adulthood.

**8.** A **family history of birth defects or mental retardation** may be indicative of an autosomal or X-linked disorder or a balanced chromosomal translocation within the family.

## BIBLIOGRAPHY

Buyse ML (ed): *The Birth Defects Encyclopedia.* Cambridge, MA, Blackwell Scientific, 1990.

Emery AEH, Rimoin DL: *Principles and Practice of Medical Genetics.* New York, Churchill Livingstone, 1983.

Gelehrter TD, Collins FS: *Principles of Medical Genetics.* Baltimore, Williams & Wilkins, 1990.

McKusick VA: *Mendelian Inheritance in Man,* 9th edition. Baltimore, Johns Hopkins University Press, 1990.

Thompson JS, Thompson MW: *Genetics in Medicine,* 5th edition. Philadelphia, WB Saunders, 1989.

Scriver CR, et al: *The Metabolic Basis of Inherited Disease,* 6th edition. New York, McGraw-Hill, 1989.

# STUDY QUESTIONS

**Directions:** Each of the numbered items or incomplete statements in this section is followed by answers or by completions of the statement. Select the **one** lettered answer or completion that is **best** in each case.

1. Each of the following clinical signs may be indicative of an inborn error of amino acid or organic acid metabolism EXCEPT

(A)  metabolic acidosis in an infant
(B)  an unusual odor of urine or sweat
(C)  vomiting and lethargy in an infant
(D)  accelerated growth in a child
(E)  mental retardation in a child

2. PKU is the most common disorder of amino acid metabolism. Which one of the following statements regarding PKU is true?

(A)  PKU is an autosomal dominant disorder
(B)  Hyperpigmentation is a common sign of PKU
(C)  Dietary management should begin within 1 month of birth to prevent mental retardation
(D)  Dietary restriction can be discontinued safely in adolescence
(E)  Heart defects are common in people with PKU

3. A child who displays loss of developmental milestones, or regression, should be investigated for

(A)  amino aciduria
(B)  neuronal storage disorder
(C)  chromosomal translocation
(D)  teratogenic exposure during fetal development

4. Maternal ingestion of significant amounts of alcohol throughout pregnancy can cause all of the following outcomes EXCEPT

(A)  a normal child
(B)  a child with developmental delay who is otherwise normal
(C)  a child with Down syndrome
(D)  a child with dysmorphic features, small size, and developmental retardation
(E)  a child who is microcephalic and small for gestational age

5. All of the following statements regarding Down syndrome are true EXCEPT

(A)  it is the most common chromosome abnormality
(B)  heart defects and gastrointestinal abnormalities occur with increased frequency
(C)  most individuals are severely or profoundly retarded
(D)  a familial balanced translocation involving chromosome 21 affects a small proportion of individuals

6. Chromosome analysis is indicated for all of the following conditions EXCEPT

(A)  suspected Down syndrome
(B)  recurrent pregnancy loss
(C)  primary amenorrhea
(D)  meningomyelocele
(E)  ambiguous genitalia

7. Although the exact etiology of Marfan syndrome is unknown, it is clinically associated with abnormalities in

(A)  connective tissue, causing aortic dilatation and loose joints
(B)  bone metabolism, causing excess bone length and width
(C)  muscle cell development, causing floppy tendons and ligaments
(D)  growth factors, causing tall stature and excess subcutaneous tissue

| | | |
|---|---|---|
| 1-D | 4-C | 7-A |
| 2-C | 5-C | |
| 3-B | 6-D | |

8. Which of the following statements regarding neural tube defects is true?

(A) Neural tube defects are produced prior to implantation of the embryo
(B) Abnormally low maternal serum AFP levels suggest the presence of a neural tube defect
(C) A single autosomal recessive gene is the most common cause of neural tube defects
(D) Parents who have had a child with a neural tube defect have an increased risk for having another child with such a defect
(E) Neural tube defects most commonly are part of a syndrome

9. Which of the following statements regarding syndromes is true?

(A) All major features of a known syndrome must be present before a diagnosis can be made
(B) Internal abnormalities often are associated with dysmorphic features in a syndrome
(C) Syndromes almost always can be recognized shortly after birth
(D) Syndromes almost always are the result of single gene mutations
(E) All syndromes have associated dysmorphic features

10. Amniocentesis is performed on a 36-year-old pregnant woman. The karyotype of the fetus is 46,XY/47,XY,+21, indicating that some of the cells have a normal karyotype and some of the cells are trisomic for chromosome 21. Which of the following statements concerning these findings is true?

(A) The fetus has Down syndrome
(B) The cause of there being two cell lines is prefertilization nondisjunction
(C) The chromosome abnormality reflects translocation
(D) The recurrence risk for this chromosome abnormality is 15%

**Questions 11–12**

A fourth-year medical student attends what is expected to be a normal delivery, and the child—a boy—is born with a unilateral cleft lip and palate.

11. What is the most important evaluation to be performed to determine the cause of the cleft lip and palate?

(A) Physical examination
(B) CT scan of the head
(C) Serum alcohol level
(D) Urine toxic screen
(E) Amino acid analysis

12. Evaluation of the newborn boy and his parents suggests a diagnosis of isolated cleft lip and palate. What is the most likely form of inheritance of this defect?

(A) Autosomal recessive
(B) Autosomal dominant
(C) X-linked
(D) Multifactorial
(E) Nongenetic (sporadic)

8-D      11-A
9-B      12-D
10-A

**Directions:** Each item below contains four suggested answers of which **one or more** is correct. Choose the answer

    **A**  if **1, 2, and 3** are correct
    **B**  if **1 and 3** are correct
    **C**  if **2 and 4** are correct
    **D**  if **4** is correct
    **E**  if **1, 2, 3, and 4** are correct

13. Macrocephaly in a young child may be the result of

(1) fragile X syndrome
(2) a benign familial characteristic
(3) mucopolysaccharidosis
(4) vascular brain damage

14. An adverse outcome resulting from a potentially teratogenic agent may be influenced by

(1) dosage of the exposure
(2) genetic susceptibility of the fetus
(3) gestational age at which the fetus is exposed
(4) interaction with other agents

**Directions:** The group of items in this section consists of lettered options followed by a set of numbered items. For each item, select the **one** lettered option that is most closely associated with it. Each lettered option may be selected once, more than once, or not at all.

**Questions 15–18**

Match each genetic disorder named below with its appropriate classification.

(A) Autosomal recessive disorder
(B) Autosomal dominant disorder
(C) X-linked disorder
(D) Multifactorial disorder
(E) Chromosome deletion disorder

15. Prader-Willi syndrome

16. Fragile X sundrome

17. PKU

18. Nonspecific isolated mental retardation

---

13-A      16-C
14-E      17-A
15-E      18-D

## ANSWERS AND EXPLANATIONS

**1. The answer is D** *[III C 3; Tables 7-1, 7-2].*
Accelerated growth rate is a rare finding in childhood and has not been associated with disorders of amino acid or organic acid metabolism. Growth retardation is a more common finding, due to disturbance in protein metabolism and utilization. Metabolic acidosis, vomiting, and lethargy in an infant suggest a disorder of amino acid or carbohydrate metabolism. An unusual odor of urine or sweat is noted in several metabolic disorders that affect children. Likewise, mental retardation may be caused by a number of these disorders (e.g., phenylketonuria, homocystinuria, mucopolysaccharidoses).

**2. The answer is C** *[III C 3 b (2)].*
Phenylketonuria (PKU) is an autosomal recessive disorder of amino acid metabolism, which is characterized by a block of conversion of phenylalanine to tyrosine. Dietary restriction should start early in infancy (by age 1 month) and be maintained throughout life, especially in women with PKU, who are at a high risk for giving birth to children with microcephaly and congenital heart disease when they are off dietary restriction. Because tyrosine is essential to the production of the pigment melanin, hypopigmentation is a common sign of PKU.

**3. The answer is B** *[VI C 3].*
Loss of previously attained developmental progress is seen in neurodegenerative disorders, most of which are genetic. These include, among others, neuronal storage disorders, mucopolysaccharidoses, demyelinating conditions, dementing disorders (e.g., Huntington's disease), and uncontrollable seizure disorders.

**4. The answer is C** *[II G 1 b, 2].*
Alcohol exposure during gestation can produce a child who has some or all of the features of the fetal alcohol syndrome, or it can have no recognizable effect. Clinical features of fetal alcohol syndrome include CNS abnormalities (e.g., intellectual defects, microcephaly), growth deficiencies, facial dysmorphisms, and other structural anomalies. Down syndrome is not known to occur at an increased rate as a result of maternal alcohol use.

**5. The answer is C** *[IV B 1].*
Down syndrome results in a characteristic pattern of dysmorphic features and mental retardation, with an increased risk for internal malformations, especially congenital heart defects and duodenal atresia. Mental retardation generally is moderate, with the average IQ being 50. While most Down syndrome is caused by nondisjunction (trisomy 21), about 1% of cases result from a familial balanced translocation. Such families have an increased risk for having another child with Down syndrome when compared with parents of children with trisomy 21.

**6. The answer is D** *[IV A 2; V B 1 b].*
Meningomyelocele is a birth defect characterized by failure of the neural tube to close distal to the brain. Neural tube defects display classic multifactorial inheritance; they are not associated with chromosome abnormalities. Conditions that are associated with chromosome abnormalities—for which chromosomal analysis is indicated—include Down syndrome, recurrent pregnancy loss, primary amenorrhea, and ambiguous genitalia.

**7. The answer is A** *[III A 2 a, b].*
Marfan syndrome is an autosomal dominant disorder of connective tissue. Major manifestations include a characteristic body habitus (i.e., long, thin digits and limbs; loose joints; scoliosis and chest deformity), aortic dilatation and mitral valve prolapse, and lens dislocation and myopia. Bone metabolism, muscle cell development, and hormone status are normal.

**8. The answer is D** *[V B 1–4].*
Neural tube defects are due to a defect of closure of the neural groove, which normally closes by 28 days gestation. Implantation occurs by 7–10 days postconception. Caudal failure to close results in anencephaly, and distal failure to close results in meningomyelocele (spina bifida), both occurring on the basis of a multifactorial disorder with two possible manifestations. The recurrence risk for neural tube defects increases with each additional first-degree relative who is affected. A couple with one affected child has a 3%–5% risk of having another child with a neural tube defect; the risk is 7%–10% after a second affected child. High maternal serum $\alpha$-fetoprotein (AFP) levels reflect an abnormal opening between the fetus and amniotic fluid and occurs in 85% of pregnancies in which a neural tube defect is present. Neural tube defects rarely are part of a syndrome.

**9. The answer is B** *[I D 2].*
Syndromes constitute recognizable patterns of internal and/or external structural and functional abnormalities with described natural history and recurrence risk. Common internal malformations include congenital heart defects, renal malformations, defects of brain development, and skeletal abnormalities (e.g., hemivertebrae). Variability among affected persons results in the absence of absolute diagnostic criteria in most cases, and although these individuals share a number of features, no specific feature or features need be present in a given affected person. The characteristic features of syndromes may evolve over time, so that many syndromes are not diagnosed until some growth and development have occurred. Syndromes can result from single gene defects, chromosomal abnormalities, teratogens, or deformations. Some syndromes do not have associated dysmorphic features.

**10. The answer is A** *[IV B 1 a (3)].*
The fetus described in the question has Down syndrome caused by a chromosome mosaic (i.e., one cell line with 46 chromosomes and two 21 chromosomes, and one cell line with 47 chromosomes and three 21 chromosomes). The mosaicism results from mitotic nondisjunction—a postzygotic event. The recurrence risk of mosaicism is negligible. The phenotype of mosaic Down syndrome is essentially the same as for full trisomy 21, although sometimes wilder. Translocation is the exchange of material between two chromosomes in a cell, not the presence of two chromosomally different cell lines.

**11–12. The answers are: 11-A, 12-D** *[V C 1 b].*
Cleft lip with or without cleft palate can result from teratogenic exposure; it can be part of the fetal alcohol syndrome; it can be inherited as a multifactorial disorder; or it can be part of an autosomal dominant, autosomal recessive, or X-linked condition. In all, more than 50 syndromes are associated with cleft lip with or without cleft palate. Physical examination will reveal whether there are any dysmorphic features or malformations suggestive of such a syndrome. CT scan of the head, serum alcohol level, and urine toxic screen might be helpful in specific situations, depending on the physical examination and history. Cleft lip with or without cleft palate is not associated with amino acid disorders.

When isolated, cleft lip with or without cleft palate is considered a multifactorial disorder, resulting from the effects of genes contributed by both parents (genetic liability) and some nongenetic (environmental) factors, which often cannot be identified.

**13. The answer is A (1, 2, 3)** *[VI C 4 a, 5].*
Microcephaly, not macrocephaly, may be caused by anoxic or vascular brain damage. Macrocephaly has many causes, including intracranial malformations or hydrocephalus (enlarged ventricles) and enlarged brain due to storage of abnormal substances within or between the nerve cells (e.g., mucopolysaccharidosis). Certain disorders have associated macrocephaly for unknown reasons, such as fragile X syndrome and neurofibromatosis. Macrocephaly also may run in families; by definition, 5% of the normal population have a head circumference greater than the ninety-fifth percentile. In these cases, there are no known associated abnormalities.

**14. The answer is E (all)** *[II A 1–5].*
Dosage is an important factor in teratogenesis; a threshold may exist below which no effect is seen, or a dose-response relationship may apply. Timing is the most critical factor, since each tissue is most susceptible to the influence of a teratogen during a few specific gestational weeks, usually while organogenesis is occurring. The genetic constitution of the fetus also determines whether the fetus is susceptible to the effect of a teratogen. Interaction with other agents may influence the effect of a teratogenic agent.

**15–18. The answers are: 15-E** *[IV D 1 d (2) (a)]*, **16-C** *[III C 2]*, **17-A** *[III B 3 b (2)]*, **18-D** *[VI D 1 b].*
Prader-Willi syndrome is a multisystem disorder characterized by dysmorphic features, obesity, short stature, and mental retardation. It is associated with a deletion of the long arm of chromosome 15, which is detectable with prometaphase analysis.

Fragile X syndrome is a common form of mental retardation that is X-linked. A marker, the so-called fragile X chromosome, is demonstrable on the distal end of the long arm of the X chromosome in folate-deficient cell culture studies performed in affected individuals. This karyotypic phenomenon is believed to be a consequence of the abnormal gene, which also causes mental retardation.

PKU is an autosomal recessive disorder of amino acid metabolism resulting from deficiency of phenylalanine hydroxylase, the enzyme that converts phenylalanine to tyrosine. If not treated with dietary restriction of phenylalanine, mental retardation results.

When no cause for mental retardation can be found and there are no associated physical or functional abnormalities, multifactorial inheritance is the most likely etiology. In this case, there is a 3%–5% empiric recurrence risk.

# 8

# Immunologic, Allergic, and Rheumatic Diseases

Mark Ballow
Milton Markowitz

**I. HOST DEFENSE SYSTEMS.** The human immune system is a dynamic network of cellular and humoral elements working in concert to allow the host to recognize foreign substances and to eliminate, neutralize, or metabolize those substances. Functions of the immune system fall into three main categories: **resistance** to microbial invasion, maintenance of **homeostasis,** and **surveillance** against transformed or malignant cells.

**A. Nonspecific (innate, nonadaptive) host defenses**

1. **Barriers** act as a front line in defense. There are two types:
   a. **Anatomic (physical)** barriers (e.g., skin, cilia, mucus)
   b. **Biochemical** barriers (e.g., lysozyme, lactoferrin, gastric acid)

2. **Cells** involved in nonspecific defense include leukocytes (neutrophils, eosinophils, basophils), mast cells, macrophages, cells of the reticuloendothelial system (RES), platelets, and natural killer (NK) cells.

3. **Plasma or soluble factors** serving in conjunction with the cellular elements of the nonspecific defense system include proteins of the complement and coagulation pathways, proteins of the kinin-kallikrein system, acute-phase proteins, and fibronectin.

4. **Factors released from cells** of the nonspecific defense system include α- and β-interferons, interleukins, lysosomal enzymes, and mediators of anaphylaxis.

**B. Specific (adaptive) host defenses** involve an adaptive (**immunogenic**) response to foreign materials, followed by specific recognition and long-term memory of the molecule (**antigen**) that caused the initial **immune response**.

1. **Humoral immunity** defends primarily against the extracellular phases of bacterial and viral infections.
   a. **Cellular elements** consist of B lymphocytes (B cells) and **plasma cells**.
   b. **Serum factors** include five classes of **immunoglobulins (antibodies):** immunoglobulin G (IgG), IgM, IgA, IgD, and IgE.

2. **Cellular immunity** defends against intracellular organisms (e.g., viruses, fungi, parasites) and provides immune surveillance against malignant cells and foreign tissue.
   a. **Cellular elements** consist of **T lymphocytes (T cells)** and their subsets.
   b. **T cell–derived factors** include lymphokines, interleukins, helper and suppressor factors, and γ-interferon.

**II. IMMUNODEFICIENCY DISORDERS.** Deficiencies of host defense systems result in an immunologic imbalance that can lead to a susceptibility to infection, an autoimmune disease, or a predisposition to malignancies.

**A. Complement disorders.** Activation of the complement system, by either the classic or the alternative pathway, leads to the generation of potent complement components, which have various biologic activities. The activated complement system is an important humoral mediator involved in inflammation and host defense. **Faulty complement activation or regulation** can lead to various disorders.

1. **Deficiency of early complement components** (C1, C4, C2) results in a symptom complex resembling systemic lupus erythematosus (SLE).

2. **C3 deficiency** results in severe pyogenic infections.

3. **Deficiency of late complement components** (C5, C6, C7, C8) results in recurrent *Neisseria* infections.

4. **Abnormalities of the alternative pathway** (factor H, factor I, properdin) may result in recurrent infections.

5. **Deficiency of complement inhibitors** (C1 esterase inhibitor, carboxypeptidase N) leads to recurrent angioedema.

B. **Phagocyte disorders** (Table 8-1)

1. **Types of defects.** Phagocyte disorders affect any one or several of the cell's functions, including:
   a. Adherence to vascular endothelium
   b. Recognition of and migration toward a chemical stimulus (chemotaxis)
   c. Phagocytosis
   d. Intracellular killing

2. **Clinical features**
   a. Affected individuals are prone to **infections** with low-grade bacteria such as *Staphylococcus aureus* and gram-negative enteric bacteria. Infections may range from mild skin lesions to severe systemic infections. Typical infections include furunculosis, organ abscess, and lymphadenitis.
   b. Patients with a **leukocyte adhesion deficiency** have defective expression of cell membrane adhesion glycoproteins (e.g., CD11, CD18) and have a history of delayed separation of the umbilical cord (> 4 weeks after birth).

C. **B cell deficiency disorders** (Table 8-2). Defects or deficiencies of B cells lead to various antibody deficiencies, or **hypogammaglobulinemias**. Patients suffer from recurrent infections.

1. **Causative agents** are most commonly **extracellular organisms,** namely pyogenic and enteric bacteria, because patients are deficient in serum opsonins (antibodies) necessary for phagocytosis. Patients with X-linked (Bruton's) agammaglobulinemia may also have problems with certain enteric viruses (e.g., polio virus, echo virus, coxsackievirus). Patients with IgA deficiency or common variable hypogammaglobulinemia are affected by *Giardia lamblia,* a gastrointestinal parasite (see Ch 9 X C).

2. **Sites of infection** include the skin, sinuses, meninges, and respiratory, urinary, and gastrointestinal tracts.

D. **T cell deficiency disorders** (Table 8-3), also known as **cell-mediated (cellular) immunodeficiencies,** result from abnormalities in T cell functions. Antibody production is also likely to be affected in patients with severe T cell abnormalities, since T cells are important immunoregulators of B cell differentiation and function.

1. **Recurrent infections** also are common in patients with cellular immunodeficiencies.
   a. **Causative agents** are **intracellular pathogens** [e.g., herpesviruses, mycobacteria, fungi (*Candida*), and protozoa (*Pneumocystis carinii, Toxoplasma*)].
   b. **Sites of infection** include a variety of sites, both local and systemic.

**Table 8-1.** Phagocyte Disorders in Children

| Disorder | Inheritance | Clinical Features | Therapy |
|---|---|---|---|
| Chronic granulomatous disease | X-linked (66%); autosomal recessive (33%) | Infections with catalase-positive bacteria and fungi affecting skin, lungs, liver; granuloma formation; NBT test is diagnostic | Antibiotics; γ-interferon |
| Myeloperoxidase deficiency | Autosomal recessive | Fungal infections (candidiasis) in deep tissues, especially in presence of diabetes | Antibiotics |
| Leukocyte adhesion deficiency | Autosomal recessive | Delayed separation of the umbilical cord; skin infections; otitis media; pneumonia; gingivitis; periodontitis | Antibiotics |
| Abnormal chemotaxis | Variable | Recurrent skin infections with staphylococci, enteric bacteria | Antibiotics |

NBT = nitroblue tetrazolium dye.

**Table 8-2.** B Cell Deficiency Disorders in Children

| Disorder | Inheritance | Clinical Features | Therapy |
|---|---|---|---|
| X-linked agammaglobulinemia (Bruton's disease) | X-linked | Recurrent pyogenic infections; infections of lungs, sinuses, middle ear, skin, CNS | Immune serum globulin; antibiotics |
| Transient hypogammaglobulinemia of infancy | Unknown | Recurrent pyogenic infections; frequent in families with other immunodeficiencies | Antibiotics; immune serum globulin (selected patients) |
| Selective immunoglobulin deficiency (IgA, IgM, IgG subclasses) | Various (IgA deficiency only); autosomal recessive; unknown | Recurrent infections of lungs, sinuses; gastrointestinal disease; allergy; frequent in families with common variable immunodeficiency | Antibiotics; immune serum globulin (IgG subclass deficiency only) |
| Immunoglobulin deficiency with increased IgM (and IgD) | X-linked; autosomal recessive; unknown | Infections of lungs, sinuses, middle ear; increased frequency of autoimmune disease | Immune serum globulin; antibiotics |
| Common variable immunodeficiency | Autosomal recessive; autosomal dominant; unknown | Infections of lungs, sinuses, middle ear; giardiasis; malabsorption; autoimmune disease | Immune serum globulin; antibiotics |
| Transcobalamin II deficiency | Autosomal recessive | Recurrent infections; megaloblastic anemia; intestinal villous atrophy; defective granulocyte bactericidal activity | Immune serum globulin; high dose of vitamin $B_{12}$ |
| X-linked hypogammaglobulinemia with growth hormone deficiency | X-linked | Recurrent pyogenic infections; short stature | Immune serum globulin |
| Functional or specific antibody deficiency with normal total immunoglobulins and normal IgG subclasses | Unknown | Recurrent sinopulmonary infections | Antibiotics; immune serum globulin |

2. **Congenital cell-mediated immunodeficiencies** represent a complex spectrum of immunodeficiencies. At one extreme are defects in lymphoid stem cell differentiation, which result in severe combined immunodeficiency disorders. At the other extreme are isolated defects that affect only cell-mediated immunity to one particular pathogen (e.g., chronic mucocutaneous candidiasis).

E. **Acquired immune deficiency syndrome (AIDS)** is a disorder associated with a profound deficiency of T cell immunity and, in children, T cell and B cell abnormalities. Although identified only in 1981, AIDS currently is the ninth leading cause of death among children age 1–4 years and the seventh leading cause of death in the 15–24 year age-group. By 1992, AIDS probably will be one of the top five leading causes of death in the 1–4 year age-group.

1. **Causative agent and risk factors.** AIDS is caused by a retrovirus called human immunodeficiency virus (HIV-1).
   a. **Transmission.** Pediatric AIDS may be acquired prenatally or later during childhood.
      (1) In most HIV-infected children, the virus is transmitted prenatally from mother to child. The efficiency of intrauterine transmission from infected mother to infant is unknown, but the rate appears to be approximately 30%–40%.
      (2) Perinatal transmission also has been suggested, as a consequence of exposure to maternal blood at the time of delivery or during breast feeding.

**Table 8-3.** T Cell and Combined T Cell and B Cell Deficiency Disorders in Children

| Disorder | Inheritance | Clinical Features | Therapy |
|---|---|---|---|
| Severe combined immuno-deficiency<br>Sporadic<br>X-linked<br>Autosomal recessive<br>With B cells and a mixed lymphocyte reaction<br>Nezelof syndrome | X-linked; autosomal recessive | Recurrent infections; wasting; chronic diarrhea; failure to thrive; graft versus host disease | Bone marrow transplantation |
| Defects of the purine salvage pathway<br>Adenosine deaminase deficiency<br>Purine nucleoside phosphorylase deficiency | Autosomal recessive | Recurrent infections; dysostosis (some adenosine deaminase deficiency); anemia and mental retardation (purine nucleoside phosphorylase deficiency) | Bone marrow transplantation; enzyme replacement therapy |
| DiGeorge anomaly (third and fourth pouch/arch syndrome) | None or unknown (embryologic defect) | Hypoparathyroidism (hypocalcemia); facial abnormalities; cardiovascular abnormalities; infections; mental deficiency (some patients); gastrointestinal tract malformation (some patients) | Thymus graft or thymic humoral factors (e.g., thymosin) |
| Chronic mucocutaneous candidiasis | Autosomal recessive | Chronic candidal infection of the skin, nails, scalp, and mucous membranes; autoimmune endocrine disorders | Topical and systemic antifungal agents; transfer factor; thymus transplantation |
| Major histocompatibility complex deficiency<br>Class I deficiency<br>Class II deficiency | Autosomal recessive | Intestinal malabsorption (class II deficiency); recurrent infections | Bone marrow transplantation |
| Ataxia-telangiectasia | Autosomal recessive | Oculocutaneous telangiectasia; progressive cerebellar ataxia; bronchiectasis; malignancy; defective chromosomal repair; raised $\alpha$-fetoprotein level | Bone marrow transplantation |
| Wiskott-Aldrich syndrome | X-linked | Eczema; thrombocytopenia; susceptibility to infections; malignancy; small defective platelets | Bone marrow transplantation; antibiotics; splenectomy |
| Immunodeficiency with short-limbed dwarfism | Autosomal recessive | Short-limbed dwarfism; lymphopenia | Immune serum globulin |

   **b. Risk factors** include:
     **(1)** A mother who is an intravenous (IV) drug abuser or a prostitute
     **(2)** A father who is an IV drug abuser or bisexual
     **(3)** History of blood transfusion or therapy with plasma-derived coagulation factors
     **(4)** For adolescents, IV drug abuse, prostitution, and sexual (especially homosexual) promiscuity

  **2. Immunologic abnormalities** associated with AIDS include:
   **a.** Decreased ratio of helper-inducer to suppressor-cytotoxic T cells (T4/T8 ratio)

      **b.** Functional impairment of T cell immunity
      **c.** Increased serum immunoglobulin levels
      **d.** Defective B cell function with impaired production of specific antibody

**3. Clinical features** of childhood AIDS may include:
   **a. Nonspecific manifestations**
      **(1)** Lymphadenopathy (90%)
      **(2)** Hepatosplenomegaly (85%)
      **(3)** Oral candidiasis (48%)
      **(4)** Failure to thrive (62%)
      **(5)** Other nonspecific findings (e.g., weight loss, fever, diarrhea, chronic eczema, hair thinning, craniofacial dysmorphia)
   **b. Infections**
      **(1) Bacterial infections** (45%), including sepsis, pneumonia, meningitis, abscess, and cellulitis (due to *Streptococcus pneumoniae, Hemophilus influenzae, Salmonella, S. aureus,* Enterobacteriaceae, or *Pseudomonas*).
      **(2) Viral infections,** including herpes simplex (6%), herpes zoster, rubeola, measles, and Epstein-Barr virus infection
      **(3) Fungal and opportunistic infections,** including *Pneumocystis carinii* pneumonia (64%), *Mycobacterium avium-intracellulare* infection (10%), *Candida* esophagitis (11%), cryptosporidiosis (6%), cryptococcosis (1%), toxoplasmosis, and tuberculosis
   **c. Central nervous system (CNS) manifestations,** including diffuse encephalopathy, cerebral atrophy, microcephaly, and intracranial calcifications
   **d. Lymphocytic interstitial pneumonitis (LIP)** [17%]
   **e. Malignancies** including primary lymphoma of the brain (2%), and Kaposi sarcoma (rare)
   **f. Other manifestations,** such as chronic active hepatitis, pancreatitis, renal disease, cardiomyopathy, parotitis, eye disease, thrombocytopenia, anemia, and coagulopathies

**4. Diagnosis** of HIV infection relies on suspicion of infection based on risk factors or clinical manifestations and attempted confirmation by serologic tests or assays that screen blood or body fluid for a viral structural protein (p24 core antigen). New laboratory techniques not yet readily available include viral culture and the polymerase chain reaction method of testing leukocytes for the HIV genome.
   **a. Symptoms** must meet the Centers for Disease Control (CDC) case definition for AIDS. Mean age of onset of symptoms is 4 months, with a range from birth to 60 months.
   **b. Serologic testing** uses enzyme-linked immunosorbent assay (ELISA) and a specific confirmatory test (e.g., the Western blot test). Serodiagnosis in infants and children is more difficult than in adults due to false positive and false negative results and the placental transfer of maternal antibodies to HIV.

**5. Prognosis.** Over 60% of children fulfilling the CDC criteria for AIDS die.
   **a.** Reported children survive a median of 9 months after diagnosis, and 75% die within 2 years.
   **b.** A mean survival of only 3 months following opportunistic infection has been reported.

**6. Therapy.** Supportive and general management includes treatment of bacterial and opportunistic infections and nutritional support.
   **a.** The role of antiretroviral therapy appears to be promising. Azidothymidine (AZT) currently is available for pediatric use.
   **b.** Certain children may benefit from prophylactic therapy for *P. carinii* pneumonia with drugs such as trimethoprim-sulfamethoxazole.
   **c.** In some children, prophylactic treatment with intravenous immune serum globulin may decrease the frequency of bacterial infections.
   **d.** HIV vaccines need further development.

**7. Prevention**
   **a.** Prevention of childhood AIDS requires decreasing the number of births to HIV-infected women through education, counseling, and serologic screening programs and the education of children and adolescents about risk behavior and safe sex practices.
   **b.** AIDS is not acquired through casual contact. The automatic exclusion from school of all children with AIDS is inappropriate and a violation of such children's legal rights. Because of widespread fears and misconceptions, the issue of confidentiality must be carefully considered.

**F. Evaluation for immunodeficiency disorders.** During examination of a patient with a suspected immunodeficiency disorder, several clues should be sought.

1. **History**
   a. **Infections.** Severe, recurrent, or persistent infections strongly suggest an immunodeficiency disorder. The following points should be investigated.
      (1) **Age at onset.** In general, the earlier the age at onset, the more serious the underlying immunodeficiency.
      (2) **Site of infection.** Serious sites of infection (as in meningitis, pneumonia, sepsis, or generalized dermatitis) suggest an underlying immunodeficiency.
      (3) **Causative agent**
         (a) Usually, infectious agents in **phagocytic dysfunction** are low-grade bacteria (e.g., *Staphylococcus, Klebsiella,* and *Serratia* species)
         (b) Infectious agents in **B cell deficiency disorders** include:
            (i) High-grade (i.e., virulent) bacteria (e.g., *S. pneumoniae* and other streptococci, *H. influenzae,* meningococci)
            (ii) *G. lamblia*
         (c) Infectious agents in **T cell deficiency disorders** include:
            (i) Viruses (e.g., herpesviruses, cytomegalovirus)
            (ii) Fungi (e.g., *Candida* species)
            (iii) Opportunistic organisms (e.g., *Pneumocystis* species, mycobacteria)
   b. **Family history.** A pedigree chart is helpful, since many immunodeficiency disorders are autosomal recessive or X-linked.
   c. **Adverse reactions** to drugs, vaccines, or blood products occur more commonly in patients with immunodeficiency disorders.

2. **Physical examination**
   a. **Growth and development.** The physical appearance is characteristic in short-limbed dwarfism and in DiGeorge anomaly. Failure to thrive is common in patients with combined T cell and B cell deficiencies.
   b. **Skin and oral mucosa** should be inspected for signs of infection (e.g., pyoderma, abscess, candidiasis). Eczema is seen in a number of immunodeficiency disorders, especially Wiskott-Aldrich syndrome.
   c. **Eyes.** Conjunctival telangiectasias occur in ataxia-telangiectasia.
   d. **Lymphatic system**
      (1) Hepatomegaly and splenomegaly may be present in patients with phagocytic defects or common variable hypogammaglobulinemia.
      (2) Other lymphoid tissues (e.g., lymph nodes, tonsils) are enlarged in some defects but are very small in others.
   e. **Cardiovascular system.** Congenital heart disease occurs in DiGeorge anomaly.
   f. **Neuromuscular system.** Ataxia may indicate ataxia-telangiectasia.
   g. **Skeletal system.** Nonspecific arthritis may be seen in Bruton's disease and other B cell immunodeficiencies.

3. **Laboratory testing.** Information about immune function can be obtained from a number of tests (Table 8-4).

**III. HYPERSENSITIVITY REACTIONS.** The same immunologic mechanisms that protect the host can cause tissue damage if they occur in exaggerated or inappropriate form.

**A. Types of hypersensitivity.** The widely accepted **Gell and Coombs classification** divides these mechanisms into four types of hypersensitivity reactions. Many immunopathologic processes are mediated by more than one type of hypersensitivity reaction.

1. **Type I (immediate-type, atopic, or reaginic) hypersensitivity reactions.** An antigen reacts with IgE antibodies, triggering the release of pharmacologic mediators (chiefly histamine) from mast cells and basophils (see also IV A 1). Examples of type I reactions include hay fever, extrinsic asthma, and anaphylactic shock.

2. **Type II (antibody-dependent cytotoxic) hypersensitivity reactions.** Antibody (usually IgG or IgM) binds to cell-associated antigens, leading to phagocytosis, killer cell activation, or complement-mediated lysis. An example of a type II reaction is autoimmune hemolytic anemia.

**Table 8-4.** Tests of Immune Competence

---

**Screening tests**
  Nonspecific tests
    Absolute granulocyte count
    Total hemolytic complement ($CH_{50}$; for primary complement deficiency)
    Nitroblue tetrazolium test of neutrophil function (for chronic granulomatous disease)
    Flow cytometry (for leukocyte adhesion molecules on surface of monocytes)

  Tests of humoral (B cell) immunity
    Quantitation of serum immunoglobulins
      Isotypes—IgG, IgM, IgA, IgE
      IgG subclasses
    Tests for functional antibodies
      Serum isohemagglutinin levels
      Patient's antibody response following immunization to diphtheria and tetanus toxoids or pneumococcal polysaccharide antigens, if older than 2 years
    Antibody response following infection to respiratory viruses
    Enumeration and phenotyping of B cells in blood

  Tests of cellular (T cell) immunity
    Absolute lymphocyte count
    Chest x-ray for thymus shadow (only in first few days of life)
    Delayed hypersensitivity skin tests to recall antigens
    Enumeration and phenotyping of T cells and T cell subsets

**Special immunologic tests**
  B cell tests
    Polyclonal B cell–induced immunoglobulin production in vitro
    Tests of immunoregulation by T cells of immunoglobulin synthesis

  T cell tests
    Lymphocyte blast transformation response to mitogens, antigens
    Mixed lymphocyte culture assays
    Tests of lymphocyte-mediated cytotoxicity

---

3. **Type III (immune complex–mediated) hypersensitivity reactions.** Complexes composed of antigen and antibody activate complement and mediate an inflammatory reaction. An example of a type III reaction is acute glomerulonephritis.

4. **Type IV (cell-mediated or delayed) hypersensitivity reactions.** Not antibody, but T cells capable of reacting with a specific antigen (**sensitized T cells**) are involved in conjunction with activated macrophages. The sensitized T cell, after binding to antigen, causes cytotoxicity either directly or through the release of lymphokines. Examples of type IV reactions include contact dermatitis and graft rejection.

B. **Role in autoimmune disease.** In most hypersensitivity reactions, the antigen is a foreign substance that the host defense mechanisms recognize as **nonself.** For unknown reasons, the body's self-recognition system sometimes goes awry, so that substances in the body's own tissues become **autoantigens,** and the stage is set for the development of an **autoimmune disease.** Autoimmune disorders usually are type II or type III hypersensitivity reactions but also may include type IV processes.

## IV. ALLERGIC DISORDERS

A. **Principles of IgE-mediated allergic disorders.** IgE originally was called **reaginic or atopic antibody,** because it was known to react with the antigens that cause symptoms in atopic individuals (i.e., persons with a familial predisposition to allergic disorders such as hay fever, asthma, and atopic eczema).

1. **Pathogenesis of IgE-mediated allergies.** In IgE-mediated allergies, IgE binds to surface receptors on **mediator cells,** thereby sensitizing the cells. When these sensitized cells come in contact with a **specific antigen,** they release substances that are **mediators** of inflammation. The mediators act rapidly on local tissues, causing the patient's symptoms. In some allergic disorders, the immediate short-lived inflammatory episode is followed 4–8 hours later by a second event that persists for 24–48 hours. **Late phase allergic reactions** contribute to the clinical manifestations and prolonged inflammation in bronchial asthma (see Ch 12 III), allergic rhinitis, urticaria, and atopic dermatitis.

   a. **Mediator cells**

      (1) **Mast cells and basophils**

         (a) **Mast cells** are the major cell type that is sensitized by IgE antibodies through the Fc receptor on the cell membrane. Two different mast cell phenotypes are found: mucosal and connective tissue mast cells.

         (b) **Basophils** also bind IgE antibody by their Fc receptor. The number of IgE receptors on basophils has been estimated to be about 400,000. Basophils comprise fewer than 0.2% of the leukocytes in the circulation.

         (c) Both mast cells and basophils are characterized by their intense **deep blue granules,** which contain several pharmacologic mediators of type I hypersensitivity reactions.

      (2) **Eosinophils** comprise 2%–5% of blood leukocytes and are characterized by heavily stained **red granules**. These cells play an important role in allergic diseases and helminthic infections. Eosinophilia is used as an indicator of atopic states.

   b. **Antigens** are molecules that induce a specific immune response, resulting in the creation of antibodies or T cells that specifically match the antigen. Antigens react with their matching antibodies or T cells. **Allergens** are antigens that cause an allergic reaction (i.e., a clinical type I hypersensitivity reaction) by eliciting IgE antibodies. Characteristics of **allergens** include the following.

      (1) Molecules larger than 70,000 daltons are too large to be allergens as they cannot cross mucosal surfaces to reach IgE-forming plasma cells.

      (2) Substances with molecular weights below 10,000 daltons are too small to link the IgE molecules on mast cells, a prerequisite for mediator release. However, smaller molecules can bind to proteins, and this **protein-hapten combination** can be allergenic.

      (3) Most allergens are **glycoproteins**.

   c. **Mechanisms of mediator release**

      (1) **Crosslinking.** When adjacent cell-bound IgE molecules become crosslinked by the specific antigen, the mast cells degranulate and release the mediators of immediate hypersensitivity.

      (2) **Other mechanisms** also lead to mast cell activation and degranulation, including:

         (a) **Complement activation products,** such as anaphylatoxins (complement components C3a and C5a)

         (b) **Drugs** (e.g., codeine, morphine), which activate mast cells by causing an influx of calcium ions

   d. **Mast cell- and basophil-derived mediators**

      (1) **Preformed mediators** found in mast cell and basophil granules include:

         (a) Histamine, which causes vasodilation, increased capillary permeability, chemokinesis, and bronchoconstriction

         (b) Heparin

         (c) Proteolytic enzymes (e.g., chymase, tryptase).

         (d) Chemotactic peptides [i.e., eosinophil chemotactic factor of anaphylaxis (ECF-A), neutrophil chemotactic factor (NCF), and platelet activating factor (PAF)]

      (2) **Newly formed mediators** in the cytoplasm of mast cells and basophils include:

         (a) Lipoxygenase pathway products [e.g., leukotriene $C_4$ ($LTC_4$), $LTB_4$, $LTD_4$, monohydroxyeicosatetranoic acid], which have various vasoactive, chemotactic, and chemokinetic actions and cause bronchoconstriction and mucus secretion

         (b) Cyclooxygenase products (e.g., prostaglandins, thromboxanes), which cause bronchial muscle contraction, platelet aggregation, and vasodilation

   e. **Late phase allergic reactions** are mediated by antigen interaction with IgE antibody and by the release of mediators from mast cells, with subsequent recruitment of leukocytes (i.e., neutrophils, eosinophils, and mononuclear cells). Corticosteroids and sodium cromolyn are important pharmacologic modifiers of the late phase response.

**2. Evaluation for allergic disorders**
  **a. History.** Information obtained can help in identifying specific allergens as well as in identifying the child's condition as allergic.
    **(1) Infections**
      **(a) Causative agents.** In allergic diseases, respiratory viruses and rhinoviruses are common agents.
      **(b) Site of infections.** Pharyngitis, sinusitus, serous otitis, and acute otitis media suggest allergy-related infections, which often are due to boggy mucous membranes and lymphoid tissue hypertrophy.
    **(2) Variations in symptoms** provide clues to the allergen. Symptoms may vary with:
      **(a) Time** (e.g., symptoms may be seasonal, perennial, monthly, diurnal, nocturnal)
      **(b) Geography** [e.g., symptoms may occur indoors, outdoors, at school or work, at home, at certain places in the home (e.g., basement, bedroom)]
      **(c) Environment** (e.g., symptoms may be induced or made worse by pets, foods, soaps, fabrics)
    **(3) Family history.** Information regarding family history of atopic disorders (e.g., asthma, rhinitis, eczema) should be sought.
  **b. Physical examination. Allergic signs and symptoms** can be classified by body system.
    **(1) Skin** (e.g., dermatitis, eczema, urticaria)
    **(2) Eyes** (e.g., pruritus, tearing, swelling)
    **(3) Ears** (e.g., fullness, popping, infection)
    **(4) Nose** (e.g., sneezing, pruritus, discharge)
    **(5) Throat** (e.g., pruritus, scratchiness or soreness, postnasal mucous discharge, cobblestoning due to lymphoid hypertrophy of posterior pharynx)
    **(6) Chest** (e.g., cough, dyspnea, wheezing, sputum production)
    **(7) Gastrointestinal tract** (e.g., diarrhea, malabsorption, food intolerance)
  **c. Laboratory testing**
    **(1) Pulmonary function testing** may be helpful (see Ch 12 I B 3 b).
    **(2) Skin testing** is based on the antigen-IgE reaction that occurs on the surface of mast cells in the skin. Usually, several potential antigens are tested at one time. Controls used for skin testing include histamine (positive) and solvent or vehicle (negative).
      **(a)** A small amount of presumed antigen is administered, as a solution, into the superficial layers of the skin by a superficial scratch (**scratch test**), by a needle-prick through a drop of the antigen solution (**prick test**), or by intracutaneous injection (**intracutaneous test**).
      **(b)** If the patient is allergic to the test substance, the patient's mast cells bind specific IgE antibody via the Fc receptor, which recognizes the substance. The IgE and test substance react, and if two IgE receptors are bridged, the patient's mast cells release histamine. The histamine causes local vasodilation and capillary permeability, producing a **wheal-and-flare reaction** at the skin test site.
    **(3) Quantitation of total and specific IgE**
      **(a) Total serum IgE levels** are determined by a paper radioimmunosorbent test (PRIST).
        **(i)** At birth, cord serum contains virtually no detectable IgE. Serum concentrations in children increase slowly, reaching adult levels at 5–7 years of age.
        **(ii)** Basal total serum IgE level is determined by complex interaction of multiple genetic and nongenetic factors.
        **(iii)** Not all atopic subjects have high IgE levels, and, conversely, not all nonatopic individuals have low IgE levels; the adult cutoff is 95 IU/ml.
      **(b) Antigen-specific IgE levels** in serum can be determined by a radioallergosorbent test (RAST). This in vitro analogue of skin testing is 10-fold less sensitive than intracutaneous skin testing.
    **(4) Provocation (challenge) testing.** A presumed allergen sometimes is administered directly to the mucosa of the target organ to identify the relationship between direct contact with the allergen and the development of symptoms.
      **(a) Route.** The oral route is used in food allergy, the nasal route in allergic rhinitis, and the bronchial route in asthma.
      **(b) Elimination diets** for the diagnosis of food allergy and food intolerance are a form of challenge testing. The patient first eats a basic diet consisting of standard nonallergenic food (the elimination diet) and then adds possible offenders to the diet one by one.

3. **Drug therapy for allergic disorders.** Drugs used to treat allergies act at various stages of the IgE-mediated reaction.
   a. **β-Adrenergic agonists and theophylline** inhibit the release of mediators from mast cells, which appears to require a fall in cyclic adenosine 3′,5′-monophosphate (cAMP).
      (1) β-Adrenergic agonists increase intracellular levels of cAMP.
      (2) Theophylline and other phosphodiesterase inhibitors prevent the breakdown of cAMP.
   b. **Cromolyn** inhibits the degranulation of mast cells and, thus, inhibits the release of histamine and other mediators.
   c. **Corticosteroids** stabilize membranes and inhibit arachidonic acid metabolism.
   d. **Antihistamines** block tissue receptors for histamine and, thus, prevent its effects.

B. **Anaphylaxis** is an acute, life-threatening systemic reaction caused by an IgE-mediated hypersensitivity reaction and characterized by urticaria, acute airway obstruction, and circulatory collapse. **Anaphylactoid reactions** are clinically identical to anaphylaxis but are due to the nonimmunologic release of mediators from mast cells and basophils.

1. **Pathogenesis**
   a. The most common **causes** are antibiotic (penicillin) injections and Hymenoptera (bee) stings, although almost any foreign substance can cause anaphylaxis.
   b. The **route** of allergen administration most commonly is parenteral. Ingestion also is common. Inhalation is less common.
   c. The **onset of anaphylaxis** occurs within a few minutes to hours after antigen exposure. Systemic manifestations are caused by the release of inflammatory mediators from mast cells and basophils.

2. **Clinical features** include:
   a. **Skin manifestations,** such as urticaria and angioedema
   b. **Respiratory manifestations,** such as edema of the larynx and epiglottis (causing hoarseness and stridor), bronchospasm, hypoxia, nasal congestion, sneezing, and rhinorrhea
   c. **Circulatory manifestations,** such as vasodilation, loss of intravascular volume, hypotension, circulatory collapse, arrhythmias, palpitations, and syncope
   d. **Gastrointestinal manifestations,** such as vomiting, diarrhea, dysphagia, and abdominal cramps
   e. **Genitourinary manifestations,** such as urgency

3. **Therapy** must be immediate.
   a. The administration of epinephrine and antihistamines is the first-line approach to the treatment of anaphylaxis.
   b. Fluid therapy and vasopressors are given for circulatory collapse to maintain blood pressure.
   c. Airway maintenance and bronchodilating drugs may be necessary.
   d. In severe anaphylaxis, corticosteroids are administered; however, these do not take effect for 6–8 hours.
   e. Oxygen should be given if the patient is cyanotic or has a low oxygen tension ($Po_2$).

4. **Prevention** involves avoidance of known antigens (e.g., drugs, foods) and the use of emergency self-treatment kits and identification bracelets.

C. **Allergic rhinitis** is a disorder of the nasal mucosa characterized by nasal blockage, rhinorrhea, sneezing, and pruritus.

1. **Pathophysiology.** Itching, sneezing, and hypersecretion are related to the effects of histamine on nerve receptors. Mast cells in the nasal mucosa also regulate the local blood flow in the mucosa by a controlled release of vasoactive mediators. Parasympathetic nerve pathways also play a major role in hypersecretion and congestion.

2. **Classification and clinical features**
   a. **Seasonal allergic rhinitis (hay fever)**
      (1) **Nasal symptoms** include congestion, pruritus, and increased mucus secretion (rhinorrhea).
      (2) **Other symptoms** include loss of the senses of smell and taste, chronic cough and clearing of the throat due to postnasal discharge, and chronic malaise and fatigue. Epistaxis, nasal or sinus polyps, and persistent serous otitis and sinusitis may also be significant problems.

      **(3) Physical findings** are characteristic.

        **(a)** Children typically show certain **facial features** such as a transverse nasal crease, dark shadows under the eyes ("allergic shiners"), and dental malocclusion.

        **(b)** The **nasal turbinates** are edematous and pale with a bluish tinge; they are covered with a thin, clear secretion.

      **(4) Nasal mucosal scrapings** show large numbers of eosinophils.

   **b. Chronic or perennial rhinitis** may have an allergic or nonallergic basis. Perennial rhinitis most often is a **vasomotor rhinitis,** which results from local autonomic imbalance.

**3. Inhalant or airborne allergens**

   **a. Pollens** constitute one of the most important groups of allergens. Ragweed, other weeds, grasses, and trees are the most common offenders.

      **(1)** To cause clinically significant sensitization, a pollen must be produced in large quantities by a common plant and must be dispersed by wind rather than by insects.

      **(2)** Seasonal occurrence varies with geographic location and time of pollination (Table 8-5).

   **b. Molds or fungi.** Spores are ubiquitous in the environment; molds are especially present in places of high humidity and warmth.

   **c. Household dust.** The principal allergen is the **dust mite**. Dust mite–sensitive patients have perennial symptoms but usually are worse in the late fall and winter.

   **d. Animal allergens.** Dander, hairs, dried saliva, and feathers are the major allergens. Cats are the most highly allergenic of the common household pets.

**4. Contributing factors**

   **a.** While **odors and fumes** are not allergens, they are primary irritants of the mucosal epithelium.

   **b.** Other contributing factors include weather conditions, temperature changes, infections, air pollution, and stress.

**5. Therapy**

   **a. Avoidance.** The most direct and safest mode of treatment is avoidance of the offending allergen, such as removal of a pet from the home. After removal of a pet from the household, it may take 4–6 months before the allergen levels are significantly reduced.

   **b. Drug therapy** is directed at preventing mast cell degranulation and blocking the effects of the released mediators.

      **(1) Antihistamines** are useful for controlling rhinorrhea and pruritus. A variety of agents are available, which fall into two main classes.

        **(a) First-generation antihistamines** include several pharmacologic groups of drugs that produce varying degrees of sedation.

        **(b) Second-generation antihistamines** are recently developed drugs that are nonsedating (they do not cross the blood-brain barrier).

      **(2) Decongestants** (oral only) are useful for reducing rhinorrhea.

      **(3) Cromolyn sodium** (topical) blocks mediator release from mast cells and is effective in both early and late phase allergic reactions.

      **(4) Corticosteroids** (topical sprays) affect mainly late phase allergic reactions.

      **(5) Atropine-like drugs** (topical sprays) are useful for vasomotor rhinitis.

   **c. Desensitization (immunotherapy)** can be useful in patients with clear-cut seasonal allergic rhinitis to the inhalant pollen allergens.

**D. Allergic diseases of the eyes and ears**

**1. Allergic (hay fever) conjunctivitis** usually is due to inhalant allergens. Patients often have other allergic disorders (e.g., rhinitis, eczema, asthma).

   **a. Clinical features** include tearing, itching, edema (chemosis), and redness of the conjunctiva. The **cornea is not involved;** thus, no scarring occurs.

**Table 8-5.** Seasonal Prevalence and Inhalant Allergens (Region—North Atlantic)

| | |
|---|---|
| Trees (oak, maple) | Late winter, early spring |
| Grasses (June, Timothy) | Spring, early summer |
| Molds (*Alternaria*) | Summer |
| Weeds (ragweed) | Late summer, early fall |
| Dust mites | Late fall, winter |

    **b. Therapy** is primarily drug therapy with combination ocular decongestant-antihistamine preparations, 4% ocular cromolyn sodium, or oral antihistamines.

  **2. Vernal conjunctivitis** is a severe bilateral inflammatory disorder that occurs mainly in the spring and summer in preadolescent boys (the male to female ratio is 3:1). The disease tends to resolve after puberty.

    **a. Clinical features** include intense itching, tearing, photophobia, and a stringy ocular mucous discharge that contains numerous eosinophils. Physical findings include giant papillae or cobblestoning of the upper tarsal conjunctiva. Unlike allergic conjunctivitis, vernal conjunctivitis **can result in corneal damage** with ulceration and scarring.

    **b. Therapy** is with 4% ocular cromolyn sodium and, if necessary, topical corticosteroids.

  **3. Involvement of the lids** can occur in patients with **atopic dermatitis** or **eczema**. Symptoms can range from a scaly, edematous, crusty exudate to keratoconjunctivitis, cataracts, or keratoconus.

  **4. Serous otitis media** and **middle ear effusions** may be allergy-related. In allergic children, adenoidal hypertrophy contributes to obstruction of the eustachian tube.

**E. Atopic dermatitis (atopic eczema).** This common pruritic skin disorder usually begins in infancy and has a chronic fluctuating course with seasonal variations. In 80% of patients, the skin problem starts in the first year of life; in up to 90%, onset is before age 5 years.

  **1. Immunologic aspects**

    **a.** Serum IgE levels are elevated in 80% of patients, and most patients have immediate skin reactivity (i.e., specific IgE antibodies) to a variety of environmental allergens.

    **b.** Atopic dermatitis often occurs in combination with other atopic diseases such as asthma or hay fever.

    **c.** The family history influences the likelihood of atopic dermatitis. If one parent is atopic, there is a 60% chance of atopy in the child; if both parents are atopic, then the incidence increases to 80%.

  **2. Clinical features**

    **a.** Atopic dermatitis is characterized by a chronic or relapsing course.

    **b.** The pruritic dermatitis has a typical morphology and distribution.

      **(1)** In infants and young children, the facial and extensor surfaces are affected. Lesions tend to be erythematous, papulovesicular, and exudative.

      **(2)** In older children, the distribution is more on the flexural surfaces, and lesions are more dry and lichenified.

    **c.** Other clinical features include cheilitis, infraorbital folds, anterior neck folds, white dermatographism and a delayed blanch response, and facial pallor associated with infraorbital darkening.

  **3. Complications** include repeated cutaneous infections and, occasionally, keratoconus. Anterior or posterior subcapsular cataracts are rare before puberty.

  **4. Therapy.** It is imperative to suppress the itch-scratch cycle by using oral antihistamines (e.g., hydroxyzine) and, if necessary, mild sedation. Skin lubricants and moisturizers are used to maintain skin hydration and prevent drying. Antibiotics may be necessary for patients with weepy lesions and pyoderma. Topical corticosteroids are used only in patients with severe atopic dermatitis.

**F. Urticaria and angioedema. Hives,** the lesions of **urticaria,** are evanescent wheals of varying size affecting the superficial layers of the epidermis and mucous membranes. **Angioedema** is similar but involves the deeper layers of the dermis and submucosal or subcutaneous tissues. In both disorders, acute evanescent lesions are more common than chronic lesions lasting 6 weeks or more.

  **1. Pathogenesis**

    **a. IgE-mediated (type I) hypersensitivity reactions** are a common cause of urticaria and angioedema. This mechanism underlies the acute urticaria commonly seen with **viral infections** and associated with parasitic, fungal, and certain bacterial infections. **Hymenoptera stings, drugs,** and certain **foods** (e.g., nuts, shellfish, eggs, milk) are other common causes of IgE-mediated urticaria and angioedema.

    **b. Immune complex disease and cutaneous vasculitis,** which are associated with activation of the complement system and the generation of anaphylatoxins, can also be associated with urticaria, angioedema, or both.

    **c. Other mechanisms** also cause urticaria and angioedema.

        **(1)** A variety of factors can cause urticaria or angioedema through the **nonspecific release of histamine** from mast cells or basophils. Morphine, codeine, and curare derivatives can act by this mechanism, as can bacterial toxins, crustacean secretions, and snake venoms. **Physical agents** also can induce urticaria by this mechanism in some people, as in dermatographism (from pressure), solar urticaria, and cold urticaria.

        **(2)** Some substances activate the **arachidonic acid pathway,** with production of leukotrienes. Examples include aspirin, food dyes [e.g., tartrazine (yellow food dye no. 5)], and preservatives (e.g., metabisulfite, methylparabens, benzoic acid).

        **(3) Complement** can also be involved in the pathogenesis of urticaria and angioedema. Radiocontrast dyes and blood transfusions can induce complement-mediated urticaria or angioedema. **Hereditary angioedema** is caused by the deficiency of C1 esterase inhibitor.

**2. Therapy**

    **a. Antihistamines.** $H_1$-receptor antagonists are the principal drug for the management of urticaria and angioedema. The choice of antihistamine depends on efficacy and tolerance. Hydroxyzine may show a slight advantage over other classic (first-generation) antihistamines. The newer antihistamines (i.e., terfenadine, astemizole) have a distinct advantage of not being able to cross the blood-brain barrier to cause sedation. Some patients with chronic urticaria unresponsive to $H_1$-receptor antihistamines may respond to therapy with both $H_1$- and $H_2$-receptor antihistamines.

    **b. Systemic corticosteroids** should be used only in patients with severe, acute urticaria and angioedema and in patients with an underlying disorder that calls for their use.

    **c. Avoidance.** In 70% of chronic urticaria cases, the etiology cannot be found, but if it can, its removal may be sufficient to resolve the urticaria and angioedema.

**G. Food allergy**

**1. Pathogenesis**

    **a.** The **foods that most commonly cause reactions** include milk, eggs, shellfish, peanuts and other nuts, cereal grains (gluten), citrus fruits, and the preservatives (metabisulfite) and dyes (yellow food dye no. 5) added to foods.

    **b.** Many adverse reactions to foods are not true food allergy (i.e., the development of IgE-mediated hypersensitivity to a food antigen). Among the many **other causes of adverse reactions to foods** are the toxic or pharmacologic effects of bacterial toxins, chemical additives, or certain food substances; nonimmunologically mediated histamine release; an inborn enzyme deficiency; psychological reactions; and intrinsic gastrointestinal disease.

**2. Clinical features.** Food allergy can be expressed through a variety of clinical symptoms.

    **a.** Some patients have abdominal symptoms, such as nausea, vomiting, abdominal pain, bloating, or diarrhea. There may be an associated swelling of the lips and tingling of the mouth or throat.

    **b.** Other patients may have different clinical symptoms, including anaphylaxis, asthma, rhinorrhea, urticaria, angioedema, and joint pain. Whether headaches, lethargy, and behavioral disturbances can be symptoms of food allergy remains controversial.

**3. Diagnosis.** The classic diagnostic tests used in allergy (e.g., RAST, skin testing) will not reliably identify a food allergy. The diagnosis of food allergy is best made by **oral challenge testing** in which the food is given in a disguised form (double-blind) and effects on the target organ (e.g., skin, lungs, intestine) are evaluated. An **elimination diet** with a gradual add-back of foods is an approach that may help in the management of food allergy as well as in diagnosis.

**4. Therapy.** Elimination or avoidance of the offending food substance from the diet is the major approach to the treatment of patients with food allergy.

**H. Allergy to stinging insects (Hymenoptera).** Allergic reactions to stinging insects (bees, yellow jackets, hornets, wasps) are mediated by IgE antibodies directed at one or more proteins in the venom of these insects. Between 0.5% and 5% of the population experience a systemic reaction following a sting, but death from insect allergy in children is very rare.

**1. Clinical features**

    **a. IgE-mediated reactions** can range from mild symptoms, such as urticaria and pruritus, to angioedema or life-threatening anaphylactic shock.

    **b. Large local reactions** that exceed 5 cm and occur within 24–72 hours after the sting are probably delayed hypersensitivity reactions.

**2. Diagnosis.** Allergy to stinging insects is identified from the history and by skin testing (or by in vitro testing with RAST), using purified venoms.

**3. Therapy** is mainly preventive. Patients should carry an emergency treatment kit containing epinephrine and antihistamines in case anaphylaxis follows an insect sting. Desensitization or immunotherapy may be helpful. Patients should avoid using perfumes and wearing brightly colored clothes, which attract stinging insects; they also should not walk barefooted outdoors.

**I. Adverse drug reactions**

**1. Pathogenesis**

    **a. Cause.** Adverse drug reactions (i.e., undesirable reactions that occur at an appropriate therapeutic dose) have many causes.

        **(1)** Fully 70%–80% of adverse drug reactions are **predictable adverse reactions** that result from the pharmacologic actions of a drug.

        **(2) Unpredictable adverse reactions** can result from immunologic hypersensitivity, from an underlying genetic susceptibility, or from idiosyncrasy. In contrast to idiosyncratic reactions, which can occur on first exposure to a drug, immunologic reactions require prior exposure or at least 7 days of continuous therapy with the drug in question.

    **b. Mechanism.** A drug hypersensitivity reaction may occur by any of the four Gell and Coombs mechanisms (see III).

    **c. Factors that may influence the development of drug allergy**

        **(1)** Few drugs are large enough molecules to serve as complete antigens. **Drugs** (or their metabolites) **that can serve as haptens** are most likely to cause sensitization.

        **(2) Topical application** causes sensitization more often than other routes of drug administration, probably because the carrier proteins for the drug haptens are readily available in the skin.

        **(3) Intermittent courses of moderate doses of a drug** are more likely to predispose to sensitization than prolonged treatment courses.

        **(4) Atopy.** Although the incidence of adverse drug reactions is the same for atopic and nonatopic patients, an atopic individual is more prone to the development of severe reactions.

**2. Clinical features**

    **a. Skin manifestations.** The skin is the most common site of drug hypersensitivity reactions and may be affected by any of the four hypersensitivity mechanisms. Drug eruptions can take many forms. Exanthematous eruptions, urticaria, angioedema, and photosensitivity are most common and are relatively mild; the less common bullous eruptions (epidermal necrolysis, Stevens-Johnson syndrome) can be fatal.

    **b. Anaphylaxis** occurs most commonly with parenteral administration.

    **c. Serum sickness** is a type III (immune complex) hypersensitivity reaction (a type I reaction may also occur). It can be induced by various drugs, notably the penicillins and related agents, as well as by the foreign protein in serum.

        **(1) Symptoms** usually develop in 7–12 days but may be accelerated (appearing in 1–3 days or even as anaphylaxis) in patients previously exposed to the drug. Symptoms include urticaria, angioedema, erythema multiforme, fever, and arthritis.

        **(2) Therapy.** Reactions can be controlled by antihistamines or, in severe cases, corticosteroids. There are no sequelae.

    **d. Other manifestations** of drug allergy include drug fever; a reaction resembling SLE; hematologic manifestations (hemolytic anemia, thrombocytopenia, purpura); asthma; hypersensitivity pneumonitis; hepatocellular damage; cholestasis; peripheral neuritis; and seizures (rarely).

**3. Examples of drug allergies**

    **a. Penicillin and its derivatives** cause many cases of allergic drug reactions.

        **(1) Mechanism.** Metabolites of penicillin are haptens and bind with proteins to form antigenic groups known as the **major determinant** [benzyl penicilloyl (**BPO**)] and several **minor determinants.**

(2) **Types of reactions**
  (a) **Anaphylaxis** is an IgE-mediated reaction to the minor determinants.
  (b) **Serum sickness or hematologic reactions** may be related to IgG, IgM, or even IgE antibodies to either the major or minor determinants.
  (c) **Other reactions** to penicillin (e.g., late or recurrent urticaria, arthralgia, late maculopapular reactions) also may be caused by either the major or minor determinants.
(3) **Semisynthetic penicillins,** the **cephalosporins,** and penicillin are similar structurally; therefore, a person who is sensitive to one of these drugs is at risk of **cross-sensitivity** to all the others.
  b. **Aspirin** can cause reactions that appear to be allergic in nature, such as urticaria, angioedema, or asthma. However, such reactions to aspirin are probably not IgE-mediated but instead may be related to inhibition of prostaglandin biosynthesis since the structurally unrelated nonsteroidal anti-inflammatory drugs (e.g., indomethacin, naproxen) can produce similar reactions.

## V. RHEUMATIC DISEASES. 
Growing evidence suggests that a number of the rheumatic diseases are **autoimmune** in nature (see III B). Other rheumatic diseases have an unknown pathogenesis but show clinically related features.

A. **Rheumatic fever** is a nonsuppurative inflammatory disease triggered by a group A β-hemolytic streptococcal infection of the upper respiratory tract. Because rheumatic fever may cause permanent damage to the heart muscle and heart valves (**rheumatic heart disease**), it is potentially serious.

1. **Incidence.** Rheumatic fever mainly affects young people from age 5 years through adolescence, with a peak occurrence at age 6–10 years. Although the incidence declined markedly in the United States prior to 1985, several recent rheumatic fever outbreaks suggest an increase in streptococcal virulence or a return of "rheumatogenic" strains of these bacteria. Rheumatic fever continues to be a major cause of heart disease in developing countries.

2. **Pathogenesis.** Autoimmune mechanisms most likely underlie the various manifestations of rheumatic fever.
  a. Antigenic cross-reactions between streptococcal cellular components and human heart tissue have been demonstrated.
  b. Cross-reactive (anti-heart) antibodies are found in rheumatic fever patients, although it is not known whether they are the cause or an effect of injury.

3. **Pathologic features.** Acute exudative and subacute proliferative cellular reactions occur mainly in connective tissue and around small blood vessels. Characteristic myocardial lesions, called **Aschoff's bodies,** are clusters of large, multinucleated cells in a mass of fragmented, swollen collagen fibers. Besides the heart, target organs include the joints, brain, and skin.

4. **Clinical features**
  a. **Polyarthritis**—usually with fever—is the presenting finding in about 75% of patients. The arthritis chiefly affects large joints, is distinctly migratory, and is painful out of proportion to objective findings. There are no sequelae.
  b. **Carditis** occurs in about 50% of the patients and may be asymptomatic. A pansystolic, blowing mitral murmur is the hallmark. Less common is a diastolic aortic murmur heard along the left sternal border. Murmurs may remain but often disappear if carditis does not recur.
  c. **Chorea** occurs in about 10% of the patients. Often insidious in onset, it causes emotional lability followed by characteristic, random jerky movements and muscle weakness. Chorea runs a self-limited course of 6–13 weeks duration, and recovery is complete.
  d. **Less common findings** include **subcutaneous nodules** (small, painless swellings found overlying bony prominences) and **erythema marginatum** (a pink, evanescent rash over the trunk).

5. **Diagnosis**
  a. **Jones criteria** (Table 8-6). The widely accepted Jones criteria classify the manifestations as **major** and **minor** according to their diagnostic usefulness.

**Table 8-6.** Revised Jones Criteria for Diagnosis of Rheumatic Fever

| Major Manifestations | Minor Manifestations | Evidence of Preceding Streptococcal Infection |
|---|---|---|
| Carditis | Clinical | Increased antistreptolysin O titer or other |
| Polyarthritis | Fever | streptococcal antibodies |
| Chorea | Arthralgia | Positive throat culture for group A |
| Erythema marginatum | Previous rheumatic fever | streptococcus |
| Subcutaneous nodules | or rheumatic heart disease | Recent scarlet fever |
| | Laboratory | |
| | Erythrocyte sedimentation rate | |
| | Leukocytosis | |
| | C-reactive protein | |
| | Prolonged P-R interval | |

    (1) The presence of two major criteria, or of one major and two minor criteria, indicates a high probability of the presence of rheumatic fever if supported by evidence of a preceding streptococcal infection.

    (2) The absence of a preceding streptococcal infection should make the diagnosis suspect, except in situations in which rheumatic fever is first discovered after a long latent period from the antecedent infection (e.g., Sydenham's chorea, low-grade carditis).

  **b. Laboratory tests**

    (1) Streptococcal antibody tests (antistreptolysin O) are useful for documenting a recent streptococcal infection, and the erythrocyte sedimentation rate and C-reactive protein test can provide evidence of an inflammatory process.

    (2) Throat culture is not very helpful, because it is usually negative by the time signs of rheumatic fever appear.

    (3) Doppler echocardiography has proven useful in identifying "silent" mitral insufficiency.

  **c. Differential diagnosis** includes other cardiac conditions (e.g., functional murmurs, congenital heart disease, viral carditis), other causes of arthritis, and other movement disorders.

  **6. Therapy**

    **a.** Once the diagnosis is established, the patient should be given 600,000–1.2 million units of penicillin G as one injection or therapeutic doses of oral penicillin for 10 days. Penicillin-allergic patients may be treated with erythromycin. Long-term prophylaxis with penicillin or erythromycin should be started thereafter to prevent streptococcal infections and recurrent attacks of rheumatic fever.

    **b.** Symptomatic treatment includes bed rest, anti-inflammatory drugs (e.g., salicylates, steroids), and, if needed, treatment of heart failure. Sedating drugs (e.g., phenobarbital, chlorpromazine, haloperidol) should be given for severe attacks of chorea.

**B. Juvenile rheumatoid arthritis (JRA)** is a chronic inflammatory disease of the joints. It begins before age 16 years, most commonly between age 1 and 4 years, and it occurs most often in girls.

  **1. Pathogenesis and pathologic features.** The etiology is unknown, but there is a strong probability that immunologic mechanisms are involved. Pathologically, inflammation of synovial membranes is followed by synovial proliferation and destruction of cartilage.

  **2. Clinical features**

    **a. Subtypes** of JRA are distinguished by the features at onset.

      (1) **Polyarticular JRA** involves five or more joints. Onset often is insidious, with low-grade fever and lethargy. There is symmetrical swelling of large joints, and small joints of the hands are often involved. Joints are frequently warm but only slightly tender.

      (2) **Pauciarticular JRA** involves one to four joints. The large joints are mainly affected, the knee most often. Generally, fever and systemic manifestations are absent. However, there is a high risk of **uveitis,** especially in girls with a positive antinuclear antibody (ANA) test.

      (3) In **systemic JRA,** illness begins with high, spiking fever, macular or papular rash, lymphadenopathy, and hepatosplenomegaly. The systemic illness often obscures the arthritis at onset.

    **b. Clinical course.** The course in all three forms is variable. Joint destruction may cause deformities, or the disease may remit with no sequelae.

3. **Diagnosis** is made from the history, the physical examination, and the exclusion of other joint disorders (e.g., rheumatic fever, other collagen vascular diseases, infectious arthritis). There are no characteristic radiographic findings in early JRA. ANA tests are useful for identifying subsets. Rheumatoid factors are not found in most cases, and, when present, are not specific for JRA.

4. **Therapy.** Anti-inflammatory drugs are prescribed in the following order of usage: salicylates, other nonsteroidal agents, and prednisone. Slower-acting drugs (e.g., gold, chloroquine, penicillamine) are indicated when anti-inflammatory drugs fail to control symptoms. Physical therapy is important.

## C. Other rheumatic diseases

1. **Systemic lupus erythematosus (SLE)** is an immunologically mediated inflammatory disease affecting multiple organ systems. It is rare in children under age 5 years and uncommon in children under age 10. SLE is seen occasionally in adolescents, particularly females.

    a. **Pathogenesis and pathologic features.** The manifestations are due to immune complex deposition in various organs (a type II hypersensitivity reaction), but why this occurs is unknown. Pathologic features consist of fibroid deposition and lupus erythematosus (LE) bodies in certain tissues (e.g., kidneys, skin, heart, brain, lungs, peripheral blood vessels).

    b. **Clincal features.** The butterfly rash across the nose and cheeks is the most characteristic sign. Nephritis may be the major presenting problem or a concomitant finding. Arthralgia is common, although severe arthritis is uncommon and deforming arthritis is rare. Other symptoms reflect involvement of other organ systems.

    c. **Diagnosis.** The appearance of the butterfly rash and the presence of LE cells in a patient with multisystem disease simplify diagnosis. ANA is present in virtually all patients, but its detection, although of diagnostic importance, is not a specific test for SLE. Testing for LE bodies is not always positive in children but is more specific than ANA testing.

    d. **Therapy.** Prednisone is given in a dosage and frequency suitable to the severity of the disease. Immunosuppressive agents can be tried for steroid-resistant patients.

2. **Dermatomyositis** is an uncommon connective tissue disease of unknown etiology characterized by inflammation of the skin and muscles. The **skin lesions** are due to perivascular infiltration by lymphocytes and histiocytes, resulting in thinning of the epidermis and dermal edema. The **muscle lesions** consist of foci of inflammation, capillary necrosis, and ischemia, causing atrophy. **Polymyositis** is the diagnosis when the disease is limited to the muscle.

    a. **Clinical features**
       (1) Onset usually is insidious, with a maculopapular rash over the joints, especially the knuckles, knees, and elbows, and a characteristic dusky discoloration and edema of the upper eyelids. Later in the disease course, pain and weakness develop symmetrically in distal muscle groups.
       (2) Less frequently, the patient presents with acute high fever and profound muscle weakness.

    b. **Diagnosis.** The typical skin rash and signs of myositis usually are diagnostic. Muscle enzymes are elevated and electromyography is indicative of myositis, but neither finding is specific. Muscle biopsy shows characteristic pathologic features.

    c. **Therapy.** Long-term corticosteroid therapy results in permanent remission in 90% of the patients.

3. **Scleroderma** is an uncommon disease of unknown etiology that occurs as a localized form (**morphea**) or even more rarely as a multisystem disorder (**progressive systemic sclerosis**). Histologic changes consist of a small artery vasculitis in the subcutaneous fat, which becomes replaced with sclerotic collagen extending into the dermis.

    a. **Clinical features**
       (1) **Morphea,** the localized form, appears as oval sclerotic plaques or linear bandlike lesions. Erythematous at first, these evolve into firm, shiny white lesions with violaceous borders.
       (2) **Progressive systemic sclerosis** presents as a diffuse hardening and tightening of the skin and subcutaneous tissues. The joints, lungs, heart, kidneys, and gastrointestinal tract may be involved.

    b. **Diagnosis.** The characteristic clinical findings usually are sufficient. Laboratory findings are essentially negative but help to exclude other collagen vascular diseases.

    c. **Therapy** is limited to symptomatic treatment.

4. **Mixed connective tissue disease** is a connective tissue disorder that combines the clinical and laboratory features of SLE, dermatomyositis, and scleroderma. Therapy is the same as that for SLE.

**D. Miscellaneous conditions with arthritis as a feature**

1. **Lyme disease** is a multisystem spirochetal infection with greatest involvement of the skin, neurologic system, and joints. The disease, transmitted by a tick, occurs primarily in the spring and summer in three areas of the United States: the Northeast, the midwestern states of Wisconsin and Minnesota, and the Pacific northwest area, including California and Oregon. However, cases have been identified in 43 states and on 6 continents.

   a. **Clinical features.** Joint and neurologic manifestations may arise weeks to months after the tick bite. The characteristic skin lesion, **erythema chronicum migrans,** is a bright red, expanding circle with a pale center that appears at the site of the bite 3–30 days after the injury.

   b. **Diagnosis.** Erythema chronicum migrans is so characteristic that its presence can be used to make the diagnosis. In the absence of this skin lesion, serologic confirmation usually is required.

   c. **Therapy.** Antibiotics can be used to treat the disease at any stage but are particularly effective in the early phase (i.e., erythema chronicum migrans), in which they can prevent further progression.

2. **Mucocutaneous lymph node syndrome (Kawasaki disease)** is a systemic **vasculitis** of unknown etiology, affecting the skin, mucous membranes, and heart.

   a. **Clinical features.** A constellation of findings occur, including spiking fever, polymorphous rash, lymphadenopathy, erythema and fissuring of the lips, induration and erythema of the hands and feet, suffused conjunctivae, arthritis, and arthralgia. Coronary arteritis may lead to infarction.

   b. **Diagnosis.** The combination of clinical features usually is diagnostic. Laboratory tests indicate an inflammatory process (e.g., elevated sedimentation rate and leukocytosis), but no specific test is available.

   c. **Therapy.** Salicylates are given in full doses during the acute phase, followed by small doses to minimize the development of late sequelae, such as coronary artery aneurysms. Giving immune serum globulin intravenously during the acute phase has recently been shown to decrease the incidence of such aneurysms.

3. **Other conditions with arthritic symptoms**

   a. **Serum sickness** (see IV I 2 c) causes a painful arthritis without heat or redness. There are no sequelae.

   b. **Henoch-Schönlein (anaphylactoid) purpura** (see also Ch 13 IV G) is a hypersensitivity reaction that causes a hemorrhagic purpuric rash over the lower half of the body, abdominal pain, periarticular pain and swelling, and hematuria. Attacks are self-limited but may be recurrent, and chronic renal disease may result. Therapy is primarily symptomatic; steroids may be useful to control pain.

   c. **Reiter's syndrome** in its classic form consists of a triad of urethritis, arthritis, and either conjunctivitis or iritis. The arthritis usually is mild and primarily affects lower extremity joints. Chronic arthritis rarely occurs. Reiter's syndrome in children may follow *Shigella* or *Yersinia* infections and is a form of **reactive arthritis.** Therapy is symptomatic.

   d. **Arthritis and psoriasis** often occur together. The psoriatic skin lesions may precede, accompany, or follow the joint symptoms. The arthritis is chronic and is indistinguishable from JRA. Dactylitis ("sausage finger") is a characteristic finding. Therapy is the same as that for JRA (see V B 4) and psoriasis.

   e. **Reactive arthritis** is the occurrence of a sterile synovial reaction to infection elsewhere in the body (e.g., due to *Shigella, Salmonella,* or *Yersinia enterolitica*).

# BIBLIOGRAPHY

Falloon J, Eddy J, Wiener L, et al: Human immunodeficiency virus infection in children. *J Pediatr* 114:1–30, 1989.

Rubinstein A: Schooling for children with acquired immunodeficiency syndrome. *J Pediatr* 109:242–244, 1986.

# STUDY QUESTIONS

**Directions:** Each of the numbered items or incomplete statements in this section is followed by answers or by completions of the statement. Select the **one** lettered answer or completion that is **best** in each case.

1. The group A β-hemolytic streptococcus may trigger an attack of acute rheumatic fever when it

(A) spreads via the bloodstream
(B) causes an upper respiratory infection
(C) lodges in the myocardium
(D) invades the joints
(E) enters through a skin infection

2. All of the following statements characterize an adverse reaction to a drug EXCEPT

(A) the reaction does not require prior exposure
(B) topical applications have a higher incidence of sensitization than other routes
(C) the incidence of adverse drug reactions is higher in atopic patients than in nonatopic patients
(D) the reaction may take the form of serum sickness
(E) the reaction may take the form of interstitial nephritis

3. Recurrent *Neisseria* infections are associated with which of the following immunodeficiency disorders?

(A) Neutrophil dysfunction
(B) Deficiency of complement component C3
(C) Deficiency of carboxypeptidase N
(D) Deficiency of complement components C5, C6, C7, and C8
(E) Deficiency of T cells

4. Acute rheumatic fever may cause which of the following disorders?

(A) Chronic joint disease
(B) Isolated pericarditis
(C) Pulmonary valve insufficiency
(D) Prolonged low-grade fever
(E) Aortic or mitral valvulitis

5. All of the following findings may occur in JRA EXCEPT

(A) uveitis
(B) high spiking fever
(C) erythema chronicum migrans
(D) enlargement of the spleen
(E) lymphadenopathy

6. The most common cause of chronic urticaria is

(A) food allergy
(B) connective tissue disease
(C) drug allergy
(D) idiopathic
(E) viral infections

7. Which of the following is a good screening test for T cell deficiency?

(A) Lymphocyte proliferative responses to antigens or mitogens
(B) Delayed hypersensitivity skin test to recall antigens
(C) $CH_{50}$
(D) NBT test

8. An anaphylactoid reaction can be caused by

(A) pollen
(B) bee venom
(C) aspirin
(D) peanuts

9. Clinical features of allergic rhinitis include all of the following EXCEPT

(A) dark shadows under the eyes
(B) erythematous nasal mucosa
(C) dental malocclusion
(D) thin, watery, nasal secretions
(E) eosinophils in the nasal secretions

| | | |
|---|---|---|
| 1-B | 4-E | 7-B |
| 2-C | 5-C | 8-C |
| 3-D | 6-D | 9-B |

10. Which of the following drugs should be given to treat late phase allergic reactions?

(A) Epinephrine
(B) Corticosteroid
(C) Atropine
(D) β-Agonist
(E) Antihistamine

11. An infant with atopic eczema is likely to present with which of the following clinical manifestations?

(A) An erythematous, papulovesicular, exudative rash
(B) Lichenified lesions on the flexural surfaces
(C) Urticaria
(D) Posterior subcapsular cataracts

12. Which of the following constitutes the safest and most direct mode of treatment for allergic rhinitis?

(A) Antihistamines
(B) Avoidance of the offending allergen
(C) Desensitization
(D) Local steroids
(E) Antibiotics

13. Signs and symptoms of seasonal allergic rhinitis might include all of the following EXCEPT

(A) nosebleeds
(B) nasal polyps
(C) loss of smell and taste
(D) thick, yellow nasal discharge

14. Immediate-type (type I) hypersensitivity reactions are mediated by

(A) complement component C3
(B) IgE antibodies
(C) neutrophils
(D) plasma cells

15. Pollens are important airborne allergens. Which of the following is a characteristic of pollens?

(A) Molecular weight greater than 70,000 daltons
(B) Dispersal largely by insects
(C) Production by flower-bearing plants
(D) Seasonal variation

**Directions:** Each group of items in this section consists of lettered options followed by a set of numbered items. For each item, select the **one** lettered option that is most closely associated with it. Each lettered option may be selected once, more than once, or not at all.

**Questions 16–20**

Match each of the following allergens with the time of year it is most likely to cause symptoms of allergic rhinoconjunctivitis in the North Atlantic region.

(A) Late summer, early fall
(B) Late fall, winter
(C) Late winter, early spring
(D) Spring, early summer
(E) Throughout the summer

16. Grass pollens

17. Ragweed pollen

18. *Alternaria* mold

19. House dust mite

20. Tree pollens

**Questions 21–24**

For each immune response listed below, choose the type of hypersensitivity reaction it represents.

(A) Type I
(B) Type II
(C) Type III
(D) Type IV
(E) Type V

21. Release of mediators from mast cells by antigen and IgE

22. Delayed cutaneous reaction to *Candida* or mycobacteria

23. Autoimmune hemolysis of red blood cells

24. Inflammation in the renal glomerulus from antigen-antibody immune complexes

| | | | | |
|---|---|---|---|---|
| 10-B | 13-D | 16-D | 19-B | 22-D |
| 11-A | 14-B | 17-A | 20-C | 23-B |
| 12-B | 15-D | 18-E | 21-A | 24-C |

**Questions 25–28**

For each immunodeficiency disorder listed below, select the infections to which a patient with that disorder is susceptible.

(A) Viral infections
(B) Infections due to high-grade virulent bacteria
(C) Both
(D) Neither

25. T cell immunodeficiency

26. Common variable hypogammaglobulinemia

27. Chronic granulomatous disease

28. Severe combined immunodeficiency

25-A        28-C
26-B
27-D

## ANSWERS AND EXPLANATIONS

**1. The answer is B** *[V A]*.
For reasons that are unclear, the upper respiratory tract is the only site of streptococcal infection preceding an attack of rheumatic fever. Skin infections due to this organism are common and may lead to nephritis but apparently not to rheumatic fever. Streptococci are not present in the heart, joints, or bloodstream in rheumatic fever or its antecedent infection.

**2. The answer is C** *[IV I]*.
The incidence of adverse drug reactions is not correlated with the atopic state of the patient; however, atopic individuals may be prone to more severe drug reactions. Immune complex reactions (e.g., serum sickness) and interstitial nephritis are among the many varieties of drug hypersensitivity reactions that can occur. Idiosyncratic drug reactions can occur on first exposure to a drug, but hypersensitivity reactions require prior exposure or at least 7 days of continuous therapy with the drug in question. Topical drug applications have a higher incidence of sensitization than other routes of drug administration, probably because the carrier proteins for drug haptens are more readily available in the skin.

**3. The answer is D** *[II A 3]*.
A deficiency of one of the late-acting complement components (i.e., C5, C6, C7, and C8) results in recurrent *Neisseria* infections, especially recurrent meningococcal meningitis and gonococcal septicemia. Deficiency of the complement component C3 results in bacterial infections, particularly with gram-negative bacteria. Neutrophil dysfunction usually results in infection with gram-positive organisms. T cell immunodeficiencies result in viral, parasitic, and fungal infections. Carboxypeptidase N deficiency is associated with recurrent angioedema.

**4. The answer is E** *[V A 4]*.
The joint manifestations of rheumatic fever have no long-term sequelae. Rheumatic fever may cause pericarditis, but only in association with myocarditis or valvulitis. The pulmonary valve rarely, if ever, is affected, in contrast to the mitral and aortic valves. Prolonged fever of unknown origin does not usually emerge as rheumatic fever.

**5. The answer is C** *[V B 2, D 1 a]*.
Erythema chronicum migrans is the hallmark skin lesion of Lyme disease; it differs from the maculopapular rashes seen in systemic juvenile rheumatoid arthritis (JRA). Other features of systemic JRA include high spiking fever, lymphadenopathy, and hepatosplenomegaly. Children with pauciarticular JRA are at risk for uveitis.

**6. The answer is D** *[IV F 2 c]*.
While it is true that urticaria can be caused by or associated with allergies to foods, connective tissue disease, drug allergy, or viral infections, in 70% of patients with chronic urticaria, an underlying etiology cannot be elucidated. The most common cause of acute urticaria, particularly in children, is viral infections.

**7. The answer is B** *[Table 8-2]*.
Several laboratory tests are available to evaluate T cell immune competence, including lymphocyte proliferative responses to antigens or mitogens and flow cytometry for T cell subsets. However, the best screening test for T cell deficiency, which can be available in any office or clinic setting, is delayed skin reactivity to recall antigens (e.g., *Candida*, tetanus). The total hemolytic complement ($CH_{50}$) is important in diagnosing congenital complement deficiencies. The nitroblue tetrazolium (NBT) test is important in the diagnosis of chronic granulomatous disease.

**8. The answer is C** *[IV H, I 3 b]*.
Reactions caused by pollen, bee venom, and peanuts all are IgE-mediated. In contrast, reactions to aspirin or aspirin-like compounds are believed to be mediated by perturbations of the arachidonic acid pathway, not IgE. These reactions are called anaphylactoid reactions, because they produce the same signs and symptoms as are seen in anaphylaxis, but they are not IgE-mediated.

**9. The answer is B** *[IV C 2 a]*.
In patients with allergic rhinitis, the nasal mucosa is not erythematous (red) but, instead, is pale and quite boggy. The pale appearance is due to edema and the presence of eosinophils in the mucosa. An erythem-

atous nasal mucosa is seen more commonly in patients with infectious rhinitis or rhinitis medicamentosa. Other physical findings in allergic rhinitis patients include dark shadows under the eyes; thin, watery, nasal secretions; and dental malocclusion.

**10. The answer is B** *[IV A 1 e]*.
Corticosteroids and cromolyn sodium are important pharmacologic agents useful in the treatment of late phase allergic reactions. Epinephrine, atropine, β-agonists, and antihistamines are useful for the early or immediate allergic phase of an IgE-mediated hypersensitivity reaction.

**11. The answer is A** *[IV E 2 b (1)]*.
Infantile eczema is characterized by a rash that is erythematous, papulovesicular, and, occasionally, exudative. In infants, the rash involves the facial and extensor surfaces. Older children or adults have lesions on the flexural surfaces, which become lichenified. Urticaria is not part of atopic eczema but is a separate atopic disorder. Posterior subcapsular cataracts take a number of years to develop and, therefore, would not be found in infants but rather in older children or adults.

**12. The answer is B** *[IV C 5]*.
Although antihistamines, local steroids, and desensitization therapy may be useful in the treatment of allergic rhinitis, the most direct and safest approach to therapy is avoiding the allergen. For example, someone who is allergic to animal dander should avoid contact with pets; this includes the removal of pets from the home.

**13. The answer is D** *[IV C 2 a]*.
Nose bleeds, nasal polyps, and loss of smell and taste all are characteristic findings in seasonal allergic rhinitis. However, the nasal discharge usually is thin, watery mucus and not a yellow discharge. A thick yellow or green nasal discharge should suggest the presence of sinusitis.

**14. The answer is B** *[III A 1]*.
Immediate type (type I) hypersensitivity reactions are mediated by IgE antibodies. Type III hypersensitivity reactions are mediated by IgG antibodies produced from plasma cells, complement, and neutrophils.

**15. The answer is D** *[IV A 1 b, C 3 a]*.
The inhalant pollen allergens vary with their season of pollination (e.g., trees pollinate in the Northeast in late winter or early spring, whereas ragweed pollinates from late summer to the first frost). In general, the allergens are less than 70,000 daltons. Structures larger than 70,000 (e.g., the pollen from pine trees) are not thought to cause allergic diseases. Plants that bear pollen allergens are from nonflowering plants and, thus, rely on wind or air currents to spread the pollen. In contrast, flowering plants (e.g., roses) depend on insects to carry pollen to other plants for reproduction and, thus, do not cause allergies.

**16–20. The answers are: 16-D, 17-A, 18-E, 19-B, 20-C** *[Table 8-5]*.
The clinical symptoms of allergic diseases such as allergic rhinitis should correlate with the time of year in which certain trees, grasses, or weeds pollinate. In the North Atlantic region, grasses pollinate in spring and early summer, ragweed pollinates in later summer and early fall, *Alternaria* pollinates throughout the summer, and trees pollinate in later winter and early spring. Identification of the inhalant allergens causing symptoms in a particular patient is helpful in formulating a suitable treatment plan. For example, the onset of symptoms of allergic rhinitis in late October or November, as the weather gets cold and the heat is turned on in a house, may suggest a hypersensitivity to house dust mites. Simple measures of environmental dust control may significantly help a patient with such an allergy. Decisions of desensitization or immunotherapy to an inhalant allergen is based on the history, seasonal nature of the symptoms, and skin test results.

**21–24. The answers are: 21-A, 22-D, 23-B, 24-C** *[III A]*.
A type I (immediate-type, atopic, or reaginic) hypersensitivity reaction is mediated by immunoglobulin E (IgE) antibodies. Antigen attaches to its specific IgE on the surface of mast cells and basophils. This triggers the release of pharmacologic mediators that produce the inflammation seen in type I hypersensitivity reactions.

A delayed cutaneous reaction to specific antigen is a type IV (cell-mediated or delayed-type) hypersensitivity reaction. Type IV hypersensitivity reactions are mediated by sensitized T cells. The T cells, after binding to antigen, release a variety of lymphokines, which results in the infiltration of tissues by mononuclear cells and lymphocytes, causing destruction of the tissue. Type IV reactions are typically seen in organ graft rejection reactions or in infections with *Mycobacterium* (tuberculosis).

The pathogenesis of many autoimmune hemolytic anemias is an antibody-dependent cytotoxic reaction, which is a type II hypersensitivity reaction. Antibody binds to a cell-membrane antigen, and, acting in conjunction with complement, causes lysis of the red cells.

Immune complex–mediated (type III) hypersensitivity reactions begin when antibody and antigens in the circulation combine to form soluble complexes. These complexes eventually filter out along basement membranes, such as the glomerular basement membrane. The deposition of these complexes on the basement membrane, together with the activation of complement, produces the inflammatory reaction that results in glomerulonephritis.

**25–28. The answers are: 25-A** *[II D 1 a],* **26-B** *[II C 1],* **27-D** *[II B 2 a; Table 8-1],* **28-C** *[II D 2; Table 8-3].* Patients with T cell immunodeficiency are primarily affected by viral and fungal infections, whereas patients with B cell abnormalities (e.g., common variable hypogammaglobulinemia) are prone to infections with high-grade virulent bacteria. Patients with chronic granulomatous disease have problems primarily with catalase-positive organisms, such as *Staphylococcus aureus* and certain gram-negative enteric bacteria. Patients born with severe combined immunodeficiency have severe defects of both cellular and humoral immunity and, therefore, are susceptible to infection with any of these microbial agents.

# 9
# Infectious Diseases

Peter J. Krause
Henry M. Feder, Jr.

**I. INTRODUCTION.** Infectious diseases are the leading cause of morbidity in infants and children, and are not, contrary to popular belief, disappearing. Since the introduction of effective vaccines, certain infections (e.g., polio, diphtheria, measles, mumps, rubella, pertussis, tetanus) have been reduced dramatically; however, only smallpox has been eradicated worldwide. In addition, other infectious diseases [e.g., hepatitis, shigellosis, Rocky Mountain spotted fever, acquired immune deficiency syndrome (AIDS)] are on the rise. Antimicrobial compounds have markedly improved the prognosis associated with many infections, but the emergence of resistant strains has required the continued development of new antimicrobial compounds. Infectious diseases that are not covered in this chapter but elsewhere in the text are as follows:

**A.** Acute infectious diarrhea (see Ch 10 V A)

**B.** Hepatitis (see Ch 10 IX C)

**C.** Genitourinary infections (see Ch 4 IV and Ch 13 VII)

**D.** Neonatal infections (see Ch 5 V F)

**E.** AIDS (see Ch 8 II E)

**F.** Lyme disease (see Ch 8 V D 1)

**G.** Tuberculosis (see Ch 12 VIII A)

**II. GENERAL PRINCIPLES OF INFECTIOUS DISEASES IN CHILDREN**

**A. Diagnostic criteria.** The diagnosis of infectious diseases in children is based on the history and physical examination, with the specific cause determined with the help of the microbiology laboratory.

1. A thorough **medical history and physical examination** usually allow the physician to make an anatomic diagnosis and a tentative conclusion regarding the cause.

2. Certain **laboratory tests** (e.g., a complete blood count, erythrocyte sedimentation rate, radiologic studies, tissue histology, skin tests) may help to support or eliminate the diagnosis.

3. **Confirmation of the etiologic agent** usually is made by culture, antigen detection, or antibody detection.

**B. Effective use of the microbiology laboratory.** Accurate microbiologic diagnosis of an infectious disease depends on appropriate specimen collection. To ensure the best result, it is important to sample the correct anatomic site prior to initiation of antibiotics, to obtain an adequate quantity of material to culture, to avoid contamination, and to deliver the specimen promptly to the laboratory.

1. **Methods of organism identification**
   a. **Microscopic examination** of specimens is performed with or without stains, depending on the nature of the organism.

**(1) Unstained specimens.** Organisms that have typical structural features (e.g., fungi, parasites) can be identified with an ordinary light microscope, without staining.

**(2) Stained specimens.** Special stains can be used to make organisms (or parts of organisms) more visible or identifiable with microscopic examination. An enormous variety of stains are available; two of the most commonly used are **Gram stain** (for classifying bacteria) and **acid-fast stain** (for identifying acid-fast microorganisms).

**b. Immunologic methods** are used to identify microbial antigens or antibodies in body fluid specimens or cultures.

**(1) Immunofluorescence** employs fluorescein-labeled antibody specific for a particular antigen. This method is used for rapid detection of viruses and bacteria.

**(2) Agglutination tests** serve to detect and quantitate agglutinins (i.e., antibodies that agglutinate cellular structures, such as bacteria). A common procedure is **latex agglutination,** in which latex beads coated with antibodies against specific bacteria are reacted with patient serum. Agglutination tests are rapid and specific and do not require living organisms.

**(3) Enzyme-linked immunosorbent assay (ELISA),** like agglutination tests, has been used to detect microbial antigens in body fluids.

**c. Culture**

**(1) Identification of bacteria or fungi** on solid or in liquid media is accomplished by noting the pattern of growth in the type of media used, colony morphology, and biochemical characteristics.

**(2) Identification of viruses** usually requires the use of tissue culture. Characteristic alterations in the morphology of the infected cells in the tissue, hemagglutination or hemadsorption of red blood cells to infected cells, and binding of specific fluorescein-labeled antibody may be used to identify the etiologic agent.

**2. Evaluation of antimicrobial activity**

**a. Antimicrobial susceptibility tests** are used to determine the effects of antimicrobial agents on the growth of the microbial isolate. Susceptibility testing is indicated for bacterial isolates that are clinically significant and should not be performed on isolates that are part of the normal flora.

**(1)** Antimicrobial susceptibility often is expressed in terms of the concentration of antibiotic needed to inhibit the growth of the microorganism, or the **minimum inhibitory concentration (MIC).** The lower the MIC, the more susceptible the organism.

**(2)** In some cases, the clinician requests both the MIC and the **minimum bactericidal concentration (MBC)** of an antimicrobial agent. (The MBC is the lowest concentration of the antibiotic that kills $\geq$ 99.9% of the microbial isolate being tested.)

**(3)** Occasionally, combinations of antibiotics are studied to determine whether the combined agents have a greater or lesser effect than that of either agent alone.

**b. Serum bactericidal test** is used to determine the effect of both the peak antibiotic level and the antimicrobial factors in the serum (e.g., antibody, complement) on the microbial isolate.

**c. Tests for β-lactamase production** by staphylococci, *Hemophilus influenzae,* and *Neisseria gonorrhoeae* are rapid and useful in treating infections due to these agents. Any organism that produces β-lactamase will be resistant to penicillin G and ampicillin.

**C. Antimicrobial therapy.** Treatment of infectious diseases primarily involves antimicrobial agents combined with supportive care. It is incumbent on any physician caring for children with infectious diseases to understand the antimicrobial spectrum, pharmacokinetics, and side effects of antimicrobial agents. A thorough understanding of supportive therapy also is necessary. Severe morbidity or death may result from inadequate supportive therapy, regardless of whether the appropriate antimicrobial agents are used. For example, a child with septic shock must have appropriate intravenous fluid management and cardiovascular and ventilatory support as well as appropriate antibiotic therapy to survive.

**1. To begin antimicrobial therapy or not.** This is the initial therapeutic question in managing a patient with an infection, the answer to which is determined by several factors.

**a. Diagnosis.** In general, the more severe the illness, the more important it is to begin antimicrobial therapy. For example, antimicrobial therapy always is begun for purulent meningitis but may be withheld for pharyngitis until further laboratory data are available.

**b. Host defense factors.** Patients with underlying immunologic defects or deficiencies (e.g., newborns) who show signs of infection are more likely to be given antibiotics than patients whose host defenses are intact.

    c. **Follow-up.** A child with pharyngitis who may not return for follow-up is more likely to be given penicillin than a child who will return for follow-up.

  **2. Antimicrobial choice.** Antimicrobial therapy is **empiric** if it is chosen on the basis of a probable clinical diagnosis and is **specific** if it is chosen on the basis of culture or antigen test results.

    a. **Antimicrobial activity** is the most important consideration in choosing an antibiotic. The spectrum should be broad enough to cover the likely pathogens if empiric therapy is begun but as narrow as possible when a specific organism is being treated.

    b. **Toxicity and side effects.** There usually are several antibiotics to choose from when treating an infection. The antibiotic with the lowest toxicity is preferred.

    c. **Cost.** Antimicrobial therapy often is expensive. The least expensive antibiotic should be used when all other factors are equal. Because of the costs of preparing and infusing drugs, a single expensive antibiotic may cost less to give by the intravenous route than a combination of two or more less expensive antibiotics.

    d. **Dosage and route.** For oral antibiotics, fewer doses each day may improve patient compliance. Pediatric dosages usually are based on body weight. Antibiotics given by mouth or intramuscularly may allow for outpatient administration, whereas intravenous antibiotics are not as easily administered on an outpatient basis.

    e. **Development of new antimicrobial agents.** New antibiotics are constantly being developed because microorganisms develop resistance to conventional antibiotics. Recently developed third-generation cephalosporins—which include cefotaxime, ceftriaxone, and ceftazidime—are often used instead of ampicillin and chloramphenicol for serious infections.

**D. Fever and fever of unknown origin**

  **1. Definitions**

    a. **Fever** has no universally recognized definition. It is not uncommon for healthy children to have a rectal temperature of 100.4° F (38° C) in the afternoon or after exercise; thus, a practical definition of fever in children is a rectal temperature above 100.4° F (38° C). Oral temperatures generally are about 1° F lower than rectal temperatures.

    b. **Fever of unknown origin** has been defined as an illness that persists for 3 or more weeks with an accompanying temperature above 101° F (38.4° C) and an uncertain diagnosis after a 1-week investigation in the hospital. Many children are admitted to the hospital with a relatively brief febrile illness without localizing findings on physical examination. Although fever of unknown origin often is the diagnosis, it is more useful clinically to classify this fever syndrome as **fever without localizing signs**.

  **2. Diagnosis.** Several general principles are important to consider when performing a workup on a child with fever of unknown origin or fever without localizing signs.

    a. The **major illnesses that cause fever in children** are infectious diseases, collagen vascular diseases, malignancies, and inflammatory bowel disease. Infectious diseases are the most common cause of fever of unknown origin in children. Children with malignancies usually do not have fever as the only manifestation of their illness.

    b. **The presence of fever must be documented.** Parents may exaggerate the actual temperature of their child, in some cases deliberately (factitious fever). The erythrocyte sedimentation rate usually is elevated in patients with fever and significant illness.

    c. Most children with fever of unknown origin have **common illnesses with uncommon presentations**. The most common infectious causes of fever of unknown origin in children are tuberculosis, brucellosis, tularemia, salmonellosis, diseases due to rickettsiae or spirochetes, infectious mononucleosis, cytomegalic inclusion disease, and hepatitis.

    d. **Continued observation** of the child, with repeated review of the history and physical examination and occasionally repeated laboratory tests, is important in helping to establish a specific diagnosis.

    e. **Young children** (younger than 2 years) **with fever and no localizing findings are at higher risk for serious infection,** including bacteremia, than older children and, consequently, should have at least a complete blood count, urinalysis, and blood culture as part of their workup. A febrile or hypothermic newborn usually receives a "septic workup" consisting of a lumbar puncture; blood, urine, and cerebrospinal fluid (CSF) cultures; and a chest x-ray.

  **3. Therapy.** Neonates and children with underlying immunodeficiency who have fever without localizing signs generally are admitted to the hospital and begun on empiric antibiotic therapy pending the results of cultures. The management of nonimmunodeficient older patients with this problem is more variable. In general, it is better to withhold antibiotics until a definitive diagnosis is made.

## III. BACTEREMIA AND SEPSIS

### A. Definitions

1. **Bacteremia** is defined as the presence of bacteria in the blood. **Occult bacteremia** is a transient, self-limited bacterial invasion of the bloodstream, without an obvious focus of infection.

2. **Sepsis** is a life-threatening bacterial invasion of the intravascular compartment, which may or may not be associated with a focus of infection. Neonatal sepsis is discussed in Chapter 5 V F 2.

### B. Occult bacteremia

1. **Incidence and etiology**
   a. Studies done in the 1960s showed that routine blood cultures in infants with febrile seizures often were positive for *Streptococcus pneumoniae* but that most of these infants had no focus of infection and recovered without therapy. Subsequent studies have shown that occult pneumococcal bacteremia is not uncommon, with the greatest risk (5%–10%) occurring in infants between the ages of 6 months and 2 years who have a temperature above 102° F (38.9° C) and leukocytosis.
   b. Other causes of occult bacteremia include *H. influenzae* type b and *Neisseria meningitidis*.

2. **Clinical features.** Signs and symptoms usually consist of a temperature of at least 102° F (39.8° C) and irritability without an obvious focus of infection. Febrile seizures have been associated with occult bacteremia.

3. **Diagnosis.** Laboratory workup consists of white blood cell count (which usually exceeds 15,000/mm³) and blood culture. Quantitative blood culture usually reveals a low titer of the causative microorganism (i.e., about 10 bacteria/ml).

4. **Therapy.** Occult pneumococcal bacteremia usually resolves spontaneously in 24–48 hours. Large controlled studies are needed to determine whether patients at greatest risk for occult bacteremia should be followed as outpatients without treatment or should be given empiric treatment with penicillin.

### C. Sepsis in infants and children

1. **Incidence and etiology.** Sepsis is uncommon in children who are older than 3 months of age and immunologically normal. The most common causative agents are *H. influenzae* type b and *N. meningitidis*. The incidence of sepsis and other illnesses due to *H. influenzae* is decreasing as a result of the development of *H. influenzae* vaccines.

2. **Clinical features.** Sepsis should be suspected in any previously healthy infant or child who develops a fever without an obvious focus of infection and appears ill. A petechial rash occurs frequently with sepsis due to *N. meningitidis* and also can occur with sepsis due to *H. influenzae* type b.

3. **Diagnosis.** Laboratory evaluation of an infant or child with suspected sepsis and no obvious focus of infection consists of white blood cell count (which usually exceeds 15,000/mm³ and demonstrates a shift to the left), chest x-ray, urinalysis, blood and urine cultures, and lumbar puncture (if clinically indicated).

4. **Therapy** for suspected sepsis in a previously healthy patient older than 3 months of age usually consists of a third-generation cephalosporin.

### D. Sepsis in the immunocompromised patient.
Defects in immune function may be congenital or acquired (see Ch 8 II) and include disorders of humoral immunity (antibody and complement defects), cellular immunity (neutrophil, monocyte, and lymphocyte defects), and structural immune mechanisms (e.g., compromised skin integrity, splenic dysfunction). One of the most commonly encountered immunocompromised patients is the cancer patient whose neutrophil count has fallen below 500/mm³ secondary to chemotherapy.

1. **Etiology.** Common causative agents include *Pseudomonas aeruginosa*, gram-negative enteric rods, and *Staphylococcus aureus*. *Staphylococcus epidermidis* is a common cause of sepsis in children with central venous or intra-arterial catheters.

2. **Clinical features.** Fever may be the only manifestation of life-threatening sepsis in immunocompromised children. These patients must be examined carefully for a focus of infection, especially in the oral and rectal areas.

3. **Diagnosis.** Laboratory evaluation includes white blood cell count, chest x-ray, and cultures of the blood, urine, and skin.

4. **Therapy.** Empiric therapy usually consists of vancomycin and ceftazidime. Alternatively, oxacillin, an aminoglycoside (e.g., tobramycin), and an antipseudomonal penicillin (e.g., ticarcillin) can be used.

## IV. CENTRAL NERVOUS SYSTEM INFECTIONS

A. **Meningitis** refers to any inflammation of the meninges. Most commonly, the term refers to an inflammation of the arachnoid membrane, the subarachnoid space (including the CSF), and the pia mater covering the brain.

1. **Classification and etiology.** There are two major classifications of meningitis—**bacterial** and **aseptic**—which usually can be distinguished on the basis of CSF characteristics.
   a. In **bacterial meningitis,** the CSF has an increased white cell count and protein level and a lowered glucose level. The cause of bacterial meningitis varies with the age of the patient.
      (1) In neonates, the most common causes are group B streptococci and *Escherichia coli.*
      (2) In infants and children, the most common causes are *H. influenzae* type b, *S. pneumoniae,* and *N. meningitidis.*
   b. In **aseptic meningitis,** the CSF does not contain bacteria and is characterized by a mildly elevated white cell count, a normal or mildly elevated protein level, and a normal glucose level. The cause of aseptic meningitis usually is viral. The most common viral causes of meningitis in infants and children are enteroviruses (e.g., coxsackieviruses, echoviruses) and mumps virus.

2. **Incidence.** Meningitis, particularly bacterial meningitis, is a common, serious infection in infants and children. The risk of a child developing bacterial meningitis in the United States by age 5 years is between 1 in 400 and 1 in 2000.

3. **Clinical features.** The early signs and symptoms of meningitis are less specific in young infants than in older children. Generally, the clinical manifestations are more severe in bacterial meningitis than in viral meningitis.
   a. **CNS involvement** manifests as severe headache, lethargy, confusion, irritability, seizures, vomiting, and bulging fontanelle.
   b. **Meningeal involvement** manifests as neck or back pain and Brudzinski's and Kernig's signs.
   c. **Nonspecific features** include fever, poor feeding, and petechial lesions (most commonly seen with meningitis due to *N. meningitidis*).

4. **Diagnosis.** Bacterial meningitis is a medical emergency; diagnostic procedures must be carried out with dispatch and therapy begun promptly. The diagnosis is made on the basis of CSF findings following **lumbar puncture**.
   a. **CSF findings in bacterial meningitis** usually include:
      (1) Increased pressure
      (2) Increased white blood cell count (100–10,000/mm$^3$), with a predominance of neutrophils
      (3) Increased protein level (> 40 mg/dl)
      (4) Decreased glucose level (< 40 mg/dl or < 66% of a simultaneously drawn blood glucose level)
      (5) Gram stain and culture positive for bacteria
      (6) Latex agglutination test positive for bacterial antigen
   b. **Contraindications to lumbar puncture.** The decision to perform a lumbar puncture is based on clinical suspicion of bacterial meningitis. Contraindications to this procedure include:
      (1) Increased intracranial pressure due to a space-occupying lesion
      (2) Shock
      (3) Respiratory failure
      (4) Bleeding diathesis

5. **Therapy** for bacterial meningitis consists of antibiotics and supportive care.
   a. **Antimicrobial therapy**
      (1) Initial therapy (prior to identification of the causative organism) is based on patient age.

        **(a)** Neonates and infants younger than 2 months usually are given ampicillin and an aminoglycoside or ampicillin and cefotaxime.

        **(b)** Infants and children older than 2 months usually are given cefotaxime, ceftriaxone, or ampicillin and chloramphenicol.

    **(2)** The duration of therapy varies but generally is 2–3 weeks in neonates and 7–10 days in older children.

  **b. Supportive care** is very important and consists of:

    **(1)** Fluid restriction to minimize cerebral edema (generally, two-thirds of the daily maintenance requirement)

    **(2)** Maintenance of intravascular volume by rapid administration of intravenous fluids if meningitis is accompanied by shock (e.g., fulminant *N. meningitidis* meningitis)

    **(3)** Anticonvulsants if seizures occur

    **(4)** Assisted ventilation if respiratory failure occurs

    **(5)** Subdural taps for evacuation of extensive subdural effusions

  **c. Corticosteroid therapy** for *H. influenzae* meningitis has been shown to improve CSF findings and decrease the incidence of hearing loss.

  **d. Follow-up care.** Children who have had meningitis should have a complete neurologic evaluation at the time of their discharge from the hospital, including a vision test, a hearing test, and a formal developmental assessment. Periodic monitoring of neurologic and developmental status should be carried out for at least 2 years.

**B. Encephalitis** is an inflammation of the brain.

  **1. Etiology.** Most cases of acute encephalitis are due to viruses, most commonly herpes simplex virus, arboviruses, and enteroviruses. The incidence of encephalitis due to common childhood infections such as measles and mumps has declined significantly with the increased use of vaccines.

    **a. Herpes simplex virus** causes encephalitis year-round and is the most common cause of sporadic acute encephalitis in the United States. Herpes simplex virus type 2 usually is the cause of encephalitis in neonates, whereas herpes simplex virus type 1 causes most cases of encephalitis in older children.

    **b. Arboviruses** cause encephalitis outbreaks during the summer, as these viruses are transmitted by insects (usually mosquitoes). Important arboviral causes of encephalitis in the United States include:

      **(1)** California encephalitis virus

      **(2)** St. Louis encephalitis virus

      **(3)** Eastern equine encephalitis virus

      **(4)** Western equine encephalitis virus

    **c. Enteroviruses** (i.e., coxsackieviruses and echoviruses) cause encephalitis outbreaks during the summer.

    **d. Viruses associated with childhood illnesses** (e.g., mumps, measles, varicella, rubella) may cause acute or postinfectious encephalitis. In postinfectious illness, the encephalitis is thought to be mediated primarily by immune mechanisms.

    **e. Epstein-Barr virus** is a rare cause of encephalitis; occasionally, encephalitis may develop during infectious mononucleosis.

    **f. Nonviral causes of encephalitis** include *Mycoplasma pneumoniae* and *Toxoplasma gondii*.

  **2. Clinical features** of encephalitis vary widely in severity but most commonly include the following symptoms.

    **a. Early signs and symptoms** are nonspecific and typical of acute systemic illness (e.g., fever, headache, vomiting, upper respiratory symptoms).

    **b. Neurologic signs and symptoms** develop abruptly. Most commonly there is a decreased level of consciousness, which may range from confusion to deep coma. Seizures, paralysis, and abnormal reflexes also are common. Increased intracranial pressure can result in papilledema.

  **3. Diagnosis.** A detailed medical history should be obtained, which should include an evaluation of all possible exposures to infected persons, insects, or animals. In addition, the following laboratory tests commonly are used to confirm the diagnosis of encephalitis; occasionally, these tests may reveal a specific infectious etiology.

    **a. Lumbar puncture and CSF examination** are essential.

      **(1)** Typical CSF findings in viral encephalitis include:

        **(a)** Increased intracranial pressure

            **(b)** Variable pleocytosis (generally 10–500 cells/mm³)
            **(c)** Increased protein level (> 40 mg/dl)
            **(d)** Normal glucose level
        **(2)** In addition, the CSF should be examined directly for bacteria and cultured for bacteria, mycobacteria, fungi, and viruses.
    **b. Brain biopsy** may be performed to obtain tissue specimens for culture and rapid viral antigen tests. The diagnosis of herpes simplex encephalitis is best confirmed by brain biopsy.
    **c. Serologic tests** (e.g., hemagglutination inhibition, complement fixation, ELISA) may be used to detect viral antibodies. The diagnosis of arboviral encephalitis is best confirmed by serologic tests.
    **d. Electroencephalograms (EEG)** and **computed tomography (CT)** and **brain scans** may reveal focal or generalized abnormalities in patients with encephalitis.

  **4. Therapy**
    **a. Antimicrobial therapy**
      **(1)** Acyclovir is the drug of choice for treatment of herpes simplex and varicella zoster encephalitis.
      **(2)** There is no specific therapy for other types of viral encephalitis.
    **b. Supportive care**
      **(1)** Patients with encephalitis should be cared for in an intensive care unit, with close cardiac monitoring and placement of an intracranial pressure transducer if intracranial pressure is moderately to severely increased.
      **(2)** Phenobarbital (5 mg/kg/24 hr) is given to prevent convulsions.
      **(3)** Severe cerebral edema can be decreased by the following methods:
        **(a)** Dexamethasone (0.5 mg/kg/24 hr), given intramuscularly
        **(b)** Mannitol (1.5–2.0 mg/kg/24 hr), given intravenously as a 20% solution
        **(c)** Lasix (1–2 mg/kg), given intravenously every 6 hours

## V. UPPER AIRWAY INFECTIONS

  **A. Otitis media,** or inflammation of the middle ear, is one of the most common infections of childhood. The characteristic feature of otitis media is a bulging, erythematous tympanic membrane with impaired mobility. Otitis media is classified as acute or chronic. The pathologic process of chronic otitis media usually is well established prior to the onset of clinical complaints. Otitis media that persists longer than several months is considered to be chronic.

    **1. Etiology**
    **a. Bacteria** are the primary agents of otitis media.
      **(1)** The most common causes in all age-groups are *S. pneumoniae* (25%–40% of cases) and unencapsulated *H. influenzae* (15%–25% of cases). In addition, gram-negative bacilli cause about 20% of otitis media in neonates; however, these bacteria rarely are found in older children with otitis media.
      **(2)** Less common causes include group A streptococci and *Branhamella catarrhalis* (acute form) and *S. aureus* and *P. aeruginosa* (chronic form).
    **b. Viruses** are not important causes of otitis media. In rare cases, respiratory syncytial virus, parainfluenza viruses, adenoviruses, and coxsackieviruses have been isolated from middle ear fluid.

    **2. Clinical features** of otitis media are variable and often nonspecific. Neonates and infants may be asymptomatic or may present with only subtle manifestations of illness (e.g., irritability).
    **a. Classic signs and symptoms of acute otitis media** include pain in one or both ears and hearing loss. A discharge may be present.
    **b. Common signs and symptoms of chronic otitis media** include hearing impairment and a foul discharge. Ear pain and fever occasionally occur and coincide with flare-ups of acute infection.
    **c. Nonspecific signs and symptoms** include fever, irritability, mild upper respiratory symptoms, vomiting, and diarrhea.

    **3. Diagnosis**
    **a. Otoscopy and tympanometry** are used to provide the basis for a diagnosis of otitis media.
      **(1)** Bulging of the tympanic membrane, as evidenced by partial or total loss of the bony landmarks, and diffuse erythema generally are accepted as reliable indications of otitis media. Erythema can result from crying and, by itself, does not establish the diagnosis.

      **(2)** Impaired mobility of the tympanic membrane is another diagnostic sign of otitis media, which can be assessed with a pneumatic otoscope.

      **(3)** Tympanic membrane compliance can be determined more objectively using a tympanometer.

   **b. Needle aspiration and culture** of the middle ear contents is the most reliable method for confirming the presence of infection and can be used to identify the causative agent. Only rarely is this procedure necessary, as in the case of a critically ill child or a child who fails to respond to standard antimicrobial therapy.

**4. Therapy**
   **a. Acute otitis media**

      **(1)** Initial treatment of acute otitis media is directed against the most commonly encountered bacteria, *S. pneumoniae* and *H. influenzae*. The drug of choice is amoxicillin, which usually is effective against both of these organisms.

      **(2)** If there is a poor response to initial therapy, alternative antibiotic regimens are used, such as amoxicillin-clavulanic acid, cefaclor, cefuroxime, cefixime, erythromycin-sulfisoxazole, or trimethoprim-sulfamethoxazole. Most clinical trials show no significant therapeutic differences among these drug regimens, but there are differences in cost, ease of administration, and side effects.

      **(3)** Patients who are not cured after a second course of antibiotics or who become severely ill may be considered for tympanocentesis to identify the offending pathogen so the most appropriate antibiotic can be used.

   **b. Recurrent otitis media.** Patients with recurrent otitis media may be placed on daily doses of an antibiotic such as sulfisoxazole for 3–6 months after the acute infection has cleared. Sulfisoxazole prophylaxis has been shown to decrease the incidence of recurrent otitis media in controlled trials.

**B. Sinusitis** is an inflammation of the mucous membrane lining the paranasal sinuses, which may be acute or chronic.

   **1. Acute and chronic forms**

      **a. Acute sinusitis** may involve one or more sinuses. Inflammation of the ethmoid sinuses (**ethmoiditis**) is most common in children, as these are the only sinuses that are fully developed at birth. The maxillary sinuses also may be involved but are not clinically important until after 18 months of age. Frontal sinusitis and sphenoidal sinusitis are rare before 10 years of age.

      **b. Chronic sinusitis** occurs following prolonged episodes of untreated or inadequately treated sinusitis that results in permanent changes in the mucosal lining of the sinus. Sterility no longer is maintained in the sinus. Although acute infectious exacerbations may occur, infection is not thought to play a major role in the symptoms of chronic sinusitis.

   **2. Predisposing factors.** Several conditions may precede sinusitis, the most common being viral upper respiratory infection, allergy (allergic rhinitis), and asthma. Other contributing factors include rapid changes in altitude, swimming, trauma, and immunologic defects.

   **3. Etiology.** Although sinusitis may be due to a viral infection or an allergy, the clinician making the diagnosis of sinusitis primarily is concerned with bacterial infection.

      **a.** The predominant microorganisms recovered from both children and adults with acute sinusitis include *S. pneumoniae,* unencapsulated strains of *H. influenzae,* and *B. catarrhalis*.

      **b.** *S. aureus* often is cultured from sinus fluid of patients with acute sinusitis, but this organism is not believed to be a major cause of sinusitis.

      **c.** Anaerobic organisms are uncommon causes of acute sinusitis.

   **4. Clinical features**

      **a.** Common symptoms of acute sinusitis in children older than 5 years are fever, facial pain, and headache. In younger children, the most common symptoms are fever, purulent nasal discharge, and daytime cough that persists longer than 10 days.

      **b.** Suggestive signs of acute sinusitis include periorbital swelling, localized tenderness to pressure, and malodorous breath.

   **5. Diagnosis** of sinusitis is complicated by the fact that the mucous membrane of the paranasal sinuses is continuous with that of the nose. As a result, even a transient viral upper respiratory infection may cause sinus membrane swelling.

a. **Radiography** is the most commonly used method for the diagnosis of acute sinusitis. The finding of air-fluid levels or complete opacity of the sinus cavity is strong evidence of acute bacterial sinusitis.
b. **Transillumination** of the sinuses may provide valuable information for the diagnosis of sinusitis in older children but not in younger ones. Opacity of the sinus cavity suggests the presence of sinusitis, whereas normal light transmission suggests the absence of infection.
c. **Sinus aspiration and culture** can provide the specific microbial etiology of sinusitis, but sinus puncture rarely is needed to confirm the diagnosis of sinusitis in children.
   (1) When aspiration is used, a Gram stain and culture of the sinus aspirate usually are obtained, although a biopsy of the sinuses also can give useful information.
   (2) Swab cultures of the anterior nares, nasal vestibule, and throat are not reliable because they do not correlate well with cultures of sinus aspirates.

6. **Therapy**
   a. **Antimicrobial therapy**
      (1) Initial treatment of acute sinusitis is directed against the most common bacterial causes, *S. pneumoniae* and *H. influenzae*. The drug of choice, therefore, is amoxicillin.
      (2) An alternative antibiotic regimen should be given in the case of apparent antibiotic failure or in the case of a patient who is allergic to penicillin or who lives in an area where ampicillin-resistant strains of *H. influenzae* abound. Alternatives include amoxicillin-clavulanic acid, cefaclor, erythromycin-sulfisoxazole, and trimethoprim-sulfamethoxazole.
   b. **Sinus irrigation or surgical drainage** of the sinuses is indicated in patients who do not respond to antimicrobial therapy and in those who develop intraorbital or intracranial complications, such as orbital cellulitis, cavernous sinus thrombosis, meningitis, and brain abscess.
   c. **Supportive care**
      (1) **Nasal decongestants** may be helpful in the supportive care of patients with acute sinusitis. These may be administered locally (by drops or spray) or orally for shrinkage of the nasal mucosa.
      (2) **Antihistamines** may be helpful in patients with associated allergic rhinitis. However, these agents may thicken purulent nasal secretions and, thus, inhibit drainage.

C. **Infections of the oral cavity. Gingivitis** and **stomatitis** refer to inflammatory disease of the gingivae (gums) and oral mucosa, respectively. Combined inflammation of the gingivae and oral mucosa is termed **gingivostomatitis**. The following discussion is limited to clinically important examples of gingivitis and stomatitis that occur in infants and children and excludes infections of the teeth and tongue.

1. **Necrotizing ulcerative gingivitis** (Vincent's disease, trench mouth) consists of necrosis and ulceration of the interdental papillae.
   a. **Incidence.** This infection is most common in adults but may also occur in children.
   b. **Etiology and pathogenesis**
      (1) Necrotizing ulcerative gingivitis results from a decreased resistance of the gingivae to infection by normal oral flora. Subgingival plaque is present in large amounts and consists of a mixture of fusiform bacilli and spirochetes.
      (2) The infection begins in an area of the gum that is in contact with plaque (the interdental papillae) and results in the punched-out, eroded papillae and purulent, gray membrane characteristically seen in these patients.
   c. **Clinical features** include gingival pain, fever, malaise, and foul-smelling breath.
   d. **Therapy**
      (1) Oral irrigation with oxidizing agents relieves the pain associated with the infection.
      (2) Antimicrobial therapy (usually penicillin G) is effective against the infection and, along with oral irrigation, generally brings prompt relief.

2. **Aphthous stomatitis** (canker sore) is a common and often recurrent oral mucosal lesion. It consists of circular, shallow ulcers that are painful and may occur anywhere on the oral mucosa, particularly the freely movable (buccal) mucosa. The lesions may occur singly or in clusters, are covered by a gray membrane, and are surrounded by a raised border of inflammation.
   a. **Etiology.** The exact cause of aphthous stomatitis is not known, but several infectious agents have been suspected.

    **b. Clinical course and therapy.** Aphthous stomatitis is a self-limited infection that heals in 1–2 weeks without treatment but tends to recur in susceptible individuals. Symptomatic therapy with saline mouthwash may be helpful in mild cases.

**3. Herpetic gingivostomatitis**
    **a. Incidence.** Herpetic gingivostomatitis is the most common type of gingivostomatitis in children. The first infection (primary infection) usually occurs within the first 5 years of life.
    **b. Etiology.** Herpes simplex virus is the causative agent. Most cases are due to herpes simplex virus type 1 rather than type 2.
    **c. Pathogenesis**
        **(1)** Primary infection affects the mouth and gums, whereas recurrent disease usually affects the lips (**herpes labialis**) and is less severe than the primary infection.
        **(2)** Recurrent illness often is precipitated by emotional stress, exposure to the sun, or another illness (e.g., pneumonia, meningitis).
    **d. Clinical features.** Painful, erythematous, edematous, and ulcerative lesions are present on the buccal mucosa, gums, and, sometimes, the hard palate and tongue. There usually is fever, often to a temperature of 105° F (40.6° C). The infection occurs after a 3- to 9-day incubation period, improves after 3–5 days, and generally resolves within 2 weeks.
    **e. Therapy.** Cold foods (e.g., ice cream) and oral fluids should be given. Viscous xylocaine (2%) can provide some pain relief. The condition may be severe enough that a child refuses to eat or drink and requires intravenous rehydration in the hospital.

**4. Herpangina.** Although herpangina has been considered a specific febrile disease, the term is more appropriately used to refer to the characteristic oropharyngeal lesions noted as one of the protean manifestations of enteroviral infections. Herpangina can occur in association with meningitis, exanthems, and other clinical presentations of the enteroviruses. **Hand-foot-and-mouth disease** is another infectious disease caused by enteroviruses, which is characterized by vesicular lesions of the anterior mouth, hands, and feet.
    **a. Etiology and incidence.** Coxsackieviruses (types A and B) and echoviruses are the causative agents. Herpangina occurs almost exclusively in the summer and fall, when enteroviruses are prevalent.
    **b. Clinical features**
        **(1)** Fever, sore throat, and pain on swallowing are the hallmarks of herpangina. The fever is of sudden onset and may reach a temperature of 106° F (41.1° C). Headache, myalgia, and vomiting also may occur at the onset of the illness.
        **(2)** The characteristic lesions are 1- to 2-mm vesicles and ulcers surrounded by an erythematous ring measuring up to 10 mm in diameter. The lesions occur in the posterior pharynx, including the anterior tonsillar pillars, soft palate, uvula, tonsils, and pharyngeal wall.
        **(3)** The fever subsides in 2–4 days, but the ulcers may persist for a period of up to 1 week.
    **c. Therapy.** No treatment is necessary other than prevention of dehydration and observation for signs of more severe enteroviral illness.

**5. Candidal gingivostomatitis. Thrush** is the term used to describe gingivostomatitis due to *Candida* species, usually *Candida albicans*.
    **a. Incidence.** Candidal gingivostomatitis is common in newborns. The condition usually clears by 3 months of age, except in severely debilitated infants. When candidal gingivostomatitis occurs after infancy, a defect of cell-mediated immunity should be considered.
    **b. Clinical features.** Grayish white lesions occur on the buccal mucosa and dorsum of the tongue. Occasionally, the gingival mucosa and posterior pharynx may be involved. If a scraping from the affected area is Gram stained, yeast forms and pseudohyphae are seen. Culture on blood agar will yield *Candida* organisms.
    **c. Therapy** consists of administering a solution of nystatin orally 4 times daily for 1 week. Retreatment sometimes is necessary.

**6. Other infections that are associated with gingivostomatitis** include syphilis, herpes zoster, histoplasmosis, actinomycosis, diphtheria, and tularemia.

**D. Streptococcal pharyngitis.** "Acute pharyngitis" refers to any of the numerous inflammatory conditions involving the pharynx. Most often it is due to a virus and occurs as a component of a generalized upper respiratory infection (e.g., the common cold). However, the most clinically significant cause of acute pharyngitis is group A β-hemolytic streptococcus. Because penicillin is effective against streptococcal but not viral pharyngitis, it is important to recognize streptococcal pharyngitis so that its symptoms can be alleviated and its complications (see V D 5) can be prevented.

1. **Epidemiology.** Streptococcal pharyngitis is one of the most common respiratory infections of childhood. Although all age-groups may be affected, the peak incidence occurs in children between the ages of 5 and 15 years. There is no sex or race predilection.

2. **Clinical features**
   a. **Symptoms** may vary widely from very mild to severe. In older children there is an abrupt onset of fever and sore throat accompanied by headache and malaise. Younger children may present with nausea, vomiting, and abdominal pain.
   b. **Physical signs** that may be seen in patients include:
      (1) Temperature above 101° F (38.4° C)
      (2) Tonsillar enlargement with exudate
      (3) Edema, erythema, and lymphoid hyperplasia of the pharynx
      (4) Tender anterior cervical lymph nodes and petechiae on the soft palate

3. **Diagnosis**
   a. **Differential diagnosis.** Acute pharyngitis may be due to a variety of pathogens, most of which are viruses.
      (1) Viruses that can cause infections that mimic streptococcal sore throat include Epstein-Barr virus, adenovirus, herpes simplex virus, enterovirus, influenza virus, parainfluenza virus, and measles virus.
      (2) Other bacterial causes of pharyngitis include *Corynebacterium diphtheriae* (rare in immunized populations), *M. pneumoniae, N. gonorrhoeae, Corynebacterium hemolyticum,* and *Chlamydia.*
   b. **Throat culture** is the primary method for the diagnosis of streptococcal pharyngitis and the most reliable means of differentiating streptococcal from viral pharyngitis.
      (1) A swab is rubbed over the tonsils and posterior pharynx, with care taken to avoid the buccal mucosa and tongue, and the swab is rolled over a blood agar plate.
      (2) Although the swab can be sent to a central laboratory, many pediatricians process their own throat cultures, with results usually available after overnight incubation. Presumptive differentiation of group A from other hemolytic streptococci is by the use of a bacitracin disk: group A hemolytic streptococci are sensitive whereas relatively few other hemolytic streptococci are sensitive to bacitracin.
   c. **Rapid diagnostic tests** recently have been developed for office use, which involve the extraction of streptococcal antigens from throat swabs so that the antigens can be identified using immunologic methods such as latex agglutination. Some of these commercial kits can secure the diagnosis within 10–60 minutes. In general, these tests are as specific but less sensitive and more expensive than throat cultures.

4. **Therapy**
   a. The treatment of choice for streptococcal pharyngitis is oral penicillin V (250 mg) given 3 times daily for 10 days. Noncompliant patients may be given a single intramuscular injection of benzathine penicillin G, which provides adequate penicillin levels for 10 days as well as local pain relief. The usual dose is 600,000–900,000 units for children younger than 12 years and 1,200,000 units for adolescents.
   b. **Penicillin-allergic patients** may be given any one of several alternative antibiotics.
      (1) Oral erythromycin is the favored alternative, which may be given in the form of erythromycin estolate (30 mg/kg/day) or erythromycin ethylsuccinate (50 mg/kg/day).
      (2) Oral cephalosporins, such as cephalexin and cefadroxil, also may be used to treat streptococcal pharyngitis but carry a 5%–10% risk of cross-reactivity in patients who are allergic to penicillin.

5. **Complications**
   a. Streptococcal pharyngitis may give rise to several **suppurative complications,** the most common of which are acute otitis media and acute sinusitis. Other suppurative complications include peritonsillar cellulitis or abscess, retropharyngeal abscess, and suppurative cervical lymphadenitis.
   b. Of even more importance, however, are the delayed **nonsuppurative complications** of streptococcal pharyngitis—acute rheumatic fever (see Ch 8 V A) and acute glomerulonephritis (see Ch 13 IV A 1).

E. **Cervical adenitis** refers to inflammation and enlargement of the lymph nodes of the neck. Swollen and tender cervical lymph nodes are common in children. In many cases the illness is self-limited (as in cervical adenitis associated with a viral infection); however, in other cases the illness requires prompt and effective treatment.

1. **Etiology.** The etiologic agents of childhood cervical adenitis are highly varied. Most cases are related to either bacterial infection of the oral cavity or other areas of the head and neck (e.g., streptococcal pharyngitis) or viral upper respiratory infection.

   a. **Common agents.** The most frequently identified agents of childhood cervical adenitis are *S. aureus* and group A streptococci; in addition, group B streptococci are common causes in neonates. Recent studies also have implicated anaerobic bacteria, which may cause cervical adenitis alone or in combination with other bacteria.

   b. **Less common agents**

      (1) **Cat-scratch disease** primarily affects children and is an important cause of cervical adenitis. The causative organism has not been definitely established, but a pleomorphic bacillus has been implicated. Transmission usually is by a cat scratch; occasionally, the skin injury is due to the scratch of a dog or other animal, a splinter, or a thorn.

      (2) Several species of **atypical mycobacteria** cause cervical adenitis in infants and young children. The most common of these are *Mycobacterium scrofulaceum* and *Mycobacterium avium-intracellulare.*

      (3) **Other agents** of childhood cervical adenitis include:

          (a) Epstein-Barr virus
          (b) *Mycobacterium tuberculosis*
          (c) *Francisella tularensis*
          (d) *S. pneumoniae*
          (e) *Yersinia pestis*
          (f) Fungi
          (g) *T. gondii*

2. **Clinical features**

   a. **General description.** Typically, a child with cervical adenitis presents with swollen, tender nodes in a single location of the neck, with reddening of the skin overlying the nodes. Bilateral involvement suggests a nonspecific or viral infection, which usually resolves spontaneously. Unilateral involvement with nodes that are more severely swollen (3–6 cm in diameter), tender, and warm suggests a pyogenic infection. Low-grade fever is an inconsistent finding.

   b. **In cat-scratch disease,** which is unilateral, the involved nodes may be quite large and in 10%–25% of cases are suppurative. Low-grade fever and a transient maculopapular rash also may be noted.

   c. **In atypical mycobacterial infection,** the cervical adenitis usually involves the submandibular or submaxillary nodes, is unilateral, and runs an indolent course. Fever and other systemic signs usually are absent.

3. **Diagnosis**

   a. **Medical history and physical examination.** The medical history of a child with cervical adenitis should include information concerning exposure to individuals with tuberculosis, contact with pets (especially cats), recent upper respiratory infections, and the duration of the lymphadenopathy. All node sites should be examined, with dimensions noted. Liver and spleen size also should be noted.

   b. **Specific diagnosis** of the cause of cervical adenitis usually is not attempted if the child has only slightly enlarged and minimally tender lymph nodes. A diagnostic workup is performed if the child has a moderate fever and systemic symptoms when first examined, if a large (> 3 cm) or fluctuant node is found, if findings suggest an unusual etiology, or if empiric antibiotic therapy has failed (see V E 4).

      (1) **Needle aspiration, incision and drainage,** or **excision and biopsy** are the most direct methods for the diagnosis of cervical adenitis. When appropriately performed, needle aspiration is a safe and accurate procedure. The aspirated material should be prepared for Gram stain, acid-fast stain, and culture.

      (2) A **tuberculin skin test** should be given to all children with cervical adenitis, even if there has been no history of exposure to tuberculosis.

      (3) **Serologic tests** may help to identify viruses (e.g., Epstein-Barr virus), bacteria (e.g., *F. tularensis, Streptococcus pyogenes),* and fungi.

      (4) **Other diagnostic tests** include:

          (a) Gram stain and culture of any primary focus of infection

**(b)** Blood culture
**(c)** Complete blood count
**(d)** Chest x-ray

**4. Therapy**

**a.** Cervical adenitis that is characterized by only slight enlargement and minimal tenderness of the lymph nodes is closely observed but otherwise untreated.

**b.** Cervical adenitis that is characterized by more severe enlargement and tenderness usually is treated first with empiric antibiotic therapy for 10–14 days.

**(1)** The preferred agents are penicillinase-resistant penicillins, such as dicloxacillin.

**(2)** Penicillin-allergic patients usually are given an oral cephalosporin or clindamycin.

**c.** If there is a poor response to empiric therapy, needle aspiration is performed. If a specific etiology is determined, appropriate therapy is as follows.

**(1)** Cervical adenitis due to *S. aureus* or group A streptococci is treated with an oral antistaphylococcal agent or oral penicillin, respectively. Excision and drainage may be necessary in severe cases.

**(2)** Cervical adenitis associated with cat-scratch disease usually is self-limited and requires only analgesics. Suppuration may occur and is managed with needle aspiration to remove pus.

**(3)** Cervical adenitis due to atypical mycobacteria is treated with excision and drainage of infected nodes. Antituberculous drug therapy alone usually is unsuccessful, although it may be used in addition to surgical excision.

**F. Croup** is a general term used to describe several acute infectious conditions involving the larynx and, to a lesser extent, the trachea and bronchi. Croup syndromes are characterized by a distinctively brassy cough combined with one or more of the following: hoarseness, inspiratory stridor, and signs of respiratory distress due to laryngeal obstruction. The following clinical entities have been described: acute infectious laryngitis, acute epiglottitis (supraglottic laryngitis), acute laryngotracheobronchitis ("viral" croup), and acute spasmodic laryngitis (spasmodic croup).

**1. Acute infectious laryngitis** is common and usually occurs in association with the common cold and influenza syndromes.

**a. Etiology.** Acute laryngitis is caused primarily by viruses, the most frequently implicated being influenza virus, rhinovirus, and adenovirus. In addition, acute laryngitis may be caused by group A β-hemolytic streptococci (*S. pyogenes*) in some cases and, rarely, by *C. diphtheriae.*

**b. Clinical features.** The illness usually is mild, with respiratory distress often absent except in young infants. In rare cases (usually with diphtheria), subglottic obstruction can be severe and result in severe inspiratory stridor, dyspnea, and respiratory arrest.

**c. Diagnosis** of acute laryngitis usually is apparent from the clinical features of the illness. Mirror examination of the larynx reveals hyperemic and edematous mucosa. A specific diagnosis sometimes can be made with a throat culture for bacteria and viruses.

**d. Therapy.** Supportive measures include resting the voice and inhaling moistened air. Antimicrobial therapy is indicated for laryngitis that is due to group A β-hemolytic streptococci or *C. diphtheriae.* For laryngitis due to *C. diphtheriae,* diphtheria antitoxin is administered in a single dose.

**2. Acute epiglottitis** is a rapidly progressive infection of the epiglottis and contiguous structures, which may cause life-threatening airway obstruction.

**a. Etiology.** Almost all cases of acute epiglottitis in children are caused by *H. influenzae* type b.

**b. Clinical features.** The abrupt onset of high fever, moderate to severe respiratory distress, and stridor in a child who is sitting forward with mouth open and drooling (due to the inability to swallow normally) are highly suggestive of acute epiglottitis.

**c. Diagnosis** must be made swiftly but in such a way as to minimize patient anxiety, as even a slight increase in restlessness may cause obstruction of the airway by the swollen epiglottis.

**(1)** **Physical examination** should be done quickly and with care to minimize anxiety. The diagnosis is based on finding a swollen, **cherry-red epiglottis**. It is essential to visualize the epiglottis with a laryngoscope or bronchoscope in an operating room, with complete cardiorespiratory support. Visualization of the epiglottis by depressing the tongue is contraindicated because of the possibility of inducing airway obstruction.

    **(2) X-ray.** In patients with mild stridor who are not acutely ill, x-ray (lateral neck views) of the nasopharynx and upper airway is useful to rule out epiglottitis.

    **(3) Culture** of the epiglottis and blood should be obtained for identification of the causative organism and its antimicrobial susceptibility pattern.

    **(4) Immunologic tests.** Rapid tests for *H. influenzae* type b antigen on serum or urine may be helpful.

    **(5) Differential diagnosis.** The major differential consideration is acute laryngotracheobronchitis. Epiglottitis has a more abrupt onset and more severe symptoms, and the usual age range is 2 years to 7 years compared with 3 months to 5 years for laryngotracheobronchitis. A complete blood count may be helpful for differentiating the two conditions; epiglottitis is characterized by leukocytosis with a marked shift to the left.

  **d. Therapy**

    **(1) Ventilatory support.** Following visual confirmation of epiglottitis, the patient should be intubated and given ventilatory support until edema subsides—usually after several days.

    **(2) Intravenous antibiotic therapy** is given for 7–10 days and is directed against *H. influenzae* type b. The agents of choice are ampicillin, a third-generation cephalosporin, or chloramphenicol, depending on the sensitivity pattern of the causative organism.

    **(3) Contraindications.** Racemic epinephrine and corticosteroids should not be given to these patients.

**3. Acute laryngotracheobronchitis** is the most common of the clinical entities termed "croup."

  **a. Etiology.** Acute laryngotracheobronchitis is caused primarily by respiratory viruses, most commonly, parainfluenza virus. Because of its viral etiology, this croup syndrome often is referred to as "**viral croup.**"

  **b. Clinical features.** Viral croup usually has a gradual onset and course. Symptoms often are worse at night and persist for several days.

    **(1)** Patients present initially with symptoms of upper respiratory infection, followed after several days by the characteristic barking cough, inspiratory stridor, and respiratory distress.

    **(2)** Fever often is low grade, but temperatures as high as 104° F (40° C) have been noted.

    **(3)** Hoarseness and aphonia are common.

  **c. Diagnosis** usually is apparent from the clinical features but can be aided by x-ray of the larynx, which reveals subglottic narrowing.

  **d. Therapy** for viral croup consists mainly of improving air exchange.

    **(1) Humidification**

      **(a)** Patients with mild illness may be treated at home with humidified air from a hot shower or bath, hot steam from a vaporizer, or "cold steam" from a nebulizer. Respiratory distress may improve within minutes, but humidification should be continued until the cough subsides—usually after 2 or 3 days.

      **(b)** Patients with moderate to severe illness should be hospitalized if any one of the following signs and symptoms is noted: cyanosis, depressed sensorium, progressive stridor, or a toxic appearance. Cold humidified oxygen should be provided, and the patient should be observed closely in case emergency intubation is needed but otherwise should be disturbed as little as possible. Arterial blood gas analysis is important to assess the adequacy of air exchange.

    **(2) Racemic epinephrine** (2.5% solution delivered by nebulizer) has been shown to improve air exchange in these patients. It should be used in moderately ill, hospitalized patients, as it may eliminate the need for intubation during the 24–48 hours when the illness is most severe.

    **(3) Corticosteroids** have been the subject of much debate but may be helpful in severe cases. A trial using dexamethasone (0.3–0.5 mg/kg given once and repeated in 2 hours) showed a shorter course in patients receiving the drug than in those who did not.

    **(4) Contraindications.** Sedatives, opiates, expectorants, bronchodilators, and antihistamines should not be given to these patients.

**4. Acute spasmodic laryngitis,** or spasmodic croup, refers to brief, repeated attacks of symptoms that are clinically similar to those of viral croup but less severe. Spasmodic croup occurs most often in children between 1 and 3 years old.

  **a. Etiology.** Spasmodic croup is believed to be caused by viruses, although important allergic and psychological factors probably contribute to the illness in some patients.

    **b. Clinical features.** Spasmodic croup is characterized by the sudden onset—usually at night—of croupy cough and respiratory stridor. The episodes generally last less than 1 day but may recur several times per year.

    **c. Therapy.** Treatment at home with humidified air generally is sufficient for this illness.

**G. Mumps** is a highly contagious, acute, generalized viral disease, the most characteristic feature of which is painful enlargement of the salivary glands—primarily the parotids. The disease is benign and resolves spontaneously; 20%–40% of infections are subclinical.

    **1. Epidemiology.** Mumps is found throughout the world and occurs year-round, although epidemics are more frequent during the winter and spring. The disease is uncommon in infants younger than 1 year; the highest incidence is in school-age children.

    **2. Etiology and pathogenesis**

      **a.** Mumps is caused by a paramyxovirus—the mumps virus—of which only one serotype has been identified. Mumps virus has been isolated from the saliva, CSF, blood, urine, and infected tissues of mumps patients.

      **b.** The virus may spread by direct contact, by airborne droplet nuclei, and by fomites that have been contaminated by saliva.

      **c.** Virus transmission generally occurs during the period 48 hours before the appearance of salivary gland swelling to 7 days after its appearance.

    **3. Clinical features**

      **a.** The incubation period varies in length from 2 to 4 weeks but usually is 16–18 days. After the incubation period, a **prodrome** of fever, anorexia, headache, and malaise may occur but is uncommon.

      **b.** Within 1 day, the illness manifests as **pain and swelling in one or both parotid glands,** from the posterior border of the mandible forward and downward. Pain and erythema often occur at the opening of the parotid duct (Stensen's duct).

        **(1)** The swelling usually peaks in 1–3 days and then resolves over a 3- to 7-day period.

        **(2)** Submandibular or sublingual gland swelling may accompany the parotitis but rarely is the only manifestation of disease.

      **c. Fever** usually is moderate, although temperatures may reach 104° F (40° C). Fever is absent in 20% of cases.

    **4. Diagnosis** often can be made on the basis of known exposure to mumps combined with characteristic symptoms and physical signs. An elevated serum amylase level due to parotid involvement and/or pancreatitis is the most useful indicator in any patient with mumps.

      **a. Definitive diagnosis** requires either culture of the virus from the saliva, urine, CSF, or blood or demonstration of a significant rise in circulating mumps antibody from the acute to convalescent stage.

      **b. Differential diagnostic considerations** include acute parotitis (due to coxsackie A virus infection or lymphocytic choriomeningitis), suppurative parotitis (due to bacterial infection), recurrent parotitis (possibly of allergic origin), and a salivary calculus.

    **5. Therapy** for mumps is entirely symptomatic and supportive.

    **6. Prevention**

      **a.** Passive prophylaxis has not been shown to be effective for preventing mumps or decreasing the incidence of complications.

      **b.** Active immunization with live attenuated mumps virus vaccine is effective for prevention of mumps and has few side effects (see Ch 1 II A 5 e).

    **7. Complications** of mumps are uncommon and usually not severe.

      **a. Meningoencephalitis** is the most frequent complication in childhood, with clinical manifestations noted in about 10% of patients. Mumps is one of the most common causes of aseptic meningitis.

      **b. Epididimo-orchitis** is rare in prepubescent boys but develops in 20%–30% of postpubertal men; it usually is unilateral. Symptoms usually occur about 8 days after parotitis develops but may occur in the absence of salivary gland infection. Approximately 50% of infected testes will show some degree of atrophy, but infertility is rare.

      **c. Pancreatitis** usually presents as epigastric pain and tenderness combined with fever, chills, and vomiting.

   **d. Unilateral deafness** occurs in 1 in 20,000 mumps patients. Hearing loss is complete and permanent. Bilateral nerve deafness due to mumps is rare.
   **e. Other complications** include oophoritis, nephritis, thyroiditis, myocarditis, arthritis, thrombocytopenic purpura, and mastitis.

**H. Infectious mononucleosis** is an acute infection characterized by fever, sore throat, lymphadenopathy, splenomegaly, atypical lymphocytosis, and the presence of heterophil antibody. Infectious mononucleosis most often affects adolescents and young adults.

1. **Etiology.** Infectious mononucleosis is caused by Epstein-Barr virus, a herpesvirus. Cytomegalovirus and *T. gondii* cause illnesses that are virtually indistinguishable from Epstein-Barr virus–induced mononucleosis.

2. **Clinical features** of infectious mononucleosis are highly variable, often being less severe in younger children than in older children, adolescents, or adults. A prodrome of malaise, fever, and headache may extend for 3–7 days before the onset of more profound symptoms.
   **a. Fever** is invariably present and may last as long as 21 days. Temperature seldom exceeds 104° F (40° C).
   **b. Pharyngitis** occurs in about 80% of patients with infectious mononucleosis and may be severe. Although group A streptococci may be cultured from these patients, the incidence of streptococcal pharyngitis in patients with infectious mononucleosis is not increased compared with normal controls.
   **c. Lymphadenopathy** usually is generalized and most often involves the posterior cervical nodes; other anatomic sites also may be affected.
   **d. Splenomegaly** is noted in most patients with infectious mononucleosis.
   **e. Rash** occurs in 10%–40% of patients overall, but it develops in almost all patients who are given ampicillin. The rash is maculopapular and generalized.
   **f. Other clinical findings** include fatigue, eyelid edema, abdominal pain, and, rarely, jaundice.

3. **Diagnosis.** Laboratory confirmation of infectious mononucleosis consists of positive serologic findings. Several serologic tests have been developed.
   **a. Paul-Bunnell-Davidsohn test** is an extension of the classic Paul-Bunnell test for the heterophil antibody characteristic of infectious mononucleosis. **Heterophil antibodies** are antibodies that can react with antigens that are different from the antigens that induced their production.
      **(1)** Heterophil antibodies in patients with infectious mononucleosis cause sheep erythrocytes to agglutinate after absorption of the test serum by guinea pig kidney cells. The antibody can reach high titers.
      **(2)** Heterophil antibodies in normal individuals and those with diseases other than infectious mononucleosis (e.g., serum sickness) may cause agglutination of sheep erythrocytes, but these antibodies are absorbed by guinea pig kidney cells, whereas those of patients with infectious mononucleosis are not.
   **b. Monospot test.** This test is a simple, rapid, and fairly sensitive heterophil antibody test. The test usually is positive within the first week of infection and remains positive for several months. False positive results are not uncommon; furthermore, only 80% of patients with Epstein-Barr virus infection have positive results. Also, for unknown reasons, children younger than 5 years with Epstein-Barr virus infection often have false negative results on Monospot testing.
   **c. Antibodies to Epstein-Barr virus.** Patients with infectious mononucleosis produce antibodies to various specific antigens, including Epstein-Barr viral capsid antigen (**VCA**), Epstein-Barr nuclear antigen (**EBNA**), and Epstein-Barr virus–induced early antigen (**EA**).
      **(1)** Antibodies to VCA—initially immunoglobulin M (IgM) followed by IgG—peak in the second or third week of illness and persist for life.
      **(2)** Antibodies to EA appear early in the course of illness and disappear 2–6 months later.
      **(3)** Antibodies to EBNA appear 3–6 months after the onset of infection and probably persist for life.

4. **Therapy.** In most cases, rest is the only treatment that is necessary; there is no specific drug therapy for infectious mononucleosis. Convalescence may take weeks to months and is relatively shorter in younger patients as compared with older patients.

**5. Complications**
   a. **Splenic rupture,** either due to trauma or occurring spontaneously, is a rare complication. Patients should be advised not to engage in any contact sports until they are fully recovered and splenomegaly has resolved.
   b. **Airway obstruction** due to tonsillar or pharyngeal hypertrophy also is rare. Treatment with corticosteroids often is effective, although tracheal intubation or tonsillectomy and adenoidectomy may be necessary in some cases.
   c. **Neurologic complications** usually are self-limited and reversible and include aseptic meningitis, encephalitis, myelitis, peripheral neuropathies, and Guillain-Barré syndrome.
   d. **Icteric hepatitis** occurs in about 5% of cases, whereas subclinical hepatitis occurs in about 20%–40%. Acute liver failure is rare.
   e. **Other rare complications** include autoimmune hemolytic anemia, thrombocytopenia, neutropenia, acute renal failure, complete heart block, myositis, pericarditis, pneumonia, acrocyanosis, and immunologic disorders (e.g., impaired cell-mediated immunity, agammaglobulinemia).

# VI. LOWER RESPIRATORY TRACT INFECTIONS

**A. Bronchiolitis** is an acute viral infection of the bronchioles.

   **1. Epidemiology.** Bronchiolitis is a common lower respiratory tract illness of children younger than 2 years (due to their small airways), with a peak incidence at 6 months of age. Most cases occur in the winter and early spring months.

   **2. Etiology.** Over 50% of cases are due to respiratory syncytial virus. Other causes include parainfluenza virus and adenovirus.

   **3. Clinical features**
   a. **Symptoms**
      (1) The onset of bronchiolitis is characterized by mild upper respiratory tract symptoms, which last several days and may be accompanied by a mild fever [temperature of 101°–102° F (38.3°–38.9° C)].
      (2) Lower respiratory tract involvement follows, with gradual development of respiratory distress (i.e., paroxysmal cough, wheezing, tachypnea, dyspnea) accompanied by irritability and decreased appetite.
   b. **Physical signs** of bronchiolitis include tachypnea, flaring of the alae nasi, and, occasionally, cyanosis. Rales and expiratory wheezes are characteristic. Hepatosplenomegaly may occur as a result of diaphragm depression due to hyperinflation of the lung.

   **4. Diagnosis** of bronchiolitis generally is made on the basis of the history (recent exposure to a child or an adult with minor respiratory illness) and physical examination. Classic, confirmatory findings on x-ray include hyperinflation and occasional scattered areas of consolidation due to atelectasis. The white blood cell count and differential usually are normal.
   a. **Diagnosis of the specific agent** of bronchiolitis can be made by rapid tests for viral antigen in the nasopharynx (especially, immunofluorescence for respiratory syncytial virus), viral cultures, or a rise in serum antibody titers.
   b. **Differential diagnostic considerations** include, most importantly, asthma as well as congestive heart failure, foreign body in the lung or trachea, pertussis, cystic fibrosis, and bacterial pneumonia.

   **5. Therapy.** The antiviral agent ribavirin can be used for treatment of severe bronchiolitis and pneumonia due to respiratory syncytial virus. Ribavirin has been shown to improve arterial oxygen tension ($Po_2$) significantly and to shorten the course of the illness.
   a. The overall mortality rate for bronchiolitis is less than 1%. In most cases, patients recover spontaneously after the first 48–72 hours of illness and do not require hospitalization or ribavirin therapy.
   b. However, in some cases—especially infants with congenital heart disease, cystic fibrosis, bronchopulmonary dysplasia, or some other underlying pulmonary disease—respiratory distress progresses rapidly and is severe enough to require that the patient be hospitalized with assisted ventilation. The mortality rate among these patients is much higher than in those with the usual case of bronchiolitis.

**(1)** Hospitalized infants are placed in an atmosphere of cold, humidified oxygen to relieve dyspnea and cyanosis. Intravenous or oral fluids are given to offset the dehydrating effects of tachypnea and anorexia.

**(2)** Ribavirin is indicated in patients with documented respiratory syncytial virus infection and severe bronchiolitis. Ribavirin is given daily by aerosol over 12–18 hours for 3–7 days.

    **c.** Special care must be taken with the use of ribavirin for patients on ventilators to prevent precipitation of the drug within the ventilator, and constant monitoring of such patients is mandatory. Pregnant health care workers should avoid caring for patients on ribavirin because of the remote possibility that the drug is a human teratogen.

    **d. Contraindications.** The use of sedatives and corticosteroids is not recommended.

**B. Pneumonia** is an inflammation of the lung parenchyma (i.e., the portion of the lower respiratory tract consisting of the respiratory bronchioles, alveolar ducts, alveolar sacs, and alveoli). There are numerous infectious causes of pneumonia, including viruses, bacteria, fungi, parasites, and rickettsiae. Although most cases of childhood pneumonia are due to viruses, antibiotics are prescribed because the precise etiology usually is not determined.

  **1. Bacterial pneumonia**

    **a. Etiology**

      **(1) Common bacterial causes** of pneumonia in children older than 3 months of age include *S. pneumoniae, H. influenzae* type b, and group A streptococcus. Group B streptococcus is a common pathogen in neonates.

      **(2) Other bacterial causes** of pneumonia in children include *S. aureus,* gram-negative enteric organisms, anaerobes, and *M. tuberculosis* (see also Ch 12 VIII A).

    **b. Clinical features.** The clinical presentation in older children (about 6 years old and older) is fairly classic and not unlike that noted in adults with pneumonia. The clinical presentation in infants and children younger than 6 years is somewhat variable.

      **(1) Older children** with bacterial pneumonia typically present first with mild upper respiratory tract symptoms (e.g., cough, rhinitis) followed by the abrupt onset of fever, tachypnea, chest pain, and shaking chills. Physical examination often reveals lateralizing chest signs, such as decreased breath sounds and rales on the affected side.

      **(2) Younger children** with bacterial pneumonia may present with nonspecific manifestations of infection including fever, malaise, gastrointestinal complaints, restlessness, apprehension, and chills. Respiratory signs may be minimal and include tachypnea, cough, grunting respirations, and flaring of the alae nasi. Signs of pneumonia also may be subtle in the young infant, with absence of rales and rhonchi.

    **c. Diagnosis**

      **(1) Laboratory findings** include a peripheral blood leukocytosis with a preponderance of neutrophils and dense, focal infiltration on chest x-ray.

      **(2) Specific diagnosis** can be made from culture or rapid testing of the blood, urine, alveolar fluid, or pleural fluid. Fluid may be obtained by lung biopsy, lung puncture, thoracentesis, transtracheal aspiration, or bronchoscopy. (Although Gram stain and culture of the sputum may help to identify the pathogen, sputum usually is difficult to obtain from children.)

    **d. Therapy.** There is no universally accepted antibiotic regimen for treatment of presumed bacterial pneumonia. In addition to the following general guidelines, such factors as age, severity of illness, presence of illness in the child's family, and results of laboratory studies must be considered when an antibiotic is chosen.

      **(1) Neonates** with pneumonia should be hospitalized and treated intravenously either with ampicillin and an aminoglycoside (e.g., gentamicin) or with ampicillin and cefotaxime or ceftazidime. In addition, hospitalized infants should receive supportive care in the form of intravenous fluids, supplemental oxygen, ventilatory support, and chest physical therapy.

      **(2) Children younger than 6 years** with mild to moderate illness can be observed closely at home and given oral amoxicillin. Children with more severe illness require hospitalization and intravenous cefuroxime, ceftriaxone, ceftazidime, or oxacillin and chloramphenicol.

      **(3) Children older than 6 years** with mild to moderate illness are given oral penicillin or, if *M. pneumoniae* is the likely cause, erythromycin. Children with severe illness are hospitalized and treated with intravenous cefuroxime, ceftriaxone, ceftazidime, or oxacillin and an aminoglycoside.

2. **Viral pneumonia**
   a. **Etiology.** A virus is the most common cause of pneumonia in children. Respiratory syncytial virus is the most common viral etiology; other common causes include parainfluenza virus, adenovirus, and enterovirus. Less common causes of pneumonia in children include rhinovirus, influenza virus, and herpesvirus.
   b. **Clinical features.** The clinical presentation of viral pneumonia, like that of bacterial pneumonia, begins with several days of rhinitis and cough followed by fever and more pronounced respiratory symptoms, such as dyspnea and intercostal retractions. In general, the symptoms of viral pneumonia are less fulminant than those of bacterial pneumonia, with lower fever and milder respiratory distress.
   c. **Diagnosis**
      (1) **Laboratory findings** include a preponderance of lymphocytes on complete blood count and diffuse, bilateral infiltrates on chest x-ray.
      (2) **Specific diagnosis** can be made by rapid tests for viral antigen (e.g., immunofluorescence) and by culturing nasopharyngeal and rectal specimens for viruses.
   d. **Therapy** for viral pneumonia at one time was limited to supportive care; however, the recent introduction of antiviral chemotherapy has allowed for specific therapy.
      (1) **Antiviral therapy**
         (a) Ribavirin is effective against both respiratory syncytial virus and influenza virus and should be used to treat severe pneumonia caused by either of these pathogens. It is administered by aerosol over a period of 5–7 days (see VI A 5 for further information regarding ribavirin therapy).
         (b) Acyclovir has been used to treat pneumonia caused by herpes simplex virus or herpes zoster virus. It is given by intravenous infusion over a period of 7–10 days.
      (2) **Supportive care** includes administration of intravenous fluids and supplemental oxygen as well as ventilatory support and chest physical therapy.

3. **Other causes of pneumonia**
   a. *M. pneumoniae* is the most common nonviral cause of pneumonia in children older than 6 years. The peak incidence of *M. pneumoniae* pneumonia is between the ages of 5 and 15 years.
      (1) **Clinical features.** In general, *M. pneumoniae* pneumonia is less severe than traditional bacterial pneumonia and often is referred to as "walking pneumonia." Hospitalization rarely is necessary.
         (a) The onset of illness is gradual; fever, headache, and malaise are experienced for 2–4 days before respiratory symptoms develop.
         (b) A nonproductive cough is the characteristic respiratory symptom. Pharyngitis also is common.
      (2) **Diagnosis**
         (a) **Laboratory findings.** The complete blood count usually is normal, but leukocytosis with a shift to the left may be noted. The chest x-ray usually is interstitial in appearance but may be focal. Cold agglutinins usually are elevated during the first week of illness but may be negative in young children.
         (b) **Specific diagnosis** is made by demonstration of a rise in antibody titer in convalescent-phase serum or by isolation of *M. pneumoniae* from sputum or throat culture.
      (3) **Therapy.** Erythromycin is the drug of choice for treatment of *M. pneumoniae* pneumonia.
   b. *Pneumocystis carinii* produces a progressive pneumonia in immunocompromised hosts, such as those with AIDS, congenital immunodeficiency, or immunosuppression caused by cancer or cancer chemotherapy.
      (1) **Clinical features.** In infants, the disease usually begins as a mild illness with low-grade fever but progresses to severe respiratory distress with cyanosis.
      (2) **Diagnosis**
         (a) The diagnosis is suggested by the typical clinical course and presentation and by a bilateral, generalized granular pattern on x-ray.
         (b) Definitive diagnosis is made by demonstration of *P. carinii* on specially stained smears from tracheal or bronchial washings, lung aspirates, or lung biopsies.
      (3) **Therapy.** Trimethoprim-sulfamethoxazole is the drug of choice for treatment of *P. carinii* pneumonia. An alternative choice is pentamidine isethionate.

**VII. EXANTHEMS** are rashes that arise as cutaneous manifestations of infectious diseases.

**A. Measles** (rubeola) is an acute, highly contagious viral disease that occurs chiefly in young children living in highly populated areas.

**1. Epidemiology.** Although measles is becoming uncommon in developed countries where vaccine is used, it continues to be a major health problem worldwide. Measles persists as a sporadic problem in the United States, despite continued efforts to eradicate the disease.

**2. Etiology.** Measles is caused by a paramyxovirus—the measles virus—of which only one serotype has been identified.

**3. Clinical features.** The clinical course of measles has three stages.
 **a.** An **incubation period** extends for 8–12 days after initial exposure to the virus; signs and symptoms are absent during this stage.
 **b.** A **prodrome** follows, consisting of malaise, fever [temperatures up to 105° F (40.6° C)], cough, coryza, and conjunctivitis. Within 2 or 3 days after the onset of symptoms, **Koplik's spots** (small, irregular red spots with central gray or bluish white specks) appear on the buccal mucosa.
 **c.** An **erythematous maculopapular rash** erupts about 5 days after the onset of symptoms. The rash begins on the head and spreads downward, lasting about 4–5 days and then resolving from the head downward.

**4. Diagnosis** usually can be made on the basis of observed characteristic clinical findings. A fourfold or greater rise in hemagglutination inhibition antibodies over 2 or 3 weeks confirms the diagnosis.

**5. Therapy** mainly is supportive.

**6. Prevention**
 **a.** A live attenuated vaccine given alone or as part of the measles, mumps, and rubella or measles and rubella vaccines is highly effective in preventing measles (see Ch 1 II A 5 e). It may provide protection if given within 72 hours of measles exposure.
 **b.** Immunoglobulin can be given to modify or prevent measles in a susceptible person if given within 6 days of exposure.

**7. Complications** are rare but may occur, especially in malnourished or immunocompromised children. Measles complications include pneumonia, encephalitis, subacute sclerosing panencephalitis, pericarditis, and hepatitis. The mortality rate is low in healthy children but may exceed 10% in malnourished children living in poor and crowded environments.

**B. Rubella** (German measles) is a viral disease that generally is innocuous when acquired postnatally; however, it can have devastating effects when a fetus is infected transplacentally during maternal infection. Prior to the development of a rubella vaccine in 1969, rubella was the most important cause of congenital infection, resulting in thousands of fetal deaths, premature deliveries, and children born with congenital defects.

**1. Etiology.** Rubella is caused by rubella virus, an RNA virus that is classified as a togavirus based on its biochemical and morphologic properties.

**2. Clinical features**
 **a. Postnatal rubella.** Clinical manifestations are absent in many cases of rubella.
  **(1)** An incubation period of 12–23 days is followed, in adults, by a prodrome of malaise, fever, and anorexia. There is **no prodrome** in children.
  **(2)** Several days after the onset of symptoms, posterior auricular, cervical, and suboccipital lymphadenopathy develops, followed by the appearance of a **maculopapular rash**. The rash begins on the face and then becomes generalized; it seldom lasts longer than 5 days. Fever may accompany the rash on the first day and then resolves.
 **b. Congenital rubella** most commonly results in deafness, cataracts, glaucoma, congenital heart disease, and mental retardation, but numerous other defects have been described. Some complications, such as a progressive encephalopathy, do not become apparent until the child is older. The risk of congenital defects increases the earlier in pregnancy that the disease occurs.
  **(1) Disease at 1–2 months gestation** is associated with a 40%–60% risk of multiple congenital defects and spontaneous abortion.

**(2) Disease at 3 months gestation** is associated with a 30%–35% risk of a single defect.
**(3) Disease at 4 months gestation** is associated with a 10% risk of a single defect.
**(4) Disease at 5–9 months gestation** occasionally is associated with a single defect.

**3. Diagnosis**
   **a. Definitive diagnosis** of rubella requires either virus isolation or serologic techniques.
      **(1)** Virus isolation can be performed in specialized laboratories, but it is difficult and time-consuming.
      **(2)** The diagnosis usually is confirmed by a fourfold or greater rise in titer of hemagglutination inhibition or complement-fixing antibodies. Congenital rubella also can be diagnosed in the neonatal period by a positive IgM antibody to rubella virus in the newborn's serum; increased IgM titer indicates recent rubella infection of the fetus, because IgM does not cross the placenta.
   **b. Differential diagnosis.** The diagnosis of rubella is difficult because the symptoms often are mild and may be confused with those of enteroviral infections, roseola, toxoplasmosis, infectious mononucleosis, mild measles, and scarlet fever.

**4. Therapy and prevention**
   **a.** Postnatal rubella usually is mild and self-limited, requiring no treatment. Treatment of congenital rubella is supportive.
   **b.** Prevention of rubella is effected by a live attenuated vaccine, which usually is given at age 15 months as part of the measles, mumps, and rubella vaccine.

**C. Roseola infantum** (exanthem subitum) is a common, acute disease of infants and young children, which is caused by herpesvirus 6.

**1. Clinical features**
   **a.** The illness usually begins with an **abrupt fever** characterized by temperatures of 103°–106° F (39.5°–41.2° C). The fever persists for 1–5 days, although the child appears well and has no physical findings to explain the fever.
   **b.** The temperature usually returns to normal by the third or fourth day of illness, and a **macular or maculopapular rash** appears on the trunk and spreads peripherally. The rash often resolves within 24 hours.
   **c.** Initially, the leukocyte count may be as high as 20,000/mm$^3$, with a shift to the left. By the second day of illness, leukopenia and neutropenia are noted.

**2. Therapy.** Most cases are benign and self-limited. No treatment is available to shorten the course of the illness or to prevent it.

**3. Complications** are uncommon, although febrile convulsions may occur. The prognosis generally is good.

**D. Erythema infectiosum** (fifth disease) is a mild, self-limited systemic illness accompanied by a distinctive rash. It occurs primarily in epidemics involving children, although adults infrequently are affected. A human parvovirus is the cause of the illness.

**1. Clinical features**
   **a.** Usually there is **no prodrome,** and fever may be absent or only low grade. Systemic symptoms occur more frequently in adults.
   **b.** The **rash** progresses through three stages.
      **(1)** The rash begins as a marked **erythema** of the cheeks, which gives a "slapped cheek" appearance.
      **(2)** An **erythematous maculopapular rash** then invades the arms and spreads to the trunk and legs, producing a reticular pattern.
      **(3)** The third stage lasts 2–3 weeks but may persist for several months, with low-grade fever. This stage is characterized by fluctuations in the severity of the rash with environmental changes.

**2. Therapy** consists of supportive measures, such as an antipruritic to relieve the itching associated with the rash.

**3. Complications** (e.g., arthritis, hemolytic anemia, encephalopathy) are rare. Parvovirus B-19 infection during pregnancy can cause fetal hydrops and death. The risk of death is less than 10% following proven maternal infection.

**E. Varicella and herpes zoster** are two different infectious diseases caused by herpes zoster virus.

**1. Definitions**

   **a. Varicella** (chickenpox) is a highly contagious disease, occurring primarily in children younger than 10 years. It usually is a mild self-limited disease in normal children but may be a severe or even fatal illness in immunocompromised children.

   **b. Herpes zoster** (shingles) represents a reactivation of herpes zoster infection, occurring predominantly in adults who previously had varicella and who have circulating antibodies. Although herpes zoster occurs in children, it is uncommon in those younger than 10 years. Herpes zoster is an acute infection characterized by crops of vesicles confined to a dermatome and often accompanied by pain in the affected dermatome.

**2. Clinical features**

   **a. Varicella**

   (1) After an incubation period ranging from 11 to 21 days, a **prodrome** begins, consisting of mild fever, malaise, anorexia, and, occasionally, a scarlatiniform or morbilliform rash.

   (2) The characteristic **pruritic rash** begins the following day, appearing first on the trunk and spreading peripherally.

   (a) The rash begins as red papules and develops rapidly into clear **"teardrop" vesicles** that are about 1–2 mm in diameter. The vesicles become cloudy, break, and form scabs.

   (b) The lesions occur in widely scattered "crops," so that several stages of the lesions usually are present at the same time. Vesicles may occur on mucous membranes.

   (3) The severity of the illness ranges from a few lesions associated with a low-grade fever, to hundreds of lesions associated with temperatures up to 105° F (40.6° C), to fatal disseminated disease in immunocompromised children.

   (4) Patients are infectious from approximately 24 hours before the appearance of the rash until all lesions are crusted, which usually occurs 1 week after the onset of the rash.

   **b. Herpes zoster**

   (1) Attacks of herpes zoster may begin with pain along the affected sensory nerve, accompanied by fever and malaise, although these symptoms are more common in adults than in children.

   (2) A vesicular eruption similar to the vesicular form of varicella then appears and, in most cases, clears in 7–14 days. The rash may last as long as 4 weeks, however, with pain persisting for weeks or months.

   (3) The lesions are infectious if there is direct contact.

**3. Diagnosis** of both varicella and herpes zoster usually is obvious from the clinical presentation.

   **a.** Early in the course of the illness, a Tzanck test should be performed on scrapings taken from the base of a vesicle. The demonstration of multinucleated giant cells with intranuclear inclusions indicates varicella, herpes zoster, or herpes simplex infection.

   **b.** The definitive diagnosis is made by positive culture from a pharyngeal swab or vesicular scraping or by demonstration of a fourfold rise in antibody titer between acute and convalescent sera.

**4. Therapy**

   **a.** Uncomplicated cases of varicella are treated with an antipruritic medication and daily bathing to reduce secondary bacterial infection.

   **b.** Immunocompromised children (e.g., those with AIDS or leukemia and those on immunosuppressive drugs) who have not had varicella and who are exposed to someone with the disease should receive prophylaxis with herpes zoster immune globulin and be observed closely. Immunocompromised patients with disseminated varicella or herpes zoster should be treated with vidarabine or acyclovir.

**5. Prevention** may soon be possible. Studies of a **varicella vaccine** indicate that it is effective for healthy children and for children with malignancies.

**6. Complications**

   **a.** The most common complications of herpes zoster infection include encephalopathy, cerebellitis, Guillain-Barré syndrome, aseptic meningitis, pneumonia, thrombocytopenic purpura, purpura fulminans, cellulitis, abscess formation, and arthritis.

   **b.** Progressive varicella—with meningoencephalitis, pneumonia, and hepatitis—occurs in immunocompromised children and is associated with a mortality rate of approximately 20%.

   **c.** Maternal varicella during the first trimester may be associated with congenital malformations.

**F. Scarlet fever** is an acute illness characterized by fever, pharyngitis, and an erythematous rash. Scarlet fever is rare in infancy. It can occur more than once in a single patient.

  **1. Etiology.** Scarlet fever results from infection with group A streptococcal strains that produce erythrogenic toxin. The disease usually is associated with pharyngeal infections but in rare cases follows streptococcal infections at other sites (e.g., wound infections, impetigo).

  **2. Clinical features**
    **a.** The **characteristic rash is erythematous** and finely punctate and blanches on pressure. It appears initially on the trunk and becomes generalized within a few hours to several days. The face is flushed with circumoral pallor, and there is increased erythema in the skin folds (**Pastia's lines**). The skin may feel rough, similar to sandpaper. The skin rash fades over 1 week followed by desquamation, which may last for several weeks.
    **b.** A **strawberry tongue** (rough, erythematous, swollen tongue) and pharyngeal erythema with exudate may be present.

  **3. Diagnosis** is made on the basis of the clinical presentation and the isolation of group A streptococci on throat culture.

  **4. Therapy** for scarlet fever is the same as that for streptococcal pharyngitis, consisting of 10 days of orally administered penicillin.

  **5. Complications.** Both suppurative (e.g., cellulitis) and nonsuppurative (e.g., rheumatic fever) complications can occur with scarlet fever, just as with streptococcal pharyngitis (see V D).

**G. Rocky Mountain spotted fever** is an acute febrile illness characterized by the sudden onset of fever, headache, myalgia, mental confusion, and rash. The disease may be severe, leading to shock and death in 5%–7% of patients even with appropriate antimicrobial therapy.

  **1. Etiology and epidemiology**
    **a.** Rocky Mountain spotted fever is a tick-borne illness caused by *Rickettsia rickettsii,* which is widespread in the United States but most predominant in the eastern coastal and southeastern states.
    **b.** The principal vectors of Rocky Mountain spotted fever are *Dermacentor andersoni*—the **wood tick** that is found in the West and is most active during the spring—and *Dermacentor variabilis*—the **dog tick** that is found in the East and is most active during the summer.
    **c.** Almost two-thirds of the cases of Rocky Mountain spotted fever occur in patients who are under 15 years of age.

  **2. Clinical features**
    **a.** The clinical onset of Rocky Mountain spotted fever is abrupt and follows an incubation period that averages about 7 days (usually 2–8 days after an infected-tick bite). Typical **initial presentations** include:
      **(1)** Fever, which lasts 2–3 weeks in untreated patients
      **(2)** Chills
      **(3)** Headache, which is generalized and severe
      **(4)** Signs of meningoencephalitis (e.g., irritability, confusion, delirium)
      **(5)** Myalgia, especially of the gastrocnemius
      **(6)** Conjunctivitis with photophobia
      **(7)** Nonpitting edema, which may be profuse
    **b.** A **characteristic rash** develops on the third to fifth day of illness. The lesions begin as rose-colored, blanching macules on the hands, wrists, feet, and ankles, which spread to involve the entire body. The rash then becomes more **papular, petechial, and eventually purpuric** if treatment is delayed.

  **3. Diagnosis** is made primarily on the basis of clinical appearance and history. (There is a history of tick bite in 60%–85% of cases.) Isolation of the organism is difficult and dangerous; serologic confirmation generally takes 7–10 days and may be delayed for 5 or more weeks if antibiotics are begun early. If a specialized laboratory is available, rapid diagnosis can be made using immunofluorescence of a skin biopsy specimen.

  **4. Therapy**
    **a.** Antibiotic therapy includes either chloramphenicol or tetracycline given until 2–3 days after the temperature returns to normal (usually a course of 5–7 days). Tetracycline is given only to children older than 8 years.
    **b.** Supportive therapy is essential for patients with serious illness, such as those with shock.

5. **Prevention** is best achieved by avoidance of tick-infested areas and by prompt removal of a tick. Ticks should be removed with forceps applied to the head, so that the contents of the tick are not squeezed into the skin.

6. **Complications** of Rocky Mountain spotted fever include focal neurologic deficits, coma, renal failure, disseminated intravascular coagulation, gangrene of the distal extremities and scrotum, pneumonia, and shock possibly leading to death.

## VIII. CARDIAC INFECTIONS

A. **Infective endocarditis** is an inflammatory disorder, mainly of the cardiac valves, which results from infection by any of several types of microorganisms, including bacteria, fungi, and rickettsiae.

1. **Etiology**
   a. Viridans streptococcus (α-hemolytic streptococcus) is the most common cause of infective endocarditis in children. However, this etiologic agent has decreased in importance since the introduction of antimicrobial therapy.
   b. *S. aureus* and *S. epidermidis* have become progressively more important causes of infective endocarditis.
   c. Enterococcus, which is a common cause of infective endocarditis in adults, rarely is implicated in childhood disease.

2. **Epidemiology.** Pediatric patients who are at greatest risk for infective endocarditis include those with congenital heart disease, those with acquired valvular heart disease, and those with prosthetic valves. Infective endocarditis is a rare disease in children without underlying heart conditions, although adolescent drug abusers and children with central venous or arterial lines demonstrate an increased risk for the disease. The relatively good oral hygiene in children may explain the lower incidence of infective endocarditis in children as compared with adults.

3. **Pathogenesis**
   a. Endocarditis develops when a jet of blood, turbulence, or trauma leads to **cardiac endothelial damage,** which serves as the nidus for bacterial infection. In most cases, oral bacteria, which intermittently invade the bloodstream, infect the damaged endothelium.
   b. **Vegetations** consisting primarily of fibrin, platelet aggregations, and bacterial masses form on the valve leaflet. They may be single or multiple and range in size from a few millimeters to several centimeters. Pieces of the vegetations may break off and cause embolization (e.g., splinter hemorrhages, Roth's spots).

4. **Clinical features**
   a. **Early manifestations.** Infants and children with early infective endocarditis may be nearly free of symptoms, with fatigue sometimes the only manifestation of disease. Fever, malaise, and weakness are common. The classic signs of endocarditis (e.g., splinter hemorrhages, changing heart murmurs) are not always evident. Other signs that may occur include cardiomegaly, splenomegaly, petechiae, weight loss, and clubbing of the fingers.
   b. **Late manifestations** of infective endocarditis classically include such skin lesions as **Roth's spots** (conjunctival or retinal hemorrhages with clear centers), **Janeway lesions** (flat hemorrhagic macules on the hands or feet), and **Osler's nodes** (pea-sized painful nodules usually on the fingers). These infrequently occur in appropriately treated patients.

5. **Diagnosis**
   a. **Laboratory findings.** The erythrocyte sedimentation rate usually is elevated but may be normal early in the course of the illness. The leukocyte count may be normal or elevated. Microscopic hematuria may occur.
   b. **Blood cultures** are critical for the diagnosis of infective endocarditis and will identify the causative agent in more than 90% of cases. It rarely is necessary to obtain more than four cultures, but at least three blood cultures should be obtained during the first 24 hours of hospitalization.
   c. **Two-dimensional echocardiography** is helpful for establishing the presence and location of vegetations. About half of all patients tested have vegetations on echocardiography.

6. **Therapy.** When untreated, this infection is almost uniformly fatal.
   a. **Antibiotic therapy** should be provided as soon as the diagnosis is confirmed. Intravenous antibiotics are given for 4 weeks, except in patients with staphylococcal endocarditis or in those with an artificial valve, in whom 6 weeks of therapy is preferred.

**(1)** Initial therapy usually consists of penicillin plus gentamicin, unless staphylococci are suspected, in which case vancomycin and gentamicin are given.

**(2)** It is imperative that the MBC is determined, since peak antibiotic levels in the serum must exceed the MBC for successful therapy.

**(3)** A serum bactericidal (Schlicter) test is recommended to document adequate antibiotic therapy. The dosage usually is adjusted to achieve a serum bactericidal titer of at least 1:8 against the causative pathogen.

    **b. Surgical intervention** (for removal of vegetations or valve replacement) may be required for patients who fail to respond to medical treatment.

**7. Complications** of infective endocarditis must be anticipated and, with early intervention, may be minimized or even prevented. Important sequelae of infective endocarditis include:

    **a. Emboli** to the brain, lungs, coronary arteries, or any peripheral artery

    **b. Mycotic aneurysms,** which are infected aneurysms of the arterial vessels in the brain

    **c. Congestive heart failure,** which usually results from valvular dysfunction

    **d. Local cardiac abscesses,** which can present as aneurysm or persistent fever

    **e. Drug reactions**

    **f. Autoimmune phenomena** (e.g., nephritis, arthritis)

    **g. Depression,** which can occur due to the prolonged hospitalization

**B. Myocarditis** is an infection of the myocardium (i.e., the muscle of the heart). It occurs infrequently in children.

**1. Etiology.** Most cases of myocarditis are caused by enteroviruses, predominantly coxsackie B virus and echovirus. Important bacterial causes include *C. diphtheriae* and *Salmonella typhi*.

**2. Clinical features** include fever, congestive heart failure, and arrhythmias. The electrocardiogram is abnormal, with ST segment depression and T wave inversion.

**3. Therapy** for patients with viral myocarditis is supportive.

**C. Pericarditis** is an inflammation of the pericardium (i.e., the fibroserous sac that contains the heart).

**1. Etiology.** The most common causes of pericarditis are bacteria, especially *S. aureus* and *H. influenzae* type b, and viruses, especially coxsackie B virus, echovirus, influenza virus, and adenovirus. Other causes include fungi and *M. tuberculosis*.

**2. Clinical features**

    **a.** Left shoulder pain and back pain, which decrease when the patient is sitting, are characteristic of pericarditis. Fever, tachypnea, tachycardia, cough, and decreased heart sounds due to pericardial fluid and pericardial friction rub also are common.

    **b.** It is important to recognize significant pericardial fluid accumulation, which can lead to cardiac tamponade. Signs of tamponade include neck vein distension on inspiration and paradoxic pulse. The essential features of paradoxic pulse are a greater than normal inspiratory decrease in arterial blood pressure and an absence of the normal inspiratory fall in venous pressure.

**3. Diagnosis**

    **a. Electrocardiographic findings** with pericarditis include a low-voltage QRS complex, ST segment changes, and T wave inversion.

    **b. Chest x-ray** reveals a rapidly increasing cardiothoracic ratio without increasing pulmonary vascular markings.

    **c. Echocardiography** allows an estimate of the amount of pericardial fluid, although false negative results may be obtained.

**4. Therapy** for severe cases of pericarditis involving cardiac tamponade consists of pericardial drainage and supportive measures such as administration of oxygen and isoproterenol. Prolonged antibiotic therapy is given for cases of pericarditis due to bacteria.

## IX. SKIN, JOINT, AND BONE INFECTIONS

**A. Skin infections**

**1. Impetigo** is a common, contagious skin infection in infants and children, which is characterized by pustular, crusted, or bullous lesions. It occurs more frequently in warm, humid weather and is transmitted from child to child by direct contact.

    **a. Etiology.** The primary causes of impetigo in children are group A β-hemolytic streptococcus (*S. pyogenes*) and *S. aureus*. In past years, *S. aureus* was the etiologic agent in roughly 10% of cases, mostly in newborns and young infants. Recent studies suggest that *S. aureus* is increasing in importance as a cause of impetigo. Occasionally, both agents can be identified.

    **b. Clinical features**

      **(1) Lesions**

        **(a)** The lesions of **vesicopustular impetigo** begin as papules that progress to vesicles and then to painless pustules measuring about 5 mm in diameter, with a thin erythematous rim. The pustules rupture, revealing a honey-like exudate, which then forms a crust over a shallow ulcerated base. While previously considered due to group A β-hemolytic streptococcus, *S. aureus* recently has been increasingly cultured from such lesions.

        **(b)** The lesions of **bullous impetigo** begin as red macules that progress to bullous (fluid-filled) eruptions on an erythematous base. These lesions range from a few millimeters to a few centimeters in diameter. After the bullae rupture, a clear, thin, varnish-like coating forms over the denuded area. Bullous impetigo generally is associated with *S. aureus*.

      **(2) Local adenopathy** is common with streptococcal impetigo.

      **(3) Fever** seldom occurs, even with extensive superficial impetigo.

    **c. Diagnosis** is made by Gram stain and positive culture of specimens obtained from the base of pustular or ulcerated lesions or of fluid obtained from bullous lesions.

    **d. Therapy.** Until recently, impetigo was treated with oral antibiotics. A new topical therapy, mupirocin, has been found to be effective in a few studies. It may be considered for use in children with mild impetigo.

      **(1)** Oral penicillin V (250 mg 3 or 4 times daily for 10 days) is the treatment of choice for more severe streptococcal impetigo.

      **(2)** Oral dicloxacillin, cephalexin, or erythromycin is indicated for staphylococcal impetigo.

      **(3)** Until culture results are available, treatment against both streptococci and staphylococci appears logical.

**2. Cellulitis** is a localized, acute inflammation of the skin characterized by erythema and warmth. The location of the infection is important, since it may arise from underlying osteomyelitis, septic arthritis, sinusitis, or deep wound infection.

    **a. Etiology and clinical features.** Most cellulitis in children is caused by group A β-hemolytic streptococcus, *S. aureus*, or *H. influenzae* type b.

      **(1) Trauma-related cellulitis.** Cellulitis that occurs following some form of skin trauma (e.g., wound, burn, surgery) usually is due to group A streptococcus or *S. aureus*.

        **(a) Erysipelas** refers to an acute infection of the skin and subcutaneous tissues, which is characterized by a sharply demarcated, firm, raised border. Group A streptococcus is the predominant cause.

        **(b)** Local trauma, with or without marked cellulitis, may give rise to **lymphangitis,** which presents as a thin line of redness from the point of trauma to the draining regional node. Group A streptococcus, again, is the primary cause.

      **(2) Cellulitis unrelated to trauma.** Cellulitis that occurs in a child who is younger than 2 years, without evidence of trauma, is most likely due to *H. influenzae* type b. *S. pneumoniae* also may cause cellulitis in this age-group.

        **(a)** *H. influenzae* type b cellulitis often has a violaceous hue. *S. pneumoniae* cellulitis may have a similar appearance.

        **(b)** Cellulitis of the face often is caused by *H. influenzae* type b. Other causes include group A β-hemolytic streptococcus, *S. aureus,* and *S. pneumoniae.*

    **b. Diagnosis**

      **(1)** Blood cultures frequently are positive in *H. influenzae* type b cellulitis.

      **(2)** Aspiration of material from the leading edge or center of the cellulitis and culture may yield the etiologic agent.

      **(3)** Culture of material that has drained from a wound associated with cellulitis is helpful for defining etiology.

    **c. Therapy.** Children with cellulitis should be hospitalized and given parenteral antibiotics, such as ceftriaxone or chloramphenicol and oxacillin, which are effective against the likely pathogens.

3. **Abscess** represents a deeper skin infection than cellulitis; in addition, it contains pus.
   a. **Etiology.** Abscesses usually are caused by *S. aureus* or group A streptococcus.
   b. **Therapy.** Treatment of superficial abscesses consists of warm compresses until they become fluctuant. Surgical drainage is necessary if spontaneous drainage has not occurred. Appropriate antibiotics are indicated.

B. **Septic arthritis** occurs when bacteria from the circulation enter the joint space. It also may occur from direct implantation of bacteria from an osteomyelitis or penetrating trauma. Septic arthritis may cause destruction of articular cartilage due to lack of normal nutrients in the synovial fluid and as a result of purulent exudate and increased pressure in the joint space. The joints usually involved are the knee (40% of cases), hip (20%), ankle (15%), elbow (15%), wrist (5%), and shoulder (5%).

1. **Etiology.** Blood cultures are positive in up to 50% of patients with septic arthritis.
   a. **Neonates.** Group B streptococcus, *S. aureus,* and enteric gram-negative rods are the most common pathogens in this age-group.
   b. **Older children.** *S. aureus* is the most common pathogen; *H. influenzae* type b also is common, especially in children younger than 6 years. Other causes include group A streptococcus, *S. pneumoniae,* and *N. meningitidis. N. gonorrhoeae* causes septic arthritis in adolescents.

2. **Clinical features.** In most children, the affected joint is warm, swollen, and very painful when moved. Septic arthritis in a young infant may present simply as fever and poorly localized pain in the affected extremity. Signs and symptoms associated with a septic hip often are subtle and, in an infant, may be limited to a limp or a fixed, flexed hip.

3. **Diagnosis**
   a. **Synovial fluid analysis.** Joint aspiration is necessary for the diagnosis of septic arthritis, and it has the additional benefit of decreasing pressure in the joint space. Gram stain and culture of the synovial fluid are obtained.
   b. **Serologic findings.** The peripheral white blood cell count usually is elevated, with a shift to the left, and the erythrocyte sedimentation rate usually is increased.
   c. **Imaging results.** X-ray frequently shows widening of the joint space. A gallium scan shows increased uptake of gallium in the involved joint.
   d. **Differential diagnosis** of septic arthritis includes other causes of monoarticular arthritis, including *M. pneumoniae, M. tuberculosis, C. albicans,* Lyme disease, toxic synovitis, trauma, juvenile rheumatoid arthritis, and Reiter's syndrome.

4. **Therapy**
   a. **Antibiotic therapy** initially should consist of broad-spectrum, parenteral antibiotics to treat the likely pathogens (i.e., oxacillin for children over 6 years of age; ceftriaxone or oxacillin and chloramphenicol for children less than 6 years of age). Antibiotics should be continued for a minimum of 3 weeks. In some cases, subsequent high-dose oral therapy can be substituted for parenteral therapy.
   b. **Drainage of the joint space** by needle aspiration or surgical excision is important to remove inflammatory material. Septic arthritis of the hip requires immediate surgical drainage, because the blood supply of the femoral head may be compromised, which carries the risk of serious sequelae.

C. **Osteomyelitis** refers to inflammation of the bone. Osteomyelitis in children occurs most frequently in the long bones of the lower extremities and, to a lesser extent, of the upper extremities.

1. **Etiology**
   a. Staphylococci and streptococci account for more than 90% of bacterial isolates in childhood osteomyelitis.
   b. *H. influenzae* type b is a frequent cause of osteomyelitis in children younger than 2 years.
   c. *Salmonella* is a common pathogen in patients with sickle cell anemia.
   d. *P. aeruginosa* is a common pathogen in patients with puncture wounds of the foot.

2. **Pathogenesis.** The tortuous course of the nutrient vessels in bone cause bacteria to be trapped in the **metaphysis**. The metaphysis is located between the **epiphysis** (growth plate) and the **diaphysis** (shaft of the bone). The epiphyseal plate prevents infection from entering the joint space in older children but not in neonates. Joint infection secondary to osteomyelitis may occur in the shoulder and hip as a result of the synovial membrane inserting distally to the epiphysis, allowing bacteria to spread directly from the metaphysis to the joint space.

### 3. Clinical features
  a. In young infants, fever may be the only manifestation of osteomyelitis.
  b. Fever and localized bone tenderness are the most common symptoms in older children. Local swelling, redness, warmth, and suppuration may occur subsequently.
  c. There is a history of minor trauma in about half of the cases.

### 4. Diagnosis
  a. **Hematologic findings**
   (1) The white blood cell count and erythrocyte sedimentation rate usually are elevated. The erythrocyte sedimentation rate is useful for monitoring therapy.
   (2) Blood cultures are positive in approximately 50% of the cases.
  b. **Imaging results**
   (1) A bone scan usually is positive 24 hours after symptoms begin and provides strong evidence of osteomyelitis.
   (2) X-ray does not become positive until 10–12 days after the onset of symptoms.

### 5. Therapy
  a. **Aspiration** of the affected site is desirable to recover the causative organism and to determine whether an abscess is present, which would require surgical drainage. Aspiration and drainage are essential if a bone abscess or an unusual organism is suspected. (An example of the latter is osteomyelitis secondary to a puncture wound, in which case *P. aeruginosa* is likely and drainage is necessary.)
  b. **Antibiotic therapy** initially should consist of a parenteral antistaphylococcal antibiotic (e.g., oxacillin), unless a gram-negative organism is suspected. Appropriate antibiotic therapy is continued for a minimum of 4 weeks. In some cases, an oral antibiotic can be substituted after 1 week of parenteral antibiotics.
  c. **Surgical drainage** is necessary in addition to antibiotics for successful treatment of bone abscess.

## X. INFESTATIONS AND COMMON PARASITIC INFECTIONS

A. **Lice.** Three types of lice infest humans: head lice, body lice, and crab lice. Head lice and body lice are quite similar in body structure and are about 2–4 mm in length. Crab lice are about 1–2 mm in length and bear a striking resemblance to crabs, with widespread pincers.

1. **Head lice.** The head louse (*Pediculus humanis* var. *capitis*) is a common problem in preschool and elementary school children. Head lice usually are confined to the fine hair of the head; they rarely infest clothing. Head lice are most common in the winter, they usually are not the result of poor hygiene, and they are not more common in children with long hair. They are spread by direct contact. The female louse lays eggs (**nits**) on hair close to the scalp, and as the hair grows, the eggs dry.
  a. **Clinical features.** Pruritus and a macular rash on the scalp occur. Head lice sometimes cause no signs or symptoms.
  b. **Diagnosis.** The discovery of nits and, less commonly, live lice usually is made by a child's parent or teacher.
  c. **Therapy.** Four effective shampoo therapies are available for head lice: malathione, pyrethrin, permethorin, and gamma benzene hexachloride. (The latter drug should be used with caution in children because of its potential for causing neurotoxicity.) A second shampooing should be done 7 days after the first application to kill hatching progeny. The lice live for only a short time on inanimate objects. Thus, washing of all clothing and bed linens is not necessary.

2. **Body lice.** The body louse (*Pediculus humanis* var. *corporis*) lives on the body and on clothing. Body lice are not endemic to the United States. They may carry typhus, trench fever, and relapsing fever.

3. **Crab lice.** The crab louse (*Phthirus pubis*) lives in pubic hair and, in rare cases, can infest hair other than pubic hair, such as eyelashes. Crab lice usually are asymptomatic but can cause local pruritus and a macular rash. Treatment consists of local application of pyrethrin or gamma benzene hexachloride.

**B. Scabies** is caused by a round mite that is 0.4 mm long and has four sets of legs. It is spread by direct contact.

   1. **Clinical features.** Scabies causes an intensely pruritic rash with pustules and burrows. The rash can be generalized or have a focal distribution; it is especially common in intertriginous areas (e.g., the folds between the fingers and toes).

   2. **Diagnosis.** Scrapings of the burrows with mineral oil can reveal the mites. However, this procedure often produces negative results, and the diagnosis usually relies on demonstration of the characteristic rash.

   3. **Therapy** consists of crotamiton (cream or lotion), sulfur ointment in petrolatum, benzyl benzoate, or gamma benzene hexachloride.

**C. Giardiasis.** *Giardia lamblia* is a parasite that is a common cause of diarrhea. It is spread from person to person or can be acquired from animal contact or from contaminated water.

   1. **Clinical features.** Diarrhea due to *G. lamblia* is characterized by watery stools without blood, mucus, eosinophils, or leukocytes. Fever is absent. A prolonged course of diarrhea accompanied by excessive abdominal gas is characteristic of giardiasis.

   2. **Diagnosis** most commonly is by identification of the parasite (trophozoite or cyst) in formed or unformed stool. The parasite also can be recovered from the duodenum if a string is passed, by mouth, into the duodenum (string test).

   3. **Therapy**
      a. Quinacrine is the drug of choice for treatment of giardiasis in children. Alternatives are metronidazole and furazolidone (a liquid preparation).
      b. The finding of *G. lamblia* eggs in the stool of an asymptomatic patient is not an indication for therapy. They are commonly identified in infants who attend day care centers.

**D. Enterobiasis,** or pinworm infestation, is a common infection in children caused by *Enterobius vermicularis*. The eggs of *E. vermicularis* are passed on hands, clothing, and house dust. Gravid females migrate at night to the perianal region to deposit their eggs.

   1. **Clinical features.** Although many symptoms have been associated with pinworm infection, the only well-documented symptom is perianal pruritus.

   2. **Diagnosis.** Eggs can be detected by pressing adhesive cellophane tape against the perianal region in the morning. Adult worms may be seen by direct inspection.

   3. **Therapy.** Mebendazole, 100 mg in a single oral dose, usually is sufficient therapy.

**E. Ascariasis,** or roundworm infestation, is caused by *Ascaris lumbricoides*. Ascariasis is a very common infection, especially in preschool and younger children.

   1. **Life cycle**
      a. Eggs are found in the soil, and humans are infected by contact with the soil. The eggs are ingested and hatch in the intestine, where they become larvae.
      b. The larvae penetrate the intestine, enter the venules or lymphatics, and subsequently reach the lungs, where they mature.
      c. Mature roundworms then migrate up the bronchioles into the pharynx, where they are swallowed and finally pass into the small intestine, and the cycle is repeated.
      d. The adult worm is 25–30 cm long.

   2. **Clinical features**
      a. Most patients are asymptomatic. Abdominal pain may occur with heavy infection.
      b. Pulmonary symptoms are rare and are due to large numbers of larvae passing through the lungs, causing cough, blood-stained sputum, eosinophilia, and pulmonary infiltrates.

   3. **Diagnosis.** Worms that appear like long, pink, earthworms are seen in the stool. Eggs are found in the stool and can be identified microscopically.

   4. **Therapy.** Pyrantel pamoate in a single dose is curative in 80%–90% of cases. The drug is well tolerated and easy to take. Mebendazole and piperazine citrate also are effective.

## BIBLIOGRAPHY

American Academy of Pediatrics Committee on Infectious Diseases: *Report of the Committee on Infectious Diseases,* 22nd edition. Elk Grove Village, IL, American Academy of Pediatrics, 1991.

Feigin RD, Cherry JD (eds): *Textbook of Pediatric Infectious Diseases,* 2nd edition. Philadelphia, WB Saunders, 1987.

Mandell GL, Douglas RG, Bennett JE (eds): *Principles and Practice of Infectious Diseases,* 3rd edition. New York, Churchill Livingstone, 1990.

Moffet HL: *Pediatric Infectious Diseases: A Problem-Oriented Approach,* 3rd edition. Philadelphia, JB Lippincott, 1989.

Remington JS, Klein JO (eds): *Infectious Diseases of the Fetus and Newborn Infant,* 3rd edition. Philadelphia, WB Saunders, 1990.

## STUDY QUESTIONS

**Directions:** Each of the numbered items or incomplete statements in this section is followed by answers or by completions of the statement. Select the **one** lettered answer or completion that is **best** in each case.

1. A 1-year-old boy is brought to the emergency room with a 10-hour history of fever and listlessness. Physical examination reveals a lethargic child with a temperature of 103° F, a respiratory rate of 35, blood pressure of 60/30, a full fontanelle, and a petechial rash. The most appropriate initial action is

(A) lumbar puncture
(B) Gram stain of the petechiae
(C) administration of intravenous fluids and antibiotics
(D) administration of corticosteroids
(E) examination of the fundi

2. A 3-year-old girl presents with a nonsuppurative and moderately tender anterior cervical lymph node that measures 2 × 4 cm. What is the most appropriate initial therapy?

(A) Amoxicillin
(B) Dicloxacillin
(C) Erythromycin
(D) Penicillin
(E) Incision and drainage

3. A previously healthy 13-year-old boy develops a mild pneumonia characterized by a nonproductive cough. The most appropriate therapy is

(A) cephalexin
(B) amoxicillin
(C) erythromycin
(D) penicillin
(E) trimethoprim-sulfamethoxazole

4. A 3-month-old infant with bronchopulmonary dysplasia is admitted to a hospital with fever, wheezing, and respiratory distress. A chest x-ray shows hyperinflation and bilateral, interstitial infiltrates. The complete blood count is normal, and a rapid test for respiratory syncytial virus is positive. Blood cultures are obtained. The most appropriate therapy is

(A) intravenous ampicillin
(B) intravenous ceftriaxone
(C) oral amoxacillin
(D) ribavirin by aerosol
(E) close observation without antibiotic use

5. A 2-year-old child is noted to have an erythematous, bulging right tympanic membrane. The two most likely bacterial causes of this illness are

(A) *Streptococcus pyogenes* and *Staphylococcus aureus*
(B) *Hemophilus influenzae* and *S. aureus*
(C) *H. influenzae* and *Streptococcus pneumoniae*
(D) *S. pneumoniae* and *S. aureus*
(E) *Branhamella catarrhalis* and *S. pyogenes*

6. A 6-month-old, lethargic infant is brought to the emergency room with a temperature of 105° F. The infant has been ill for 12 hours and is not responsive. Chest x-ray, urinalysis, and CSF are normal. The complete blood count shows a white count of 37,000, with 50% neutrophils and 40% bands. The patient is treated with ceftriaxone for presumed sepsis. Among the following microorganisms, the one most likely to cause sepsis in this infant is

(A) *Staphylococcus epidermidis*
(B) *Listeria monocytogenes*
(C) *Pseudomonas aeruginosa*
(D) *Hemophilus influenzae* type b
(E) *Staphylococcus aureus*

1-C      4-D
2-B      5-C
3-C      6-D

7. All of the following statements regarding the diagnosis of sinusitis in children are true EXCEPT

(A) common symptoms of acute sinusitis in young children include fever, purulent nasal discharge, and persistent daytime cough for longer than 10 days
(B) evidence of bilateral maxillary sinus membrane swelling on sinus x-ray confirms the diagnosis of acute bacterial sinusitis
(C) transillumination of the sinuses may provide valuable information for the diagnosis of sinusitis in older children
(D) sinus puncture seldom is needed to confirm the diagnosis of sinusitis
(E) swab cultures of the throat are not reliable for the diagnosis of sinusitis

**Directions:** Each item below contains four suggested answers of which **one or more** is correct. Choose the answer

A    if **1, 2, and 3** are correct
B    if **1 and 3** are correct
C    if **2 and 4** are correct
D    if **4** is correct
E    if **1, 2, 3, and 4** are correct

8. Microbiology laboratory techniques that are useful for determining the correct type and dosage of an antimicrobial agent against a bacterial isolate include

(1) latex agglutination
(2) susceptibility tests
(3) ELISA
(4) tests for β-lactamase production

9. True statements about head lice infestation include

(1) head lice are spread by direct contact
(2) head lice live for long periods on fomites
(3) diagnosis usually is made by identifying nits (dry eggs)
(4) children with long hair are more commonly affected

10. A 6-month-old boy is brought to the emergency ward with a 1-day history of fever and lethargy. Abnormal physical findings consist of a temperature to 102° F and irritability on flexion of the neck. A lumbar puncture reveals an abnormally elevated number of leukocytes and gram-negative coccobacilli on Gram stain. Appropriate management of this patient consists of

(1) parenteral ceftriaxone
(2) parenteral gentamicin
(3) fluid restriction
(4) phenobarbital

**Directions:** Each group of items in this section consists of lettered options followed by a set of numbered items. For each item, select the **one** lettered option that is most closely associated with it. Each lettered option may be selected once, more than once, or not at all.

**Questions 11–14**

Match each skin infection described below with the microorganism most likely to be the cause of the infection.

(A) Enteric gram-negative bacillus

(B) *Hemophilus influenzae* type b

(C) *Staphylococcus aureus*

(D) *Neisseria meningitidis*

(E) Group A streptococcus

11. Cellulitis with a raised, firm, well-demarcated border

12. Cellulitis with lymphangitis

13. Violaceous cellulitis associated with high fever

14. Bullous impetigo

**Questions 15–19**

For each exanthematous rash described below, select the infectious disease it best characterizes.

(A) Measles

(B) Rubella

(C) Erythema infectiosum

(D) Varicella

(E) Rocky Mountain spotted fever

15. Maculopapular rash that begins on the head and spreads downward

16. Rash that begins as a marked erythema of the cheeks

17. Vesicular rash that appears in "crops"

18. Petechial rash that begins on the wrists and ankles

19. Maculopapular rash that is associated with posterior auricular, cervical, and suboccipital lymphadenopathy

| | | |
|---|---|---|
| 11-E | 14-C | 17-D |
| 12-E | 15-A | 18-E |
| 13-B | 16-C | 19-B |

## ANSWERS AND EXPLANATIONS

**1. The answer is C** *[IV A 4 b, 5 a (1) (a), b (2)].*
This patient presents with classic findings of meningococcal sepsis and meningitis. Although the diagnosis of meningitis and the microbiologic etiology of the illness can be established by examination of cerebrospinal fluid (CSF), a lumbar puncture should be deferred until the patient's condition is stabilized. The blood pressure indicates that the child is in shock. Initial efforts, therefore, should be focused on maintaining intravascular volume by administration of fluids. Intravenous antibiotics also should be administered promptly (preferably after a blood culture is obtained), and, in this case, an appropriate choice would be a third-generation cephalosporin.

**2. The answer is B** *[V E 4 b].*
Inflammation and enlargement of the lymph nodes of the neck, or cervical adenitis, is a common problem in children. Appropriate treatment of cervical adenitis depends on the causative microorganism and the presence or absence of pus. Initial therapy for a nonsuppurative node of moderate size and tenderness usually consists of an oral antistaphylococcal antibiotic (e.g., dicloxacillin) for treatment of *Staphylococcus aureus* and group A streptococcus, the most likely etiologies. Erythromycin would be a logical choice in a penicillin-allergic child, but it is not as effective against *S. aureus* as dicloxacillin. Neither amoxicillin nor penicillin usually is effective against *S. aureus*. Incision and drainage are indicated only when the nodes contain pus.

**3. The answer is C** *[VI B 1 d (3), 3 a (3)].*
The most common nonviral causes of pneumonia in children who are older than 6 years are *Mycoplasma pneumoniae* and *Streptococcus pneumoniae*. Pneumonia due to *M. pneumoniae* generally is milder than that due to traditional bacteria, with a gradual onset of illness that is characterized by fever, headache, malaise, and a nonproductive cough. The clinical picture described in the question, therefore, is consistent with *M. pneumoniae* pneumonia, for which the treatment of choice is erythromycin. Cephalexin, amoxicillin, penicillin, and trimethoprim-sulfamethoxazole would be effective treatment for *S. pneumoniae* pneumonia but not for *M. pneumoniae* pneumonia.

**4. The answer is D** *[VI A 5 b].*
This infant has evidence of severe bronchiolitis, pneumonia, and respiratory syncytial infection—conditions that call for treatment with aerosolized ribavirin. Bronchiolitis is an acute viral infection of the bronchioles, which is common in infants younger than 2 years. Clinical features include cough, wheezing, tachypnea, and dyspnea. Hyperinflation of the lungs typically is evident on chest x-ray. Complete blood count often is normal, reflecting a viral etiology. Over 50% of cases are caused by respiratory syncytial virus, identified by rapid immunoflourescence In most cases, patients recover spontaneously and do not require hospitalization or specific therapy. However, severe infection is more common among children with underlying pulmonary disease (e.g., bronchopulmonary dysplasia). In such cases, hospitalization is necessary and therapy includes oxygen, fluids, and possibly intubation with assisted ventilation. Aerosolized ribavarin is indicated for severe infection due to respiratory syncytial virus.

**5. The answer is C** *[V A 1 a (1)].*
This child presents with otitis media—one of the most common infections of childhood. The characteristic feature of otitis media is a bulging, erythematous tympanic membrane with impaired mobility. Bacteria are the primary agents of otitis media. The most common causes in all age-groups are *S. pneumoniae* (25%–40% of cases) and unencapsulated *Hemophilus influenzae* (15%–25% of cases). Less common causes include group A streptococcus, *Branhamella catarrhalis*, and, for chronic otitis media, *S. aureus* and *Pseudomonas aeruginosa*.

**6. The answer is D** *[III C 1].*
Although sepsis is uncommon in children who are older than 3 months and immunologically normal, it should be suspected in any child who develops a fever without an obvious focus of infection and appears ill. White cell count often is elevated and demonstrates a shift to the left. For children older than 2 months, the most common causes of sepsis are *H. influenzae* type b and *Neisseria meningitidis*. Therapy usually consists of a third-generation cephalosporin, such as ceftriaxone.

**7. The answer is B** *[V B 5].*
Since the mucous membrane of the paranasal sinuses is continuous with that of the nose, even transient

viral upper respiratory infections may cause sinus membrane swelling, which appears as hazy densities on sinus x-ray. A unilateral air-fluid level or complete opacification of a sinus cavity strongly suggests acute bacterial sinusitis. For this reason, sinus x-rays should be reviewed with an experienced radiologist.

**8. The answer is C (2, 4)** *[II B 2].*
Antimicrobial susceptibility tests and tests for β-lactamase production are two commonly used microbiology laboratory methods for determining antimicrobial activity of a bacterial isolate. Antimicrobial susceptibility often is expressed in terms of the minimum inhibitory concentration (MIC) and minimum bactericidal concentration (MBC) of an antimicrobial agent. The MIC and MBC indicate the degree to which a microorganism is susceptible to an antimicrobial agent and, thus, are useful for determining the type and dosage of an antibiotic to use. Tests for β-lactamase production are valuable for treating infectious diseases due to certain microorganisms (e.g., *H. influenzae*), as any organism that produces β-lactamase will be resistant to penicillin antibiotics. Latex agglutination and enzyme-linked immunosorbent assay (ELISA) are microbiology laboratory methods used primarily to detect bacterial antigen in body fluids.

**9. The answer is B (1, 3)** *[X A 1].*
The head louse (*Pediculus humanis* var. *capitis*) is common in preschool and elementary school children. The lice usually live in the fine hair of the head and are not more common in long-haired children. Head lice are spread from person to person and do not survive long on fomites. Lice infestation usually causes pruritus but may be asymptomatic; the diagnosis often is first suspected by parents who discover nits in their child's hair.

**10. The answer is B (1, 3)** *[IV A 5 a, b].*
This infant has bacterial meningitis, the therapy for which consists of appropriate antibiotics and supportive care. The most likely cause of bacterial meningitis in a 6-month-old infant is *H. influenzae* type b, and the gram-negative coccobacilli observed on Gram stain of the cerebrospinal fluid (CSF) from this infant strongly suggest this organism. Approximately 15%–30% of *H. influenzae* type b isolates are resistant to ampicillin. However, ceftriaxone resistance is very rare; therefore, this agent is appropriate for treatment of bacterial meningitis that is likely due to *H. influenzae* type b. An aminoglycoside such as gentamicin has poor activity against *H. influenzae* type b. Supportive care for all children with meningitis should include fluid restriction to minimize intracranial pressure. Phenobarbital is a supportive measure that is indicated only for children who have had seizures as a result of the meningitis.

**11–14. The answers are: 11-E** *[IX A 2 a (1) (a)],* **12-E** *[IX A 2 a (1) (b)],* **13-B** *[IX A 2 a (2)],* **14-C** *[IX A 1 b (1) (b)].*
Cellulitis is a localized, acute inflammation of the skin characterized by redness, warmth, and tenderness. Most cellulitis in children is caused by group A streptococcus or *S. aureus; H. influenzae* type b is the cause in a few cases. Cellulitis that is characterized by a sharply demarcated, firm, raised border is called erysipelas; group A streptococcus is the predominant cause of this infection. Cellulitis that is associated with painful red streaks along the course of lymph vessels (lymphangitis) also is caused primarily by group A streptococcus. Cellulitis that occurs with fever and is characterized by violaceous (purple) discoloration of the skin is most likely due to *H. influenzae* type b.
Impetigo is a contagious skin infection characterized by crusted, bullous or pustular lesions. The primary agents of impetigo are group A streptococcus and *S. aureus.* The lesions of classic staphylococcal (bullous) impetigo typically begin as red macules that progress to bullous lesions, which rupture and form a clear, thin, varnish-like coating over the denuded area. Vesicopustular impetigo has traditionally been considered due to group A streptococcus; the lesions begin as papules that progress to vesicles and then to pustules, which eventually rupture and form thick crusts.

**15–19. The answers are: 15-A** *[VII A 3 c],* **16-C** *[VII D 1 b],* **17-D** *[VII E 2 a (2)],* **18-E** *[VII G 2 b],* **19-B** *[VII B 2 a (2)].*
The characteristic rash of measles begins on the head and spreads down the body, becoming generalized. It is erythematous and maculopapular but becomes confluent as it progresses. The rash lasts 4 or 5 days and then resolves—from the head downward.
The rash of erythema infectiosum begins as a marked erythema of the cheeks, which gives a "slapped cheek" appearance. An erythematous, maculopapular rash then appears on the extremities and often has a lace-like appearance. It may be morbilliform, confluent, or annular. The rash often disappears and recurs, seemingly with fluctuations in environmental conditions.
The characteristic, pruritic rash of varicella usually appears first on the trunk and then becomes generalized. The rash begins as erythematous papules and progresses rapidly to vesicles that are 1–2 mm in

diameter, which subsequently crust. The lesions occur in "crops," so that different stages of the rash are present simultaneously.

The rash of Rocky Mountain spotted fever initially appears on the hands, wrists, feet, and ankles and spreads to involve the skin of the rest of the body. The lesions are macular, 1–4 mm in diameter, and rose-colored, but they can become petechial and then purpuric if treatment is delayed.

The rash of rubella, like that of measles, is maculopapular, begins on the face, and moves down the body. It is less pronounced than the rash of measles. It is accompanied by lymphadenopathy in the posterior auricular, cervical, and suboccipital chains.

# 10
# Gastrointestinal Diseases

William R. Treem
Jeffrey S. Hyams

**I. INTRODUCTION.** Gastrointestinal problems are extremely common in infants and children and represent the second most common reason, following respiratory infection, for seeking medical care. The differential diagnosis and treatment of routine gastrointestinal symptoms (e.g., abdominal pain, vomiting, diarrhea) often are quite different than in adults. At times, gastrointestinal symptoms may represent a nonspecific manifestation of serious infections such as pneumonia, meningitis, or pyelonephritis. The limited ability of the young child to describe her symptoms may make diagnosis more difficult. Subtle alterations in gastrointestinal function may adversely affect growth while causing minimal symptoms. Only careful examination of the child's growth curve may alert the physician to the possibility of underlying gastrointestinal disease.

## II. DISORDERS OF THE ESOPHAGUS

**A. Gastroesophageal reflux** is the most common esophageal problem in infancy. Some degree of gastroesophageal reflux occurs in normal adults and children, but it is especially common in young infants, occurring in up to 50%. Gastroesophageal reflux is regarded as a manifestation of a developmental variation in gastrointestinal motility that will resolve as the infant matures. All pediatricians and parents have witnessed the regurgitation of small amounts of formula by normal babies after feedings. When this regurgitation is unusually severe, persists beyond 12 months of age, or is associated with complications, it is deemed pathologic and warrants appropriate diagnostic testing and medical and, occasionally, surgical management.

1. **Pathophysiology.** Many factors contribute to the maintenance of the antireflux barrier, including an increased intrinsic basal tone of the lower esophageal sphincter (LES).
   a. **Low resting tone of the LES** is associated with reflux in a small group of children, primarily those who are neurologically impaired or who have some other underlying cause of esophageal dysfunction (e.g., a large hiatal hernia, a collagen vascular disease, a previous tracheoesophageal fistula repair). More commonly, however, LES pressure is normal in infants with gastroesophageal reflux. Thus, the concept of relaxation of the LES at inappropriate moments or a failure of adaptation of the LES to increases in intragastric pressure created by crying, straining at stool, diaper changes, or positional changes has been invoked to explain gastroesophageal reflux.
   b. **Other contributing factors** include:
      (1) Delayed gastric emptying
      (2) Impaired esophageal motility
      (3) Gastric distension
      (4) Loss of extrinsic mechanical factors that maintain the antireflux barrier, such as the crural diaphragm and the cardioesophageal angle of His (oblique angle at which the esophagus enters the stomach)

2. **Clinical features**
   a. **Vomiting**
      (1) The most frequent symptom in infants is effortless, painless vomiting. This may occur soon after or up to several hours after a feeding and will usually be described as multiple episodes of small amounts of curdled formula rolling out of the mouth. Occasionally, vomiting may be described as forceful, causing confusion with symptoms of pyloric stenosis.

**(2)** In the older child, a tendency to vomit easily, heartburn, dysphagia, rumination, and halitosis may occur.

**(3)** The vomiting is always nonbilious.

**b. Complications.** Persistent gastroesophageal reflux can lead to a number of complications.

**(1) Esophageal complications**

**(a)** Esophagitis (resulting in symptoms of irritability, excessive crying, and hematemesis)

**(b)** Strictures (resulting in dysphagia)

**(c)** Epithelial metaplasia or Barrett's esophagus (possibly premalignant)

**(2) Systemic complications**

**(a)** Failure to thrive (due to lost calories or anorexia secondary to esophagitis)

**(b)** Anemia (due to blood loss) and iron deficiency

**(c)** Hypoproteinemia (due to mucosal damage and protein loss)

**(3) Respiratory complications**

**(a)** Aspiration (resulting in nocturnal cough, bronchospasm, or recurrent pneumonia)

**(b)** Apnea-bradycardia episodes (secondary to laryngospasm, vagal reflexes, or both)

**3. Diagnosis** of gastroesophageal reflux is based on the history, physical examination, and exclusion of anatomic abnormalities that may predispose to the clinical features of reflux. The following tests are necessary only when the diagnosis is in doubt or when the presentation is dominated by one of the complications of gastroesophageal reflux and a causal link between reflux and that complication (e.g., apnea, bronchospasm) is sought.

**a. Barium swallow and upper gastrointestinal x-ray** has high false negative and false positive rates, which diminish its usefulness; however, it is the best test for eliminating other anatomic causes of vomiting.

**b. Esophageal pH monitoring.** The best test for assessing gastroesophageal reflux is prolonged (18–24 hours) pH monitoring. This study should be reserved for patients presenting with apnea, bronchospasm, or failure to thrive in whom reflux is suspected as the underlying cause.

**c. Radionuclide scanning.** Gastroesophageal reflux may be detected and gastric emptying may be quantitated by adding technetium 99m ($^{99m}$Tc) to formula or milk and scanning.

**d. Esophageal manometry** is used to measure resting LES pressure, the response of the LES to a swallow, peristalsis in the body of the esophagus, and functioning of the upper esophageal sphincter (UES).

**e. Endoscopy with esophageal biopsy.** Endoscopy allows direct visualization of esophageal mucosa, and biopsies may show microscopic evidence of esophagitis, even if the mucosa appears grossly normal.

**4. Therapy**

**a. Simple measures.** Most infants with gastroesophageal reflux can be treated conservatively with simple measures while awaiting maturation of upper gastrointestinal motility and resolution of symptoms.

**(1) Positioning.** Infants should be positioned prone with the head of the crib elevated 30° for sleep and for 1 hour after feedings. Older children should sleep with the head of the bed elevated. The infant seat has not been shown to be useful in preventing reflux and may even be harmful if the infant slumps down in the seat with his knees pressing against his abdomen. Other positions that increase intra-abdominal pressure, such as diaper changes with the infant on his back and his legs up, also may provoke reflux episodes.

**(2) Dietary changes**

**(a)** Frequent, smaller feedings of formula thickened with 2 tsp/oz of cereal may aid infants with gastroesophageal reflux. Older children should eat smaller, more frequent meals and abstain from eating for at least 1 hour before bedtime.

**(b)** Fatty foods, alcohol, and caffeine-containing liquids may aggravate reflux and should be eliminated.

**(c)** Changing formulas is discouraged, as it sends mixed messages about potential food allergy. Cow's milk and soy protein allergy are distinct entities and should only be suspected if the vomiting is accompanied by diarrhea, heme-positive stool, an eczematoid rash, and a strong family history of allergy, asthma, or eczema.

b. **Medication.** Drug intervention is reserved for patients whose emesis has persisted without improvement after 12 months of age, patients whose emesis has worsened between 6 and 12 months of age, and patients who have developed complications.

(1) **Antacids** primarily neutralize gastric acid and thereby decrease esophageal irritation when gastroesophageal reflux occurs.

(2) **Histamine₂ (H₂)-receptor blockers** (e.g., cimetidine, ranitidine, famotidine) are longer acting than antacids and are a more convenient means of reducing gastric acidity, but they have potential side effects.

(3) **Omeprazole,** an inhibitor of the $H^+$-$K^+$-ATPase pump in the parietal cell, is a very effective suppressor of gastric acidity and is effective in treating reflux-induced esophagitis.

(4) **Prokinetic agents** (e.g., metoclopramide, bethanechol) increase LES tone and promote gastric emptying and, thus, may decrease gastroesophageal reflux. However, both drugs have side effects and may not be well tolerated in some patients. Cisapride, a new agent, appears to be as effective and has less side effects.

c. **Surgery** is indicated for patients who have failed medical therapy, patients with life-threatening or severely debilitating complications, and patients with esophageal stricture or Barrett's esophagus. Surgical procedures are designed to reestablish esophagogastric competence. The most commonly used procedure is the Nissen fundoplication, during which part of the gastric fundus is wrapped around the distal esophagus to create a high-pressure zone to resist gastroesophageal reflux. Side effects (e.g., gastric distension, dysphagia, diarrhea) may occur but usually are transient.

d. **Adjunctive nutritional therapy** consists of constant nasogastric tube feedings at a regulated rate either around-the-clock or for 8–12 hours overnight. This is particularly useful in infants with failure to thrive who are not tolerating intermittent small volume feedings by mouth. Adjunctive nutritional therapy offers the advantage of providing high-calorie formulas in a small steady volume during sleep, when reflux usually is markedly decreased.

B. **Achalasia.** Primary disorders of esophageal motility—other than those contributing to gastroesophageal reflux—are rare. The most common of these is achalasia, which is a disorder of unknown etiology characterized by lack of esophageal peristalsis and failure of a hypertonic LES to relax adequately with swallowing.

1. **Clinical features.** Most children with achalasia are older than 5 years at the time of presentation, although the disorder has been reported in infancy.

a. **Dysphagia** for both solid and liquid foods is the cardinal symptom.

b. **Other symptoms** include slow eating, regurgitation of undigested food, weight loss, substernal pain, and respiratory symptoms such as nocturnal cough due to aspiration of esophageal contents.

2. **Diagnosis**

a. **Barium swallow** usually demonstrates a widened, tortuous esophagus with a narrowed distal "beak." Sometimes, even on a plain film, an air-fluid level in the esophagus may be seen.

b. **Esophageal manometry** is necessary to document lack of peristalsis, an abnormally high LES pressure, and incomplete LES relaxation with swallowing.

c. **Endoscopy** is used to exclude other causes of distal esophageal disease.

3. **Therapy.** Although medical therapy (i.e., calcium channel blockers) may occasionally improve symptoms, disruption of the LES by pneumatic dilatation or surgery usually is required.

C. **Structural abnormalities**

1. **Tracheoesophageal fistula**

a. **Clinical features.** A congenital tracheoesophageal fistula may not cause difficulty until the child is several months of age or older, if it is not associated with esophageal atresia. Under this circumstance, however, the child may present with coughing, especially with feedings, and with recurrent pneumonia due to aspiration.

b. **Diagnosis.** To detect this H-type tracheoesophageal fistula, the radiologist must ensure that the esophagus is adequately distended on barium swallow.

c. **Therapy** is surgical ligation of the lesion.

   **2. Congenital strictures** usually occur at the junction of the middle and distal thirds of the esophagus and result in dysphagia. This lesion must be differentiated from the more common peptic stricture due to gastroesophageal reflux or strictures secondary to caustic ingestions. **Congenital webs** present in a similar manner.

**D. Esophageal damage by exogenous agents**

   **1. Caustic agents** are common accidentally ingested materials in children. Strong alkali solutions (e.g., lye) used as drain cleaners are most dangerous. Less damaging are ammonia cleaning solutions, bleaches, and dishwasher detergents. Acids and caustic liquids tend to cause more damage to the stomach than to the esophagus. The early presence or absence of oral burns or dysphagia does not predict the presence or degree of esophageal damage from caustic agents.

     **a. Clinical features**

       **(1) Acute.** There may be burns of the hands, face, and oral cavity; local pain; drooling; dysphagia, stridor or dyspnea; abdominal and chest pain; and shock if there is mediastinal penetration.

       **(2) Chronic.** Stricture formation may develop 2–4 weeks after ingestion and cause persistent dysphagia.

     **b. Diagnosis**

       **(1)** A chest x-ray can detect evidence of perforation and mediastinitis.

       **(2)** Endoscopy should be performed within 24 hours to document esophagitis and its extent.

       **(3)** A barium swallow is performed 1–2 weeks after ingestion and sequentially to detect and note progression of stricture.

     **c. Therapy**

       **(1)** No attempt should be made to induce vomiting or to neutralize the caustic agent.

       **(2)** Water or other neutral fluids may be administered carefully to dilute the caustic agent initially.

       **(3)** Intravenous fluids are necessary.

       **(4)** The cardiorespiratory status should be monitored carefully.

       **(5)** Corticosteroids may prevent stricture formation but are contraindicated if there has been perforation.

       **(6)** Antibiotics may be administered, particularly if there is suspicion of perforation or if corticosteroids have been administered.

       **(7)** Esophageal dilatation or even reconstructive surgery may be needed.

   **2. Foreign bodies.** The esophagus is the most difficult portion of the gastrointestinal tract to navigate, and objects whose progression is arrested in the esophagus should be expeditiously removed so that respiratory complications and esophageal ulceration and perforation do not occur. Children with esophageal foreign bodies (e.g., coins) will not always have symptoms of dysphagia, drooling, or chest discomfort. If there is clinical suspicion, a chest x-ray should be taken to rule out a radiopaque foreign body.

## III. DISORDERS OF THE STOMACH

**A. Pyloric stenosis** is an important cause of gastric outlet obstruction and vomiting in approximately 1 in every 500 infants. It frequently affects more than 1 child in a family, with a male to female ratio of 4:1. Symptoms generally begin between 2 and 4 weeks of age, although in 5% of cases they are present shortly after birth.

   **1. Clinical features**

     **a. Projectile nonbilious vomiting** is the cardinal feature and is seen in virtually all patients.

     **b.** Constipation and poor weight gain may be observed when the diagnosis is delayed.

     **c.** Although metabolic alkalosis is commonly seen secondary to the persistent vomiting, normal serum electrolytes never exclude a diagnosis of pyloric stenosis.

   **2. Diagnosis**

     **a.** The palpation of a firm, mobile, nontender, olive-shaped mass in the right hypochondrium or epigastrium in the appropriate clinical setting confirms the diagnosis.

     **b.** Visible peristaltic waves traveling from left to right across the abdomen may be seen.

     **c.** If a pyloric mass cannot be palpated, ultrasonographic or radiographic evaluation should be performed.

**3. Therapy.** Pyloromyotomy is the preferred surgical approach once fluid and electrolyte abnormalities have been adequately corrected.

**B. Gastritis** is frequently found in association with peptic ulcer disease in children. Recent evidence has suggested that the microorganism ***Helicobacter pylori*** may be an important contributing factor to gastric inflammation. Other causes may include allergies, aspirin, alcohol, nonsteroidal anti-inflammatory agents, corrosive ingestions, and radiation.

  **1. Clinical features** include abdominal pain and tenderness (usually epigastric), nausea, vomiting, and, occasionally, overt bleeding.

  **2. Diagnosis** of gastritis may be difficult since a barium study of the stomach usually is unrevealing in this disorder. If the clinical picture warrants investigation (i.e., if there is severe pain or bleeding), endoscopy can be performed. Specific histochemical stains should be performed on gastric biopsy tissue to identify *H. pylori*.

  **3. Therapy**
     **a.** If the gastritis is secondary to ingestion of aspirin or another drug, that medication should be discontinued and a brief (1- to 2-week) course of antacids or an $H_2$-blocker should be initiated.
     **b.** If the gastritis is associated with frank ulcerative disease, a 6-week course of antacids or an $H_2$-blocker is indicated. If *H. pylori* is identified in biopsy specimens, additional therapy with bismuth subsalicylate suspension, amoxicillin, and possibly metronidazole should be given for 2–3 weeks.

**C. Peptic ulcer disease.** In children younger than age 6 years, ulcers are found with equal frequency in boys and girls, a gastric location is as common as a duodenal one, and a precipitating event (e.g., drugs, stress) is common. In children older than 6 years of age, ulcers are most frequently found in boys and are more common in the duodenum.

  **1. Clinical features**
     **a.** In **neonates, bleeding and perforation** from a gastric ulcer usually are the first indications that an ulcer is present. Frequently, these infants have other underlying problems, such as sepsis or respiratory distress.
     **b. Older infants and toddlers** frequently present with **vomiting and poor eating**. Bleeding also is common and is seen with equal frequency in primary (idiopathic) and secondary (e.g., stress) ulcers.
     **c.** In **older children, pain** becomes a more important feature and may persist for some time before the child receives medical attention. Although many patients have "classic" ulcer pain relieved by eating, it is not uncommon for some children to claim that eating makes their pain worse. Either overt or occult **bleeding** is seen in about half of school-age children with ulcer disease.

  **2. Diagnosis.** Endoscopic evaluation of the upper gastrointestinal tract is the preferred diagnostic modality because of its superior sensitivity in detecting pathology compared to contrast radiography. Endoscopy also allows for tissue biopsy and evaluation of patterns of inflammation (e.g., allergic versus peptic) and possible infection (e.g., *H. pylori*).

  **3. Therapy.** If the ulcer is thought to be secondary to an underlying illness, the predisposing factors must be addressed. The management of the ulcer itself has historically been directed against gastric acid, either through neutralization (via antacids) or suppression of secretion (via $H_2$-receptor antagonists). The goal of either modality is the maintenance of gastric pH at or above 5. New, possibly cytoprotective, agents (e.g., sucralfate) are being evaluated for treatment of ulcers.
     **a. Medications**
        **(1) Antacids.** In the acutely ill patient, antacids can be administered either orally or through a nasogastric tube at a dose of 0.5 ml/kg every 1–2 hours.
        **(2) $H_2$-receptor antagonists.** Ranitidine (2–3 mg/kg every 12 hours orally, 1–1.5 mg/kg every 8 hours intravenously) and cimetidine (7.5–10 mg/kg every 6 hours orally or intravenously) have been used in the pediatric population. Since ranitidine does not inhibit the cytochrome $P_{450}$ hepatic enzyme system as does cimetidine, its use may be preferred when additional medications are being used.
     **b. Duration of therapy.** A 6-week course of therapy is recommended. Up to one-third of children with primary peptic ulcers suffer at least one recurrence. The recurrence rate is especially high in adolescents.

   **c. Dietary restrictions** probably are unnecessary, although elimination of substances that increase gastric acid secretion (e.g., alcohol, caffeine) is advisable.

## IV. GASTROINTESTINAL HEMORRHAGE.
Bleeding from the gastrointestinal tract is a common and, occasionally, life-threatening condition in infants and children. Usually, a careful history and physical examination, as well as consideration of the patient's age, will suggest the most likely etiologies. However, attempts to make a specific diagnosis should be made only after the patient's cardiovascular status (pulse, blood pressure, and so forth) has been adequately stabilized.

**A. Diagnosis.** The diagnostic approach in the patient with suspected gastrointestinal bleeding involves three sequential steps.

   **1. Did the patient actually bleed?**
      **a.** Food coloring can cause vomit and stools to turn red, and bismuth and iron may make stools black.
      **b.** Confirmation of the presence of heme protein by a test such as Hemoccult II (guaiac) is essential.

   **2. Did the bleeding originate in the upper or the lower tract?**
      **a.** Hematemesis suggests a site proximal to the ligament of Treitz.
      **b.** If the clinical picture is unclear, gastric aspiration should be performed.
         **(1)** A gastric aspirate positive for blood is highly specific for upper tract bleeding.
         **(2)** A negative aspirate suggests lower tract bleeding but cannot exclude an upper tract source that has stopped bleeding or a duodenal lesion with no reflux of blood back into the stomach.

   **3. What is the specific source of the bleeding?** A variety of noninvasive and invasive techniques may identify the source of the bleeding.
      **a. Radiologic evaluation**
         **(1)** A plain film of the abdomen may exclude bowel obstruction and free intra-abdominal gas.
         **(2)** Barium studies are contraindicated in the actively bleeding child as they generally are insensitive and will make other diagnostic tests difficult. A barium enema may be the first diagnostic test if intussusception (see VII A 3) is suspected.
         **(3)** Bleeding scans involving injection of $^{99m}$Tc pertechnetate-labeled red blood cells may detect very slow rates of bleeding. $^{99m}$Tc pertechnetate injected intravenously may detect ectopic gastric mucosa in the case of Meckel's diverticulum.
         **(4)** Angiography may be used to detect bleeding sites in more difficult cases.
      **b. Endoscopy**
         **(1)** In up to 90% of upper tract bleeding, esophagogastroduodenoscopy detects the site of hemorrhage.
         **(2)** Sigmoidoscopy should be the first diagnostic study in patients with suspected colonic bleeding. Abnormal colonic mucosa will immediately alert the clinician to an infectious or other type of inflammatory process (e.g., ulcerative colitis) or possibly identify a structural lesion (e.g., a polyp). If inspection of the entire colon is indicated, colonoscopy may be performed.

**B. Therapy**

   **1. Cardiovascular resuscitation** should be vigorous in the presence of orthostatic hypotension. With massive bleeding, whole blood (or a combination of packed cells and fresh frozen plasma) should be given to maintain intravascular volume. Once bleeding has stopped, packed cells alone may be given. Vitamin K (1 mg per year of age up to 10 mg), platelets, and plasma should be given as needed to correct any coagulopathy.

   **2. Treatment of upper tract lesions**
      **a. Mucosal lesions** of the upper tract should be treated with antacids or $H_2$-receptor antagonists.
      **b. Esophageal varices** may be treated with a variety of techniques, including the following.
         **(1)** Vasopressin infusion may be used to decrease splanchnic blood flow. A bolus of 0.3 units/kg up to a maximum of 20 units is given over 20 minutes, followed by a continuous infusion of 0.2–0.4 units/1.73 $m^2$/min.

**(2)** Variceal obliteration may be accomplished by direct variceal injection of a sclerosant solution such as 5% morrhuate sodium.

**(3)** Surgery to decompress the portal system can be performed, but with the emergence of variceal sclerosis, it will be used less frequently.

**3. Treatment of lower tract lesions** is dependent on the specific lesions causing the bleeding (e.g., surgery is used for Meckel's diverticulum).

# V. DIARRHEAL DISORDERS

**A. Acute infectious diarrhea** remains a leading cause of morbidity and mortality throughout the world.

**1. Diarrhea as a result of bacterial pathogens** (e.g., *Escherichia coli, Campylobacter, Salmonella, Shigella, Yersinia*)

   **a. Pathogenic mechanisms**
   **(1)** Toxin production (e.g., *Vibrio cholerae*)
   **(2)** Adherence to the intestinal mucosa with a local cytolytic effect (e.g., enteroadherent *E. coli*)
   **(3)** Invasion (e.g., *Shigella*)

   **b. Clinical features.** Bacterial diarrhea may present as either a cholera-like picture caused by bacterial toxins or a dysentery-like picture with bloody stools associated with invasive bacteria.

   **c. Diagnosis** is dependent on isolation of the particular organism by stool culture. A Gram stain of the stool may reveal leukocytes, and this is generally indicative of an invasive pathogen.

   **d. Therapy** with antibiotics is not always needed.
   **(1)** Salmonellal gastroenteritis should not be treated with antibiotics unless it is accompanied by septicemia, because it may prolong fecal excretion of this organism.
   **(2)** If symptoms associated with other bacterial pathogens have abated by the time of diagnosis, treatment generally is unnecessary.
   **(3)** Drugs that slow intestinal motility (e.g., diphenoxylate hydrochloride) should never be used in cases of bacterial diarrhea.

**2. Diarrhea as a result of viral pathogens**
   **a. Rotavirus** is the primary viral pathogen associated with diarrhea in children. It is a 70-nm, double-stranded, segmented RNA virus.
   **(1) Epidemiology.** Rotavirus is found worldwide, generally in children from 6 months to 2 years of age, and is most common during the cooler months of the year.
   **(2) Pathogenesis.** Rotavirus infects and destroys only the mature villous cells of the small intestine, not small intestinal crypt cells or colonic epithelial cells. Functionally immature crypt cells predominate, and abnormalities in electrolyte and carbohydrate absorption ensue.
   **(3) Clinical features** are seen after a 48- to 72-hour incubation period and include a predictable sequence of fever, vomiting, and subsequent diarrhea. Upper respiratory symptoms are common.
   **(4) Diagnosis.** Specific diagnosis can be made with a commercially available enzyme-linked immunosorbent assay (ELISA).
   **(5) Therapy** is supportive, and oral rehydration usually is successful. Lactose intolerance is seen in approximately 50% of infants suffering rotavirus infection and may last for several weeks.

   **b. Norwalk agent,** a 27-nm virus, is the prototype of a larger group of viruses that are associated with outbreaks of gastroenteritis. It is found more commonly in older children than in infants. After a 48-hour incubation period, vomiting alone, diarrhea alone, or both may be seen. Therapy is supportive and similar to that for rotavirus infection.

   **c. Enteric adenovirus** (serotypes 40, 41) has been increasingly recognized as a cause of diarrhea in young children. Clinically this infection resembles that seen with rotavirus, although the diarrhea may last somewhat longer (mean duration 5–6 days). Infection is seen year-round.

**3. Diarrhea as a result of protozoal pathogens**
   **a.** *Giardia lamblia* is a protozoan parasite that occurs either in active trophozoite form in the small bowel or as cysts, the form more commonly identified in feces.

    **(1) Epidemiology.** Ingestion of water contaminated with *G. lamblia* cysts is the usual mode of spread, but venereal transmission has also been described.

    **(2) Pathogenesis.** Significant intestinal epithelial cell injury usually is seen.

    **(3) Clinical features.** One to three weeks following ingestion, affected individuals experience cramping, abdominal distension, flatulence, and diarrhea. Many individuals may remain asymptomatic.

    **(4) Diagnosis** is made by careful examination of several fresh stool specimens for trophozoites or cysts. Rarely, duodenal intubation with tissue biopsy and fluid sampling may be required.

    **(5) Therapy.** Several drugs may be used for a 1-week course, including metronidazole, quinacrine, and furazolidone. Transient lactose malabsorption is common.

  **b. *Entamoeba histolytica*** may also exist in either a trophozoite or cyst form.

    **(1) Epidemiology.** Transmission is by the fecal-oral route and is associated with the ingestion of cysts. Infection is most common in areas with poor sanitation. Venereal transmission also is possible.

    **(2) Pathogenesis.** Ameba trophozoites invade colonic epithelium and exert a cytopathic effect.

    **(3) Clinical features.** Patients with dysenteric colitis have fever, numerous bloody stools, and cramping. Extraintestinal spread is common and may result in formation of a hepatic abscess.

    **(4) Diagnosis.** Ameba trophozoites can be identified upon stool examination. Serologic testing occasionally is useful.

    **(5) Therapy** is drug treatment via metronidazole.

**B. Food-associated diarrhea**

  **1. Protein sensitivity**

    **a. Celiac disease,** also called **gluten-sensitive enteropathy,** is an important, albeit decreasingly frequent, cause of chronic diarrhea in children.

      **(1) Pathogenesis. Gliadin,** a part of the protein gluten, is the substance associated with the small intestinal damage. Surface epithelial cells are destroyed, the villi become blunted or flat, and the crypts hypertrophy. Brush border enzyme levels are greatly decreased.

      **(2) Clinical features.** Most children develop symptoms between 9 and 24 months of age.

        **(a)** Diarrhea is the most common symptom.

        **(b)** Failure to thrive is frequently seen.

        **(c)** Vomiting is more common in younger patients.

        **(d)** There is abdominal distension.

        **(e)** Affected children often are irritable.

        **(f)** Short-stature, iron-resistant anemia, and rickets may be seen in older children.

      **(3) Diagnosis.** The definitive diagnosis of gluten-sensitive enteropathy can be made only with three sequential small intestinal biopsies showing flattened mucosa at presentation, recovery of villi after a gluten-free diet for 12 months, and flattening again upon gluten rechallenge.

      **(4) Therapy** for gluten-sensitive enteropathy is the provision of a gluten-free diet. Restriction of lactose as well as vitamin and iron supplementation may be necessary for several weeks to months as the small intestinal mucosa heals.

    **b. Cow's milk and soy protein intolerance (allergic enterocolitis)**

      **(1) Pathogenesis.** The precise mode by which these dietary proteins may cause disease is unknown. Sensitization may occur de novo (i.e., without any known precipitating event) or following a bout of acute infectious enteritis. Variable mucosal abnormalities may be found in the stomach, small bowel, and colon. Thirty percent of infants sensitive to cow's milk protein also are sensitive to soy protein.

      **(2) Clinical features.** Most symptoms develop in the first 3 months of life.

        **(a)** Vomiting and diarrhea are most commonly seen and in rare cases may persist for weeks to months.

        **(b)** Rectal bleeding may be seen if allergic colitis is present.

        **(c)** Edema secondary to excessive enteric protein loss may be dramatic and often is associated with anemia.

        **(d)** Rhinorrhea, wheezing, and eczema occasionally may be seen and frequently are accompanied by eosinophilia and an elevated serum immunoglobulin E (IgE) level. Anaphylaxis rarely is observed but may be life-threatening.

**(3)** **Diagnosis** generally is made empirically after symptoms resolve following elimination of the suspected dietary antigen.

**(4)** **Therapy.** Elimination of the offending dietary antigen usually is curative, although severely affected infants may take weeks to months to recover and may require intravenous alimentation until the intestinal mucosa heals.

 **c. Breast milk intolerance**

  **(1)** **Pathogenesis.** Some infants appear to react to antigenic material ingested via breast milk. At times this material appears to reflect the maternal diet, and cow's milk protein fractions have been isolated from breast milk. At other times maternal dietary features appear unimportant.

  **(2)** **Clinical features** generally develop in the first several weeks of life and include:

   **(a)** Diarrhea (frequently bloody)

   **(b)** Vomiting

   **(c)** Irritability

  **(3)** **Diagnosis** generally is based on the dietary history and exclusion of infectious agents. Rectal biopsy may reveal an intense eosinophilic infiltrate.

  **(4)** **Therapy.** Initial treatment is restriction of maternal ingestion of cow's milk protein. If this is not successful or if the infant's symptoms are severe, provision of a protein hydrolysate formula is indicated.

 **d. Other food-induced small bowel disturbances** have been associated with goat's milk, eggs, fish, and poultry.

**2. Carbohydrate intolerance** is a very common cause of diarrhea in childhood.

 **a. Pathogenesis.** Dietary carbohydrate is processed by several enzymes, beginning with amylase (which metabolizes starch) and ending with the brush border enzymes lactase, sucrase, isomaltase, and glucoamylase. Any process—congenital or acquired—that diminishes the activities of these enzymes may lead to carbohydrate malabsorption.

 **b. Clinical features.** Diarrhea, vomiting, flatulence, borborygmi, and cramping may be present; however, blood is not seen in the stool.

 **c. Diagnosis**

  **(1)** Breath hydrogen testing is the most accurate diagnostic test.

  **(2)** Stool pH and examination of stool for reducing substances (e.g., lactose, glucose, fructose) are less helpful in making the diagnosis, but a stool pH less than 5 and the presence of reducing substances suggest carbohydrate malabsorption.

  **(3)** Intestinal biopsy with direct assay of brush border enzyme activity rarely is needed.

 **d. Therapy** is restriction of the offending carbohydrate. Lactase enzyme now is commercially available and may be ingested along with lactose-containing foods to lessen symptoms. Yogurt and aged cheeses may be well-tolerated even by lactose-intolerant individuals. If lactose restriction is severe and prolonged, calcium supplementation is needed.

**C. Intractable diarrhea of infancy** is an uncommon problem but one that may have life-threatening consequences. Multiple disease states may be responsible for this clinical entity.

 **1. Pathogenesis.** Some infants have a specific defect in pancreatic, hepatic, or intestinal function, which can readily explain the cause of their diarrhea. Unfortunately, a significant number of infants with intractable diarrhea have no readily identifiable underlying disease.

  **a.** Current knowledge suggests that some children may suffer a series of important pathogenetic events, which include:

   **(1)** Mucosal injury of the small bowel caused by an unrecognized infection or allergy

   **(2)** Malnutrition, which results from the malabsorption associated with the intestinal mucosal injury

   **(3)** Delayed healing of the mucosal injury and depressed immunity, which result from the malnutrition

  **b.** Others appear to suffer intestinal injury on an autoimmune basis.

 **2. Clinical features**

  **a.** Diarrhea is severe and often persists even when the patient is given nothing by mouth **(secretory diarrhea)**.

  **b.** Vomiting is common.

  **c.** Fluid, electrolyte, and enteric protein losses may be excessive, resulting in dehydration, acidosis, hyponatremia, hypokalemia, hypoalbuminemia, and edema.

  **d.** Severe failure to thrive is evident.

3. **Diagnosis.** A systematic approach to diagnose readily treatable conditions must be made. This includes:
   a. Culture of stool, urine, and blood
   b. Stool examination for blood, leukocytes, pH, reducing sugars, ova, and parasites
   c. Assessment of renal and hepatic function
   d. Sweat test for cystic fibrosis
   e. Immunologic evaluation
   f. Small intestinal biopsy and sigmoidoscopy
   g. Radiologic evaluation (e.g., upper gastrointestinal series, barium enema)

4. **Therapy.** If the underlying condition permits specific treatment, that treatment should be given. In most cases of idiopathic intractable diarrhea, the primary treatment is nutritional support.
   a. Central venous hyperalimentation frequently is required and should be instituted early to reverse the patient's severely catabolic state.
   b. Elemental formulas are required when enteric nutrition is initiated. These usually need to be given slowly by continuous infusion through a nasogastric tube.

**D. Chronic nonspecific diarrhea, or irritable bowel syndrome,** is the most common cause of chronic diarrhea in otherwise healthy children.

1. **Pathogenesis.** Although the precise pathogenesis of chronic nonspecific diarrhea is unknown, alterations in gastrointestinal motility are thought to be of primary importance. A number of additional factors have been noted to increase symptoms, including:
   a. Chilled foods or fluids
   b. Excessive fluid intake, especially of fruit juices
   c. A low-fat, high-carbohydrate diet
   d. Stress and anxiety

2. **Clinical features.** Chronic nonspecific diarrhea usually manifests between age 9 and 36 months.
   a. Diarrhea is variable in severity and may occur up to six times each day. Occasionally, normal or even hard stools are seen.
   b. Undigested food, particularly vegetables, and mucus frequently are observed in the stools.
   c. Abdominal cramping may be present.
   d. Activity and appetite usually are normal, and growth generally is unaffected.

3. **Diagnosis** is based on a compatible clinical history and the exclusion of other disorders (e.g., carbohydrate malabsorption, chronic infection).

4. **Therapy.** Frequently no treatment other than parental reassurance is needed. Symptoms usually resolve spontaneously by 3–4 years of age. Specific measures that can be of help include:
   a. Decreasing fluid intake, particularly fruit juices, and providing high-fat foods to slow gastric emptying
   b. Increasing fiber intake through the use of bulking agents
   c. Pharmacologic intervention, although rarely required, including the use of cholestyramine and loperamide

**VI. INFLAMMATORY BOWEL DISEASE** is a generic term generally used to refer to two chronic disorders of intestinal inflammation—**ulcerative colitis** and **Crohn's disease**.

**A. Epidemiology.** Recent studies suggest a modest increase in the incidence of Crohn's disease and perhaps a mild decrease in the incidence of ulcerative colitis over the past decade. Up to 30% of newly diagnosed cases of inflammatory bowel disease occur in individuals less than 20 years of age.

**B. Pathogenesis.** A number of genetic and environmental factors may be contributory.

1. **Immunologic.** A variety of immunologic abnormalities have been noted in patients with inflammatory bowel disease, including anticolon antibodies and lymphocytes cytotoxic to intestinal cells. It is not clear whether these phenomena are primary or secondary.

2. **Infectious.** No infectious agent has been reproducibly isolated and thought to be causative in patients with inflammatory bowel disease. Recently, a new strain of atypical mycobacteria has been isolated from intestinal tissue of some patients with Crohn's disease.

3. **Psychological.** Despite numerous theories on the so-called colitis personality, no consistent psychological abnormalities have been found preceding disease onset in patients with inflammatory bowel disease.

4. **Multifactorial.** It is likely that a variety of factors as detailed above are important. Genetic predisposition to inflammatory bowel disease may be a crucial factor.

C. **Histologic features.** Considerable overlap may be seen in the anatomic and histologic distribution of inflammation in ulcerative colitis and Crohn's disease.

1. **Ulcerative colitis.** Disease is limited to the colon.
   a. Mucosal inflammation predominates, but, in severe disease, inflammation may involve the submucosa. Inflammation is diffuse; it is not in a segmental distribution.
   b. Crypt abscesses are common in active disease.

2. **Crohn's disease.** Anatomic distribution is quite variable. In children, disease is ileocolic in 60%, involves the small intestine in 30%, and involves the colon in only 10%.
   a. Intestinal inflammation frequently is transmural, although it may be limited to the mucosa. Segmental distribution of inflammation is common.
   b. Fibrosis is transmural, and strictures are common.
   c. Granulomas are observed in up to 30% of patients.
   d. Internal or external fistula formation, or both, is observed in up to 40% of patients.

D. **Clinical features**

1. **Ulcerative colitis**
   a. **Diarrhea** is a constant feature of ulcerative colitis and frequently contains mucus and blood.
   b. **Abdominal cramping** usually occurs prior to and during defecation.
   c. **Toxic megacolon** is a severe complication of fulminant ulcerative colitis.
   d. **Carcinoma of the colon** is a significant complication of chronic disease. After 10 years of disease, there is a cumulative risk of 1%–2% per year for the development of carcinoma.
   e. **Extraintestinal complications**
      (1) Arthritis, which usually is nondeforming and may involve any joint but especially the large joints in the lower extremity
      (2) Ankylosing spondylitis, which is seen rarely and which is more common in patients who are HLA-B27–positive
      (3) Skin manifestations, including erythema nodosum and pyoderma gangrenosum
      (4) Ophthalmologic manifestations, including uveitis, episcleritis, and recurrent iritis, which are rare in children
      (5) Aphthous stomatitis
      (6) Hepatic complications, including fatty liver, chronic active hepatitis, and sclerosing cholangitis
      (7) Thrombophlebitis
      (8) Fever

2. **Crohn's disease**
   a. **Diarrhea** is a frequent but not a universal finding. Rectal bleeding is observed in 30%–40% of cases.
   b. **Abdominal pain** tends to be more severe than that in ulcerative colitis, may be diffuse, and frequently is worse in the right lower quadrant.
   c. **Anorexia, poor weight gain, and delayed growth** may be seen in up to 40% of patients.
   d. **Extraintestinal manifestations** are common in patients with Crohn's disease and may include all the problems listed for ulcerative colitis (see VI D 1 e).

E. **Diagnosis** relies on a complete history and physical examination as well as the following studies.

1. **Laboratory studies**
   a. **Hematologic.** Anemia is common and usually is associated with iron deficiency. Megaloblastic anemia may also be seen secondary to folate and vitamin $B_{12}$ deficiency. An elevation of the erythrocyte sedimentation rate is seen in about 50% of cases of ulcerative colitis and in 80% of cases of Crohn's disease.
   b. **Biochemical.** Hypoalbuminemia is common in individuals with severe symptoms and is

often exacerbated by poor nutritional intake. Acute-phase reactant concentrations are elevated. Serum aminotransferase levels are increased if hepatic inflammation is a complicating feature.

**2. Endoscopy.** Flexible sigmoidoscopy should be performed before barium studies are attempted. Upper tract lesions are common in Crohn's disease and may require endoscopic evaluation for diagnosis.

**3. Radiographic evaluation**
   **a.** A double-contrast barium enema gives better definition of mucosal detail than does a single-contrast study.
   **b.** An upper gastrointestinal series with small bowel follow-through is used to diagnose gastric and small bowel disease.

**F. Differential diagnosis.** A number of conditions may present with signs and symptoms suggestive of idiopathic inflammatory bowel disease, including:

**1.** Appendicitis

**2.** Enteric infection (e.g., *Campylobacter, Salmonella, Shigella, Yersinia, Amoeba*)

**3.** Pseudomembranous colitis (antibiotic-associated diarrhea) secondary to *Clostridium difficile* infection

**4.** Hemolytic-uremic syndrome

**5.** Henoch-Schönlein purpura

**6.** Radiation enterocolitis

**7.** Eosinophilic gastroenteritis

**G. Therapy**

**1. Medication**
   **a.** Sulfasalazine is the mainstay of treatment in mild to moderate ulcerative colitis and Crohn's disease involving the colon. It has no efficacy in Crohn's disease involving the small bowel. In patients who are allergic to sulfasalazine, 5-aminosalicylate (the active moiety) can be administered orally via newer carrier molecules or as an enema preparation.
   **b.** Corticosteroids remain the most efficacious therapy, particularly in severe disease and in Crohn's disease involving the small bowel. As daily corticosteroid therapy can inhibit growth, attempts should be made to use alternate-day therapy when possible.
   **c.** Metronidazole currently is used to treat severe perirectal fistulae in patients with Crohn's disease.
   **d.** 6-Mercaptopurine is now being used in patients with severe Crohn's disease who are dependent on high doses of corticosteroids. It may permit reduction of the steroid dosage.
   **e.** Diphenoxylate and loperamide may be used for symptomatic relief but never in the presence of severe symptoms.

**2. Nutrition**
   **a.** Since anorexia and increased nutrient losses through stool are common in children with inflammatory bowel disease, adequate calories and protein are essential. A variety of techniques may be used and often are effective in reversing growth retardation, including:
      **(1)** Oral supplements
      **(2)** Nasogastric tube feedings
      **(3)** Central venous hyperalimentation
   **b.** Vitamin and mineral (particularly iron) supplementation may be required.

**3. Surgery**
   **a. Ulcerative colitis**
      **(1) Indications**
         **(a)** Fulminant colitis with severe blood loss or toxic megacolon
         **(b)** Intractable disease with a high-dose steroid requirement, steroid toxicity, growth failure, or invalidism
         **(c)** Colonic dysplasia
      **(2) Procedure.** Ileoanal-endorectal pull-through procedures after colectomy and mucosal proctectomy are the methods of choice and eliminate the need for a permanent ileostomy.

**b. Crohn's disease**
   **(1) Indications**
      **(a)** Hemorrhage
      **(b)** Obstruction
      **(c)** Perforation
      **(d)** Intractability
      **(e)** Severe fistula formation
      **(f)** Ureteral obstruction
      **(g)** Growth retardation (if medical measures are unsuccessful)
   **(2) Procedure.** In general, conservatism is warranted since removal of the diseased bowel is not curative in Crohn's disease. After segmental resection, recurrence rates of about 50% have been reported.

# VII. ABDOMINAL PAIN

## A. Acute pain

1. **Approach to the patient with acute abdominal pain.** The most urgent consideration in evaluating a child with acute abdominal pain is to determine whether there is an underlying cause requiring surgery. Most causes of abdominal pain in children do not require surgical treatment, although such causes of pain are more common in children younger than 2 years. Sources of pain outside the abdominal cavity (e.g., lower lobe pneumonia) must be considered in the evaluation.
   a. **Important causes of abdominal pain possibly requiring surgery (the "acute abdomen")**
      **(1)** Intestinal obstruction due to malrotation and volvulus, intussusception, strangulated hernia, or adhesions
      **(2)** Appendicitis, Meckel's diverticulitis, or an abdominal abscess
      **(3)** Toxic megacolon
      **(4)** Perforated duodenal ulcer or perforation of intestine secondary to another process
      **(5)** Cholecystitis
      **(6)** Rupture of the spleen or other organ due to trauma
   b. **Clinical features suggesting a cause requiring surgery**
      **(1)** Vomiting, especially if it is bilious or feculent
      **(2)** Sudden onset of abdominal distension
      **(3)** Absent bowel sounds or high-pitched sounds suggestive of intestinal obstruction
      **(4)** Abdominal signs of peritonitis (e.g., rigidity, guarding, rebound tenderness)
   c. **Important causes of acute abdominal pain not requiring surgery**
      **(1)** Enteritis; colitis of any cause
      **(2)** Henoch-Schönlein purpura, hemolytic-uremic syndrome, and other types of vasculitis
      **(3)** Fecal impaction
      **(4)** Hepatitis
      **(5)** Pancreatitis
      **(6)** Vaso-occlusive crisis of sickle cell anemia
      **(7)** Primary peritonitis
      **(8)** Mesenteric adenitis
      **(9)** Urinary tract infection or urinary calculi
      **(10)** Extra-abdominal causes (e.g., pneumonia, osteomyelitis, acute neurologic processes)
      **(11)** Unusual causes [e.g., porphyria, familial Mediterranean fever, diabetic ketoacidosis, lead poisoning, Kawasaki's disease (gallbladder hydrops)]

2. **Appendicitis in infancy and childhood.** Appendicitis is the **most common indication for acute abdominal surgery in childhood**. Appendicitis occurs more frequently in children between 10 and 15 years of age. Less than 10% of patients are under 5 years old.
   a. **Pathogenesis.** Bacterial invasion of the appendix occurs, especially if the lumen is obstructed by a fecalith, parasite, or lymph node.
   b. **Clinical features**
      **(1)** Classically, fever, vomiting, anorexia, and diffuse periumbilical pain develop. Subsequently, pain and abdominal tenderness localize to the right lower quadrant as the parietal peritoneum becomes involved.
      **(2)** The incidence of perforation and diffuse peritonitis is high, especially in a child under 2 years of age when diagnosis may be delayed.

**(3)** Atypical presentations are common in childhood.
**(4)** Certain bacterial infections (e.g., *Campylobacter, Yersinia*) may be associated with right lower quadrant pain and tenderness and may mimic appendicitis.
  c. **Diagnosis** of appendicitis should be established clinically by history and by a physical examination (including a rectal examination to detect tenderness or a mass). Laboratory tests may help confirm the diagnosis.
  **(1)** The white blood cell count is only moderately elevated in uncomplicated appendicitis.
  **(2)** A plain film of the abdomen may demonstrate a fecalith or other nonspecific abnormalities.
  **(3)** Occasionally, a barium enema may be useful.
  d. **Therapy.** When the diagnosis of appendicitis cannot be ruled out after a period of close observation, laparotomy and appendectomy are indicated.
  e. **Prognosis.** The mortality rate is very low unless perforation has occurred.

**3. Intussusception** is the invagination of one part of the intestine into another. It is **one of the most common causes of intestinal obstruction in infancy**.
  a. **Pathogenesis.** Most intussusceptions are ileocolic.
  **(1)** In patients beyond the neonatal period but under the age of 2 years (the period of peak incidence), no lead point of the intussusception is typically found. A previous viral infection may cause hypertrophy of the Peyer's patches or mesenteric nodes, which are hypothesized to play a role in intussusception.
  **(2)** A specific lead point is identified in only about 5% of cases, but it should be sought in neonates or in children over 5 years of age. Recognizable causes of the intussusception include Meckel's diverticulum, an intestinal polyp, lymphoma, or a foreign body. Meckel's diverticulum usually presents as melena unassociated with abdominal pain or intussusception.
  **(3)** As a result of impaired venous return, the affected bowel may swell, become ischemic and necrotic, and perforate.
  b. **Clinical features**
  **(1)** Bouts of irritability and colicky pain start suddenly. Vomiting is common. Rectal bleeding may occur but only rarely in the form of the classic "currant jelly" stools (i.e., stools containing red blood and mucus).
  **(2)** The degree of lethargy demonstrated by the child may be striking.
  **(3)** A tubular mass is palpable in about half of the patients.
  c. **Diagnosis**
  **(1)** A plain abdominal film may show a paucity of gas in the right lower quadrant or evidence of obstruction.
  **(2)** A barium enema demonstrates a coiled-spring appearance to the bowel, which is diagnostic.
  d. **Therapy**
  **(1)** **Hydrostatic reduction** by careful barium enema performed by an experienced radiologist is successful in about 75% of cases. Peritoneal signs, however, are an absolute contraindication to this procedure.
  **(2)** **Surgery** is indicated when hydrostatic reduction is inappropriate or unsuccessful.
  e. **Prognosis.** The immediate recurrence rate is about 15%. When a specific lead point is present, the recurrence rate is higher.

**B. Chronic pain.** Chronic abdominal pain is a frequent problem in children (see Ch 3 VI). Most often, no specific cause can be documented. Two particularly vexing problems are infantile colic and irritable bowel syndrome.

**1. Infantile colic** is observed in up to 15% of normal newborn infants.
  a. **Pathogenesis.** Despite hundreds of years of observation, the cause of infantile colic remains unknown. Postulated important factors have included abnormal mother-infant interaction, protein allergy, hormonal imbalances, and increased sensitivity to colonic distension.
  b. **Clinical features** of infantile colic include:
  **(1)** Pulling up of legs during paroxysms, often with a change in facial color to bright red
  **(2)** Difficulty with defecation despite soft stools
  **(3)** Inconsolability

c. **Diagnosis**
   (1) A clinical diagnosis is based on a characteristic history and a normal physical examination.
   (2) Other causes of irritability (e.g., protein allergy, hernia, gastroesophageal reflux) must be excluded.
d. **Therapy.** Parental support is the mainstay of therapy. Rocking machines or increased dietary fiber may be helpful.
e. **Prognosis.** In over 80% of cases, symptoms abate by 4–5 months of age.

2. **Irritable bowel syndrome** may represent the most common cause of chronic abdominal pain, yet it is probably the least characterized.
   a. **Pathogenesis.** The precise pathogenesis of irritable bowel is unknown, but abnormal intestinal (primarily colonic) motility has been described. In addition, increased sensitivity to colonic distension appears to be common in these patients.
   b. **Clinical features**
      (1) Abdominal cramping is a cardinal feature of irritable bowel syndrome and may be described in virtually any part of the abdomen. It frequently is paroxysmal and severe.
      (2) Stool consistency may frequently vary from hard to loose.
      (3) Nausea, diaphoresis, and light headedness occasionally are seen.
      (4) Anxiety often provokes an attack.
   c. **Diagnosis**
      (1) A clinical diagnosis is based on a characteristic history and a normal physical examination.
      (2) Other disorders (e.g., lactose intolerance, inflammatory bowel disease, giardiasis) must be excluded.
   d. **Therapy** consists of:
      (1) Reassurance that, while symptoms are frequent, they do not suggest a life-threatening disease
      (2) Dietary fiber supplementation
      (3) Anticholinergic medications (e.g., dicyclomine)
      (4) Psychotherapy (if stress frequently exacerbates symptoms)
   e. **Prognosis.** Little is known about the natural history of irritable bowel syndrome in children, although clinical experience suggests that the problem may persist for intervals of months to years.

**VIII. CONSTIPATION** can be defined as a decrease in the frequency or fluidity of bowel movements. Less than three bowel movements per week is considered abnormal. Most constipated children have no underlying disorder, and treatment can be directed solely at the symptom. Formal evaluation is reserved for cases beginning at birth and those that are intractable to standard symptomatic treatment.

A. **Pathogenesis**

1. **Functional or simple constipation** occurs in the absence of an organic cause. In a normal child, constipation may result simply from an episode of painful defecation, difficulties during the period of toilet training, inattention to the urge to defecate because of involvement in other activities, or discomfort with toilet facilities in school. Frequently, a family history of constipation may be elicited. Inadequate fiber in the diet also may play a role.

2. **Specific causes**
   a. **Structural lesions,** including anal fissure, anterior ectopic anus, stenosis of the bowel, inflammatory proctitis, and extrinsic lesions causing bowel obstruction
   b. **Neuromuscular disorders,** such as spinal cord defects, disorders of smooth muscle, and Hirschsprung's disease (see VIII E)
   c. **Medications,** particularly opiates and anticholinergic agents
   d. **Metabolic causes,** including hypothyroidism, hypercalcemia, hypokalemia, uremia, pregnancy, and disorders causing dehydration
   e. **Toxins,** particularly chronic lead intoxication
   f. **Infection** with *Clostridium botulinum* in infants (infant botulism)

**B. Clinical features**

1. **Pattern of defecation.** A detailed history of the pattern of defecation may be difficult to obtain. Even a history of regular bowel movements does not exclude constipation if evacuation is incomplete. Large stools and stool-withholding behavior may be mistaken for straining to defecate.

2. **Accompanying symptoms** include pain, abdominal distension, and flatulence. Occasional symptoms include rectal bleeding, poor appetite, enuresis, and a history of urinary tract infection. Rectal prolapse may rarely be seen with defecation.

3. **Encopresis.** In cases of long-standing constipation, children may become incontinent of liquid stool and be thought to have diarrhea. This "overflow incontinence" is called encopresis and is present in more than 50% of children with long-standing constipation (see Ch 3 II B).

**C. Diagnosis**

1. Physical examination of the abdomen may reveal distension or palpable fecal masses. The perianal area should be examined for congenital or acquired abnormalities, including trauma. Digital rectal examination is necessary to evaluate the sphincter and estimate the amount of stool in the ampulla.

2. When no underlying disorder is identified by history and physical examination, a favorable response to treatment supports the diagnosis of functional constipation.

3. Treatment failure or relapse should prompt investigation of an underlying disorder with appropriate radiographic and serologic studies.

**D. Therapy for functional constipation.** An individualized, multifaceted treatment program should be designed.

1. **Medications** are continued until a regular pattern of defecation is established and then are slowly tapered.
   a. In infants, short-term or intermittent treatment with glycerin suppositories may be rewarding. Excessive milk or cow's milk protein formula (> 32 oz/day) should be avoided, and juices such as apple or pear juice may be helpful. Extra fiber in the form of barley malt extracts or methylcellulose also may help.
   b. In older children, mineral oil or mild laxatives such as senna derivatives commonly are used.
   c. In cases of severe constipation, a period of aggressive treatment including enemas (otherwise to be avoided) may be required.
   d. A balanced polyethylene glycol–electrolyte solution administered by the oral or nasogastric route is safe, prompt, and effective in cleansing the bowel and may avoid prolonged use of enemas or the need for manual disimpaction.

2. **Other measures**
   a. **High-fiber diet** and fiber supplements
   b. Reinforcement of **regular toilet use**
   c. **Psychological evaluation,** which may be necessary to address emotional factors resulting in voluntary withholding

**E. Hirschsprung's disease** is an uncommon developmental disorder (incidence is 1 in 5000) resulting in constipation.

1. **Pathogenesis.** In children with Hirschsprung's disease, progenitor cells destined to become the ganglion cells of the submucosal and myenteric plexuses fail to complete their distal bowel migration in the colon. As a result, the abnormally innervated distal colon remains tonically contracted and obstructs the flow of feces. In approximately 75% of cases, the aganglionic segment is limited to the **rectosigmoid,** but the entire colon may be involved.

2. **Clinical features**
   a. In most cases, the onset of symptoms occurs in the first month and the diagnosis is made in the first 3 months of life. The neonate classically has delayed passage of meconium and then develops evidence of obstruction with poor feeding, bilious vomiting, and abdominal distension.
   b. In the older child, failure to thrive may be seen as well as intermittent bouts of intestinal obstruction and even enterocolitis with bloody diarrhea and, occasionally, bowel perforation, sepsis, and shock.

3. **Diagnosis**
   a. **Rectal examination** may reveal a narrowed high-pressure zone in continuity with the sphincter, and stool may not be palpable.
   b. **Plain x-rays** may show gaseous distension of proximal bowel but no gas or feces in the rectum.
   c. **Barium enema** may demonstrate a transition zone between the narrowed abnormal distal segment and the dilated normal proximal bowel.
   d. **Anal manometry** demonstrates failure of the internal anal sphincter to relax with balloon distension of the rectum.
   e. **Rectal biopsy** revealing **no ganglion cells** and **hypertrophied nerve trunks** is necessary for the diagnosis.

4. **Therapy.** Initial treatment usually is a diverting colostomy. Subsequently, at 6 months or 1 year, the aganglionic segment is removed and the remaining colon is anastomosed to the anorectal region.

# IX. LIVER DISEASE

A. **General principles.** Certain unique aspects of liver disease in infancy and childhood must be considered before specific hepatic disorders can be evaluated.

   1. **Estimation of liver size.** In healthy children under the age of 2 years, both the liver and spleen are usually palpable below the costal margins due to the relatively large size of these organs at this age. Standards have been established for liver span as measured by percussion in the midclavicular line in older children.

   2. **Reaction to hepatic injury in infancy. Jaundice** is the most important manifestation of a variety of hepatic insults in infancy. **Hypoglycemia** occurs early in the course of hepatic injury.

   3. **Key elements of the history**
      a. The **family history** is especially important in the consideration of metabolic liver disease.
      b. Illness or **exposure during pregnancy** may suggest a vertically transmitted (i.e., from mother to infant) infectious cause of hepatitis.
      c. A **dietary history** is crucial in the diagnosis of hepatic disease resulting from the failure to metabolize galactose or fructose.

   4. **Diagnostic tests.** The serum **alkaline phosphatase** level usually is elevated in children with obstructive or inflammatory hepatic lesions. Care must be used, however, in the interpretation of the concentration in infancy and adolescence. Because of rapid growth at these ages, the level of serum alkaline phosphatase from bone is elevated, and other enzymes, such as **γ-glutamyl transpeptidase (GGT),** must be used to evaluate cholestasis.

B. **Neonatal obstructive jaundice.** Direct hyperbilirubinemia in the neonate is never "physiologic" and, therefore, should always be thoroughly investigated. Direct hyperbilirubinemia is defined as a direct bilirubin greater than 2 mg/dl or greater than 20% of the total bilirubin (see also Ch 5 V C).

   1. **Differential diagnosis** (Table 10-1). Direct hyperbilirubinemia in the neonate is a medical emergency and must be expeditiously investigated to avoid permanent liver damage. The key distinction in the neonatal period is between **intrahepatic** and **extrahepatic** causes of direct hyperbilirubinemia. Extrahepatic causes require prompt surgical therapy to relieve obstruction and reconstitute bile flow from the liver. Certain intrahepatic metabolic causes can be effectively treated by dietary therapy and some intrahepatic infectious causes can be specifically treated with antimicrobial agents.
      a. **Tests for specific causes of neonatal cholestasis**
         (1) Serum tests, including total and direct bilirubin, aminotransferase and GGT levels, complete blood count, titers of TORCH organisms (see Ch 7 II B), VDRL, hepatitis B surface antigen (HBsAg), $\alpha_1$-antitrypsin level and phenotyping, amino acids, blood culture (if clinically indicated), serum albumin, prothrombin time (PT), and partial thromboplastin time (PTT)
         (2) Urine tests, including urinalysis, reducing substances, urine culture, and organic and amino acids
         (3) Sweat test

**Table 10-1.** Causes of Direct Hyperbilirubinemia with Cholestasis (Obstructive Jaundice in the Infant)

| | Intrahepatic Causes | | |
| Extrahepatic Causes | Infectious | Metabolic | Miscellaneous |
| --- | --- | --- | --- |
| Biliary atresia | Cytomegalovirus | Galactosemia | Neonatal hepatitis |
| Choledochal cyst | Toxoplasmosis | Hereditary fructose | Alagille syndrome |
| Common duct stenosis | Rubella | intolerance | Byler disease |
| Common duct stone | Herpesvirus | Tyrosinemia | Zellweger syndrome |
| Obstructing tumor | Coxsackievirus | $\alpha_1$-Antitrypsin defi- | Trisomy (17, 18, 21) |
| Bile/mucous plug | Echovirus | ciency | Hypopituitarism |
| Spontaneous perfora- | Syphilis | Cystic fibrosis | Hepatic hemangio- |
| tion of the common | Hepatitis B | Niemann-Pick disease | matosis |
| duct | Epstein-Barr virus | Gaucher's disease | TPN-induced chole- |
| | Urinary tract infection | Glycogen storage disease | stasis |

TPN = total parenteral nutrition.

(4) Abdominal ultrasound to rule out a choledochal cyst or common duct stone
(5) Radionuclide biliary imaging study to document patency of the extrahepatic biliary system
(6) Liver biopsy
**b. Differentiation of intrahepatic and extrahepatic idiopathic causes** (Table 10-2)
(1) Often the tests for neonatal cholestasis reveal no specific etiology. In fact, **neonatal hepatitis** and **biliary atresia** are the most common causes of persistent direct hyperbilirubinemia. No serum test, including aminotransferases, GGT, bilirubin, α-fetoprotein (AFP), or lipoprotein X, reliably distinguishes between these two entities. Further testing is directed at distinguishing these two entities, including percutaneous liver biopsy.
(2) In spite of testing, it often is necessary to perform a laparotomy and intra-operative cholangiography to accurately delineate the presence or absence of the extrahepatic biliary system.

**2. Therapy**
**a. Neonatal hepatitis.** The treatment for neonatal hepatitis and for other causes of nonsurgically remediable prolonged cholestasis is supportive. It includes:
(1) Administration of bile acid binding resins (cholestyramine) and phenobarbital to increase bile flow
(2) Fat-soluble vitamin (A, D, E, K) supplementation
(3) Supplementation of the diet with medium-chain triglycerides that do not require bile acids for assimilation
**b. Biliary atresia**
(1) **Surgical management.** In less than 20% of patients, there are identifiable proximal hepatic bile ducts that can be anastomosed to the bowel. In most patients, a portoenterostomy must be created between the cut surface of the liver at the porta hepatis and the bowel (Kasai procedure).
(2) **Timing of operation.** Successful drainage of the biliary tract occurs most frequently when the operation is performed before the infant is 60 days old.
(3) **Complications** of surgery include failure to establish bile flow, loss of bile flow due to further injury to bile ducts, and ascending cholangitis.

**3. Prognosis**
**a. Neonatal hepatitis**
(1) In most patients, the cholestasis resolves over the first year of life with no sequelae.
(2) A few infants develop progressive liver disease and cirrhosis, with its complication of ascites, portal hypertension, esophageal varices, and liver failure. These children may be candidates for liver transplantation.
**b. Biliary atresia**
(1) Without surgical correction, biliary cirrhosis and its complications supervene, and most patients die in the first 2 years of life.
(2) After successful portoenterostomy, with normalization of serum bilirubin, the 5-year survival rate is 60%–90%.

**Table 10-2.** Features of Intrahepatic and Extrahepatic Neonatal Obstructive Jaundice

| Intrahepatic Causes | Extrahepatic Causes |
|---|---|
| **Clinical features** | **Clinical features** |
| Prematurity | Full-term |
| Small for gestational age | Appropriate size for gestational age |
| Familial incidence (15%–20%) | No familial incidence |
| Ill appearance | Well appearance |
| Intermittently acholic stool | Completely acholic stool |
| Hepatosplenomegaly | Splenomegaly rare before age 3 weeks |
| Liver not hard | Liver firm to hard |
| Associated abnormalities | Associated abnormalities |
| Alagille syndrome | Polysplenia |
| Peripheral pulmonic stenosis or | Cardiovascular malformations |
| pulmonic stenosis | Malrotation of gut |
| Vertebral anomalies | |
| Posterior embryotoxon | |
| **Laboratory features** | **Laboratory features** |
| GGT > 10 times normal | GGT < 10 times normal |
| Gallbladder seen on ultrasound | No gallbladder or rudimentary gallbladder |
| Excretion into small bowel with radionuclide | seen on ultrasound |
| biliary scan | No excretion into small bowel with radio- |
| 24-hr duodenal fluid collection shows pigment | nuclide biliary scan |
| (especially after feeding) | 24-hour duodenal fluid collection shows no |
| | pigment |
| **Liver biopsy findings** | **Liver biopsy findings** |
| Bile ducts normal or decreased | Bile duct proliferation and inflammation |
| Minimal fibrosis | Portal fibrosis |
| Giant cell transformation | Giant cell transformation in about 25% of |
| Hepatocellular necrosis | cases |
| Lobular disarray | Bile lakes |
| Portal inflammation | Bile plugs in portal ducts |
| Cholestasis | Cholestasis |

GGT = γ-glutamyl transpeptidase.

    **(3)** Liver transplantation now is showing promise as treatment for patients with biliary atresia for whom attempts at corrective surgery fail. The 5-year survival rate for liver transplant recipients having biliary atresia is about 70%.

  **C. Acute viral hepatitis** (Table 10-3)

    **1. Diagnosis.** Typically, children with acute viral hepatitis have elevated serum aminotransferase levels (sometimes to more than 2000 U/L) and elevated serum bilirubin levels, although many cases are anicteric. In severe cases, hepatic synthesis of clotting factors may be affected, with resulting prolongation of PT.

      **a. Hepatitis A ("infectious" hepatitis).** The diagnosis of acute hepatitis A is established by the finding of hepatitis A antibodies of the IgM class (IgM antibody is present for 1–3 months; IgG antibody is long lasting).

      **b. Hepatitis B ("serum" hepatitis)**

        **(1)** The standard marker for hepatitis B is the presence of surface antigen (HBsAg). The presence of antibodies directed against HBsAg usually indicates immunity.

        **(2)** IgG antibodies directed against hepatitis B core antigen (HBcAg) may indicate acute infection, chronic infection, or past infection. IgM antibodies against HBcAg are more indicative of acute infection.

      **c. Hepatitis C ("transfusion-related" hepatitis).** Both radioimmune and enzyme-linked assays for circulating viral antibodies to hepatitis C virus (HCV) have recently been developed.

        **(1)** Anti-HCV antibody is a marker for hepatitis C, not for immunity, and may be delayed in appearance for up to 6–12 months after infection.

**Table 10-3.** Comparison of Viral Hepatitis Types A, B, C, and D

| | Hepatitis A | Hepatitis B | Hepatitis C | Hepatitis D |
|---|---|---|---|---|
| **Virus** | RNA | DNA | RNA | Defective RNA* |
| **Age-group** | Primarily young | All ages | All ages | All ages |
| **Onset** | Abrupt | Insidious | Insidious | Insidious, fulminant |
| **Incubation** | 30–38 days | 41–180 days | 35–140 days | Variable† |
| **Transmission** | | | | |
| Feces | + | − | − | − |
| Semen | − | + | ? | + |
| Saliva | − | + | − | − |
| Transfusion | − | + | + | + |
| Needlestick | − | + | + | + |
| Drug abuse | − | + | + | + |
| Dialysis | − | + | + | + |
| Sexual contact | + | + | ? | + |
| Household contact | + | − | − | − |
| Mother-infant | − | + | + | + |
| Secondary cases | Common | Rare | Rare | Rare |
| **Symptoms** | | | | |
| Anorexia | Common | Common | Common | Common |
| Nausea, vomiting | Common | Common | Common | Uncommon |
| Fever | Common before jaundice | Uncommon | Uncommon | Uncommon |
| Jaundice | Uncommon in children | More common | Uncommon | More common |
| Rash, arthritis | Rare | Common | Rare | Rare |
| **Outcome** | | | | |
| Severity | Mild | Mild to severe | Intermediate | Mild to severe |
| Mortality | Low (< 1%) | Low (1%–3%) | Low (1%–3%) | Low to moderate |
| Chronic hepatitis | No | Yes (5%–10%) | Yes (30%–50%) | Yes |
| Chronic carrier | No | Yes | Yes | Yes |
| Liver cancer | No | Yes | Yes | ? |

*Replicates and causes hepatitis only in patients who concurrently are infected with hepatitis B virus (HBV).

†Incubation period typical of hepatitis B if infection with delta virus is simultaneous. Incubation period short (35 days) if hepatitis D is superimposed on chronic HBV carrier state.

      **(2)** Anti-HCV antibody persists in chronic hepatitis C but eventually disappears after recovery from acute hepatitis C.

   **d. Hepatitis D (delta hepatitis)**

      **(1)** Delta antigen in the serum is only briefly detectable (first 2 weeks of the disease). Antibodies to delta virus (anti-HDV) become detectable in more than 90% of cases within 3–8 weeks of acute hepatitis D.

      **(2)** The highest titers of anti-HDV (> 1:1000) are found in chronic hepatitis D.

  **2. Therapy.** No specific therapy exists for acute viral hepatitis. Strict bedrest is not necessary, but vigorous activity should be avoided.

  **3. Prognosis.** The prognosis is excellent for full recovery from nonfulminant hepatitis A. Ten percent of patients with hepatitis B develop chronic active or chronic persistent hepatitis.

  **4. Prevention**

    **a. Hepatitis A.** Family members, children and staff exposed at day-care centers, and sexual contacts should receive **immune globulin** (0.02 ml/kg) within 2 weeks of contact.

    **b. Hepatitis B**

      **(1) Hepatitis B immune globulin.** After sexual, percutaneous, or mucosal exposure, contacts should receive hepatitis B immune globulin (0.06 ml/kg). The dose should be repeated in 1 month.

**(2) Hepatitis B vaccine** is effective in infants as well as in older children and has few side effects. The vaccine is recommended for residents and staff of institutions for the retarded, family contacts of chronic carriers, and other high-risk populations including all health care workers engaged in patient care or in contact with laboratory specimens from patients, seronegative homosexual men, intravenous drug abusers, prisoners, dialysis patients, and recipients of high-risk blood products (e.g., hemophiliacs).

**(3) Prophylaxis in infants.** Infants of women who are serum HBsAg-positive in the third trimester of pregnancy—especially if they are also positive for hepatitis B e antigen (HBeAg), which is the marker for infectivity—should receive 0.5 ml of hepatitis B immune globulin and 0.5 ml of hepatitis B vaccine at birth, with doses of the vaccine repeated at 1 and 6 months of age. Infants of women in high-risk groups (Southeast Asian refugees) should receive hepatitis vaccine even if the serologic status of the mother is unknown at the time of delivery.

**(4) Postexposure prophylaxis.** Hepatitis B vaccine may soon be recommended for sexual contacts of HBsAg-positive individuals, those exposed to HBsAg-positive blood via needlestick exposure, and individuals infused with high-risk blood products. Accelerated induction of protective antibody levels may be facilitated by an accelerated vaccine schedule of injections at 0, 2, and 6 weeks postexposure.

**(5) Booster doses.** Antibodies to HBsAg that are generated by exposure to the vaccine diminish with time. Boosters are recommended at age 5 for those vaccinated in infancy. Adults who expect to be continuously exposed to hepatitis B should consider a booster 5–10 years after the initial series of innoculations.

**D. Fulminant hepatitis** is severe acute hepatitis resulting in progressive liver failure and hepatic encephalopathy.

**1. Etiology**
   **a. Viral infection.** Fulminant hepatitis may follow hepatitis A or hepatitis B, although this is rare. Non-A, non-B hepatitis may account for many of the "idiopathic" causes of fulminant disease. Delta hepatitis superimposed on chronic hepatitis B may convert a stable or chronic persistent hepatitis B patient to one with severe chronic active or even fulminant hepatitis.
   **b. Metabolic causes.** Tyrosinemia, galactosemia, and fructose intolerance in the neonate may lead to fulminant hepatitis; Wilson's disease may lead to this condition in the older child.
   **c. Hepatotoxic drugs** can cause fulminant hepatic failure via overdosage (e.g., acetaminophen) or an idiosyncratic, hypersensitivity reaction to a normal dose of the drug (e.g., halothane, phenytoin).
   **d. Plant toxins** also have been implicated (e.g., *Amanita phalloides* mushrooms).

**2. Clinical features**
   **a.** Early symptoms include persistent anorexia, progressive jaundice, and mental status changes.
   **b.** On sequential physical examinations, a shrinking liver size despite a worsening clinical status may be noted as well as hyperventilation and the development of ascites.
   **c.** Laboratory tests reflect hepatic failure, indicated by vitamin K–resistant coagulopathy, hypoglycemia, hypoalbuminemia, low blood urea nitrogen (BUN), low cholesterol, and high blood ammonia levels.
   **d.** Agitation, stupor, and eventually coma with diffuse slowing of activity on electroencephalogram (EEG) are seen.

**3. Complications**
   **a.** Gastrointestinal bleeding
   **b.** Secondary infection
   **c.** Renal dysfunction
   **d.** Increased intracranial pressure (ICP)

**4. Therapy.** The use of sedatives (especially benzodiazepines) and barbiturates should be avoided.
   **a. Supportive care** consists of:
      **(1)** Maintenance of fluid and electrolyte balance with correction of hyponatremia and hypokalemia
      **(2)** Correction of hypoglycemia and hypophosphatemia

(3) Use of fresh-frozen plasma to correct clotting abnormalities when there is clinical evidence of bleeding

(4) Endotracheal intubation and assisted ventilation as required by deepening coma

(5) Treatment of ICP, including ICP monitoring and the use of mannitol

**b. Measures to minimize encephalopathy.** Treatment involves measures to lower serum ammonia levels by decreasing protein available as substrate and eliminating ammonia-producing bacteria in the bowel, including:

(1) Restriction of oral and intravenous protein

(2) Use of cathartics

(3) Oral or nasogastric administration of neomycin or lactulose

**c. Heroic measures.** Interventions such as plasmapheresis, exchange transfusion, charcoal hemoperfusion, and dialysis alone have not improved survival rates. However, as adjunctive measures to stabilize and maintain a patient prior to liver transplantation, they appear to have a definite role.

**d. Liver transplantation.** Small series of patients (including children) with fulminant hepatic failure have been transplanted with a 50%–60% survival rate. This compares favorably with the 20%–40% survival rate previously obtained with intensive conservative management.

**E. Chronic hepatitis** can be defined as an inflammatory process of the liver lasting longer than 6 months. The distinction between chronic persistent and chronic active hepatitis is made pathologically.

**1. Chronic persistent hepatitis**

**a. Pathology.** The inflammatory reaction is limited to the portal zone, and there is little or no fibrosis.

**b. Etiology.** Chronic persistent hepatitis is usually due to persistent hepatitis B or non-A, non-B hepatitis.

**c. Clinical features.** Malaise or anorexia, which fails to resolve after a bout of acute hepatitis, is common. There may be mild hepatomegaly.

**d. Laboratory findings.** Usually the only abnormality is a mild elevation of the serum aminotransferase levels.

**e. Prognosis.** The prognosis for complete resolution without treatment is very good. Only rarely is there progression to chronic active hepatitis.

**2. Chronic active hepatitis**

**a. Pathology.** The inflammatory reaction is not limited to the portal area, and fibrosis may occur in areas of necrosis.

**b. Etiology.** In addition to viral infection, chronic active hepatitis may be caused by drugs or associated with Wilson's disease or inflammatory bowel disease. Some cases are idiopathic or ascribed to autoimmune mechanisms.

**c. Clinical features.** Almost all patients have jaundice and hepatosplenomegaly. Ascites, digital clubbing, cutaneous stigmata of chronic liver disease, and arthritis also may occur.

**d. Laboratory findings**

(1) The serum bilirubin level is elevated but is usually less than 5 mg/dl. The serum aminotransferase levels are typically elevated at least 10-fold. Of the plasma proteins, serum albumin is low and gamma globulin is elevated.

(2) About 25% of patients have detectable levels of serum HBsAg. Serum HBsAg-negative patients may have antinuclear antibodies (ANA), antismooth muscle antibodies, antiliver-kidney-microsomal antibodies, or other serologic evidence of autoimmune disease.

(3) Hypersplenism may result in anemia, leukopenia, and thrombocytopenia.

**e. Therapy and prognosis**

(1) Until recently, there was no effective therapy for HBsAg-positive patients with chronic hepatitis. Treatment with recombinant interferon alfa, either alone or following a brief course of prednisone, currently is under study and shows promising results.

(2) About 75% of HBsAg-negative patients have a biochemical response to prednisone or a combination of prednisone and azathioprine. The 5-year survival rate is approximately 70%.

(3) Liver transplantation may be necessary in patients who develop cirrhosis, with its attendant complications (e.g., portal hypertension, esophageal varices, ascites, liver failure).

**F. Metabolic liver disease.** The metabolic diseases affecting liver function are numerous and varied in presentation. For example, $\alpha_1$-antitrypsin deficiency can present in the neonatal period as cholestasis and in the older child as cirrhosis. The remainder of this section focuses on two metabolic liver diseases of particular importance to the pediatrician—$\alpha_1$-antitrypsin deficiency and Wilson's disease.

**1. $\alpha_1$-Antitrypsin deficiency**
   **a. Pathogenesis**
   **(1)** $\alpha_1$-Antitrypsin is a **serum protease inhibitor** synthesized in the liver. Codominant alleles dictate the type and concentration of $\alpha_1$-antitrypsin inherited.
   **(2)** Deficiency of $\alpha_1$-antitrypsin is due to homozygous inheritance of the z-type $\alpha_1$-antitrypsin gene. This results in low serum $\alpha_1$-antitrypsin levels and an abnormally slow-moving protein (PiZZ protein) on acid-starch electrophoresis when compared with the normal protein (PiMM).
   **(3)** Liver disease results from a defect in secretion of the PiZZ protein and accumulation of abnormal $\alpha_1$-antitrypsin in hepatocytes.
   **b. Clinical features**
   **(1)** About 5%–10% of PiZZ individuals develop neonatal cholestasis. Jaundice resolves in most cases. Occasionally, severe disease causes death in the first year of life. Breast-feeding in early infancy appears to confer some protection against liver damage due to inherent antiproteases in human breast milk.
   **(2)** Older infants and children may present with failure to thrive, hepatomegaly, or cirrhosis.
   **(3)** In the adolescent and adult, the deficiency may cause early pulmonary disease (emphysema).
   **c. Diagnosis**
   **(1)** There are low serum levels of $\alpha_1$-antitrypsin (usually less than 100 mg/dl) and an abnormal protein phenotype (PiZZ).
   **(2)** Liver biopsy shows characteristic eosinophilic cytoplasmic granules in periportal hepatocytes.

**2. Wilson's disease** (see also Ch 17 IX B 1) is a treatable autosomal recessive disorder that should be considered in the differential diagnosis of any liver disease in the school-age child.
   **a. Pathogenesis.** Organ damage is due to toxicity from copper deposition. Although levels of the copper-binding protein ceruloplasmin are low in 95% of patients, the exact mechanism underlying Wilson's disease is not known.
   **b. Clinical features.** Wilson's disease has many unusual modes of presentation, and there often is a delay in diagnosis.
   **(1) Liver disease** is the primary mode of presentation in the pediatric age-group. Liver disease rarely is clinically evident before age 5 years; the presentation may include an episode of acute hepatitis, fulminant hepatitis, chronic hepatitis, or cirrhosis.
   **(2) Neurologic symptoms** (e.g., tremor, dysarthria, loss of fine motor control, seizures) usually occur when the child is over 10 years of age. Personality changes may be striking.
   **(3)** Coombs'-negative **hemolytic anemia** occurs.
   **(4)** There is renal involvement, usually a **Fanconi-like syndrome**.
   **(5)** Corneal deposition of copper causes the formation of characteristic **Kayser-Fleischer rings**.
   **c. Diagnosis**
   **(1)** Kayser-Fleischer rings are pathognomonic when present (a slit lamp may be required to see them).
   **(2)** The ceruloplasmin level usually is low in Wilson's disease, but it may be low in other disorders as well. A level exceeding 30 mg/dl excludes Wilson's disease.
   **(3)** Patients with Wilson's disease have elevated urine copper excretion ($> 100$ μg/24 hr in symptomatic patients).
   **(4)** Quantification of liver copper by biopsy demonstrates levels greater than 250 μg/g dry weight.
   **(5)** Studies of incorporation of radioactive copper into ceruloplasmin occasionally are necessary if the above tests fail to distinguish Wilson's disease from other disorders with elevated concentrations of hepatic copper and urine copper excretion.
   **d. Therapy**
   **(1) Dietary restrictions.** Chocolate, nuts, shellfish, mushrooms, and other foods rich in copper should be avoided.

(2) **Life-long treatment with chelating agents** is necessary. Such agents include D-penicillamine, trientine (if penicillamine is not tolerated), and oral zinc (to reduce intestinal copper absorption and help maintain negative copper balance).

e. **Prognosis.** The prognosis is excellent with early treatment. However, fulminant hepatitis continues to be associated with a poor prognosis.

**G. Reye syndrome** is characterized by encephalopathy and acute liver dysfunction, with fatty infiltration of the liver and kidney in individuals who are usually between 3 months and 16 years of age. The incidence has dropped dramatically in the last 8 years corresponding to the association of the disease with **aspirin ingestion** and subsequent warnings.

1. **Etiology**
   a. Reye syndrome may follow a viral infection, typically influenza or varicella.
   b. Rarely, it has been associated with toxins, including aflatoxin $B_1$ (from a fungus) and hypoglycin A (from unripe akee fruit).

2. **Pathophysiology.** A basic defect in energy metabolism on a cellular level exists. Electron micrographs demonstrate a derangement of mitochondria.

3. **Clinical features**
   a. After an apparent viral illness, pernicious vomiting develops.
   b. Subsequently, mental status changes occur—confusion and agitation, then stupor and coma.
   c. Infants may have seizures or apneic episodes.

4. **Diagnosis**
   a. **Serum tests.** Serum aminotransferase levels always are elevated. Serum ammonia levels usually are elevated, and the prothrombin time is prolonged. The bilirubin is less than 3 mg/dl.
   b. **Liver biopsy** reveals microvesicular fat but no acute inflammatory reaction.
   c. **Differential diagnosis**
      (1) Other causes of central nervous system dysfunction (e.g., meningitis, toxic ingestion) must be excluded.
      (2) Inborn errors of metabolism, including urea cycle defects and defects in fatty acid oxidation, can be confused with Reye syndrome particularly in infants and young children.

5. **Therapy** for Reye syndrome is **supportive**. Increased ICP must be monitored and treated aggressively.

6. **Prognosis.** The overall fatality rate is approximately 20%. Rapid progression to deeper levels of coma and an ammonia level greater than 300 μg/dl imply a poor prognosis.

**H. Liver transplantation.** Orthotopic liver transplantation has become the accepted therapy for end-stage liver disease and metabolic liver disease in children. Well over 500 pediatric liver transplants were performed in the United States in the 1980s.

1. **Major indications** for liver transplantation in children include:
   a. Biliary atresia (particularly after an unsuccessful Kasai procedure)
   b. $\alpha_1$-Antitrypsin deficiency
   c. Tyrosinemia, Wilson's disease, and other inborn errors of metabolism
   d. Cryptogenic cirrhosis and chronic active hepatitis
   e. Fulminant hepatitis

2. **Postoperative management.** Chronic immunosuppression with cyclosporine, prednisone, and azathioprine is necessary to prevent rejection.

3. **Prognosis.** Five-year survival rates are approximately 70%.

4. **Long-term complications** of liver transplantation and chronic immunosuppression include:
   a. Nephrotoxicity and hypertension
   b. Susceptibility to infection, including viral (e.g., Epstein-Barr virus, cytomegalovirus), *Pneumocystis carinii*, bacterial, and fungal infections
   c. Biliary strictures, obstruction, or leak
   d. Predisposition to malignancy, especially lymphoma and lymphoproliferative syndromes
   e. Growth impairment if high doses of corticosteroids are required

## X. DISORDERS OF THE PANCREAS

### A. Pancreatic insufficiency

1. **Cystic fibrosis** is the major cause of pancreatic insufficiency in the United States, Canada, and western Europe. The general aspects of cystic fibrosis and its pulmonary complications are discussed in Chapter 12 IV. The following discussion focuses on pancreatic insufficiency and other gastrointestinal manifestations of cystic fibrosis.
   a. **Pancreatic disease due to cystic fibrosis**
      (1) **Pancreatic insufficiency.** Of patients with cystic fibrosis, 85%–90% have evidence of exocrine pancreatic dysfunction.
         (a) **Pathogenesis.** Abnormally viscid pancreatic secretions lead to plugging of ducts and eventual autodigestion of ducts and acinar tissue.
         (b) **Clinical features**
            (i) Malnutrition and failure to thrive may begin in the first few months of life.
            (ii) Steatorrhea occurs, and stools are bulky, foul-smelling, and pale and greasy in appearance.
            (iii) Complications due to malabsorption of fat-soluble vitamins or calcium may occur (e.g., hemorrhagic diathesis, rickets, neurologic abnormalities).
         (c) **Diagnosis** is made on the basis of the following:
            (i) Quantitative determination of fecal fat excretion
            (ii) Duodenal intubation and pancreozymin-secretin stimulation to assay enzymes and bicarbonate produced by the pancreas
            (iii) New tests using artificial substrates of pancreatic enzymes
         (d) **Therapy** consists of:
            (i) Pancreatic extracts given before meals to supplement enzyme activity
            (ii) A balanced but high-caloric diet
      (2) **Pancreatitis.** Recurrent pancreatitis may occur in some patients who retain some pancreatic exocrine function.
   b. **Other gastrointestinal and hepatic disorders associated with cystic fibrosis**
      (1) Meconium ileus presenting with neonatal intestinal obstruction due to abnormal meconium [see Ch 12 IV C 2 c (1)]
      (2) Intestinal impaction in older children
      (3) Intussusception
      (4) Rectal prolapse
      (5) Liver disease, including neonatal cholestatic syndrome, fatty liver, and focal biliary fibrosis (in older children), which may progress to biliary cirrhosis
      (6) Abnormal gallbladder function and cholelithiasis

2. **Other conditions associated with pancreatic insufficiency** include:
   a. **Malnutrition,** which is the most common cause of childhood pancreatic insufficiency worldwide.
   b. **Schwachman-Diamond syndrome** (pancreatic insufficiency and bone marrow dysfunction)
   c. **Isolated enzyme defects**

### B. Pancreatitis

1. **Etiology.** A variety of factors may lead to activation of pancreatic enzymes, causing autodigestion and inflammation of the pancreas. Such factors include:
   a. Abdominal trauma (or surgery)
   b. Infections (e.g., mumps and other viruses, mycoplasmas)
   c. Biliary obstruction
   d. Congenital anomalies of the pancreatic ducts (e.g., pancreas divisum)
   e. Drugs
   f. Systemic diseases (e.g., collagen vascular disease, hyperlipidemia, hypercalcemia)
   g. Cystic fibrosis
   h. Penetrating duodenal ulcer
   i. Unidentified factors (30% of cases are idiopathic, some of these factors may be familial)

2. **Clinical features**
   a. More than 75% of patients have epigastric pain, which may radiate to the back and is frequently exacerbated by eating.

    **b.** Nausea and vomiting are common.

    **c.** On examination, the abdomen is slightly distended and is tender on palpation. Bowel sounds are diminished.

    **d.** Severe cases may result in shock.

**3. Diagnosis**

    **a.** The serum amylase and lipase levels are elevated.

    **b.** Calculation of the amylase-creatinine clearance ratio may help distinguish pancreatitis from other causes of an elevated level of serum amylase.

    **c.** Abdominal ultrasound may demonstrate decreased density of the pancreas, but it is basically insensitive.

**4. Complications** include:

    **a.** Hypocalcemia

    **b.** Hyperglycemia

    **c.** Pseudocyst formation, which occurs in 5% of patients and is heralded by an epigastric mass and recurrent pain (pseudocysts are easily detected and monitored by ultrasound)

    **d.** Pancreatic phlegmon, with a potential for secondary bacterial infection and abscess formation

    **e.** Peritonitis

**5. Therapy** is aimed at minimizing pancreatic stimulation and includes:

    **a.** Nothing by mouth

    **b.** Nasogastric suction for all patients but those with the mildest cases

    **c.** Administration of adequate intravenous fluids and electrolytes with appropriate hemodynamic monitoring of patients with severe cases

    **d.** Meperidine for pain

    **e.** With recovery, gradual introduction of a high-carbohydrate, low-fat diet

    **f.** Surgical drainage, which eventually may be needed for pseudocysts

**6. Prognosis**

    **a.** Fulminant hemorrhagic pancreatitis has a high mortality rate.

    **b.** Episodes may recur if the cause is not identified and remedied.

## STUDY QUESTIONS

**Directions:** Each of the numbered items or incomplete statements in this section is followed by answers or by completions of the statement. Select the **one** lettered answer or completion that is **best** in each case.

1. All of the following individuals should receive the hepatitis B vaccine EXCEPT

(A) infants born to women who test positive for HBsAg
(B) patients with hemophilia
(C) patients requiring chronic hemodialysis
(D) children in a classroom with a child who is a hepatitis B carrier
(E) technicians working in a blood bank

2. Although the etiology is not precisely known, several pathophysiologic factors are believed to contribute to gastroesophageal reflux in neurologically normal children. Such factors include all of the following EXCEPT

(A) a chronically low resting LES pressure
(B) delayed gastric emptying
(C) relaxation of the LES at inappropriate times
(D) increased intragastric or intra-abdominal pressure during certain maneuvers
(E) abnormal esophageal peristalsis

3. The most important piece of historic information that may distinguish a child with Hirschsprung's disease from one with functional constipation is

(A) a pattern of defecation of less than 1 stool per week
(B) the presence of fecal soiling
(C) a history of infrequent bowel movements dating back to the first weeks of life
(D) a history of rectal prolapse
(E) a history of fecal impaction requiring enemas to relieve the obstruction

4. All of the following clinical findings are diagnostic of fulminant hepatic failure EXCEPT

(A) prolonged prothrombin time and partial thromboplastin time
(B) respiratory alkalosis
(C) serum aminotransferase levels more than 10 times normal
(D) mental status changes
(E) hyperammonemia

5. Characteristics of hepatitis D include all of the following EXCEPT

(A) it affects the same groups of individuals who are at high risk for hepatitis B
(B) it is the major cause of transfusion-related hepatitis
(C) it is caused by an RNA virus
(D) it may adversely affect the course of infection in a hepatitis B carrier
(E) the delta virus antigen rarely is detected because of its short life in the circulation

6. All of the following conditions are causes of acute pancreatitis in childhood EXCEPT

(A) abdominal trauma
(B) mumps
(C) cholelithiasis
(D) cystic fibrosis
(E) Schwachman-Diamond syndrome

7. A 16-year-old girl complains of frequent abdominal pain of 6 months duration. The pain usually is periumbilical, often is exacerbated by eating, and frequently is associated with nausea. All of the following conditions would be included in the differential diagnosis EXCEPT

(A) lactose intolerance
(B) peptic ulcer disease
(C) irritable bowel syndrome
(D) chronic pancreatitis
(E) Meckel's diverticulum

8. All of the following signs and symptoms are indicative of rotavirus infection in young children EXCEPT

(A) vomiting followed by watery diarrhea
(B) blood in the stool
(C) temperature above 38° C
(D) upper respiratory symptoms
(E) lactose malabsorption

| | | |
|---|---|---|
| 1-D | 4-C | 7-E |
| 2-A | 5-B | 8-B |
| 3-C | 6-E | |

9. Gastroesophageal reflux may give rise to all of the following conditions in a 4-month-old infant EXCEPT

(A) fever of unknown origin
(B) recurrent pulmonary infiltrates
(C) iron deficiency anemia
(D) the onset of asthma-like symptoms
(E) failure to thrive

**Directions:** Each item below contains four suggested answers of which **one or more** is correct. Choose the answer

A  if **1, 2, and 3** are correct
B  if **1 and 3** are correct
C  if **2 and 4** are correct
D  if **4** is correct
E  if **1, 2, 3, and 4** are correct

10. After a viral upper respiratory infection, a 1-year-old boy suddenly becomes irritable and draws his legs up to his abdomen as if in pain. After several minutes, the symptoms partially subside, although the child seems rather lethargic and is not interested in eating. When the child vomits and has another episode of pain, he is brought to the emergency ward by his parents. On arrival at the hospital, the mother notes that her child has passed a bloody stool. On physical examination, the child is indeed lethargic, and a sausage-like mass is palpable in the right upper quadrant. Conclusions that can be drawn from this history include

(1) if untreated, the child might develop necrotic bowel, and perforation and peritonitis could ensue
(2) most likely, this process is the result of an underlying defect in the bowel
(3) a carefully performed barium enema may be both diagnostic and therapeutic
(4) the cause of the patient's lethargy is probably unrelated to the abdominal process

11. A 5-week-old infant has developed persistent jaundice with pale stools. The direct fraction of the serum bilirubin is 4 mg/dl. An exhaustive evaluation has failed to identify a specific cause for the cholestasis. Which of the following tests would be most helpful in distinguishing between the two most common idiopathic causes of the cholestatic syndrome, which are neonatal hepatitis and biliary atresia?

(1) Measurement of serum aminotransferase levels
(2) Abdominal ultrasound
(3) Serum $\alpha$-fetoprotein determination
(4) Radionuclide biliary excretion study

9-A
10-B
11-C

**Directions:** Each group of items in this section consists of lettered options followed by a set of numbered items. For each item, select the **one** lettered option that is most closely associated with it. Each lettered option may be selected once, more than once, or not at all.

## Questions 12–16

Listed below are clinical features that are useful in the diagnosis of liver disease in the school-age child. For each clinical feature, select the diagnosis that is most appropriate.

(A) $\alpha_1$-Antitrypsin deficiency
(B) Wilson's disease
(C) Autoimmune chronic active hepatitis
(D) None of the above

12. Kayser-Fleischer rings on slit lamp examination

13. Eosinophilic cytoplasmic inclusions in hepatocytes on liver biopsy

14. Urine copper excretion greater than 100 μg/ 24 hr

15. ANA on serum evaluation

16. Abnormal protein phenotype (PiZZ) on serum evaluation

## Questions 17–21

Listed below are tests that are useful in the diagnosis of chronic diarrheal disorders. Match each test with the disorder for which it is indicated.

(A) Celiac disease
(B) Antibiotic-associated diarrhea
(C) Cystic fibrosis
(D) Ulcerative colitis
(E) Rotavirus infection

17. Stool *Clostridium difficile* toxin

18. Flexible sigmoidoscopy

19. Small intestinal biopsy

20. Sweat test

21. ELISA

| | | | |
|---|---|---|---|
| 12-B | 15-C | 18-D | 21-E |
| 13-A | 16-A | 19-A | |
| 14-B | 17-B | 20-C | |

## ANSWERS AND EXPLANATIONS

**1. The answer is D** *[IX C 4 b].*
Hepatitis B is spread only via contaminated blood products and sexual intercourse; thus, it is very unlikely that a child who is a carrier of hepatitis B will infect any of his classmates. Several studies have indicated that there is a very low infectivity rate of normal children in a classroom with a hepatitis B carrier, and so there is no current recommendation to vaccinate these children. Infants born to women who test positive for hepatitis B surface antigen (HBsAg), however, are at particularly high risk for acquiring hepatitis B, either at the time of birth or soon after. Thus, all infants born to mothers who are HBsAg-positive should receive hepatitis B vaccine. Patients with hemophilia who are multiply transfused with blood and clotting factor concentrates also are in a high-risk group, as are patients who are on chronic hemodialysis. Technicians working at a blood bank, as well as operating room personnel and emergency room personnel in hospitals, all should be vaccinated.

**2. The answer is A** *[II A 1].*
Lower esophageal sphincter (LES) pressure is measured via esophageal manometry. Such measurements in neurologically normal children with gastroesophageal reflux rarely show a low resting LES pressure. Currently, it is thought that relaxation of the LES at inappropriate times accounts for episodes of reflux in these children. Contributing factors include increased intragastric or intra-abdominal pressure and delayed gastric emptying. In addition, failure to clear acid from the distal esophagus secondary to abnormal esophageal peristalsis may play a role in perpetuating gastroesophageal reflux.

**3. The answer is C** *[VIII E 2].*
The most important piece of historic information suggesting Hirschsprung's disease is a history of constipation and infrequent bowel movements dating back to birth. Classically, children with Hirschsprung's disease do not have fecal soiling, in contrast to children with functional constipation and encopresis. Rectal prolapse is seen in approximately 3% of children with functional constipation. Fecal impaction is seen in both Hirschsprung's patients and patients with functional constipation and does not distinguish between the two conditions. Some children with functional constipation defecate extremely infrequently (less than 1 stool per week). It is extremely rare for a child with functional constipation to have had this problem in the first few weeks of life. Usually, functional constipation becomes a clinical problem after the first several months or even after the first year of life, when there is a change of diet to milk and table foods.

**4. The answer is C** *[IX D 2 c].*
Patients with fulminant hepatic failure can have extremely high serum aminotransferase levels (> 10,000 U/L), or they can have levels that are surprisingly low (as is true in children with fulminant hepatic failure associated with metabolic liver disease). Thus, the degree of serum aminotransferase elevation is not helpful in the diagnosis of fulminant hepatic failure. A decrease in the synthesis of clotting factors causes a prolongation of the prothrombin and partial thromboplastin times (PT and PTT). Early stages of hepatic encephalopathy are characterized by central hyperventilation and a respiratory alkalosis. Hepatic encephalopathy resulting in first irritability and then delirium, stupor, and coma is the sine qua non of hepatic failure. Hyperammonemia caused by the failure of the liver to metabolize ammonia to urea always is associated with hepatic failure.

**5. The answer is B** *[IX C 1; Table 10-3].*
The major cause of transfusion-related hepatitis in the United States is hepatitis C (non-A, non-B hepatitis). The virus that causes hepatitis D is a defective RNA virus: The virus can infect only cells that already are infected with hepatitis B. Hepatitis D has been implicated in the worsening of hepatitis B; it may convert a silent carrier of hepatitis B into a patient with chronic active disease or a patient with chronic active hepatitis into a patient with cirrhosis and hepatic failure. The incidence of fulminant hepatic failure is higher in patients with both hepatitis D and hepatitis B than in those with hepatitis B alone. Usually, only antibody to delta virus can be detected in the circulation, because the circulating antigen has a very short half-life.

**6. The answer is E** *[X A 2 b, B 1].*
Schwachman-Diamond syndrome is an important cause of pancreatic insufficiency, not acute pancreatitis. Cystic fibrosis also is an important cause of pancreatic insufficiency. However, early in the course of cystic fibrosis when some exocrine pancreatic function is still present, the viscous pancreatic secretions

may obstruct the pancreatic ducts, resulting in pancreatitis. Trauma and viral infections are frequent causes of pancreatitis in children. Although disease of the biliary tract, especially cholelithiasis, is a common factor in adults, it only rarely causes pancreatitis in children.

**7. The answer is E** *[VII A].*
A Meckel's diverticulum is associated with pain only on rare occasions. If the diverticulum acts as a lead point in an intussusception, acute, severe pain is observed. Rarely, diverticulitis may occur and may also lead to abdominal pain. Lactose intolerance, peptic ulcer disease, irritable bowel syndrome, and chronic pancreatitis all may be associated with chronic postprandial abdominal pain.

**8. The answer is B** *[V A 2 a].*
Since rotavirus infection is limited to the surface epithelial cells of the small intestine, rectal bleeding is never associated with it. Typically, the patient develops fever and vomiting, which are followed by watery diarrhea. Rhinorrhea, red tympanic membranes, and pharyngeal erythema are common. About 50% of children with rotavirus infection develop temporary lactose malabsorption.

**9. The answer is A** *[II A 2].*
Persistent gastroesophageal reflux can lead to a variety of complications, but fever is not a likely development. Recurrent aspiration of gastric contents may result in recurrent pulmonary infiltrates in a child with severe gastroesophageal reflux. Chronic esophagitis can lead to gastrointestinal blood loss and chronic iron deficiency anemia. It may also lead to decreased oral intake and failure to thrive secondary to dysphagia and anorexia. The onset of wheezing or "asthma" before age 6 months should suggest possible gastroesophageal reflux–induced bronchospasm. Most children with atopic disease resulting in bronchospasm or asthma do not have significant symptoms at such an early age.

**10. The answer is B (1, 3)** *[VII A 1, 3].*
This case history is classic for intussusception. In a child who is beyond the neonatal period but younger than 5 years of age, a preexisting intestinal lesion serving as a lead point is very unusual. The degree of lethargy at the time of presentation may be striking, even if complications have not occurred. With time, the blood supply to the obstructed bowel may become compromised, with resulting necrosis and perforation. A barium enema should demonstrate a coiled-spring appearance of the affected colon, and hydrostatic reduction under fluoroscopy can usually be accomplished. The presence of peritoneal signs, however, are an indication for immediate laparotomy.

**11. The answer is C (2, 4)** *[IX B 1 a, b].*
No serologic test reliably distinguishes between neonatal hepatitis and biliary atresia. The finding of a normal-sized gallbladder on ultrasound makes biliary atresia very unlikely. Excretion of radionuclide into the intestine excludes the diagnosis of biliary atresia. Frequently, however, liver biopsy or even exploratory laparotomy eventually is required to secure the diagnosis.

**12–16. The answers are: 12-B** *[IX F 2 c]*, **13-A** *[IX F 1 c]*, **14-B** *[IX F 2 c]*, **15-C** *[IX E 2 d]*, **16-A** *[IX F 1 c].*
Wilson's disease is characterized by a defect in copper metabolism. As a result, copper accumulates in various tissues, including the liver, brain, kidney, and cornea. Accumulation in Descemet's membrane of the cornea produces the Kayser-Fleischer ring, which is pathognomonic of Wilson's disease. Associated with Wilson's disease is a decrease in the serum concentration of the copper-binding protein, ceruloplasmin; a ceruloplasmin level of 30 mg/dl or more excludes the diagnosis. In untreated Wilson's disease, urinary excretion of copper is elevated, almost always to more than 100 $\mu$g/24 hr. Some elevation in copper excretion may also be observed in other chronic liver diseases.

$\alpha_1$-Antitrypsin is a serum glycoprotein that serves as a protease inhibitor. Deficiency of $\alpha_1$-antitrypsin is due to homozygous inheritance of the z-type $\alpha_1$-antitrypsin gene. This causes low $\alpha_1$-antitrypsin levels and the presence of an abnormally slow-moving protein (PiZZ protein) on acid-starch electrophoresis. In approximately 5%–10% of infants who are homozygous for deficiency of this protease inhibitor, clinical neonatal liver disease develops with some children going on to end-stage liver disease within the first decade of life. Liver biopsy reveals eosinophilic cytoplasmic inclusions, which represent $\alpha_1$-antitrypsin immunoreactive material.

Autoimmune chronic active hepatitis is characterized by the presence of antinuclear antibodies (ANA) and antismooth muscle antibodies in the serum.

**17–21. The answers are: 17-B** *[VI F 3]*, **18-D** *[VI E 2]*, **19-A** *[V B 1 a (3)]*, **20-C** *[X A 1; Ch 12 IV]*, **21-E** *[V A 2 a (4)].*
Antibiotic-associated diarrhea (pseudomembranous colitis) is common in pediatric patients and may oc-

cur in up to 10%–15% of children given certain antibiotics, particularly ampicillin. While generally self-limited, the diarrhea can be severe and prolonged and usually is associated with *Clostridium difficile* toxin. Ulcerative colitis always involves the rectum, which can be inspected easily and biopsied during flexible sigmoidoscopy. A diagnosis of celiac disease relies on small bowel biopsy evidence of severe villous atrophy and crypt hyperplasia in a patient on a gluten-containing diet. Cystic fibrosis is characterized by an elevation in sweat chloride (to more than 60 mEq/L), detected by sweat test. Enzyme-linked immunosorbent assay (ELISA) is used to detect rotavirus antigen in stool.

# 11
# Cardiovascular Diseases

Leon Chameides, Daniel J. Diana
Harris B. Leopold, Daniel A. Kveselis

## I. EVALUATION OF THE CARDIOVASCULAR SYSTEM

### A. History

1. **Cyanosis**
   a. Peripheral cyanosis (i.e., bluish discoloration around the mouth and over the eyelids but not of the mucous membranes) is normal in infants.
   b. Cyanosis of the mucous membranes is diagnostic of a right-to-left shunt; however, it may be subclinical and is sometimes present only with exertion.

2. **Other factors relevant to cardiac function** include shortness of breath, exercise intolerance, dyspnea on exertion, feeding difficulty in infants, and disturbances in growth.

3. **Familial disorders.** Some cardiovascular problems (e.g., hyperlipidemia, hypertension) may be familial.

4. **Chest pain** is common in the pediatric age-group, particularly in adolescents, but it **rarely is of cardiac origin**. Analysis of specific features (e.g., quality, distribution, relationship to level of activity) helps to distinguish anginal pain from pain due to more benign causes.

### B. Physical examination

1. **General observations**
   a. **Abnormal weight** as compared to normal growth curves may indicate the presence of cardiac disease.
   b. **Other important observations** include cyanosis and clubbing of the fingers and toes (which indicate a right-to-left shunt) and signs pointing to a syndrome or genetic disorder that includes congenital heart disease (Table 11-1).

2. **Pulses.** The presence and quality of peripheral pulses should be noted. It is important to palpate both brachial arteries simultaneously for timing and volume. If both are of equal volume, a brachial and femoral artery should be palpated simultaneously to rule out a coarctation of the aorta. The quality and timing of the femoral pulse should be noted; the pulse may appear delayed if the arteries are filled via collateral vessels.

3. **Blood pressure** should be measured over the brachial and popliteal arteries with a cuff that has a bladder approximately two-thirds the size of the extremity and that completely covers its circumference. The diastolic pressure is recorded at the disappearance of the Korotkoff sounds.

4. **Precordial palpation.** A thrill or "palpable murmur" defines an area of maximal turbulence.

5. **Cardiac auscultation**
   a. **Heart sounds**
      (1) The **first heart sound ($S_1$)** may be single or split.
      (2) The **second heart sound ($S_2$)** is split during inspiration; abnormally wide splitting occurs with right ventricular overload, right ventricular conduction delay, and prolonged right ventricular emptying (Table 11-2).
         (a) The **pulmonary component** of $S_2$ is accentuated in pulmonary hypertension.
         (b) The **aortic component** of $S_2$ is accentuated in systemic hypertension or if the aortic valve is close to the chest wall, as in transposition of the great arteries.

**Table 11-1.** Cardiovascular Manifestations of Selected Congenital Disorders

| Disorder | Cardiovascular Manifestation |
|---|---|
| Marfan syndrome | Aortic aneurysm, aortic valve insufficiency, mitral valve prolapse and regurgitation |
| Glycogen storage disease | Hypertrophic cardiomyopathy |
| Down syndrome | Endocardial cushion defect |
| Turner syndrome | Aortic coarctation |
| Noonan syndrome | Pulmonary valve stenosis, aortic valve stenosis |
| Williams syndrome | Supravalvular aortic stenosis |
| Trisomy 18 syndrome | Ventricular septal defect |
| Rubella syndrome | Patent ductus arteriosus |

  **(3)** A **third heart sound ($S_3$)** usually is normal in children but may represent a pathologic condition if associated with other abnormal findings.
  **(4)** A **fourth heart sound ($S_4$)** always is abnormal in children.
 **b. Clicks**
  **(1) Ejection clicks** occur shortly after $S_1$; they originate from the opening of a stenotic but mobile semilunar valve or from sudden distension of an enlarged or hypertensive pulmonary artery.
  **(2) Mid- or late-systolic clicks** indicate prolapse of the mitral or tricuspid valve.
 **c. Murmurs**
  **(1) Functional murmurs** (i.e., physiologic sounds of turbulence) are almost universally present at some time during childhood and often are characteristic of a particular age-group (Table 11-3; see also Ch 1 IV C 5 c).
  **(2) Pathologic murmurs** may occur during systole or diastole.
   **(a) Systolic murmurs**
    **(i)** Murmurs beginning with $S_1$ are called regurgitant murmurs. They are caused by insufficiency of and regurgitation through the atrioventricular (AV) valves or by left-to-right flow through a ventricular septal defect. Regurgitant murmurs that extend through systole are referred to as pansystolic, or holosystolic, murmurs.
    **(ii)** Murmurs beginning after isovolumic contraction are referred to as ejection murmurs; they coincide with the opening of the semilunar valves. Ejection murmurs are caused by aortic or pulmonary valve stenosis but may be functional.
    **(iii)** Murmurs also may begin late in systole. These murmurs are associated with mitral valve prolapse.
   **(b) Diastolic murmurs** beginning with $S_2$ are due to semilunar valve regurgitation; those beginning in mid-diastole are caused by impaired flow across the AV valves.

**C. Laboratory evaluation**

 **1. Chest x-ray** permits evaluation of heart size, status of the pulmonary vasculature (i.e., normal, diminished, or increased), and sites of cardiac structures and other viscera (see III).

 **2. Electrocardiography.** The electrocardiogram (ECG) permits diagnosis of cardiac dysrhythmias; it also reflects anatomic changes (e.g., ventricular or atrial hypertrophy) that develop in patients with cardiac disease and indicates the presence of myocardial ischemia.

 **3. Echocardiography** permits systematic evaluation of cardiac structure and function; flow can be evaluated by means of Doppler ultrasonography and by color flow mapping.

**Table 11-2.** Evaluation of Abnormally Wide Splitting of $S_2$

| Mechanism | Diagnosis |
|---|---|
| Increased right ventricular pressure | Pulmonary valve stenosis |
| Increased right ventricular volume | Atrial septal defect, anomalous pulmonary venous return, pulmonary valve regurgitation, ventricular septal defect |
| Right ventricular conduction delay | Right bundle branch block |
| Premature left ventricular emptying | Mitral valve regurgitation, ventricular septal defect |

**Table 11-3.** Functional Murmurs

| Murmur | Approximate Age | Timing | Origin |
|---|---|---|---|
| Peripheral pulmonary stenosis (PPS) | Newborn | Systolic ejection | Bifurcation of pulmonary artery |
| Vibratory (Still's) | 3–8 years | Systolic ejection | Unknown |
| Carotid bruit | 3–8 years | Systolic ejection | Carotid artery |
| Venous hum | 3–8 years | Continuous | Jugular vein and superior vena cava |
| Pulmonary flow | 6–18 years | Systolic ejection | Pulmonary valve |

   4. **Cardiac catheterization** allows measurement of intracardiac and intravascular pressures and determination of pressure gradients across the cardiac valves.
      a. **Blood analysis of oxygen content and saturation** permits detection of the presence and size of left-to-right and right-to-left shunts; cardiac output and systemic and pulmonary vascular resistances can also be calculated.
      b. **Selective angiography** permits the visualization of cardiac and vascular anatomy. In certain situations, therapeutic intervention with the catheter is possible.

## II. FETAL AND NEONATAL CIRCULATION. Patency of three structures—the foramen ovale, ductus arteriosus and ductus venosus—distinguishes the cardiovascular anatomy of the fetus.

   **A. Normal physiology** (see also Ch 5 I B 1 a)

   1. **Fetal circulation**
      a. Fetal blood is oxygenated in the **placenta** and then enters the umbilical vein.
         (1) One portion of the oxygenated blood perfuses the liver and proceeds to the inferior vena cava via the hepatic veins.
         (2) Another portion enters the ductus venosus, which empties directly into the inferior vena cava.
      b. Together with venous return from the lower part of the body, this blood flows into the **right atrium**.
         (1) Two-thirds is shunted, via the foramen ovale, to the left atrium, left ventricle, and ascending aorta.
         (2) The remainder joins the venous return from the upper part of the body and enters the right ventricle and pulmonary artery. A small portion (< 10%) of this blood enters the lungs, and the remainder, because of high pulmonary vascular resistance and low systemic vascular resistance, crosses the ductus arteriosus to the descending aorta.

   2. **Transition to neonatal circulation**
      a. At birth, the infant's first breaths cause an increase in arterial oxygen tension ($Po_2$); this lowers pulmonary vascular resistance, resulting in increased pulmonary blood flow. The increased pulmonary venous return to the left atrium causes the pressure to rise, resulting in functional **closure of the foramen ovale**.
      b. Systemic vascular resistance is increased by the elimination of the low-resistance vascular circuit of the placenta at birth.
      c. **Closure of the ductus arteriosus** occurs shortly after birth, first functionally and then anatomically.
      d. The neonatal circulation, with the ventricles working in series, thus is established.

   3. **Normal changes in pulmonary vascular resistance.** Pulmonary vascular resistance is inversely related to the diameter of the small pulmonary arterioles.
      a. In the fetus, high pulmonary vascular resistance is maintained by constriction of the muscular tunica media of these arterioles.
      b. The arterioles begin to dilate after birth, and the tunica media gradually atrophies. (In the average adult, cardiac output can increase fourfold without affecting pulmonary artery pressure.)

   **B. Abnormalities of the pulmonary circulation**

   1. **Persistence of the fetal circulation.** Pulmonary vascular resistance can remain high after birth if constriction of the arteriolar lumina by a pathologic process occurs (e.g., due to hypoxemia, acidosis, or some unidentified factor). The resultant pulmonary hypertension leads to right-to-left shunting at the ductus or foramen ovale.

**2. Other arteriolar abnormalities**

**a. Anatomic changes.** If stimuli to pulmonary arteriolar constriction, such as pulmonary or venous hypertension, continue into infancy, the media remains thickened instead of atrophying with age. Progressive pathologic changes may develop in a small number of infants and children, including cellular intimal proliferation, fibrosis of the intima and media, angioma formation, and arteriolitis.

**b. Physiologic changes.** A rise in pulmonary vascular resistance causes a diminution in left-to-right shunting (e.g., through a patent ductus or ventricular septal defect) and then, as pulmonary vascular resistance surpasses systemic resistance, a reversal of the shunt. Once fibrosis of the arterioles occurs, the process is irreversible. The combination of an irreversibly high pulmonary vascular resistance (culminating in pulmonary vascular obstructive disease) and a right-to-left shunt is known as the **Eisenmenger reaction**.

## III. POSITION OF CARDIAC STRUCTURES

### A. Cardiac situs

**1.** In **levocardia,** the apex of the heart points to the left, as is normal. In the presence of viscerocardiac discordance (i.e., transposition of other viscera), the likelihood of congenital heart disease is high.

**2.** In **dextrocardia,** the apex of the heart points to the right. There can be viscerocardiac concordance (i.e., a mirror-image arrangement) or discordance (i.e., dextrocardia with situs solitus).

### B. Viscera and atria (Figure 11-1)

**1.** In **situs solitus** (i.e., the normal situs), the liver is on the right and the stomach is on the left. The right atrium usually is on the same side as the liver.

**2.** In **situs inversus,** there is a mirror-image transposition of the abdominal organs: the liver is on the left and the stomach on the right. The right atrium usually is located on the left.

**3.** In **ambiguous situs,** the visceral situs is uncertain; the liver is midline without a dominant lobe. This often is associated with asplenia or polysplenia and severe congenital cardiac abnormalities.

**C. Ventricles** (Figure 11-2). In the embryonic formation of the heart, the cardiac tube usually loops to the right (**dextro-,** or **D-**), so that the right ventricle, derived from the bulbus cordis, develops to the right of the left ventricle. If the tube loops to the left (**levo-,** or **L-**), ventricular inversion results. Position of the ventricles is best evaluated by angiography.

**D. Great arteries** (Figure 11-3). The pulmonary valve normally is anterior to and to the left of the aortic valve. In each of the ventricular loops (**D-** OR **L-**), the great artery relationships can be normal (i.e., solitus with **D**-ventricular loops or inversus with **L**-ventricular loops) or transposed (i.e., the aortic valve is anterior).

**1.** In a **D**-ventricular loop with **D**-transposition of the great arteries, the aortic valve is anterior to and to the right of the pulmonary valve.

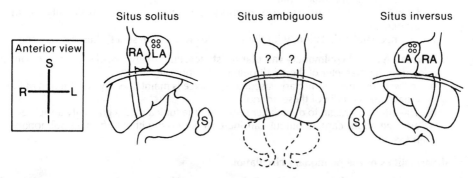

**Figure 11-1.** Visceroatrial situs. *S* = superior; *I* = inferior; *R* = right; *L* = left; *RA* = right atrium; *LA* = left atrium; *S* = spleen. (Adapted from Paul MH: Transposition of the great arteries. In: *Heart Disease in Infants, Children, and Adolescents.* Edited by Moss AJ, Adams FH. Baltimore, Williams & Wilkins, p 529, 1968.)

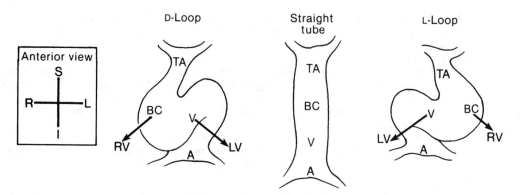

**Figure 11-2.** Cardiac looking. *S* = superior; *I* = inferior; *R* = right; *L* = left; *TA* = truncus arteriosus; *BC* = bulbus cordis; *V* = ventricle; *A* = atrium; *RV* = right ventricle; *LV* = left ventricle. (Adapted from Paul MH: Transposition of the great arteries. In: *Heart Disease in Infants, Children, and Adolescents.* Edited by Moss AJ, Adams FH. Baltimore, Williams & Wilkins, p 529, 1968.)

2. In an L-ventricular loop (ventricular inversion) with L-transposition of the great arteries, the aortic valve is anterior to and to the left of the pulmonary valve.

3. The concordance between great artery transposition and ventricular looping is approximately 90%; a D- great artery transposition almost always is associated with a D-ventricular loop.

**E. Notation.** Codes can be used to describe the various configurations of the cardiac structures. For example, **SDD** denotes situs solitus (the right atrium probably is on the right), a D-ventricular loop (the right ventricle is on the right), and a D-transposition of the great arteries (the aorta and pulmonary artery are transposed, with the aortic valve anterior to and to the right of the pulmonary valve).

## IV. CONGENITAL STRUCTURAL DISORDERS

### A. General considerations

#### 1. Etiologic considerations

a. The cause of congenital heart disease is usually unknown in individual cases; evidence points to a **multifactorial etiology,** with the insult probably occurring in the first 8 weeks gestation.

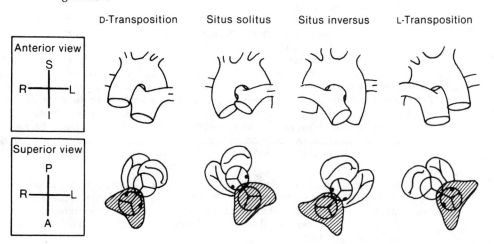

**Figure 11-3.** Relationships between the great arteries and the semilunar (i.e., aortic and pulmonary) and atrioventricular (i.e., mitral and tricuspid) valves. *Crosshatching* indicates distal conal myocardium. *S* = superior; *I* = inferior; *R* = right; *L* = left; *P* = posterior; *A* = anterior. (Adapted from Paul MH: Transposition of the great arteries. In: *Heart Disease in Infants, Children, and Adolescents.* Edited by Moss AJ, Adams FH. Baltimore, Williams & Wilkins, p 529, 1968.)

     **b.** Most congenital heart lesions are **sporadic**. However, their incidence is slightly higher in families that include one member with such an abnormality; there are families with several affected members.

     **c.** Congenital heart disease has been associated with several different **teratogenic factors**.

          **(1) Medications** that are known or suspected cardiovascular teratogens include thalidomide, folic acid antagonists, dextroamphetamine, anticonvulsants, lithium, and estrogens.

          **(2) Excessive maternal alcohol ingestion** has been associated with the development of congenital heart defects.

          **(3) Maternal infection.** Antenatal **rubella** has proven to be teratogenic. There is also evidence that maternal **cytomegalovirus** and **coxsackievirus infections** may cause congenital cardiovascular abnormalities.

  **2. Clinical considerations**

     **a.** Congenital heart disease is a **component of several syndromes** (see Table 11-1; see also Ch 7 I D 2, 3).

     **b.** Children with turbulent cardiac abnormalities are susceptible to the **development of endocarditis** whenever transient bacteremia is likely (e.g., with dental procedures or with surgery involving the respiratory, gastrointestinal, or genitourinary tract).

**B. Atrial septal defect (ASD)**

  **1. Description.** ASD (persistent patency of the interatrial septum) can occur high in the septum (**sinus venosus defect**), in the midportion (**ostium secundum defect**), and low in the septum primum (**ostium primum defect, or partial endocardial cushion defect**). The right ventricle and the pulmonary artery usually are enlarged.

  **2. Pathophysiology.** Greater right than left ventricular compliance and low pulmonary vascular resistance result in a left-to-right shunt at the atrial level, thus increasing flow across the tricuspid and pulmonary valves.

  **3. Clinical features.** Childhood ASD usually is not associated with symptoms. Occasionally, there is a history of slow weight gain and frequent lower respiratory infections.

  **4. Diagnosis**

     **a. Physical examination.** The precordium is hyperdynamic, and a right ventricular heave is present. A systolic ejection murmur in the pulmonic area and a mid-diastolic rumble in the lower right sternal area reflect the increased flow across the pulmonary and tricuspid valves. $S_2$ is widely and constantly split.

     **b. Laboratory evaluation**

          **(1) Chest x-ray.** The heart and main pulmonary artery segment are enlarged; pulmonary vascularity is increased.

          **(2) ECG.** Right-axis deviation often is seen in secundum defects. The hallmark of a primum defect is an extreme left-axis deviation. Right ventricular hypertrophy is represented by an rsR′ in the right precordial leads.

          **(3) Echocardiogram.** The right ventricle is enlarged, and the septum often moves in a paradoxical fashion. The defect usually can be visualized on a two-dimensional study. Color flow mapping demonstrates the direction of flow and AV valve competence.

          **(4) Cardiac catheterization.** The presence and size of a left-to-right shunt are indicated by an increase in oxygen saturation at the atrial level. Pressure in the pulmonary artery is normal or slightly elevated, and a flow-pressure gradient may be present across the pulmonary valve. Severe pulmonary hypertension is rare in children. Mitral regurgitation often is found in ostium primum defects.

  **5. Therapy**

     **a. Medical management.** Bacterial endocarditis prophylaxis is not necessary in secundum defects but is indicated in primum defects if mitral valve regurgitation is present.

     **b. Surgical closure** of both a secundum and a primum defect can be accomplished with minimal risk. Selected secundum atrial defects are being closed experimentally with a device in the catheterization laboratory.

**C. Ventricular septal defect (VSD)**

  **1. Description.** VSD (persistent patency of the interventricular septum) is the most common congenital heart disorder, accounting for 26% of all congenital cardiac lesions. A VSD may be single or multiple and may be found anywhere along the septum; it is most common in the membranomuscular portion.

**2. Pathophysiology**
   **a.** In small defects, the size of the shunt is determined by resistance at the defect; small defects result in small shunts. If the defect is large, both the size and direction of the shunt are determined by the relative resistances in the pulmonary and systemic circuits.
   **b.** As long as pulmonary vascular resistance is lower than systemic resistance, the shunt is left-to-right. If pulmonary vascular resistance rises above systemic resistance, the shunt reverses.
   **c.** Large defects tend to result in pulmonary hypertension, whereas in small defects pulmonary vascular dynamics remain normal.
   **d.** The sizes of the left atrium and left ventricle are directly proportional to the size of the left-to-right shunt. Right ventricular enlargement occurs when pulmonary vascular resistance increases.
   **e.** Pulmonary hypertension may lead to the development of pulmonary vascular obstructive disease (Eisenmenger reaction) and reversal of the shunt.

**3. Clinical features.** Symptoms are related to the size of the shunt.
   **a.** If the defect is small, no symptoms are present.
   **b.** If the defect is large and pulmonary vascular resistance is not significantly elevated (as in a large left-to-right shunt), growth failure, congestive heart failure, and repeated lower respiratory infections may occur.
   **c.** If the defect is large and pulmonary vascular resistance is very high (i.e., Eisenmenger reaction), shortness of breath, dyspnea on exertion, chest pain, and cyanosis may occur.

**4. Diagnosis**
   **a. Physical examination**
      **(1)** A left-to-right shunt produces turbulence during isovolumic contraction, and the murmur begins with $S_1$. The murmur usually is harsh and is best heard at the midsternal or lower left sternal border; it ends in midsystole in small defects and extends to $S_2$ in large left-to-right shunts. In the latter, a mid-diastolic rumble of relative mitral stenosis also is heard.
      **(2)** As pulmonary vascular resistance increases, the diastolic murmur disappears, the systolic murmur becomes shorter, and the pulmonary component of $S_2$ increases in intensity.
      **(3)** In the presence of pulmonary vascular obstructive disease, a right ventricular heave, ejection click, short systolic ejection murmur, diastolic murmur of pulmonary valve insufficiency, and loud $S_2$ are heard.
   **b. Laboratory evaluation**
      **(1) Chest x-ray**
         **(a)** In small defects, the chest x-ray may be normal or show mild cardiomegaly and a slight increase in pulmonary vascularity.
         **(b)** In large left-to-right shunts, cardiomegaly, increased pulmonary vascularity, and enlargement of the left atrium and ventricle are seen. As a rule, the size of the heart is proportional to the magnitude of the left-to-right shunt. As pulmonary vascular resistance rises and the left-to-right shunt decreases, the heart and the distal pulmonary arteries become smaller but the proximal pulmonary arteries enlarge.
      **(2) ECG**
         **(a)** In small defects, the ECG is normal.
         **(b)** In large left-to-right shunts, left atrial, left ventricular, or biventricular hypertrophy is seen. Right ventricular hypertrophy predominates when pulmonary vascular resistance is high.
      **(3) Echocardiogram.** Chamber size can be determined and moderate to large defects can be identified with a two-dimensional study. Doppler ultrasonography and color flow mapping can localize defects that are too small for two-dimensional resolution.
      **(4) Cardiac catheterization.** Measurement of intracardiac and intravascular oxygen content can define the degree and direction of shunting. Pulmonary arterial pressure can be measured and pulmonary and systemic vascular resistances calculated. Left ventricular angiography defines the interventricular septum and can show the size as well as the number of defects.

**5. Therapy**
   **a. Medical management.** Bacterial endocarditis prophylaxis is indicated. Congestive heart failure is treated.
   **b. Surgical management.** A large VSD should be repaired before pulmonary vascular changes become irreversible. Small defects do not require surgical repair.

## D. Patent ductus arteriosus (PDA)

1. **Description.** The ductus arteriosus connects the pulmonary artery and descending aorta; it varies in size. The left atrium and left ventricle are enlarged in direct proportion to the magnitude of the left-to-right shunt. The right ventricle is enlarged only in the presence of pulmonary hypertension.

2. **Pathophysiology**
   a. The **direction of flow** through a large PDA depends on the relative resistances in the pulmonary and systemic circuits. As long as the former is lower than the latter, a left-to-right shunt is present. If pulmonary resistance rises above systemic resistance, a right-to-left shunt develops. In small PDA, the size of the ductus limits the left-to-right shunt.
   b. The **size of the shunt** depends on the size of the PDA and the relative resistances in the two circuits. If the PDA is large, pulmonary vascular obstructive disease (Eisenmenger reaction) may develop.

3. **Clinical features.** Symptoms are related to the size of the defect and the direction of flow. A small PDA causes no symptoms. A large one with a large left-to-right shunt may result in congestive heart failure, slowed growth, and repeated lower respiratory tract infections. Reversal of flow as a result of high pulmonary vascular resistance causes shortness of breath, dyspnea on exertion, and cyanosis.

4. **Diagnosis**
   a. **Physical examination**
      (1) Pulse volume is related to the volume of the left-to-right shunt. If the flow is small, pulses are normal. In a large shunt, bounding pulses, representing an aortic diastolic runoff, are palpated.
      (2) The murmur is continuous: It begins after $S_1$, peaks with $S_2$, and trails off in diastole. If pulmonary vascular resistance rises, first the diastolic murmur and subsequently the systolic murmur become softer and shorter, and $S_2$ increases in intensity.
   b. **Laboratory evaluation**
      (1) **Chest x-ray.** Heart size, pulmonary vascularity, and left atrial and left ventricular size all are directly related to the magnitude of the left-to-right shunt. In a small PDA, the x-ray may be normal. If the PDA and left-to-right shunt are large, cardiomegaly and left heart enlargement are pronounced.
      (2) **ECG.** The ECG is normal if the PDA is small. Left ventricular or biventricular hypertrophy is seen if the left-to-right shunt is large. Right ventricular hypertrophy predominates in the presence of increased pulmonary vascular resistance.
      (3) **Echocardiogram.** The PDA sometimes can be visualized on a two-dimensional study. Doppler ultrasonography shows diastolic turbulence in the pulmonary artery and diastolic runoff in the aorta. Color flow mapping will demonstrate the direction of the flow. If the shunt is large, the left atrium and ventricle are enlarged.
      (4) **Cardiac catheterization.** A step-up in pulmonary arterial oxygen saturation may be seen, and the PDA often can be traversed with the catheter. Angiography with selective injection in the descending aorta shows the ductal anatomy well.

5. **Therapy**
   a. **Medical management.** Bacterial endocarditis prophylaxis is necessary as long as the ductus remains patent. Indomethacin often is effective in closing a PDA in the premature infant.
   b. **Surgical management.** Division or ligation of the ductus is curative. On an experimental basis, ductal closure may be achieved in the catheterization laboratory and in selected cases may become the preferred method of therapy in the future.

## E. Ductus-dependent lesions are those abnormalities involving either systemic or pulmonary blood flow dependence on patency of the ductus arteriosus

1. **Lesions involving systemic flow dependence**
   a. **Hypoplastic left-heart syndrome**
      (1) **Description.** This syndrome is a continuum of anomalies that are characterized by underdevelopment of the aortic root, aortic valve, left ventricle, and mitral valve. The aortic valve usually is atretic; mitral atresia also is possible. The ascending aorta often measures only a few millimeters, and a coarctation often is present. The right atrium and right ventricle usually are dilated.

**(2) Pathophysiology.** Since there is no antegrade aortic flow, systemic flow is ductus dependent. Systemic and pulmonary venous return mix at the atrial level (i.e., there is an obligatory left-to-right atrial shunt). Because pulmonary vascular resistance is high, flow is directed through the ductus to the aorta, with retrograde coronary artery perfusion.

**(3) Clinical features** usually are evident in the first few days of life; symptoms of severe congestive heart failure and vascular collapse occur as the ductus arteriosus closes.

**(4) Diagnosis**

    **(a) Physical examination.** Poor systemic perfusion is characterized by mottling of the skin. Pulses are poor or totally absent, and tachypnea, dyspnea, grunting, and agonal respirations may be present. Hepatomegaly, diffuse rales, a gallop rhythm with a loud $S_2$, and a nonspecific systolic murmur are additional findings.

    **(b) Laboratory evaluation**

        **(i) Chest x-ray** shows cardiomegaly, often with pulmonary congestion or edema.

        **(ii) ECG** often is normal for age.

        **(iii) Echocardiogram** is diagnostic; it defines the configuration and size of the various structures. Doppler ultrasonography and color flow mapping define the direction of blood flow.

**(5) Therapy**

    **(a) Medical management** is palliative, directed at preserving systemic perfusion [prostaglandin $E_1$ ($PGE_1$) is infused to maintain patency of the ductus], providing ventilatory support, and correcting acidosis.

    **(b) Surgical management.** Corrective surgery is not feasible.

        **(i)** The **Norwood procedure** has allowed some children to survive infancy. The first stage involves anastomosis of the main pulmonary artery to the hypoplastic aorta, ligation of the distal main pulmonary artery, creation of a shunt between a systemic and pulmonary artery, and creation of an ASD. The second stage involves a modified Fontan operation.

        **(ii)** Another proposed alternative is neonatal cardiac transplantation.

**b. Complex coarctation syndromes**

    **(1) Description.** The constriction of the aorta almost invariably is located at the junction of the ductus arteriosus with the aortic arch, just distal to the subclavian artery. The constriction may be discrete or diffuse and usually is associated with isthmic narrowing and a contraductal shelf.

        **(a)** Complex coarctation syndromes often are symptomatic in infancy, owing to the high frequency of associated anomalies (e.g., PDA in 66% of cases, VSD in 30% of cases).

        **(b)** Isolated (simple) coarctation (see IV I) often is asymptomatic in infancy.

    **(2) Pathophysiology.** As the ductus constricts in the neonatal period, obstruction increases at the coarctation site, leading to increased left ventricular afterload with subsequent left ventricular dysfunction, pulmonary hypertension, and congestive heart failure. If the coarctation is very severe and there has been insufficient time for the development of collateral vessels, blood flow to sites distal to the coarctation is markedly decreased.

    **(3) Clinical features.** Symptoms, if present in infancy, are those of low cardiac output and congestive heart failure (e.g., irritability, lethargy, poor feeding, inadequate growth).

    **(4) Diagnosis**

        **(a) Physical examination** reveals signs of low cardiac output and poor perfusion. Findings include ashen color, skin mottling, decreased or absent lower extremity pulses, gallop rhythm, single loud $S_2$, a nonspecific and often low-pitched systolic murmur, and hepatomegaly. Differential cyanosis in the presence of a patent ductus may be difficult to recognize.

        **(b) Laboratory evaluation**

            **(i) Chest x-ray** in the symptomatic infant shows cardiomegaly and pulmonary congestion.

            **(ii) ECG** often shows right ventricular hypertrophy with strain.

            **(iii) Echocardiogram** is useful in localizing and visualizing the coarctation and any associated anomalies. Doppler ultrasonography allows estimation of a pressure gradient.

            **(iv) Cardiac catheterization** with angiography allows further definition of the lesions.

**(5) Therapy**
  **(a) Medical management.** In the newborn with shock, therapy is directed at unloading the left ventricle and improving systemic flow by administering $PGE_1$ to dilate the ductus arteriosus. In addition, inotropic agents are given to improve left ventricular function, diuretics are given to decrease preload, and acidosis is treated.
  **(b) Surgical management.** Obstruction usually can be relieved surgically (see IV I 5 b).
  **c. Critical aortic stenosis**
    **(1) Description.** Isolated aortic valvular stenosis rarely causes symptoms in infancy but, if critical, can lead to profound and intractable congestive heart failure. The aortic valvular tissue is rigid and thickened with varying degrees of commissural fusion. The valve most often is bicuspid but may be unicuspid with an eccentric small opening. Annular hypoplasia almost always is present in the neonatal period; often, left ventricular hypoplasia and endocardial fibroelastosis also are found.
    **(2) Pathophysiology.** The small opening increases left ventricular afterload and end-diastolic pressure. Decreased myocardial perfusion during diastole may result in myocardial ischemia and consequent dysfunction.
    **(3) Clinical features.** Symptoms are those of low cardiac output and congestive heart failure and include lethargy, irritability, poor feeding, and varying degrees of respiratory failure.
    **(4) Diagnosis**
      **(a) Physical examination.** Infants have poor skin perfusion, indicated by mottling and ashen color. Peripheral pulses are weak or absent. Auscultation may reveal an ejection click and a systolic ejection murmur, but these may be absent if cardiac output is sufficiently depressed. The liver is enlarged, and there are signs of pulmonary venous congestion (e.g., tachypnea, dyspnea, rales).
      **(b) Laboratory evaluation**
        **(i) Chest x-ray** findings are nonspecific and include cardiomegaly and pulmonary congestion.
        **(ii) ECG** may show right ventricular hypertrophy and, occasionally, left ventricular hypertrophy. Evidence of myocardial ischemia may be present.
        **(iii) Echocardiogram** is diagnostic. The site of the lesion, the degree of obstruction, and the size and function of the left ventricle can be determined.
        **(iv)** At **cardiac catheterization,** the pressure gradient can be measured, but the low output causes underestimation of the degree of obstruction. The major benefit of angiography is the definition of associated arch anomalies.
    **(5) Therapy**
      **(a) Medical management.** Hemodynamic stabilization is attempted with inotropic agents and diuretics. Acid-base imbalances are corrected and ventilatory problems treated. Reopening of the ductus arteriosus by $PGE_1$ infusion may be beneficial.
      **(b) Surgical management.** Aortic valvotomy under direct vision can be performed, although it is associated with a high mortality rate. Balloon angioplasty is being attempted, but experience to date is limited.

**2. Lesions involving pulmonary flow dependence**
  **a. Hypoplastic right-heart syndromes**
    **(1) Description of types**
      **(a) Pulmonary atresia with intact ventricular septum** is a relatively rare anomaly.
        **(i)** In 80% of cases, the pulmonary valve alone is involved and forms an imperforate membrane. In 20% of cases, there is associated infundibular hypoplasia.
        **(ii)** Right ventricular development is variable, ranging from normal (10% of cases) to extremely hypoplastic (50% of cases).
        **(iii)** A patent foramen ovale or true ASD also is present.
      **(b) Tricuspid atresia** is a rare anomaly characterized by atresia of the tricuspid orifice (which often is identifiable only as a dimple), accompanied by a patent foramen ovale or true ASD. Three major types are:
        **(i)** Atresia with normally related great arteries and with or without VSD (70% of cases)
        **(ii)** Atresia with D-transposition of the great arteries and VSD (23%)
        **(iii)** Atresia with L-transposition of the great arteries (7%)

**(2) Pathophysiology.** In both pulmonary atresia with intact ventricular septum and tricuspid atresia, a right-to-left atrial shunt is obligatory, with mixing of systemic and pulmonary venous return. Pulmonary blood flow is dependent on a PDA and—in tricuspid atresia—on the size of the VSD (if present) and associated ventricular outflow obstruction.

**(3) Clinical features.** Severe cyanosis is present in the neonatal period.

**(4) Diagnosis**

    **(a) Physical examination.** Cyanosis usually is present.

        **(i)** In **pulmonary atresia** with intact ventricular septum, a single $S_2$ is present, and a continuous murmur of a PDA and/or a regurgitant murmur of tricuspid insufficiency may be heard.

        **(ii)** Findings in **tricuspid atresia** are more variable and depend on the size of the VSD and on pulmonary blood flow. If pulmonary blood flow is minimal, the VSD is very small, or associated pulmonary atresia is present, the findings may be identical to those in pulmonary atresia with intact ventricular septum. If the VSD is large and pulmonary blood flow is increased, signs of congestive heart failure and a harsh VSD murmur prevail.

    **(b) Laboratory evaluation**

        **(i) Chest x-ray** shows a variable heart size—although the heart usually is not markedly enlarged—and diminished pulmonary vascular markings.

        **(ii) ECG** in both pulmonary and tricuspid atresia shows right atrial enlargement and decreased forces over the right ventricle. In addition, left-axis deviation is seen in tricuspid atresia.

        **(iii) Echocardiogram** is diagnostic and demonstrates the anatomic defect. Doppler evaluation and color flow mapping can define the direction of blood flow.

        **(iv) Cardiac catheterization** and angiography confirm the anatomy and allow quantification of pulmonary blood flow. In pulmonary atresia with intact ventricular septum, right ventricular pressure may be suprasystemic.

**(5) Therapy**

    **(a) Medical management.** $PGE_1$ infusion maintains patency of the ductus, thereby preserving pulmonary blood flow. At cardiac catheterization, a balloon atrial septostomy is performed if the atrial communication is inadequate.

    **(b) Surgical management.** Initially, the aim is to maintain adequate pulmonary blood flow via a systemic artery–pulmonary artery shunt. In pulmonary atresia with intact ventricular septum, a pulmonary valvotomy also is performed to decompress the right ventricle, if the right ventricle is adequate in size.

**b. Pulmonary atresia with VSD**

**(1) Description.** In this defect, which is the extreme expression of tetralogy of Fallot (see IV F), obstruction of right ventricular outflow and a large ventricular septal defect often are accompanied by hypoplasia of the pulmonary arteries.

**(2) Pathophysiology.** Pulmonary blood flow is dependent on a PDA or on collateral flow to the pulmonary arteries. A ventricular right-to-left shunt is obligatory.

**(3) Clinical features.** Severe cyanosis is present and is inversely related to pulmonary blood flow.

**(4) Diagnosis**

    **(a) Physical examination.** A right ventricular heave may be present. $S_2$ is single, and a continuous murmur of the ductus or collateral vessels may be heard.

    **(b) Laboratory evaluation**

        **(i) Chest x-ray** reveals normal heart size, diminished pulmonary vascular markings, and a concavity in the area of the pulmonary artery. A right aortic arch often is present.

        **(ii) ECG** shows right-axis deviation and normal neonatal right ventricular forces.

        **(iii) Echocardiogram** is diagnostic and demonstrates the anatomic defect. Doppler evaluation and color flow mapping can define the direction of flow.

        **(iv)** At **cardiac catheterization,** right and left ventricular pressures are equal. Angiography further defines the anatomy, including the source and adequacy of pulmonary blood flow and size of the pulmonary arteries.

**(5) Therapy**

    **(a) Medical management.** $PGE_1$ infusion maintains patency of the ductus and, therefore, preserves pulmonary blood flow.

    **(b) Surgical management.** The initial aim is to assure adequate pulmonary blood flow by creation of a systemic artery–pulmonary artery shunt. Eventually, complete correction often is possible through closure of the VSD and replacement of the right ventricular outflow with a graft.

## F. Tetralogy of Fallot

1. **Description.** This is the most common cyanotic congenital cardiac abnormality, accounting for 10% of all congenital cardiac lesions.
   a. The primary lesion appears to involve underdevelopment of the infundibulum, leading to:
      (1) Variable right ventricular outflow tract obstruction (pulmonary stenosis)
      (2) Dextroposition of the aorta (override of the ventricular septum)
      (3) Ventricular septal defect (VSD)
      (4) Right ventricular hypertrophy
   b. A right aortic arch is not uncommon, and hypoplasia of the pulmonary arteries often is present to varying degrees.

2. **Pathophysiology.** Of the four components of tetralogy of Fallot, only the VSD and the right ventricular outflow obstruction are physiologically important. This combination equalizes right and left ventricular pressures; the magnitude of the right-to-left shunt depends on the degree of right ventricular obstruction.

3. **Clinical features.** Major manifestations reflect the degree of hypoxemia, which is governed by the severity of right ventricular outflow obstruction. Signs include cyanosis, squatting posture, hyperpnea, and dyspnea on exertion. Hypoxemic spells consist of irritability, hyperpnea, and increasing cyanosis; syncope may occur. These spells often are paroxysmal and may be fatal; they are not necessarily related to the severity of the obstruction.

4. **Diagnosis**
   a. **Physical examination**
      (1) Cyanosis is variable and, in some cases, may be absent (acyanotic tetralogy).
      (2) Digital clubbing and hyperpnea at rest are directly related to the degree of cyanosis.
      (3) A right ventricular heave is present, $S_2$ often is single, and a harsh systolic ejection murmur is heard along the sternal border, its length and loudness being inversely proportional to the degree of outflow obstruction.
   b. **Laboratory evaluation**
      (1) **Chest x-ray.** The heart size is normal. The apex is uptilted, and a concavity is noted in the pulmonary segment, giving the heart the appearance of a boot. The pulmonary vascular markings are diminished according to the severity of outflow obstruction. The aortic arch is right-sided in 25%–30% of cases.
      (2) **ECG** shows right-axis deviation and right ventricular hypertrophy.
      (3) The two-dimensional **echocardiogram** is diagnostic; it demonstrates the location and size of the VSD, the outflow obstruction, the size of the pulmonary annulus, and the degree of aortic override. Doppler analysis makes it possible to approximate pressure gradients, and color flow mapping demonstrates the direction of the flow through the VSD.
      (4) **Cardiac catheterization** is useful in measuring the degree of desaturation and the pressures in the ventricles and aorta. Angiography is used to evaluate the pulmonary and coronary arteries, the ventricular septal defect, and the nature of the right ventricular outflow obstruction.

5. **Therapy**
   a. **Medical management**
      (1) Bacterial endocarditis prophylaxis is necessary. Oral hygiene must be maintained.
      (2) Hypoxemic spells are treated by placing the child in a knee-chest position to increase systemic vascular resistance and to diminish right-to-left shunting. Morphine sulfate is given to depress the respiratory center, and oxygen is administered. β-Adrenergic blocking agents and α-adrenergic agonists (e.g., phenylephrine) also have been useful.
   b. **Surgical management**
      (1) **Palliative surgery.** A temporary increase in pulmonary blood flow can be obtained by the creation of a systemic artery–pulmonary artery shunt. The most common shunts are the **Blalock-Taussig operation** (i.e., anastomosis of the subclavian artery to a pulmonary artery branch) and the **modified Blalock-Taussig operation** (i.e., interposition of a tubular graft between the subclavian and pulmonary arteries).

**(2) Corrective surgery** consists of closing the VSD and resecting the right ventricular outflow obstruction, enlarging the area—if necessary—with a patch.

## G. Persistent truncus arteriosus

1. **Description.** A rare abnormality accounting for 1%–4% of congenital cardiac defects, persistent truncus arteriosus results when conotruncal septation does not proceed normally. A single trunk exits from the heart, and there is a large VSD. Anatomic classification is based on the exit site of the pulmonary arteries from the trunk. In the most common type, a short main pulmonary artery segment originates from the trunk. Truncal valve anatomy is variable; the valve often is stenotic or insufficient. A right aortic arch is present in 25% of cases.

2. **Pathophysiology.** Pulmonary and systemic venous return is ejected into the common trunk. Pulmonary blood flow is determined by the size of the pulmonary arteries, the presence of pulmonary artery stenosis, and pulmonary vascular resistance.

3. **Clinical features.** Symptoms depend on the status of pulmonary blood flow and truncal valve integrity.
   a. Early in life, the high pulmonary vascular resistance limits pulmonary blood flow. Cyanosis may occur without decompensation, unless significant truncal valve insufficiency is present.
   b. As the pulmonary vascular resistance falls, there is an increase in pulmonary blood flow, leading to symptoms of congestive heart failure (e.g., failure to thrive, irritability, poor feeding, tachypnea, dyspnea).

4. **Diagnosis**
   a. **Physical examination**
      (1) If pulmonary blood flow is very high, physical findings may mimic those of a large PDA with congestive heart failure.
      (2) If pulmonary blood flow is meager, the findings may be similar to those seen in severe tetralogy of Fallot.
      (3) Additionally, an ejection click and—if truncal valve insufficiency is present—a diastolic murmur may be heard.
   b. **Laboratory evaluation**
      (1) **Chest x-ray.** Heart size is related to pulmonary blood flow. The main pulmonary artery segment is concave, and a right aortic arch may be seen. Pulmonary vascularity usually is increased but may be diminished.
      (2) **ECG** reveals biventricular hypertrophy and left atrial enlargement if pulmonary blood flow is increased. If pulmonary blood flow is decreased, right ventricular hypertrophy is seen.
      (3) **Echocardiogram** is diagnostic, permitting visualization of the VSD and the origin of the pulmonary arteries. Doppler ultrasonography and color flow mapping demonstrate truncal valve stenosis or insufficiency.
      (4) **Cardiac catheterization** and angiography are useful in confirming the diagnosis and visualizing the pulmonary arteries. Pressure in the ventricles is equalized, and pulmonary vascular resistance can be calculated.

5. **Therapy**
   a. **Medical management** involves treatment of congestive heart failure.
   b. **Surgical management.** Correction is possible by closing the VSD, so that the trunk is included in the left ventricle, and by interposing a conduit between the right ventricle and pulmonary arteries, which are disconnected from the trunk.

## H. Aortic and subaortic stenosis

1. **Description**
   a. In **aortic stenosis,** the valvular tissue is thickened and often is rigid. Most commonly, the valve is bicuspid, with a single fused commissure and an eccentric orifice.
   b. In **subaortic stenosis,** a membranous diaphragm or fibrous ring encircles the left ventricular outflow tract just beneath the base of the aortic valve.

2. **Pathophysiology.** The pressure gradient between the left ventricle and aorta during systolic ejection is directly proportional to the square of the blood flow. Left ventricular end-diastolic pressure may be elevated if left ventricular function is impaired or if hypertrophy is severe enough to reduce compliance.

3. **Clinical features.** Symptoms often are absent, even if obstruction is fairly severe. When they occur, symptoms are related to diminished cardiac reserve (fatigability and exertional dyspnea) or to inadequate coronary blood flow to meet the needs of the hypertrophied left ventricle (angina). Syncope—due to inability of the left ventricle to increase output to maintain cerebral blood flow—may occur with exercise.

4. **Diagnosis**
   a. **Physical examination**
      (1) A harsh systolic ejection murmur is heard at the right base and—in valvular stenosis—is preceded by an ejection click that is heard best at the lower left sternal border.
      (2) A systolic thrill often is felt in the jugular notch, and a diastolic murmur of aortic regurgitation—heard best at the midleft sternal border—is a finding in both valvular and subvalvular stenosis.
   b. **Laboratory evaluation**
      (1) **Chest x-ray.** Poststenotic dilatation of the ascending aorta is present in valvular, but not subvalvular, stenosis.
      (2) The resting **ECG** may show left ventricular hypertrophy, but correlation with the severity of the stenosis is lacking. Left ventricular ischemia, shown by ST depression and T wave inversion, is indicative of severe stenosis, but its absence does not exclude it. Exercise ECG is a more reliable indicator of the pressure gradient.
      (3) **Echocardiogram.** The lesion and the degree of hypertrophy are demonstrated by a two-dimensional study. Doppler ultrasonography can reliably predict the transvalvular gradient and the presence of insufficiency.
      (4) With **cardiac catheterization,** the site and degree of obstruction may be assessed, and the valve area calculated.

5. **Therapy**
   a. **Medical management.** Bacterial endocarditis prophylaxis is indicated. Avoidance of competitive sports in all but the mildest cases usually is recommended.
   b. **Surgical management**
      (1) In selected patients with aortic valve stenosis, open valvotomy is currently the treatment of choice. Balloon angioplasty has been performed as an experimental procedure and in the future may supplant open valvotomy. Restenosis of the valve is not uncommon, as is an increase in regurgitation.
      (2) In subvalvular stenosis, resection of the subaortic membrane is accomplished.

**I. Coarctation of the aorta**

1. **Description.** Coarctation of the aorta accounts for 8% of congenital heart defects. It is twice as common in males as it is in females. When it occurs in a female, Turner syndrome must be considered (see Ch 7 IV C 1). The obstruction usually is located in the descending aorta, just opposite the ligamentum arteriosum. It may coexist with tubular hypoplasia of the aortic arch. The aortic valve is bicuspid in more than 50% of cases. Mitral valve abnormalities (stenosis and/or regurgitation) may be present.

2. **Pathophysiology.** Coarctation represents a mechanical obstruction between the proximal and distal aorta. The proximal aortic pressure and left ventricular afterload are elevated, whereas the distal aortic pressure is low. Collateral vessels, usually involving the internal mammary and the intercostal arteries, develop in response to the pressure differential.

3. **Clinical features.** Congestive heart failure develops in infancy in approximately 10% of cases. Most children are asymptomatic; leg cramps, headaches, and chest pain occur only rarely (see also IV E 1 b).

4. **Diagnosis**
   a. **Physical examination**
      (1) Signs typically seen in the older infant include weak, delayed, or absent femoral pulses compared to upper extremity pulses, upper extremity hypertension, and blood pressure differential between the arm and leg. These signs may not be present in the newborn whose ductus arteriosus is patent.
      (2) Flow across the coarctation or via collateral vessels may produce a systolic ejection murmur heard at the apex, left sternal border, and interscapular area. Collateral pulsations are felt around the scapula. If the aortic valve is bicuspid, an ejection click is heard.

b. **Laboratory evaluation**
  (1) **Chest x-ray.** In older children, soft tissue densities consisting of the aortic knob and the dilated descending aorta may form a "3"; the same structures indent the barium-filled esophagus to form an "E." Notching of the fourth through eighth ribs, caused by erosion from collateral vessels, may be seen in children older than age 5 years.
  (2) **ECG** may be normal or show left ventricular hypertrophy.
  (3) **Echocardiogram.** The coarctation may be visualized from the suprasternal notch approach. Left ventricular function and associated abnormalities may be evaluated.
  (4) **Cardiac catheterization.** The aortic pressure gradient can be measured. Aortography allows visualization of the lesion and evaluation of the adequacy of collateral vessels.

5. **Therapy**
  a. **Medical management.** Bacterial endocarditis prophylaxis is indicated, and treatment of hypertension may be necessary.
  b. **Surgical management.** Surgical repair can be accomplished in one of several ways, including resection with end-to-end anastomosis, subclavian flap angioplasty, patch repair, and graft repair. Balloon angioplasty has been performed with varying results.

## J. Pulmonary stenosis

1. **Description.** Pulmonary stenosis accounts for 5%–8% of congenital heart defects. The pulmonary commissures are fused, the valve is domed and has a small central opening, and there is poststenotic dilatation of the main pulmonary artery. The valve is occasionally bicuspid and is dysplastic in 10% of cases.

2. **Pathophysiology.** To maintain cardiac output, right ventricular pressure rises. In severe stenosis, right ventricular end-diastolic pressure may increase. A consequent increase in right atrial pressure may open the foramen ovale and cause a right-to-left shunt.

3. **Clinical features.** Most patients are asymptomatic. Severe to critical pulmonary stenosis may cause exertional dyspnea, fatigability, and exertional chest pain. Congestive heart failure is unusual except in infants with critical stenosis.

4. **Diagnosis**
  a. **Physical examination**
    (1) An ejection click, the loudness of which varies with respiration, and a harsh systolic ejection murmur are present at the upper left sternal border.
    (2) In severe stenosis, a thrill and right ventricular heave are palpable, the pulmonary component of $S_2$ is diminished, the ejection click merges with $S_1$, and the murmur becomes longer and louder.
    (3) If the stenosis is critical, cyanosis and an $S_4$ gallop may be found.
  b. **Laboratory evaluation**
    (1) **Chest x-ray.** Heart size and pulmonary vascularity usually are normal, but the pulmonary artery segment is prominent. In critical stenosis, cardiomegaly and diminished pulmonary blood flow may be seen.
    (2) **ECG.** The degree of right-axis deviation and right ventricular hypertrophy correlates well with right ventricular pressure and, therefore, with severity of the stenosis. An R wave of 20 mm or greater in lead $V_1$ is indicative of systemic right ventricular pressure.
    (3) **Echocardiogram.** Findings depend on the degree of stenosis. Right ventricular hypertrophy, dilatation, doming of the pulmonary valve, and poststenotic dilatation of the pulmonary artery can be seen. Doppler ultrasonography accurately predicts the transvalvular gradient.
    (4) **Cardiac catheterization.** Right ventricular function, anatomy of the pulmonary valve, and the transvalvular gradient can be accurately assessed. In mild stenosis, right ventricular pressure usually is less than 50% of systemic pressure; in moderate stenosis, it is 50%–80% of systemic pressure; and in severe stenosis, it is greater than 80% of systemic pressure.

5. **Therapy**
  a. **Medical management.** Bacterial endocarditis prophylaxis is necessary. Percutaneous balloon angioplasty of the pulmonary valve may be performed at the time of cardiac catheterization.
  b. **Surgical management.** Indications for pulmonary valvotomy include right ventricular pressure greater than 80% of left ventricular pressure, presence of symptoms in patients in

whom right ventricular pressure is greater than 60% of left ventricular pressure, cyanosis, and congestive heart failure. Pulmonary valve insufficiency of varying degree is produced both by surgical and by balloon opening of the valve.

### K. D-Transposition of the great arteries

1. **Description.** This lesion, also known as **simple transposition (SDD),** accounts for 5% of congenital heart defects and is more common in males. The configuration is as follows: The aorta arises from the right ventricle anteriorly and to the right of the pulmonary artery, which arises posteriorly from the left ventricle. Associated abnormalities may include VSD, PDA, pulmonary stenosis, or a combination of these. When D-transposition occurs with other abnormalities, it is referred to as **complex transposition**.

2. **Pathophysiology.** Systemic (unoxygenated) blood is recirculated through the body, and pulmonary venous (oxygenated) blood is recirculated through the lungs. A lesion that allows mixing of the systemic and pulmonary circulations (e.g., ASD, VSD, PDA) is necessary for survival.

3. **Clinical features.** Cyanosis is present from birth, the degree varying with the associated mixing lesion. In the absence of a natural or created communication between the two circulations, congestive heart failure develops within the first month of life.

4. **Diagnosis**
   a. **Physical examination.** In the absence of mixing lesions, there is pronounced cyanosis, a right ventricular heave, and a single loud $S_2$; a soft flow murmur occasionally is heard.
   b. **Laboratory evaluation**
      (1) **Chest x-ray.** Slight cardiomegaly and a narrow base produced by the anterior-posterior arrangement of the great arteries gives the heart an egg shape. Pulmonary vascularity is increased or normal.
      (2) **ECG** is normal in the newborn; however, right-axis deviation and right ventricular hypertrophy eventually are seen.
      (3) **Echocardiogram** shows the anterior-posterior arrangement of the great arteries, the chamber from which they originate, and the presence of associated abnormalities.
      (4) **Cardiac catheterization.** Right ventricular pressure is systemic. Left ventricular pressure may be systemic in the newborn but decreases with a decline in pulmonary vascular resistance. Angiography confirms the anatomy and indicates the direction of blood flow. Balloon atrial septostomy (**Rashkind procedure**) allows the creation of an ASD, through which the mixing of oxygenated and deoxygenated blood can occur.
      (5) **Arterial blood gas analysis** shows severe hypoxemia ($Po_2$ is often in the low 20s); increasing the ambient $Fio_2$ to 100% does not significantly alter the arterial $Po_2$. Without corrective surgery, compensatory polycythemia develops even after an adequate balloon atrial septostomy has been performed. A hematocrit in the high 50s or low 60s is not uncommon.

5. **Therapy**
   a. **Medical management.** Correction of acidosis, hypoglycemia, and hypocalcemia in the neonatal period improves myocardial function. Creation of an ASD by balloon atrial septostomy may be lifesaving. Iron supplementation often is required to prevent iron deficiency anemia.
   b. **Surgical management.** Two surgical approaches have been employed.
      (1) The **arterial switch procedure** with **coronary artery reimplantation** must be performed in the neonatal period and involves moving the arteries, but not the valves, into their "normal" position.
      (2) Alternatively, an **atrial switch procedure**—such as the **Senning** or the **Mustard** operation—is performed in the first year of life. This allows systemic venous blood to enter the left ventricle and, therefore, the pulmonary artery, and the pulmonary venous blood to enter the right ventricle and, therefore, the aorta.

### L. L-Transposition of the great arteries

1. **Description.** L-Transposition of the great arteries accounts for less than 1% of all congenital heart disease. The configuration is as follows: The great arteries are transposed, with the aortic valve anterior to and to the left of the pulmonary valve. In 98% of cases, the bulboventricular loop has developed to the left, leading to inversion of the ventricles. The anatomic right ventricle is on the left, and the anatomic left ventricle is on the right (SLL). The AV valves are also

inverted; the mitral valve leads into the anatomic left ventricle and the tricuspid valve into the anatomic right ventricle. Atrial position is unaffected. Associated abnormalities are common and may include AV conduction block, VSD, pulmonary stenosis, and left-sided AV (i.e., tricuspid) valve insufficiency.

2. **Pathophysiology.** The combination of transposition of the great arteries and inversion of the ventricles leads to a physiologically corrected circulation. (This lesion is also called **"corrected" transposition.**) Systemic venous return flows via the mitral valve to the right-sided left ventricle and is ejected into a posterior pulmonary trunk; pulmonary venous return flows via the tricuspid valve to the left-sided right ventricle and from there to the anterior aorta. This "corrected" circulation may be altered by associated defects.

3. **Clinical features.** Symptoms primarily reflect the associated defects.
   a. A large VSD produces symptoms of a large left-to-right shunt, including congestive heart failure in infants.
   b. Severe pulmonary stenosis associated with a VSD produces symptoms of a right-to-left shunt (i.e., cyanosis, dyspnea), similar to those seen in tetralogy of Fallot.
   c. Left-sided (tricuspid) valve regurgitation may produce tachypnea, dyspnea, cough, and other signs of pulmonary venous congestion.
   d. Complete heart block may be associated with syncope and clinical evidence of low cardiac output.

4. **Diagnosis**
   a. **Physical examination**
      (1) In the absence of associated defects, the only physical finding that gives a hint of the underlying lesion is a loud single $S_2$.
      (2) If a VSD is present, the findings are similar to those noted in VSD (see IV C 4 a).
      (3) When severe pulmonary stenosis is associated with a large VSD, the findings are those of tetralogy of Fallot (see IV F 4 a).
      (4) Left atrioventricular valve (tricuspid valve) insufficiency is indistinguishable from severe mitral valve regurgitation.
   b. **Laboratory evaluation**
      (1) **Chest x-ray**
         (a) Since the left heart border is formed by the ascending aorta, it is straight or slightly convex.
         (b) Cardiomegaly, pulmonary hyperflow, and left atrial enlargement are seen in the presence of a large VSD.
         (c) If severe pulmonary stenosis coexists with a VSD, the heart size is normal, and pulmonary vascularity is diminished.
         (d) Severe left-sided AV valve regurgitation results in an enlarged left atrium and evidence of pulmonary venous congestion.
      (2) **ECG.** Inversion of the septum causes reversal of initial depolarization, indicated by deep Q waves in leads II, III, and aVF and in the right precordial leads. Varying degrees of AV block may be seen.
      (3) **Echocardiogram** demonstrates ventricular structure, great vessel location, and associated defects. Doppler ultrasonography indicates AV valve regurgitation and predicts the severity of pulmonary stenosis.
      (4) **Cardiac catheterization.** In the absence of associated abnormalities, right-sided left ventricular pressure is low, and left-sided right ventricular pressure is systemic. Oxygen saturations and pressures are modified by associated defects, which are accurately delineated by angiography.

5. **Therapy**
   a. **Medical management** is determined by the presence of associated cardiac defects. Measures include treatment of congestive heart failure and conduction disturbances and implementation of bacterial endocarditis prophylaxis.
   b. **Surgical management**
      (1) Palliative systemic artery–pulmonary artery shunts relieve cyanosis produced by diminished pulmonary blood flow associated with VSD and severe pulmonary stenosis.
      (2) Pacemaker implantation in symptomatic bradycardia, surgical repair of VSD and pulmonary stenosis, and annuloplasty or replacement of a severely regurgitant left-sided AV valve also are surgically feasible.

## M. Abnormalities of the pulmonary veins

1. **Total anomalous venous return**
   a. **Description.** In this defect, the pulmonary veins are not incorporated into the left atrium. Instead, they carry oxygenated blood to the right atrium either directly or indirectly through venous channels. There are four possible routes:
      (1) **Supracardiac** (50% of cases)—blood drains into the innominate vein and thence to the superior vena cava or directly to the superior vena cava
      (2) **Cardiac** (20% of cases)—blood drains into the coronary sinus or directly into the right atrium
      (3) **Infracardiac,** also known as **infradiaphragmatic** (20% of cases)—blood drains into the portal or hepatic vein and thence into the inferior vena cava
      (4) **Mixed** (10% of cases)—blood returns to the heart via a combination of the above routes
   b. **Pathophysiology**
      (1) There is an obligatory right-to-left shunt, usually via a stretched foramen ovale or an ASD. The pulmonary blood flow depends on pulmonary venous resistance.
      (2) Obstruction of pulmonary venous flow may exist with all routes but is most common in the infracardiac route.
         (a) If obstruction is severe, the pressure in the pulmonary veins and arteries is high, pulmonary blood flow is low, and systemic arterial blood is markedly desaturated.
         (b) If there is no obstruction, pulmonary blood flow is high, pressures are only mildly elevated, and arterial blood is only mildly desaturated.
   c. **Clinical features.** Symptoms depend on the degree of pulmonary venous obstruction. In severe obstruction, the classic presentation is that of an intensely cyanotic newborn with tachypnea and dyspnea. If no obstruction is present, desaturation may be subclinical, and symptoms are those of pulmonary hyperflow.
   d. **Diagnosis**
      (1) **Physical examination**
         (a) If pulmonary venous flow is obstructed, there is a right ventricular heave and a loud narrowly split $S_2$, a gallop rhythm but usually no murmur.
         (b) If pulmonary venous flow is unobstructed, the findings are similar to those of a high-flow ASD, including prominent and active precordium with a right ventricular heave, clinical cardiomegaly, wide and fixed split $S_2$ with a loud pulmonary component, systolic ejection murmur at the upper left sternal border with wide radiation, and mid-diastolic rumble at the lower left sternal border.
      (2) **Laboratory evaluation**
         (a) **Chest x-ray.** Cardiomegaly with increased pulmonary blood flow is present in unobstructed anomalous venous return. In the supracardiac type, the base of the heart may appear widened by dilated veins, and the entire silhouette may have a "snowman" or "figure 8" appearance. In obstructed venous return, the heart size is normal, and diffuse pulmonary edema may be difficult to distinguish from hyaline membrane disease.
         (b) **ECG** indicates right-axis deviation and right ventricular hypertrophy.
         (c) **Echocardiogram.** The right side of the heart and the pulmonary artery are enlarged; left-sided structures may be relatively small. The echocardiogram indicates that the pulmonary veins do not enter the left atrium. The coronary sinus may be enlarged if the veins drain into it; in the infracardiac type, the common pulmonary vein may be seen behind the left atrium with the communicating vein traversing the diaphragm. Such anomalies can be subtle and easily missed. Color flow mapping is helpful in evaluating the direction of flow.
         (d) **Cardiac catheterization.** Because of mixing, oxygen saturation is similar in all chambers and arteries. Saturation is highest if sampling is performed near the drainage site of the pulmonary veins. Pulmonary pressure is proportional to the degree of venous obstruction. Pulmonary arteriography defines the pulmonary venous drainage.
   e. **Therapy**
      (1) **Medical management.** Congestive heart failure is treated. If pulmonary edema is present, mechanical ventilation may be necessary.

**(2) Surgical management.** Surgical redirection of the pulmonary veins into the left atrium can be accomplished in all four types of this defect.

**2. Partial anomalous venous return**

   **a. Description.** In this defect, most of the pulmonary veins drain normally into the left atrium, but one or several veins drain abnormally. Most frequently, the right upper pulmonary vein drains into the superior vena cava. Often a sinus venosus ASD also is found.

   **b. Pathophysiology.** There is a left-to-right shunt, similar to that seen in ASD.

   **c. Clinical features** (see IV B 3)

   **d. Diagnosis** (see IV B 4 for discussion of typical findings on physical examination, chest x-ray, and ECG)

      **(1) Echocardiogram.** A sinus venosus ASD may be seen, and occasionally, the anomalous pulmonary vein can be identified.

      **(2) Cardiac catheterization** [see also IV B 4 b (4)]. Pulmonary artery angiography may be needed to identify the anomalous pulmonary vein.

   **e. Therapy**

      **(1) Medical management** (see IV B 5 a)

      **(2) Surgical management.** The anomalous pulmonary vein can be surgically redirected into the left atrium at the time of closure of the ASD.

# V. ACQUIRED STRUCTURAL DISORDERS

**A. Rheumatic heart disease** (see also Ch 8 V A) is a sequela of single or multiple episodes of acute rheumatic fever. **Mitral insufficiency** is the most common lesion, followed by **aortic insufficiency**. **Mitral stenosis** is less common and usually is the end result of multiple attacks of acute rheumatic fever. Least common is **aortic stenosis**. The tricuspid and pulmonary valves virtually never are affected. Symptoms are proportional to the degree of valvular damage.

**B. Kawasaki disease** (see also Ch 8 V D 2). Cardiac effects may include pericarditis, myocarditis, and transient rhythm disturbances. However, it is the development of **coronary artery aneurysms,** with their potential for occlusion or rupture, that makes the disease life threatening. Coronary artery aneurysms develop during the subacute phase (eleventh to twenty-fifth day) in about 30% of cases, but regress in most patients. Early therapy with gamma globulin appears to decrease the incidence of coronary artery aneurysms. Low-dose salicylate therapy lessens the likelihood of late aneurysms. Echocardiography is used to assess ventricular function and to visualize pericardial fluid and coronary artery aneurysms.

**C. Endocarditis** (see also Ch 9 VIII A) usually occurs on the low-pressure side of a turbulence-producing lesion (e.g., VSD, semilunar valve stenosis, AV valve regurgitation, semilunar valve regurgitation). It does not usually occur with abnormalities that do not produce turbulence (e.g., ASD). Bacterial endocarditis prophylaxis includes good dental hygiene and preventive dental care; antibiotic prophylaxis should be instituted when the potential for bacteremia exists in children with turbulent cardiac defects.

**D. Coronary artery disease** is rare in childhood, but the atherosclerotic process appears to begin early in life. There is evidence that progression of atherosclerosis is adversely influenced by genetic factors (e.g., familial hypercholesterolemia; see Ch 16 II B 1) and lifestyle (e.g., cigarette smoking, high-cholesterol, high-saturated-fat diet). Since many lifetime habits are formed during childhood, an opportunity exists to influence young people to adopt healthful ones.

# VI. FUNCTIONAL HEART DISORDERS

**A. Myocarditis** (inflammation of the myocardium) is most commonly of **infectious** etiology (see also Ch 9 VIII B). **Noninfectious** inflammatory lesions are primarily associated with collagen vascular diseases. Some patients may be asymptomatic, and the diagnosis is made only by observing changes in the ST segment and T wave on serial ECGs. Others may manifest congestive heart failure, low cardiac output, and rhythm disturbances, which may be fatal or lead to congestive cardiomyopathy.

**B. Cardiomyopathy**

1. **Congestive cardiomyopathy**
   a. **Description.** Congestive, or **dilated,** cardiomyopathy is characterized by myocardial dysfunction and ventricular dilatation. Although it usually is a primary disorder, it may be associated with neuromuscular disease (e.g., Duchenne muscular dystrophy) or result from drug toxicity (e.g., doxorubicin).
   b. **Pathophysiology.** Failure of the left ventricle causes an increase in end-diastolic volume, which results in increases in left atrial, pulmonary venous, and pulmonary capillary pressures.
   c. **Clinical features.** Initially, dyspnea on exertion is present. As left ventricular failure progresses, small increases in left ventricular volume occur, followed by marked increases in left pulmonary capillary pressure. This results in orthopnea, paroxysmal nocturnal dyspnea, and bronchospasm. Eventually, right heart failure, characterized by dependent edema, occurs.
   d. **Diagnosis**
      (1) **Physical examination.** In advanced stages, blood pressure may be low and pulse pressure narrow; pulsus alternans may be present. Other findings may include a right ventricular heave, a prominent $S_3$ and gallop rhythm, a loud pulmonic closure sound, and a murmur of mitral or tricuspid regurgitation.
      (2) **Laboratory evaluation**
         (a) **Chest x-ray** is useful in evaluating heart size, left atrial size, pulmonary congestion, and pleural fluid.
         (b) **ECG** defines rhythm disturbances. Left ventricular hypertrophy and nonspecific or ischemic changes in the ST segment and T wave also may be seen.
         (c) Left ventricular function can be assessed by **echocardiography, radionuclide studies,** and if necessary, **cardiac catheterization**. Myocardial biopsy may be helpful in defining the pathologic process.
   e. **Therapy** is directed at improving left ventricular function with inotropic agents and at unloading the left ventricle with vasodilators. Diuretics are helpful in decreasing preload, and antiarrhythmic medications are used to control potentially fatal rhythm disturbances. In the event of clinical deterioration, cardiac transplantation may be needed.

2. **Hypertrophic cardiomyopathy**
   a. **Description.** This disorder, also known as **idiopathic hypertrophic subaortic stenosis** and **hypertrophic obstructive cardiomyopathy,** is an autosomal dominant genetic disorder with a high degree of penetrance, in which the septum is thickened out of proportion to the left free ventricular wall.
   b. **Pathophysiology.** In the thickened, stiff left ventricle, systolic function is well preserved, but diastolic function is compromised. Thickening of the septum may result in left ventricular outflow obstruction, and abnormal motion of the mitral valve may produce regurgitation.
   c. **Clinical features.** Symptoms include dyspnea on exertion, which occurs when cardiac output does not increase with exercise; chest pain, due to myocardial ischemia; and syncope. Death may result from rhythm disturbances.
   d. **Diagnosis**
      (1) **Physical examination.** The pulse often is biferious (double peaked) as ejection is interrupted by septal obstruction. A forceful left ventricular impulse may be present, and an $S_3$ or $S_4$ may be audible at the apex. Murmurs indicating mitral regurgitation or left ventricular outflow obstruction may be heard; the latter is exaggerated by the Valsalva maneuver, which increases the left ventricular outflow gradient.
      (2) **Laboratory evaluation**
         (a) **ECG** defines rhythm disturbances and often shows left-axis deviation, left ventricular hypertrophy, and changes in the ST segment and T wave.
         (b) **Echocardiogram** is diagnostic; it allows measurement of the septum, the free wall of the left ventricle, and the diastolic left ventricular cavity as well as assessment of systolic anterior motion of the mitral valve. Doppler ultrasound and color flow mapping allow evaluation of mitral valve regurgitation.
   e. **Therapy** is aimed at preventing fatal arrhythmias and at decreasing stiffness of the left ventricle with negative inotropic medications, such as calcium channel blocking and β-adrenergic blocking agents. Avoidance of competitive sports is indicated because of the risk of sudden death with exertion.

## VII. RHYTHM ABNORMALITIES (see also Ch 6 II C 2 g)

**A. Isolated premature beats** may originate from either the atrium or ventricle.

1. **Premature atrial beats** are characterized by an abnormally shaped P wave that occurs prematurely, a normal QRS complex, and no compensatory pause. Premature atrial beats are benign.

2. **Premature ventricular beats** are characterized by a wide QRS complex, no relationship between the P wave and the QRS complex, an inverted T wave, and a full compensatory pause. Premature ventricular beats usually are benign, unless they are multiform, increase with exercise, or are associated with a prolonged QT interval or with cardiomyopathy.

**B. Supraventricular tachycardia** usually is caused by a reentrant mechanism. It often is paroxysmal. A bypass tract (**Wolff-Parkinson-White syndrome**) sometimes is present. The heart rate is uniformly rapid, often greater than 220 beats/min. Infants may develop signs of low cardiac output within hours.

**C. Complete heart block** denotes loss of conduction from the atria to the ventricles and the existence of an idioventricular pacemaker. It is associated with a slow heart rate. Congenital heart block may be caused by maternal antibodies formed in mothers with collagen vascular diseases [particularly systemic lupus erythematosus (SLE)]; these antibodies cross the placenta and produce fibrosis of the conduction system. Symptoms and natural history are related to the width of the QRS complex and the heart rate.

## STUDY QUESTIONS

**Directions:** Each of the numbered items or incomplete statements in this section is followed by answers or by completions of the statement. Select the **one** lettered answer or completion that is **best** in each case.

1. Premature ventricular beats are most likely benign if they

(A) are unifocal
(B) increase with exercise
(C) are associated with a prolonged QT interval
(D) are associated with cardiomyopathy

2. Severe pulmonary stenosis is characterized by all of the following features EXCEPT

(A) increased right ventricular pressure
(B) exertional dyspnea and fatigability
(C) a right-to-left shunt
(D) a loud pulmonary component of $S_2$
(E) right ventricular hypertrophy on ECG

3. Which of the following statements about acquired structural heart disorders is FALSE?

(A) Coronary artery aneurysms develop in about 30% of cases of Kawasaki disease
(B) Kawasaki disease with coronary artery aneurysms can be fatal
(C) The atherosclerotic process leading to coronary artery disease begins in childhood
(D) Bacterial endocarditis usually occurs on the low pressure side of a turbulence-producing lesion
(E) Tricuspid insufficiency is the most common valve abnormality in rheumatic heart disease

4. In levocardia with L-transposition of the great arteries, all of the following are true EXCEPT

(A) the anatomic left ventricle is to the right of the anatomic right ventricle
(B) the pulmonary artery arises from the anatomic left ventricle and the aorta arises from the anatomic right ventricle
(C) the aortic valve is anterior to and to the left of the pulmonary valve
(D) the defect produces intense cyanosis
(E) AV conduction block is a recognized associated abnormality

5. Which of the following features is NOT a characteristic of pulmonary atresia with intact ventricular septum?

(A) Ductus-dependent pulmonary blood flow
(B) Normal right ventricular development
(C) An obligatory right-to-left atrial-level shunt
(D) A single $S_2$
(E) Decreased pulmonary vascularity

6. Lesions involving either systemic or pulmonary blood flow dependence on patency of the ductus arteriosus include all of the following EXCEPT

(A) total anomalous pulmonary venous return
(B) pulmonary atresia with intact ventricular septum
(C) critical aortic stenosis
(D) hypoplastic left-heart syndrome
(E) pulmonary atresia with ventricular septal defect

7. Which of the following statements about coarctation of the aorta is FALSE?

(A) The obstruction usually is opposite the ductus or ligamentum arteriosum
(B) More than 50% of patients have an associated bicuspid aortic valve
(C) Left ventricular afterload and proximal aortic pressure are elevated
(D) A blood pressure differential is present between upper and lower extremities
(E) The "E" and "3" signs are best seen on echocardiogram

8. All of the following statements concerning D-transposition (simple transposition) of the great arteries are true EXCEPT

(A) the aortic valve is to the right of the pulmonary valve
(B) the aortic valve is posterior to the pulmonary valve
(C) right ventricular pressure is high
(D) severe hypoxia is present
(E) a balloon atrial septostomy should be performed as the first step in treatment

| | | |
|---|---|---|
| 1-A | 4-D | 7-E |
| 2-D | 5-B | 8-B |
| 3-E | 6-A | |

9. Which of the following features is NOT a characteristic of aortic stenosis?

(A) A thickened aortic valve
(B) Ventricular hypertrophy
(C) Frequent symptoms
(D) A harsh systolic ejection murmur
(E) A systolic ejection click

10. Which of the following statements about total anomalous pulmonary venous return is FALSE?

(A) An atrial obligatory right-to-left shunt is present
(B) Pulmonary venous obstruction is most common in the infradiaphragmatic type
(C) The supracardiac type is most common
(D) Cyanosis is most severe when the pulmonary veins are severely obstructed
(E) When the pulmonary veins are not obstructed, the heart size is normal

**Directions:** Each group of items in this section consists of lettered options followed by a set of numbered items. For each item, select the **one** lettered option that is most closely associated with it. Each lettered option may be selected once, more than once, or not at all.

**Questions 11–14**

Match each group of cardiac lesions listed below with the sign or symptom that is commonly associated with it.

(A) Cyanosis
(B) Mid-diastolic rumble
(C) Single $S_2$
(D) Widely split $S_2$
(E) Chest pain

11. Mitral regurgitation, VSD, ASD

12. ASD, right bundle branch block, mitral regurgitation

13. VSD with high pulmonary vascular resistance, aortic stenosis

14. D-Transposition of great arteries, total anomalous pulmonary venous drainage with severe pulmonary venous obstruction, pulmonary atresia

**Questions 15–17**

Match each group of cardiac lesions listed below with the finding that is commonly associated with it.

(A) Right aortic arch
(B) Obligatory right-to-left shunt
(C) Left-to-right shunt
(D) Regurgitant systolic murmur

15. Tetralogy of Fallot, truncus arteriosus, pulmonary valve atresia with VSD

16. VSD, PDA, ASD

17. Total anomalous pulmonary venous return, tricuspid atresia, pulmonary valve atresia with intact ventricular septum

| | | |
|---|---|---|
| 9-C | 12-D | 15-A |
| 10-E | 13-E | 16-C |
| 11-B | 14-A | 17-B |

## ANSWERS AND EXPLANATIONS

**1. The answer is A** *[VII A 2].*
Uniform premature ventricular beats are benign in childhood, since they do not degenerate into ventricular tachycardia or ventricular fibrillation. However, if they are multiform, increase with exercise, or are associated with a prolonged QT interval or cardiomyopathy, they may degenerate into a lethal arrhythmia and must be investigated further.

**2. The answer is D** *[IV J 4 a (2)].*
The pulmonary component of the second heart sound ($S_2$) is diminished in severe pulmonary stenosis. In severe cases of this defect, the pulmonary valve is immobile. A pressure gradient is present across the valve, resulting in a high right ventricular pressure but a low pulmonary artery pressure. The loudness of the pulmonary component of $S_2$ is directly related to pulmonary artery pressure and, therefore, is soft. In severe pulmonary stenosis, right ventricular end-diastolic pressure may increase, causing the right atrial pressure to increase and eventually result in a right-to-left shunt. Severe pulmonary stenosis may cause exertional dyspnea, fatigability, and exertional chest pain. The degree of right ventricular hypertrophy on electrocardiogram (ECG) correlates with the severity of stenosis.

**3. The answer is E** *[V A].*
Rheumatic heart disease is a sequela of acute rheumatic fever. Mitral insufficiency and aortic insufficiency are the most common lesions; mitral stenosis and aortic stenosis are less common. The tricuspid and pulmonary valves are almost never involved in rheumatic heart disease. Kawasaki disease is a severe exanthematous illness with a constellation of symptoms. The cardiac effects of Kawasaki disease include pericarditis, myocarditis, transient rhythm disturbances, and—most importantly—life-threatening coronary artery aneurysms, which develop in about 30% of cases. Although coronary artery disease is rare in childhood, the atherosclerotic process begins very early in life. Bacterial endocarditis is an infection of the endocardium, which usually occurs on the low-pressure side of a turbulence-producing lesion.

**4. The answer is D** *[IV L 1, 2].*
In levocardia with L-transposition, there is ventricular inversion and transposition of the great arteries. Thus, the anatomic right ventricle is to the left of the anatomic left ventricle, the aorta arises from the anatomic right ventricle, and the pulmonary artery arises from the anatomic left ventricle. The aortic valve is anterior to and to the left of the pulmonary valve. In the absence of associated abnormalities, the circulation is physiologically corrected in levocardia with L-transposition of the great arteries; thus, there are no symptoms. One of the well-recognized associated abnormalities is atrioventricular (AV) conduction block.

**5. The answer is B** *[IV E 2 a (1) (a), (2), (4)].*
Right ventricular development is normal in only 10% of cases of pulmonary atresia with intact ventricular septum. In more than 50% of cases, the right ventricle is severely hypoplastic. Associated infundibular hypoplasia is present in 20% of cases. Pulmonary atresia with intact ventricular septum is characterized by an obligatory right-to-left shunt and ductus-dependent pulmonary blood flow. Physical examination reveals a single $S_2$, and chest x-ray shows diminished pulmonary vascular markings.

**6. The answer is A** *[IV M 1 a–c].*
Total anomalous pulmonary venous return is a defect characterized by systemic blood flow that is dependent on a right-to-left shunt at the atrial level. In both critical aortic stenosis and hypoplastic left-heart syndrome, systemic perfusion is dependent on patency of the ductus arteriosus. In pulmonary atresia—with or without ventricular septal defect—pulmonary flow is dependent on a patent ductus arteriosus.

**7. The answer is E** *[IV I 4 b (1)].*
The "E" and "3" signs that are characteristic of coarctation of the aorta are best seen on chest x-ray, not echocardiogram. The "3" is formed by soft tissue densities consisting of the aortic knob and the dilated descending aorta. The same structures indenting the barium-filled esophagus form an "E" on x-ray. Coarctation of the aorta usually is located in the descending portion, just opposite the ligamentum arteriosum. The aortic valve is bicuspid in more than 50% of cases. Coarctation is associated with increases in the proximal aortic pressure and left ventricular afterload and a decrease in the distal aortic pressure. A blood pressure differential between upper and lower extremities is a typical sign.

**8. The answer is B** *[IV K 1].*
In D-transposition (also called simple transposition) of the great arteries, the aortic valve is to the right and anterior to the pulmonary valve. Since the right ventricle is a systemic ventricle, its pressure is high. A balloon atrial septostomy creates an interatrial communication to ameliorate the severe hypoxia that is present in this anomaly. This procedure should be performed as soon as the diagnosis has been confirmed.

**9. The answer is C** *[IV H 3].*
During childhood, symptoms of aortic stenosis are infrequent, even if stenosis is severe. Because the left ventricle has a marked ability to hypertrophy, compensating for the pressure load, the affected individual can remain symptom-free for many years. Valvular degeneration, fibrosis, and calcification—which occur in adulthood—lead to rigidity of the valve and eventual development of angina, effort syncope, and heart failure. Physical examination reveals a harsh systolic ejection murmur preceded by an ejection click.

**10. The answer is E** *[IV M 1 d (2) (a)].*
In total anomalous pulmonary venous return, heart size is directly related to pulmonary blood flow; if the pulmonary veins are not obstructed, cardiomegaly with increased pulmonary blood flow is present. Since both systemic and pulmonary venous return are to the right side, systemic flow is dependent on an obligatory right-to-left shunt. Cyanosis is directly related to the degree of pulmonary venous obstruction, which is most commonly seen in the infradiaphragmatic type. In 50% of cases of total anomalous venous return, blood drains into the innominate vein and, thence, to the superior vena cava (supracardiac type).

**11–14. The answers are: 11-B** *[IV B 4 a, C 4 a],* **12-D** *[I B 5 a (2); IV B 4 a; Table 11-2],* **13-E** *[IV C 3 c, H 3],* **14-A** *[IV E 2 a (3), K 3, M 1 c].*
A mid-diastolic rumble may be heard in mitral regurgitation, ventricular septal defect (VSD), and atrial septal defect (ASD). In mitral regurgitation, the rumble results from increased flow across the mitral valve. In high flow VSD, it is caused by increased volume returning to the left atrium and, therefore, the left ventricle. In ASD, the mid-diastolic rumble is caused by increased flow across the tricuspid valve.

The S$_2$ can be widely split because of delay in pulmonary valve closure (as occurs in ASD and right bundle branch block) or from early closure of the aortic valve (as occurs in mitral valve regurgitation).

Chest pain in children most often is benign, but angina can occur in aortic stenosis and in VSD with pulmonary vascular obstructive disease.

Cyanosis is the most dramatic clinical finding in D-transposition of the great arteries, in total anomalous pulmonary venous drainage with severe pulmonary venous obstruction, and in pulmonary atresia.

**15–17. The answers are: 15-A** *[IV E 2 b (4) (b) (i), F 1 b, G 1],* **16-C** *[IV B 2, C 2 b, D 2 a],* **17-B** *[IV E 2 a (2), M 1 b (1)].*
A right aortic arch is seen in congenital conotruncal abnormalities, which include tetralogy of Fallot, persistent truncus arteriosus, and pulmonary valve atresia with VSD. Left-to-right shunts are present in VSD, PDA, and ASD. Since both the systemic and the pulmonary venous return are to the right side in total anomalous pulmonary venous return, there is an obligatory right-to-left shunt to provide a systemic output. In tricuspid or pulmonary valve atresia, there is no outlet from the right side except as an atrial right-to-left shunt.

# 12
# Pulmonary Diseases

Michelle M. Cloutier
David A. Schaeffer

## I. GENERAL PRINCIPLES OF PULMONARY DISEASE IN CHILDREN

### A. Lung development

**1. Prenatal lung development** (see also Ch 5 V A 1)

**a.** The **lung bud** arises as a pouch from the primitive foregut at 22–26 days gestation. The **bronchial tree** develops between 5 and 16 weeks gestation by continuous budding and branching of the airways. Airway branching ends at 16 weeks; further growth occurs by an increase in diameter and length but not by an increase in airway number.

**b.** Insults to the lung before 16 weeks gestation decrease both airway number and subsequent alveolar growth and number. Insults after 16 weeks affect only alveolar number and growth.

**2. Postnatal lung development.** Approximately 60 million primitive alveoli exist at birth. The lung grows most rapidly in alveolar number during the first 2 years. The growth rate decreases thereafter, until the adult number of approximately 375 million alveoli is reached at age 8–12 years.

### B. Common pathologic features of pulmonary disease.
Of the 69 million children under age 17 years in the United States, 23% (15.9 million) have chronic disease, and 16% (11 million) have chronic pulmonary disease.

**1. Underlying pathologic process.** Most lung diseases in children are classified as obstructive or restrictive.

**a. Obstruction** (i.e., airway narrowing) may be due to intraluminal secretions, edema or inflammation of the airway wall, hypertrophy or contraction of the bronchial smooth muscle, or extrinsic compression.

**b. Restriction** [i.e., impaired lung expansion (volume)] may be due to decreased lung compliance (stiff lungs), atelectasis or pneumothorax causing lung collapse, neuromuscular disease, or disorders of the chest wall.

**2. Pathophysiology**

**a. Hypoxemia** (i.e., deficient oxygenation of blood) most commonly is caused by ventilation-perfusion abnormalities but also may be due to intracardiac or intrapulmonary shunts, diffusion problems, or hypoventilation.

**b. Hypercapnia** (i.e., excess carbon dioxide in blood) most commonly is caused by primary hypoventilation [due to upper airway obstruction, neuromuscular weakness, or central nervous system (CNS) depression] but also may be seen with increased lower airway obstructive disease and associated ventilation-perfusion mismatch, shunts, and impaired diffusion.

**3. Pathogenetic factors**

**a.** The **small airways** of the child result in high airway resistance and put the child at great risk for developing obstructive lung disease. Males are affected more frequently and more severely than females, in part because the peripheral airways in males under age 5 years are smaller than those in females.

**b.** The young child **lacks specific immunity** and is relatively defenseless against invading microorganisms.

**c.** In children, most pulmonary disease has a **single cause,** whereas in adults, pulmonary disease is apt to be multifactorial in etiology.

**C. Evaluation of pulmonary disease**

1. **History.** Many pulmonary diseases are missed or misdiagnosed. Therefore, a careful history should be obtained, focusing on the following questions.

   a. **Is the disorder acute, chronic, or recurrent?** The physician must determine whether the condition is acute and self-limited, chronic (i.e., with symptoms occurring daily for more than 4 weeks), or recurrent (i.e., with disease-free intervals). With chronic or recurrent disorders, the parents may not remember each episode clearly, but they usually can recall—in reasonably good detail—the first time the problem arose.

   b. **Is the disorder immediately or eventually life-threatening?**

      (1) Cyanosis, respiratory distress, or severe stridor—regardless of cause—indicates severe difficulty and the need for immediate action.

      (2) Problems such as progressive weight loss or a progressive pulmonary opacification imply a serious long-term outlook.

   c. **What are the symptoms?** Specific pulmonary symptoms should be sought, such as:

      (1) The presence of a cough and its characteristics

      (2) Labored or noisy breathing and its interference with activities

      (3) The presence of wheezing, chest pain, sputum production, or foul breath

   d. **What factors affect the severity of symptoms?** It is important to identify factors that improve or worsen symptoms. Reactive airway disease is suggested when symptoms are exacerbated by changes in weather, viral infections (e.g., common colds), exercise, laughing or crying, or exposure to allergens.

   e. **Have any tests been performed?** The physician should determine which tests have been performed, where they were given, and what the results were.

   f. **Have any treatments been given?** Parents should be asked about the types of therapy the child has previously received, the dosages used, the duration of therapy, and the response of symptoms to treatment.

   g. **Is there a family history of pulmonary disease?** A family history of a similar problem or of any type of respiratory disease should be identified.

2. **Physical examination**

   a. **Respiratory rate** (Table 12-1) is the best indicator of pulmonary function in young infants. However, the respiratory rate is influenced by activity when the child is awake. Therefore, the most reliable and reproducible rate is the **sleeping respiratory rate**.

   b. **Effort of breathing** is a guide to pulmonary dysfunction.

      (1) **Grunting** is a sign of loss of lung volume. It is frequently found in neonatal respiratory distress syndrome and pulmonary edema. In older children, it is frequently a sign of chest pain and suggests an acute pneumonic process with pleural involvement.

      (2) **Chest retractions**

         (a) **Intercostal retractions** are a sign of increased lung stiffness or increased work of breathing due to airway obstruction.

         (b) **Subcostal retractions** are a sign of hyperinflation and a flattened diaphragm due to small airway obstruction.

      (3) **Flaring of the alae nasi** (dilated nostrils) is a sign of increased airway resistance.

      (4) **Head-bobbing** is a sign of dyspnea in an exhausted or sleeping infant; the head bobs forward owing to neck flexion with each inspiration.

   c. **Breath sounds** also are informative.

      (1) **Crackles** are heard primarily on inspiration. The sound is produced by the opening of small airways that closed on the previous breath.

      (2) **Wheezing** is produced by partial airway obstruction. It usually is expiratory in origin but can be inspiratory when the airway obstruction is fixed and rigid, as in airway

**Table 12-1.** Normal Respiratory Rates in Children

| Age | Breaths/Minute |
| --- | --- |
| Newborn | 30–75 |
| 6–12 months | 22–31 |
| 1–2 years | 17–23 |
| 2–4 years | 16–25 |
| 4–10 years | 13–23 |
| 10–14 years | 13–19 |

edema. Wheezing usually is a sign of asthma, but it can occur in any pulmonary disease when the airflow is through a sufficiently narrowed orifice.

    **(3)** **Stridor** is a harsh, primarily inspiratory sound produced by laryngeal or tracheal obstruction to breathing.

    **(4)** **Rales** is a broad term that can mean any abnormal breath sound. The term is used less now than in the past.

    **(5)** **Rhonchi** are sonorous sounds produced by secretions in large airways.

  **d. Anatomic changes** of significance include the following.

    **(1)** **Clubbing of the fingers** is due to lifting of the nail base by tissue proliferation on the dorsal surface of the terminal phalanx.

      **(a)** As a sign of pulmonary disease in children, clubbing most often is caused by cystic fibrosis. Pulmonary abscess, empyema, some neoplasms, and, occasionally, bronchiectasis not associated with cystic fibrosis also can produce clubbing.

      **(b)** Nonpulmonary causes of clubbing include congenital cyanotic heart disease, subacute bacterial endocarditis, biliary cirrhosis, chronic ulcerative colitis, and regional enteritis.

    **(2)** **A change in tracheal position** is useful in detecting a mediastinal shift and an inequality between the two sides of the chest, suggesting a pneumothorax or atelectasis.

    **(3)** **A change in thoracic configuration.** A **barrel chest deformity** suggests hyperinflation and overdistension of the lungs due to chronic airway obstruction.

**3. Laboratory studies**

  **a. Imaging procedures**

    **(1)** **Chest x-ray** is indicated if pulmonary disease is suspected. An x-ray of the sinuses may be helpful in sinus disease. Neck films are informative in upper airway obstruction.

    **(2)** **Fluoroscopy** is useful for dynamic studies (e.g., to evaluate diaphragmatic movements or the cause of stridor) and for guiding invasive procedures (e.g., thoracentesis).

    **(3)** **Ultrasonography** can be used instead of fluoroscopy when evaluating diaphragmatic motility, confirming pleural effusion, and guiding thoracentesis.

    **(4)** **Contrast studies** of value include barium swallow, bronchogram, pulmonary arteriogram, and thoracic aortogram.

    **(5)** **Radionuclide lung scans** are valuable in the evaluation of pulmonary ventilation and perfusion.

    **(6)** **Computed tomography (CT) scanning** of the chest is useful in differentiating among pulmonary lesions that cannot be distinguished on chest x-ray (e.g., to differentiate a collapsed lung from a mediastinal mass or pleural fluid from a consolidated lung). Chest CT scanning may also show the extent of cystic lesions and bronchiectasis not visualized on routine chest x-rays.

  **b. Pulmonary function tests** are used to evaluate obstructive, restrictive, and diffusion abnormalities in pulmonary function. They cannot diagnose specific diseases.

    **(1)** **Commonly used tests** in children are **spirometry, flow-volume curves,** and **lung volumes**.

      **(a)** Tests can be performed before and after inhalation of a bronchodilating agent (to determine whether abnormalities are reversible) or before and after exercise (as a challenge to elicit airway obstruction). Exercise testing is also used to evaluate cardiopulmonary fitness.

      **(b)** Testing requires a child who can cooperate by taking a deep breath to total lung capacity and then exhaling completely. Therefore, the tests cannot be performed in most children under age 7 years, in most retarded children, or in children with tracheostomies.

    **(2)** **Less commonly used tests** in children include maximal voluntary ventilation, diffusing capacity of the lung ($D_L$co), and closing volume.

  **c. Blood gas analysis**

    **(1)** **Arterial oxygen tension ($Po_2$)** is a sensitive indicator of overall pulmonary function. The arterial $Po_2$ in combination with **arterial carbon dioxide tension ($Pco_2$)** provides information about the adequacy of alveolar gas exchange.

    **(2)** **Capillary pH and $Pco_2$.** Obtaining a sample of arterial blood may be difficult [e.g., in neonates with respiratory distress syndrome (hyaline membrane disease)]. In such cases, an alternative is to determine the pH and $Pco_2$ of capillary blood and to monitor oxygen saturation by pulse oximetry, a noninvasive technique.

**d. Tests for specific situations**
  **(1)** In children suspected of having **asthma,** helpful tests include serum immunoglobulin E (IgE) level, the presence of eosinophils in a nasal smear, and total circulating eosinophil level. Antigen-specific IgE levels in serum can also be determined.
  **(2)** In children suspected of having **cystic fibrosis,** sweat testing for chloride levels is diagnostic (see IV D 1).
  **(3)** In children suspected of having **immunodeficiency disorders** (a number of which present as chronic lung disease), immunoglobulin levels and IgG subclass levels can be determined (see Ch 8 II).
  **(4)** Serum drug levels can be useful for assessing the **adequacy of drug therapy** (e.g., with theophylline).
  **(5)** In infants who have had a significant episode of **apnea,** who are siblings or half-siblings of children who have died from **sudden infant death syndrome (SIDS),** who are **unstable, premature infants,** or who have **unexplained bradycardia,** pneumography may be helpful.
    **(a)** In this study, heart rate and rhythm and respiratory pattern are recorded during sleep or over a 12-hour period. Pneumography can be combined with other monitoring procedures, such as oxygen saturation or electroencephalography.
    **(b)** Pneumograms can help to distinguish between apnea and periodic breathing. They can also identify various cardiac arrhythmias, including heart rate lability and bradycardia.
**e. Endoscopic procedures**
  **(1)** **Laryngoscopy** is useful in patients with stridor or laryngeal disorders. Older children may often be examined indirectly by mirror, but infants may require direct laryngoscopy under sedation or general anesthesia.
  **(2)** **Bronchoscopy** may be performed as either a flexible or rigid technique.
    **(a)** **Flexible bronchoscopy** is useful for dynamic airway studies in patients with stridor or airway obstruction and for obtaining culture specimens. It is performed under local sedation and can be done on an outpatient basis.
    **(b)** **Rigid bronchoscopy** is used in foreign body removal and other airway surgery. It requires general anesthesia and usually is performed by a surgeon.
**f. Thoracentesis** is used to obtain pleural fluid for culture and analysis.

## II. ACUTE RESPIRATORY FAILURE

**A. Definition.** Respiratory failure (pulmonary insufficiency) exists when the patient has hypoxemia (i.e., arterial $Po_2$ below 50 mm Hg) while breathing 50% oxygen, with or without associated hypercapnia (i.e., arterial $Pco_2$ above 50 mm Hg).

**B. Etiology.** Acute respiratory failure can be caused by many disorders. Classifying the possible causes helps to pinpoint the underlying pathophysiology and, thus, to direct appropriate management in an individual case. Representative examples of the many causes are as follows.

  **1. Obstructive disorders causing acute respiratory insufficiency**
    **a. Upper airway obstruction** can result from anomalies (choanal atresia, Pierre Robin syndrome, laryngeal webs, subglottic stenosis, vascular rings), aspiration of gastric secretions or a foreign body, infections (epiglottitis), allergic laryngospasm, or growths (tumors, cysts, tonsillar and adenoidal hypertrophy).
    **b. Lower airway obstruction** can result from anomalies (bronchomalacia, lobar emphysema), aspiration (due to tracheoesophageal fistula, pharyngeal incoordination), infection (pertussis, bronchiolitis, pneumonia), or inflammation and bronchospasm (asthma, bronchopulmonary dysplasia).

  **2. Restrictive disorders causing acute respiratory insufficiency**
    **a. Restrictive disorders of the lung parenchyma** include pulmonary hypoplasia, respiratory distress syndrome (hyaline membrane disease), pneumothorax, hemorrhage, pulmonary edema, and pleural effusion.
    **b. Restrictive chest wall disorders** include diaphragmatic hernia, absent ribs, thoracic dystrophy, abdominal distension, kyphoscoliosis, traumatic flail chest, myasthenia gravis, muscular dystrophy, and obesity.

3. **Disorders causing inefficient alveolar-capillary gas transfer**
    a. **Disorders that cause diffusion defects** include pulmonary edema, interstitial fibrosis, collagen disorders, *Pneumocystis carinii* pneumonia, sarcoidosis, and desquamative interstitial pneumonitis. Adult respiratory distress syndrome (ARDS) may be seen in children with shock, sepsis, and near-drowning.
    b. **Disorders that depress the respiratory center** include cerebral trauma, CNS infection, sedative overdoses, severe asphyxia, and tetanus.

## C. Clinical features

1. **Pulmonary features**
    a. Infants and children with acute respiratory failure show tachypnea, altered depth and pattern of respiration, chest retractions, nasal flaring, cyanosis, and diaphoresis.
    b. Breath sounds may be decreased or absent, or the child may be grunting or wheezing.

2. **Neurologic features.** Because of the brain's sensitivity to hypoxemia, headache, restlessness, irritability, seizures, or even coma may develop.

3. **Cardiac features** include hypotension and bradycardia. Severe or prolonged insufficiency can cause heart failure and pulmonary edema.

## D. Therapy depends on the degree of hypoxemia, the arterial $Pco_2$ and pH values, and the underlying pathophysiology. Ultimate recovery requires correction of the underlying cause of respiratory failure.

1. **Oxygenation** should be at the lowest concentration of oxygen that will provide an adequate arterial $Po_2$ (above 60 mm Hg). Too high an oxygen concentration can cause pulmonary edema, atelectasis, or, in neonates, retinopathy of prematurity. Intubation may be necessary to provide continuous positive airway pressure for refractory hypoxemia.

2. **Securing a patent airway** may call for removal of bronchial secretions and use of bronchodilating agents, as well as intubation or mechanical ventilation.
    a. **Endotracheal or nasotracheal intubation** may be sufficient in upper airway obstruction. Placement of the tube should be verified promptly by auscultation and chest x-ray.
    b. **Humidifying the air** helps to reduce viscous bronchial secretions.

3. **Intubation and positive-pressure ventilation** may be required for an elevated arterial $Pco_2$ with respiratory acidosis.

# III. ASTHMA

## A. Definition. Asthma is a reversible airway obstruction caused by increased responsiveness of the airways (bronchial hyperreactivity) to various stimuli.

## B. Incidence. Asthma is the most common chronic lung disease of children, affecting 5%–8% of all children.

1. Before puberty, twice as many boys are affected, but at puberty the incidence of asthma in girls increases.

2. Asthma is more severe in young children because they are more prone to viral infections (i.e., colds) and because the proportionately smaller airway size increases airway resistance.

3. Asthma rarely is fatal but causes 30–40 deaths in children each year.

## C. Triggering mechanisms of increased airway hyperreactivity are many.

1. **Respiratory viral infections** are the most common triggers in young children. Common agents include rhinovirus, respiratory syncytial virus, and parainfluenza virus.

2. **Air pollutants,** especially ozone, sulfur dioxide, and cigarette smoke, are common triggers.

3. **Allergens** include house dust, animal danders, molds, and pollens of ragweed and other grasses (see Ch 8 IV).

4. **Foods** are seldom a cause but, when implicated, include chocolate, shellfish, nuts, and (very rarely) milk.

5. **Exercise**-induced symptoms are very common.

6. **Emotions** play a major role in asthma. They can trigger attacks. Also, symptoms are frequently exacerbated by laughing or crying.

**D. Pathophysiology.** Every asthma attack has three **components:** bronchospasm, mucus production, and edema and inflammation of the airway mucosa. The components that predominate at any one time during an attack vary.

**E. Clinical features.** The reversible airway obstruction manifests as slowing of forced expiration. Resulting symptoms—which may occur singly or in any combination—include cough, chest tightness, wheezing, and dyspnea (tachypnea in young children). Symptoms may change in severity both spontaneously and as a result of therapy, making frequent clinical reassessment necessary. Hypoxemia results from airway obstruction, and arterial $Po_2$ continues to drop as the attack occurs. Initially, due to hyperventilation, arterial $Pco_2$ is low. During severe attacks, $Pco_2$ will subsequently rise as hypoventilation and respiratory failure ensue.

**F. Diagnosis**

1. **Clinical diagnosis.** A description of the child's typical recurrent symptoms often is diagnostic. Diagnosis is more difficult when symptoms are atypical (e.g., chronic cough without wheezing or dyspnea) or when asthma begins in infancy.

2. **Differential diagnosis.** All that is needed to produce a wheeze is sufficient air flow through a sufficiently narrow orifice. Therefore, wheezing episodes can occur in many diseases. Those likely to be confused with asthma include bronchiolitis, cystic fibrosis, tracheomalacia, pertussis, bronchiectasis, tuberculosis with enlarged lymph nodes, foreign body aspiration, airway tumors (adenoma, carcinoid), congestive heart failure, and $\alpha_1$-antitrypsin deficiency.

**G. Therapy**

1. **Management of the acute attack**
    a. **Emergency therapy**
       (1) Inhaled bronchodilators (e.g., isoetharine, albuterol) are rapidly effective and have minimal side effects in most patients.
       (2) If these drugs are not readily available, epinephrine or terbutaline may be given subcutaneously.
       (3) The patient who fails to respond to the above measures may be given aminophylline intravenously.
       (4) Failure to respond to inhaled, subcutaneous, or intravenous therapy is an indication for hospital admission. By definition, this is **status asthmaticus**.
    b. **In-hospital therapy**
       (1) Drugs given are intravenous aminophylline, an aerosolized bronchodilator (albuterol, isoetharine), and an intravenous steroid (e.g., methylprednisolone).
       (2) Laboratory work on admission should include arterial blood gas analysis to check the patient's $Pco_2$ and $Po_2$. A chest x-ray is advisable, although this has not been shown to alter therapy.
       (3) Oxygen is necessary to correct hypoxemia.

2. **Maintenance therapy.** Three approaches are used in the management of asthma.
    a. **Avoidance** is the simplest, most direct treatment: If cats cause wheezing, they should be avoided. However, in many households this is easier said than done.
    b. **Desensitization** may be helpful when certain allergens (e.g., ragweed) cannot be avoided, but such immunotherapy is not a panacea.
    c. **Drugs** are the keystone of therapy. Drugs used include bronchodilators, corticosteroids, and cromolyn.
       (1) **Bronchodilators**
          (a) **Xanthine drugs** (theophylline and its derivatives) are effective bronchodilators but have significant side effects and a narrow window of effectiveness. Bronchodilation is directly related to the serum concentration, and blood levels are used to guide therapy and to monitor toxicity.
             (i) **Side effects** (irritability, hyperactivity, abdominal pain, tachycardia, hematemesis, seizures) can be minimized by beginning with a small dose and increasing it slowly.

        **(ii) Preparations.** There are numerous rapid-release and slow-release theophylline preparations. Fixed combinations and preparations containing alcohol or sugar should be avoided.

     **(b) $\beta_2$-Adrenergic agonists** include isoetharine, albuterol (salbutamol), terbutaline, epinephrine, isoproterenol, and metaproterenol.

        **(i) Side effects.** Albuterol and terbutaline are the most $\beta_2$-specific and, thus, cause less severe tachycardia and jitteriness than occur with epinephrine.

        **(ii) Oral preparations.** As oral tablets or liquids, metaproterenol is short-acting; terbutaline and albuterol are medium-acting.

        **(iii) Inhaled $\beta_2$-adrenergic agonist bronchodilators** can be administered by air compressor with nebulizer (for young children or patients in significant respiratory distress) or by a metered-dose inhaler (MDI). **Spacers** also can be used in young children. These holding chambers allow young children to use an MDI without needing to coordinate activation of the MDI with inhalation. Failure to respond to an MDI usually is due to improper technique. Overuse can diminish the effectiveness of aerosolized bronchodilators (tachyphylaxis). Out of the hospital, they should not be used more often than six times per 24 hours.

   **(2) Corticosteroids** have significant side effects, when used for long periods. They are extremely effective, however, as short-term therapy (usually 3–5 days) for status asthmaticus. Moreover, low-dose (preferably alternate-day) steroid therapy can be very effective for patients whose asthma cannot be controlled with theophylline or with inhaled or oral $\beta_2$-adrenergic agonists. Inhaled steroids administered by MDI may permit further decreases in oral steroid dosage and generally do not cause side effects.

   **(3) Cromolyn** is a mast cell stabilizer that inhibits pulmonary histamine release. It is given to prevent, not treat, asthma attacks. Cromolyn is administered three to four times per day by air compressor with nebulizer or by MDI. It has virtually no side effects.

**IV. CYSTIC FIBROSIS.** The most common lethal inherited disease of whites, cystic fibrosis has an incidence of 1 in 1600 live births and an estimated carrier rate of 1 in 20. Covered in this chapter are the general aspects of cystic fibrosis and its pulmonary complications. Pancreatic insufficiency and other gastrointestinal manifestations of cystic fibrosis are covered in Chapter 10 X A 1.

  **A. Definition.** Cystic fibrosis is a disease of the exocrine glands that causes viscid secretions. The gastrointestinal and respiratory systems are most commonly and most severely affected.

  **B. Underlying defect**

    **1.** Cystic fibrosis is inherited as an **autosomal recessive trait**. The gene that causes cystic fibrosis is located on chromosome 7, and in 70% of patients there is an absence of three phenylalanines. The abnormal protein that the gene encodes for has been identified and named the **cystic fibrosis transmembrane regulator protein**.

    **2.** The defect in cystic fibrosis is thought to be a **blocked or closed chloride channel** in the cell membrane of epithelial cells. This blockage traps chloride ions inside the cell and draws sodium ions and water into the cell. This process results in dehydration of mucous secretions.

  **C. Clinical features** of cystic fibrosis vary considerably in nature and severity.

    **1. Most common and most severe manifestations**

      **a. Respiratory insufficiency** occurs eventually in all patients and is due to abnormal mucous gland secretion in the airways, producing airway obstruction and secondary infection, cough, dyspnea, bronchiectasis, and pulmonary fibrosis.

      **b. Malabsorption** of fats and protein due to pancreatic insufficiency and abnormal mucous gland secretions in the gastrointestinal tract occurs in 85% of patients (see Ch 10 X A 1), producing fatty stools, vitamin deficiencies, failure to gain weight, and retarded growth.

    **2. Other manifestations and complications**

      **a. Electrolytes in sweat.** Concentrations of sodium and chloride in sweat are abnormally high in all patients. This can lead to heat intolerance and a hyponatremic hypochloremic metabolic alkalosis.

      **b. Respiratory complications**

        **(1)** Hemoptysis is a common complication.

**(2)** The incidence of pneumothorax is increased in adolescents and adults.

**(3)** Cor pulmonale is a late complication.

**c. Other intestinal problems**

**(1)** **Meconium ileus,** in which abnormally viscid meconium completely obstructs the ileum, occurs in 10% of all infants born with cystic fibrosis.

**(2)** A comparable fecal obstruction (meconium ileus equivalent) can occur in older children as a result of dietary indiscretion or insufficient enzyme replacement therapy.

**(3)** Rectal prolapse is a relatively common complication; less common is intussusception.

**d. Reproductive effects**

**(1)** Virtually all men with cystic fibrosis are sterile, due to congenital obliteration of the vas deferens.

**(2)** Women with cystic fibrosis produce thick, spermicidal cervical mucus and have reduced fertility.

**e. Hepatic effects.** Focal biliary cirrhosis is present in 25% of all patients and is occasionally severe enough to produce portal hypertension and esophageal varices.

**f. Pancreatic effects**

**(1)** Abnormal glucose tolerance is present in 25%–75% of all patients.

**(2)** Type II diabetes may develop in 1%–2% of all patients.

**g. Nasal effects**

**(1)** Chronic sinusitis with opacification of the sinuses occurs in all patients.

**(2)** Nasal polyposis occurs in 5% of all patients.

**h. Musculoskeletal effects.** Hypertrophic osteoarthropathy develops in some patients. This condition of unknown etiology consists of periostitis and arthritis, producing joint pain, edema, and decreased activity.

**D. Diagnosis.** Diagnostic criteria for cystic fibrosis include a positive sweat test, typical pulmonary manifestations, typical gastrointestinal manifestations, and a positive family history.

**1.** The **sweat test** is positive if the chloride concentration of sweat exceeds 60 mEq/L. Normal sweat chloride values are below 40 mEq/L.

**a.** The test must be done correctly. The method of choice is quantitative pilocarpine iontophoresis by the Gibson and Cooke method or the Westcort method.

**b.** False positive results can occur in nephrogenic diabetes insipidus, hypothyroidism, mucopolysaccharidosis, adrenal insufficiency, ectodermal dysplasia, severe malnutrition, and anorexia nervosa.

**2.** Evidence of **meconium ileus** is virtually diagnostic of cystic fibrosis. Failure to pass a stool in the first 24 hours of life, combined with small bowel obstruction (usually in the area of the ileocecal valve) and evidence of a microcolon, strongly suggest meconium ileus.

**3.** Without evidence of meconium ileus, **a high index of suspicion** is required to make the diagnosis. The initial presentation may be subtle and often is missed. Any of the following initial signs and symptoms should suggest the possible need for a confirmatory sweat test.

**a. Respiratory signs and symptoms** include a chronic cough; recurrent pneumonia and atelectasis; hyperinflation; digital clubbing; persistent crackles on lung auscultation; the presence of *Pseudomonas aeruginosa, Staphylococcus aureus,* and, in infants, *Klebsiella* or *Escherichia coli* in sputum; hemoptysis; and nasal polyposis.

**b. Gastrointestinal signs and symptoms** include steatorrhea, chronic diarrhea, rectal prolapse, biliary cirrhosis, cholecystitis, and meconium ileus equivalent.

**c. Other signs and symptoms** include failure to thrive, hyponatremic hypochloremic metabolic alkalosis, and the symptom complex of hypoproteinemia, anemia, and edema in infants.

**E. Therapy**

**1. Treatment of respiratory problems**

**a. Antibiotics** are given either continuously or intermittently to prevent or treat pulmonary bacterial infection.

**(1)** **Oral therapy** usually consists of antistaphylococcal drugs (e.g., dicloxacillin), cephalosporins, trimethoprim-sulfamethoxazole, and chloramphenicol.

**(2)** **Aerosolized therapy** is used to decrease chronic lung infection and reduce the need for hospitalization.

(3) **Intravenous therapy** lasting 10–21 days may be needed for established infections. Usually, an aminoglycoside (e.g., tobramycin) and either a semisynthetic penicillin (e.g., piperacillin) or third-generation cephalosporin (e.g., ceftazidime) are given.

b. **Other drugs.** Oral and inhaled **bronchodilators** are used frequently, and the **mucolytic** acetylcysteine sometimes is given. The use of **steroids** to reduce inflammation is being investigated.

c. **Chest physiotherapy** (breathing exercises, postural drainage with or without chest percussion) is used to aid the clearance of viscid secretions. Some evidence suggests that regular vigorous **exercise** may produce the same benefit as chest physiotherapy.

2. **Treatment of digestive problems**
   a. **Pancreatic enzymes** (freeze-dried extracts of animal pancreas) are given before each meal or snack. The dosage is adjusted on the basis of growth and stool pattern.
   b. **A high-calorie, high-protein diet** should be provided. For anorectic children, an oral or parenteral supplement may be needed to improve caloric consumption.
   c. **Vitamin supplementation** is given, especially the fat-soluble vitamins A, E, and K.
   d. **Stool softeners** are often helpful.
   e. **Antacids and H$_2$-receptor antagonists** are sometimes used to decrease gastric acidity and to improve the effectiveness of enzyme therapy.

3. **Treatment of complications**
   a. **Meconium ileus** usually requires surgery, although the obstruction sometimes can be cleared by instilling an enema composed of radiocontrast agent (meglumine diatrizoate) or acetylcysteine under fluoroscopic guidance.
   b. **Meconium ileus equivalent** usually can be relieved with enemas of soapsuds, acetylcysteine, or meglumine diatrizoate.
   c. **Pneumothorax** usually is treated by closed-tube thoracostomy if it is symptomatic or large. Persistent leaks require procedures such as sclerosis or pleural stripping and abrasion.
   d. **Hemoptysis** is treated with vitamin K and antibiotics. If bleeding is severe or life-threatening, embolization of the bleeding vessel may be tried.

F. **Prognosis.** The outlook for cystic fibrosis patients has improved significantly over the past 20 years, and mean life expectancy has reached 25 years of age. Most patients (95%) die of respiratory failure; others die of liver failure or other complications. Some individuals with cystic fibrosis do live into the fifth or sixth decade of life.

# V. BRONCHOPULMONARY DYSPLASIA

A. **Definition.** Bronchopulmonary dysplasia is a chronic pulmonary disease of infants that is characterized by the need for oxygen therapy beyond 28 days of life and by a characteristic series of changes in the lung on x-ray. Bronchopulmonary dysplasia follows neonatal respiratory failure and is especially likely to occur after oxygen and mechanical ventilation therapy for hyaline membrane disease in a preterm infant. It also may occur in term infants after acute lung injury (e.g., pneumonia, meconium aspiration, diaphragmatic hernia).

B. **Pathogenesis**

1. **Important pathogenetic factors** in bronchopulmonary dysplasia include:
   a. **Oxygen toxicity** from prior oxygen therapy at a concentration fraction of inspired oxygen (Fio$_2$) exceeding 0.8
   b. **Barotrauma** from mechanical ventilation with high airway pressure

2. **Other factors** that may play a pathogenetic role include prematurity, fluid overload, damage caused by severe pulmonary disease, and a familial predisposition to asthma.

C. **Pathology.** The two most prominent features are:

1. **Diffuse alveolar injury** with endothelial cell damage, resulting in interstitial pulmonary edema and fibrosis

2. **Necrotizing bronchiolitis** with smooth muscle hypertrophy, resulting in areas of atelactasis and emphysema

D. **Clinical features** include retractions, tachypnea, wheezing, and cyanosis, especially with stress. Some infants show poor lung compliance, pulmonary edema, and pulmonary hypertension.

**E. Diagnosis**

1. **Pulmonary physical examination** should emphasize the sleeping respiratory rate, the signs of the effort of breathing, and auscultation to determine the presence of crackles and wheezes.

2. **A baseline chest x-ray** should be taken, to delineate acute findings versus chronic changes.
   a. In the acute stage, there is near-total lung opacification on x-ray.
   b. In the chronic stage, x-rays show thickened fibrotic markings and cystic changes.

3. **Blood gas analysis** is important. However, the stress of obtaining an arterial specimen can produce significant hypoxemia in these infants, and oximetry plus capillary blood gas analysis may be preferable.

4. **Electrocardiography** and **echocardiography** help to identify the presence of cor pulmonale.

**F. Therapy**

1. **Oxygen** probably is the most important therapy in these infants. Oxygen is delivered by nasal cannula or feeding tube to maintain an oxygen saturation greater than 90% and to minimize the work of breathing. Some infants may require mechanical ventilation.

2. **Diuretics.** Infants with pulmonary edema or with respiratory crackles, marked elevations in $P_{CO_2}$, and persistent hypoxemia frequently benefit from diuretic therapy. Furosemide may cause nephrocalcinosis and should be avoided if possible.

3. **Bronchodilators.** Theophylline and $\beta_2$-adrenergic agents, both inhaled and oral, improve bronchospasm, decrease the work of breathing, and may improve oxygenation.

4. **Dietary supplements.** Infants with bronchopulmonary dysplasia require more calories than other infants, in part because of a higher basal metabolic rate and in part because of increased work of breathing. Increasing the caloric density of the formula or supplementing the diet with glucose polymers or medium-chain triglycerides often is sufficient, but some infants require nasogastric feedings or parenteral hyperalimentation for adequate growth.

**G. Prognosis**

1. **Short-term prognosis**
   a. Most infants, even those with severe bronchopulmonary dysplasia, will get better with time, and by age 5 years their pulmonary function may be similar to that of age-matched children. However, these patients may require oxygen for 6–12 months after hospital discharge, and in early childhood they may have some evidence of small airway obstruction.
   b. Many infants have hyperreactive airways and may require hospitalization for acute viral infections. During childhood these infants have a greater risk of asthma.

2. **Long-term prognosis** is not known since patients who were among the first reported cases are only now approaching adulthood. However, the marked pulmonary damage that occurs during the phase of rapid lung growth may predispose affected infants to chronic lung disease in adult life.

**VI. APNEA OF INFANCY** (see also Ch 5 V A 4 b)

**A. Definition.** In infants, apnea is the cessation of breathing for longer than 20 seconds or for any duration if it is associated with pallor, limpness, cyanosis, or bradycardia and if it requires vigorous stimulation for resuscitation. Apnea is a common symptom of disease in infants, not a disease itself.

1. **SIDS** (sudden infant death syndrome) is the sudden and unexpected death of an infant whose history or postmortem examination cannot demonstrate a specific cause of death. SIDS is the leading cause of death in infants in the first year of life. Although probably not the major cause of SIDS, apnea may account for 5%–20% of SIDS deaths.

2. **ALTE** (apparent life-threatening event) is an episode of apnea associated with color change (pallor or cyanosis), marked change in muscle tone (usually limpness, rarely rigidity), or choking and gagging. Observers usually fear the child will die and intervene with vigorous stimulation or cardiopulmonary resuscitation.

**B. Types of apnea and their causes**

1. **Central apnea.** When there is no central neurologic drive to breathe, there is no chest wall or abdominal movement. There are several factors that lead to central apnea. It also may be idiopathic and may occur in infants with a positive family history of SIDS. Causes of central apnea include the following:
   a. Prematurity (see Ch 5 V A 4 b)
   b. Medications given to mother or infant
   c. Infections, either bacterial or viral
   d. Anemia
   e. Cardiac arrhythmias (especially Wolff-Parkinson-White syndrome)
   f. Seizures
   g. Gastroesophageal reflux or aspiration (vagally mediated)
   h. Hypoglycemia
   i. Central alveolar hypoventilation
   j. Bronchopulmonary dysplasia

2. **Obstructive apnea.** When airway obstruction results in apnea, chest wall and abdominal movements will be present in the absence of airflow at the nose and mouths. Causes of obstructive apnea include the following:
   a. Macroglossia (e.g., Down syndrome, hypothyroidism, or Pierre Robin syndrome)
   b. Enlarged tonsils and adenoids
   c. Posterior pharyngeal muscle incoordination (e.g., from cerebral palsy or trauma)
   d. Laryngospasm
   e. Cleft lip repair
   f. Achondroplasia
   g. Obstructed tracheostomy

3. **Mixed apnea.** A combination of central and obstructive apnea can occur. It usually begins with central apnea followed by airway obstruction.

**C. Evaluation of the infant with apnea**

1. **History.** In this important part of the evaluation, questions to be answered include the following.
   a. Was the child really apneic?
   b. Was the child asleep or awake?
   c. Were there rhythmic movements suggesting a seizure?
   d. What was the relationship to feeding?
   e. Was there mucus or vomitus in the mouth or nose?
   f. Was the child pale, limp, or cyanotic?
   g. How long was the child apneic?
   h. Did the apnea resolve on its own, and, if not, what intervention was needed?

2. **Physical examination.** Special attention should be paid to the neurologic and cardiac examinations as well as to the airway examination.

3. **Laboratory studies.** Depending on the suspected cause of the apnea and the findings on history and physical examination, the following tests may be useful:
   a. Arterial blood gas analysis
   b. Electroencephalography, both standard and during sleep
   c. Cranial ultrasonography
   d. Electrocardiography
   e. Chest x-ray
   f. X-ray of airway or bronchoscopy
   g. Barium swallow or gastrointestinal pH probe
   h. Various blood studies (e.g., complete blood count, electrolytes, calcium, blood sugar, blood cultures)
   i. Pneumography

**D. Therapy**

1. **Treatment of hypoventilation and airway obstruction.** Hypoventilation may require the use of a ventilator, and airway obstruction may call for tracheostomy.

**2. Other treatments of apnea** depend on its cause. Examples follow.
   **a.** Obstructing tonsils should be removed.
   **b.** Anemia or arrhythmias should be corrected.
   **c.** Seizures should be treated with anticonvulsants.
   **d.** Apnea due to bradycardia may be helped by the stimulant effects of theophylline or atropine.
   **e.** If the infant with gastroesophageal reflux is not helped sufficiently by an upright position and by adding cereal to thicken the formula, metoclopramide may be tried.

**3. Home monitoring.** Evaluation of the child with apnea may not identify a cause. Use of a home monitor may be recommended if the apneic episode is felt to be significant and if a recurrence could be potentially fatal (e.g., an ALTE).
   **a.** The home monitor sets off an alarm when apnea or bradycardia is detected. Families learn how to respond to an alarm and resuscitate their infant if necessary.
   **b.** Home monitoring has a significant negative impact on a family, however, and should not be recommended lightly.

# VII. CONGENITAL MALFORMATIONS that cause respiratory problems during the neonatal period are discussed in Chapter 5 V A 2. The following discussion is focused on those congenital malformations that do not cause symptoms until after the neonatal period or that have late complications.

**A. Laryngomalacia (infantile larynx).** This congenital disorder is the most common cause of stridor in infancy. The larynx appears disproportionately small and the supporting structures may be abnormally soft.

**1. Clinical features**
   **a.** Stridor begins within the first 4 weeks of life and is accentuated by increased ventilation (e.g., from crying or excitement) or by upper respiratory infections.
   **b.** Stridor usually resolves by age 12 months but may recur with respiratory infections until about age 3 years.

**2. Diagnosis** is by fiberoptic bronchoscopy or direct laryngoscopy.

**3. Therapy** usually is not needed. Rarely, tracheostomy is required when stridor occurs in association with failure to thrive or in infants with life-threatening apnea or airway obstruction.

**B. Vascular rings.** Congenital anomalies of the aortic arch or its branches can create a ring around the airway that compromises respiration.

**1. Types.** Vascular anomalies most likely to compress the trachea are:
   **a.** A right aortic arch with a left ligamentum arteriosum or patent ductus arteriosus
   **b.** A double aortic arch
   **c.** An anomalous innominate or left carotid artery
   **d.** A pulmonary artery sling

**2. Clinical features**
   **a.** Many of these infants present with stridor.
   **b.** Other respiratory symptoms can include raucous respirations, intercostal retractions, tachypnea, and dyspnea with prolonged exhalation; opisthotonos may make breathing easier.
   **c.** Respiratory symptoms may become worse with feeding.

**3. Therapy** is surgical correction of the anomaly.

**C. Tracheoesophageal fistula** (see also Ch 10 II C 1). Children born with a tracheoesophageal fistula are prone to develop chronic pulmonary disease, particularly tracheomalacia, airway hyperreactivity, or bronchiectasis. Chronic aspiration is believed to be a major factor resulting from uncoordinated esophageal peristalsis.

**D. Bronchogenic cyst.** This congenital cyst lined with bronchial epithelium usually is found in the mediastinum.

**1. Clinical features.** Symptoms result if the cyst compresses the airway or if the cyst becomes infected and suppurates through a tracheobronchial communication.

**2. Therapy** is surgical removal of the cyst.

**E. Pulmonary sequestration.** A cystlike mass of nonfunctioning lung tissue, which lacks normal communication with the tracheobronchial tree, sometimes develops in the embryo, most often within the left lower lobe, but at times entirely outside the lungs. The nonfunctioning sequestration is nourished by systemic arteries.

**1. Clinical features**
   **a.** Infection can result if a fistula develops between the sequestration and either the airway or the digestive tract.
   **b.** Children usually present with a history of recurrent, persistent, progressive pulmonary sepsis in the form of pneumonitis or lung abscess.

**2. Diagnosis**
   **a.** Chest x-ray usually shows a density in the region of the sequestration, with displacement of the bronchovascular markings.
   **b.** Contrast bronchography shows the sequestration as an area that fails to fill, outlined by bronchi that are filled. Aortography will delineate the anomalous arterial supply from the aorta.

**3. Therapy** is surgical removal of the sequestration.

**F. Pulmonary arteriovenous fistula.** A direct intrapulmonary connection between the pulmonary artery and vein, without an intervening capillary bed, produces an intrapulmonary right-to-left shunt. The fistula usually occurs in the lower lobes and is frequently small enough to be missed.

**1. Clinical features.** When the shunt is severe enough to be symptomatic, children present with dyspnea, cyanosis, clubbing, hemoptysis, epistaxis, and exercise intolerance. Generalized telangiectasia is seen in 50% of these patients.

**2. Diagnosis**
   **a.** Pulmonary arteriovenous fistula is suggested by laboratory tests showing polycythemia and oxygen desaturation at rest and during exercise and by x-rays showing homogeneous, noncalcified pulmonary density with irregular, sharp margins.
   **b.** The diagnosis is confirmed by venous cineangiography with full chest x-rays, which may not only delineate the offending fistula but may also uncover smaller fistulas that were not suspected.

**3. Therapy.** Symptomatic children with localized disease should undergo surgical correction.

## VIII. OTHER PULMONARY DISEASES.

Other pulmonary diseases not discussed in this chapter but found elsewhere in the book include aspiration of foreign bodies (see Ch 2 VI), aspiration of hydrocarbons (see Ch 2 IX E 4), drowning (see Ch 2 IV), upper and lower respiratory tract infections (see Ch 9 V B, D, F; VI), and pulmonary neoplasms (see Ch 15 I D 3 b).

**A. Pulmonary tuberculosis**

**1. Incidence**
   **a.** Childhood tuberculosis accounts for about 4% of all new cases of tuberculosis each year, and the mortality rate is highest in infants and adolescents.
   **b.** Susceptibility to infection is increased in children with chronic illness or malnutrition.

**2. Etiology and pathogenesis**
   **a.** The etiologic agent is *Mycobacterium tuberculosis* and, in children, is frequently transmitted by an adult family member. Infrequently, the organism is transmitted transplacentally via seeded amniotic fluid.
   **b.** The primary lesion occurs in the lung in 95% of cases of tuberculosis. Following inhalation, tubercle bacilli spread to regional lymph nodes and then to other lymph nodes, with healing of the primary focus.

**3. Clinical features and laboratory findings**
   **a. Initial (primary) tuberculosis.** A 2- to 10-week incubation period follows the initial infection.
      **(1) Presenting symptoms** usually are minimal and include a temperature that is slightly elevated (to 102° F) but persistent (lasting 2–3 weeks), weight loss, fatigue, irritability, and malaise. Initially, a chest x-ray may appear normal. Some patients are completely asymptomatic.

      **(2)** As the disease progresses, **x-ray findings** of pulmonary infiltration with hilar lymph node enlargement are evident. Mediastinal lymph node involvement is common and may result in bronchial obstruction, with labored breathing, a harsh cough, and tachypnea.

      **(3)** Tuberculous **pleurisy,** often a late complication, is marked by pleuritic pain, fluid in the chest, cough, and decreased breath sounds.

  **b. Reactivation (adult or chronic) tuberculosis.** Many cases of pulmonary tuberculosis are due to reactivation of *M. tuberculosis* after a long period of latency. Early lesions become encapsulated and then liquefy, spreading bacteria throughout the lungs.

      **(1) Symptoms.** A dry cough progresses to a productive cough that starts with mucoid sputum, changing to become mucopurulent and then blood-streaked. Other symptoms (e.g., low-grade fever, weight loss, night sweats) may be mild and overlooked initially; however, they progressively become more severe.

      **(2) Chest x-ray** reveals a well-defined, homogeneous shadow commonly located in the upper lobes.

**4. Diagnosis.** In childhood tuberculosis, important diagnostic points include:
  **a.** A history of contact with the disease
  **b.** A positive **tuberculin skin test,** with induration of 9 mm or more developing 48–72 hours after intracutaneous injection of **purified protein derivative (PPD)** tuberculin
  **c.** Recovery of *M. tuberculosis* in sputum or gastric washings

**5. Therapy.** Because tubercle bacilli readily develop drug resistance, at least two drugs are given concomitantly in tuberculosis. For childhood tuberculosis, isoniazid (INH) and streptomycin are used.

**6. Prophylaxis**
  **a. Routine tuberculin testing** is recommended for all children (see Table 1-3).
  **b. Chemoprophylaxis with INH** is recommended if the tuberculin test is positive and there is no evidence of disease. INH prophylaxis also is important for tuberculin-positive children undergoing prolonged therapy with corticosteroids or other immunosuppressants.
  **c. Prophylaxis with bacille Calmette-Guérin (BCG) vaccine** is used in countries where the incidence of tuberculosis is high.

**B. Desquamative interstitial pneumonitis (DIP).** In this order, macrophages, lymphocytes, and related cells accumulate in the interstitial tissue, followed by epithelial hyperplasia in alveoli and bronchioles. DIP is one of the few restrictive lung diseases of children. The etiology is unknown but it most likely is immunologic.

**1. Clinical features.** Dyspnea is the most common feature. Other symptoms include fatigue, anorexia, weight loss, cyanosis, and digital clubbing. Copious crackles are audible on auscultation, particularly at lung bases.

**2. Laboratory findings**
  **a.** The chest x-ray shows a typical ground-glass appearance at the bases.
  **b.** Blood counts may show leukocytosis, eosinophilia, and low concentrations of immunoglobulins.
  **c.** Pulmonary function tests reflect the restrictive lung disease and decreased diffusing capacity.
  **d.** Blood gas analysis reveals arterial hypoxemia and hypocapnia (hypercapnia is a late finding).

**3. Therapy** is supportive. Once infectious pneumonitis has been ruled out, corticosteroids may be tried, but they are not always effective.

**C. Pulmonary hemosiderosis.** This uncommon disease is characterized by an abnormal accumulation of iron (as hemosiderin) in the lungs as the result of bleeding into the lungs. The etiology in most cases is unknown; in some cases, especially in young children, the disease is related to ingestion of cow's milk.

**1. Clinical features and diagnosis**
  **a.** Recurrent pulmonary symptoms include cough, hemoptysis, dyspnea, wheezing, and cyanosis.
  **b.** Blood counts show a hypochromic, microcytic iron deficiency anemia.

    **c.** The chest x-ray is variable. Some patients show only transient infiltrates; others show massive parenchymal involvement with atelectasis, emphysema, and lymphadenopathy.

    **d.** Gastric aspirates or bronchial washings show the presence of hemosiderin-laden macrophages.

    **e.** Lung biopsy is necessary if the diagnosis is in doubt.

**2. Therapy.** Blood transfusions are given to correct the anemia. Corticosteroids may prove helpful. Milk-sensitive children benefit from a milk-free diet. If other measures fail, deferoxamine, a parenteral chelating agent, may be tried.

## STUDY QUESTIONS

**Directions:** Each of the numbered items or incomplete statements in this section is followed by answers or by completions of the statement. Select the **one** lettered answer or completion that is **best** in each case.

1. The most common chronic lung disease in children is

(A) asthma
(B) bronchopulmonary dysplasia
(C) cystic fibrosis
(D) pulmonary sequestration
(E) desquamative interstitial pneumonitis

2. The best indicator of cystic fibrosis is

(A) a positive family history of cystic fibrosis
(B) the presence of digital clubbing
(C) a sweat test with a chloride concentration of 70 mEq/L
(D) bronchiectasis on a chest x-ray

3. A 3-year-old girl presents with a history of recurrent pneumonia. On physical examination, wheezing and crackles are heard, and digital clubbing is evident. The most likely diagnosis is

(A) pulmonary sequestration
(B) bronchopulmonary dysplasia
(C) cystic fibrosis
(D) asthma
(E) laryngomalacia

4. A 4-year-old child presents with a history of chronic left lower lobe pneumonitis. On contrast bronchography, the area involved with the pneumonitis does not fill while the area around it does fill. The most likely diagnosis is

(A) asthma
(B) pulmonary sequestration
(C) cystic fibrosis
(D) bronchopulmonary dysplasia
(E) bronchogenic cyst

5. All of the following statements about asthma are correct EXCEPT

(A) its severity remits or exacerbates with or without therapy
(B) it is a disease of airway hyperreactivity
(C) it can be triggered by viral infections, exercise, or emotions
(D) the presence of wheezing is diagnostic
(E) inhaled sympathomimetics are effective therapy

6. Each of the following studies would be helpful in the evaluation of an infant with bronchopulmonary dysplasia EXCEPT

(A) sleeping respiratory rate
(B) oxygen saturation
(C) chest x-ray
(D) sweat test
(E) ECG

7. Components of acute asthma attack include all of the following EXCEPT

(A) bronchospasm
(B) subglottic edema
(C) edema of the airway mucosa
(D) inflammation of the airway mucosa
(E) mucus hypersecretion

8. A 4-month-old boy is brought to the emergency room. His parents report that the child stopped breathing at home, turned blue around his lips, and felt limp. After vigorous shaking of the infant and several mouth-to-mouth breaths, his color returned to normal and he resumed breathing. This infant's condition is best described as

(A) obstructive apnea
(B) central apnea
(C) apparent life-threatening event
(D) pneumonia
(E) congestive heart failure

---

| 1-A | 4-B | 7-B |
|-----|-----|-----|
| 2-C | 5-D | 8-C |
| 3-C | 6-D |     |

9. In the evaluation of a 2-year-old child with x-ray documentation of recurrent pneumonia, all of the following tests would be indicated EXCEPT

(A) immunoglobulin analysis
(B) complete blood count
(C) sweat test
(D) sputum culture
(E) pulmonary function tests

**Directions:** The group of items in this section consists of lettered options followed by a set of numbered items. For each item, select the **one** lettered option that is most closely associated with it. Each lettered option may be selected once, more than once, or not at all.

**Questions 10–14**

Match each pulmonary indication for imaging study with the appropriate procedure.

(A) Chest x-ray
(B) Chest CT scanning
(C) Barium swallow
(D) Chest ultrasonography

10. To evaluate an infant with apnea

11. To rule out diaphragmatic paralysis

12. To evaluate a child with chronic cough and wheezing

13. To differentiate a mediastinal mass lesion from a collapsed lung

14. To guide needle thoracentesis to sample a pleural effusion

---

9-E        12-A
10-C       13-B
11-D       14-D

## ANSWERS AND EXPLANATIONS

**1. The answer is A** *[III B].*
Chronic lung disease is the most common of the chronic diseases in children, and asthma is the most common of the chronic lung diseases. Asthma affects 5%–8% of all children in the United States.

**2. The answer is C** *[I C 3 d (2); IV D].*
A positive sweat test (i.e., sweat chloride level greater than 60 mEq/L) is diagnostic of cystic fibrosis. Children without cystic fibrosis have values below 40 mEq/L. While a positive family history of cystic fibrosis, the presence of digital clubbing, and evidence of bronchiectasis by chest x-ray may suggest cystic fibrosis, the sweat test is diagnostic.

**3. The answer is C** *[IV D 3 a].*
In children with a history of pulmonary disease, the presence of digital clubbing suggests cystic fibrosis until proven otherwise. Asthma, pulmonary sequestration, laryngomalacia, and bronchopulmonary dysplasia are not associated with clubbing.

**4. The answer is B** *[VII E 2 b].*
A pulmonary sequestration is a cystlike mass of nonfunctioning lung tissue, which most often is located in the left lower lobe. Children present with a history of chronic pneumonitis. Bronchography shows the sequestration as an area that does not fill with contrast, outlined by bronchi that are contrast-filled. Aortography demonstrates the anomalous arterial supply.

**5. The answer is D** *[III F 2].*
Although a clinical feature of asthma, wheezing also can occur in many other diseases, including cystic fibrosis, pertussis, foreign body aspiration, and bronchiolitis. Asthma is a disease characterized by airway hyperreactivity to a variety of stimuli, including upper respiratory infections, exercise, and emotions. The symptoms of asthma show remissions and exacerbations with or without therapy. $\beta_2$-Adrenergic agonists are effective bronchodilating therapy, which can be administered orally, by air compressor with nebulizer, or by a metered-dose inhaler (MDI).

**6. The answer is D** *[V E].*
The sweat test is used in the diagnosis of cystic fibrosis but is not helpful in assessing children with bronchopulmonary dysplasia. In the evaluation of children with bronchopulmonary dysplasia, the sleeping respiratory rate, oxygen saturation (obtained by oximetry), and chest x-ray all give valuable information. The severity of the lung disease is also assessed by the rate of growth and the number of calories needed to produce good growth. The electrocardiogram (ECG) is helpful when looking for signs of right ventricular hypertrophy secondary to pulmonary hypertension from chronic hypoxemia.

**7. The answer is B** *[III D].*
Subglottic edema is the major problem in children with croup and the underlying cause of stridor in these patients. Neither subglottic edema nor stridor is commonly seen during an asthma attack, which typically has three components: bronchospasm, mucus production, and edema and inflammation of the airway mucosa.

**8. The answer is C** *[VI A 2, B].*
An apparent life-threatening event (ALTE) is an episode of apnea associated with marked change in color and muscle tone, such that an observer typically believes the infant will die without vigorous stimulation or resuscitation. Central apnea is cessation of breathing without respiratory effort, whereas obstructive apnea is cessation of airflow at the mouth and nose with continued respiratory effort. Apnea may be a symptom of many diseases in infants and should be labeled an ALTE only if no cause can be found. Sudden infant death syndrome (SIDS) is the death of an infant without adequate explanation by history or autopsy examination. Less than 10% of infants who die of SIDS have had a prior ALTE.

**9. The answer is E** *[I C 3 b (1) (b)].*
Sweat testing, immunoglobulin analysis, complete blood count, and sputum culture are helpful in evaluating children with suspected lung disease. Pulmonary function tests require a child's cooperation in taking a deep breath to total lung capacity and then exhaling completely. Therefore, such tests cannot be performed successfully on a 2-year-old child. Such tests can sometimes be done on a research basis using a different technology.

**10–14. The answers are: 10-C, 11-D, 12-A, 13-B, 14-D** *[I C 3 a].*
A barium swallow or gastrointestinal pH probe may be useful in evaluating the possibility of gastrointestinal reflux as a cause of apnea in an infant.

Chest ultrasonography is useful for evaluating diaphragmatic motility. It also can be used to distinguish pleural effusion from adjacent lung and to guide needle thoracentesis. With chest ultrasonography, the high levels of radiation exposure associated with chest fluoroscopy are avoided.

Chest x-ray is indicated in the evaluation of a child with chronic cough and wheezing, to rule out chronic pneumonia, atelectasis, and hyperinflated lungs. In a child with asthma, increased peribronchial lung markings and air trappings are signs of chronic, poorly treated disease.

Computed tomography (CT) scanning of the chest helps to differentiate among pulmonary lesions of differing radiographic densities that cannot be distinguished on chest x-ray (e.g., a collapsed lung versus a mediastinal tumor). CT scanning of the chest also is useful in determining the extent of pulmonary cysts and in detecting signs of bronchiectasis.

# 13
# Renal Diseases
Thomas L. Kennedy

## I. GENERAL PRINCIPLES OF RENAL DISEASE IN CHILDREN

**A. Introduction.** Renal disease and dysfunction generally are considered in terms of the kidney's role in filtration and excretion of nitrogenous waste. An equally important consideration, however, is the kidney's role in fluid and electrolyte balance, in blood pressure regulation, in acid-base homeostasis, and as an endocrine organ elaborating many hormones (e.g., erythropoietin, prostaglandins, renin, vitamin D, kinins). Other important aspects of renal disease in childhood are the limitations of normal function that exist at birth and the growth and maturational changes that occur through infancy and childhood.

**B. Evaluation of renal function**

1. **Urinalysis,** although not totally specific or sensitive, is a useful, noninvasive indicator of renal function and disease. Urine bags may be used to collect urine, or urine may be squeezed from a diaper for dipstick analysis.

   a. **Urine concentration and dilution** may be measured by specific gravity or osmolality. Specific gravity may be determined using a refractometer, which requires only a drop of urine. Although it generally correlates well with urine osmolality, urine specific gravity measures the density of the solution and is disproportionately increased by high molecular weight substances (e.g., protein, glucose).

      (1) Maximally diluted urine has a specific gravity of 1.002 (osmolality of 50 mOsm/kg).

      (2) Maximally concentrated urine has a specific gravity of 1.035 (osmolality of 1200 mOsm/kg).

      (3) Urine that is neither diluted nor concentrated (isosthenuria) has a specific gravity of 1.010 (osmolality of 300 mOsm/kg).

   b. **Urine dipsticks**

      (1) The dipstick technique provides a general estimate of **acidity** and indicates the presence or absence of **albumin, glucose, ketones, urobilinogen, bilirubin,** and **blood** (including free hemoglobin or myoglobin).

      (2) Other available dipsticks indicate **pyuria** (leukocyte esterase) or **gram-negative infection** (with organisms that convert urinary nitrates to nitrite).

   c. **Urine microscopy.** A urine specimen (preferably a fresh one) is centrifuged, and the sediment is examined for **cells, casts, crystals,** and **bacteria.**

      (1) **Bacteria.** It is difficult to distinguish infecting organisms from contaminants or amorphous material (e.g., phosphates, urates). A careful **Gram stain,** however, may help to identify bacteria. Also, significant bacteriuria may occur in the absence of pyuria, and pyuria may occur with acute illness in the absence of infection. Therefore, a **culture** must be obtained to confirm the diagnosis of a urinary tract infection.

      (2) **Cells.** The **morphology** of red cells in urine may help to distinguish glomerular bleeding from blood loss elsewhere in the urinary tract. Crenated, dysmorphic red cells in fresh urine suggest a glomerular origin. These are best seen using **phase-contrast microscopy** on **Wright's stain** of the urine.

      (3) **Casts** of compacted red cells extracted from the tubular lumen (**RBC casts**) are the result of glomerular bleeding and usually are diagnostic of glomerulonephritis. **Leukocyte casts** occasionally are seen in pyelonephritis and interstitial nephritis. **Hyaline casts** and **granular casts** are not diagnostic of renal disease and may occur in sediment from children with oliguria of any cause.

**(4) Crystals** of many varieties may be present in the urine. They rarely are diagnostic of disease. In fact, they reflect factors such as the amount and concentration of solute and solubilizers and urinary pH and osmolarity. An exception is the hexagonal **cystine** crystal, which is diagnostic of cystinuria.

2. **Tests of glomerular function** use timed urine collections. Ideally, urine should be collected over 24 hours, but 8- to 12-hour collections are acceptable.
   a. **Glomerular filtration rate (GFR).** Generally, endogenous **creatinine clearance** is used to measure GFR.
      **(1)** The **normal GFR** in children age 2 years or older is 120 ml/min/1.73 m$^2$.
      **(2)** When timed urine collections are difficult to obtain (e.g., in the young child), GFR can be estimated using the formula

$$\text{creatinine clearance} = \frac{K \ (\text{height in cm})}{\text{serum creatinine (mg/dl)}}$$

   where K = 0.45 in infants less than 1 year old, 0.55 in infants over 1 year old, 0.33 in low birth weight infants, and 0.7 in adolescent males.
   b. **Urinary protein excretion**
      **(1) Total urinary protein** should be less than 150 mg/24 hr, or less than 4 mg/m$^2$/hr. Because timed collections may be difficult to obtain, a random urine specimen may be used to estimate proteinuria.
      **(2) Protein to creatinine ratio** should be less than 0.2. A ratio exceeding 3.5 suggests nephrotic proteinuria.

3. **Tests of renal tubular function**
   a. **Concentrating, diluting, and acidifying capacity.** Useful information is provided by tests that determine the kidney's capacity to concentrate, dilute, and acidify the urine. Renal concentrating capacity is easiest to assess. This is accomplished by a well-monitored overnight fluid deprivation test with determination of acute weight loss, urine output, and maximum urine specific gravity.
   b. **Reabsorptive capacity**
      **(1)** Tubular dysfunction is suggested by **detection of compounds in the urine that normally are reabsorbed completely by the renal tubules**. Such substances include glucose, amino acids, and $\beta_2$-microglobulin.
      **(2)** The **tubular reabsorption of phosphate (TRP)** can be calculated using a small serum sample and random urine specimen. The TRP normally is greater than 85%. It is determined as

$$\text{TRP} = 1 - \frac{\text{urine phosphate} \times \text{serum creatinine}}{\text{serum phosphate} \times \text{urine creatinine}} \times 100\%$$

4. **Tests of bladder function and anatomy**
   a. **Cystometry.** Bladder function may be assessed using the urodynamic test, cystometry. Because it is an invasive procedure that uses catheters, rectal pressure balloons, and needle electrodes and because it requires patient cooperation, cystometry is not employed frequently. It is indicated in the evaluation of a child who has difficulty voiding (e.g., overflow incontinence, urine retention). The test provides a profile of intravesical volume, pressure, and contractility.
   b. **Cystoscopy** is the most direct method of visualizing the urethra and bladder. Because cystoscopy is invasive, requires general anesthesia, and adds little to other imaging techniques, it has little usefulness in children.

5. **Imaging procedures**
   a. **Ultrasonography** is the least invasive and most useful renal imaging technique for pediatric **anatomic imaging**. However, it cannot assess renal function and cannot readily determine mild to moderate renal scarring.
      **(1)** Ultrasonography provides information on kidney location, size, shape, and consistency. It is useful to assess kidney growth serially. It can diagnose obstruction, malformations, cysts, calcifications, and tumors.
      **(2)** It is safe, and, because the equipment is portable, it can be performed on the most critically ill patients.
      **(3)** When combined with color Doppler imaging, blood flow in the renal artery and renal vein can be evaluated.

    **b. Intravenous pyelography (IVP, excretory urography)** has been the standard anatomic renal imaging technique, but it is not an adequate test of renal function.

        **(1)** IVP remains a useful procedure for identifying dilated calices (**caliectasis**) in the child with urinary tract infection.

        **(2)** In a cooperative child, **voiding cystourethrography** can be performed at the end of the IVP procedure to evaluate the morphology and function of the bladder and, in boys, the urethra.

        **(3) Risks and contraindications.** The radiocontrast material that must be injected can provoke allergic reactions or acute renal failure. Because of poor or absent visualization of the kidney, IVP should not be used in patients with renal insufficiency or in newborns.

    **c. Retrograde voiding cystourethrography.** In this procedure, the contrast material is instilled by urethral catheter, and the bladder is visualized using fluoroscopy. The test defines the presence and magnitude of vesicoureteral reflux and provides information about the anatomy of the bladder and urethra.

    **d. Radionuclide scanning** is a useful test of renal function. Although it involves the intravenous injection of a radiolabeled tracer, radiation exposure is low—the gonadal dose is about 10% that of IVP.

        **(1) Evaluation of renal function.** Renal scanning can provide an estimate of total renal function, including GFR [with the use of technetium 99m ($^{99m}$Tc)-labeled diethylenetriamine pentaacetic acid] as well as tubular function [with the use of iodine 131 ($^{131}$I)-labeled *o*-iodohippurate]. It can also quantitate the contribution of each renal unit to total function. When images are obtained in the first seconds after the tracer is injected, information regarding renal blood flow may be obtained.

        **(2) Evaluation of vesicoureteral reflux.** Radionuclide scanning can be used to provide cystograms in the assessment of vesicoureteral reflux.

            **(a)** For cystography alone, the tracer is instilled directly into the bladder by catheter. For cystography in conjunction with a renal scan, it is given by intravenous injection.

            **(b)** The major advantage of radionuclide cystography over standard radiographic cystography is the much lower gonadal radiation dose (less than 5% that of standard cystography). This is important since the child with reflux frequently needs serial cystograms.

            **(c)** The major disadvantages of radionuclide cystography are its relatively poor structural delineation and its inability to evaluate the urethra.

        **(3) Evaluation of kidney infection.** Recently, the use of technetium-labeled dimercaptosuccinic acid (**DMSA**), a tracer that is localized to tubular cells of functioning nephrons, has been recommended as an aid to the diagnosis of renal parenchymal infection.

    **e. Other imaging techniques** have specialized, limited uses in imaging the urinary tract in children. These include arteriography, digital subtraction angiography, computed and positron-emission tomography (CT, PET), and magnetic resonance imaging (MRI).

  **6. Renal biopsy** is the definitive study for **histologic diagnosis** of renal disease. It provides tissue for examination by light, immunofluorescent, and electron microscopy.

    **a. Procedure.** Renal biopsy usually is performed as a percutaneous closed procedure under fluoroscopic or ultrasonic guidance. In infants, renal biopsy is most safely carried out as an operative procedure under general anesthesia. For other patients, sedation and analgesia may be adequate.

    **b. Risks and contraindications.** The risks of the procedure include obtaining insufficient tissue for diagnosis, causing bleeding or infection, and creating an arteriovenous fistula within the kidney. Contraindications to a percutaneous biopsy include bleeding disorders and the presence of a single kidney.

**C. Common presenting signs of renal disease**

  **1. Hematuria** (blood in the urine) may be gross or microscopic.

    **a. Causes.** Virtually any congenital anomaly, injury, or inflammatory disease of the kidney or urinary tract may cause hematuria.

        **(1)** Isolated hematuria generally does not suggest a bleeding disorder or coagulopathy.

        **(2)** Isolated microscopic hematuria is relatively common and generally is not indicative of serious renal disease. Microscopic hematuria in association with proteinuria, however, is more likely to be a sign of significant renal disease.

**(3)** A common cause of microscopic hematuria in childhood is **idiopathic hypercalciuria,** which may be documented by a timed urine collection (normal urine calcium is less than 4 mg/kg/day) or a random urine sample for calcium to creatinine ratio (normally less than 0.2).

**b. Evaluation**

**(1)** **Gross inspection** of the urine and the **urine dipstick test** for blood may be useful in the diagnosis of hematuria, but **microscopic examination** of a fresh urine specimen is most important. Microscopic hematuria is considered significant if it is persistent and there are five or more red cells per high-power field. Urine that is brown or tea-colored suggests glomerular bleeding; a more specific indicator is the presence of crenated, dysmorphic red blood cells or red cell casts.

**(2)** Persistent, unexplained microscopic hematuria or a single episode of gross hematuria should be evaluated by **ultrasonography** to exclude abnormalities such as obstruction, renal cysts, or Wilms' tumor.

**2. Proteinuria** refers to protein in the urine.

**a. Causes**

**(1)** Most commonly, asymptomatic proteinuria discovered in a random urine specimen is the protein excreted by some individuals when ambulatory and active. This **postural proteinuria** occurs in 5%–10% of children and young adults.

**(a)** Since it disappears when the patient is recumbent, it is identified by comparing the first morning urine with urine obtained later in the day.

**(b)** Although isolated postural proteinuria is a harmless finding, patients with significant renal disease may also show increased proteinuria in the upright position.

**(2)** Heavy proteinuria indicates **glomerulopathy.** Proteinuria that exceeds 960 mg/m²/day defines the protein loss associated with **nephrotic syndrome.**

**b. Evaluation.** The **urine dipstick** is specific for albumin and does not detect tubular glycoproteins or globulins. **Sulfosalicylic acid precipitation** estimates total urinary protein.

**3. Oliguria** is defined as a urine output less than 250 ml/m²/day.

**a. Causes.** Oliguria is frequently a manifestation of **acute renal failure,** but it may also occur as an appropriate renal response to **hypovolemia** and **hypotension (prerenal oliguria).**

**b. Evaluation**

**(1)** Differentiation of oliguric renal failure from prerenal oliguria (appropriate renal salt and water retention) is often evident from the **history and physical examination.**

**(2)** When volume depletion is suspected, differentiation is aided by response to an adequate **fluid challenge** with an intravascular volume expander, such as isotonic saline infusion (20 ml/kg given over 30–60 minutes).

**(3)** The following **laboratory tests** may also help to differentiate prerenal oliguria from renal failure.

**(a)** The **blood urea nitrogen (BUN) to serum creatinine ratio** may be elevated (the normal ratio is 10:1 to 20:1; in prerenal oliguria the ratio exceeds 40:1) because urea is reabsorbed with water in prerenal states.

**(b)** Also helpful is a **random urine sodium concentration,** which is very low (< 20 mEq/L) in prerenal oliguria but usually high (> 50 mEq/L) in renal failure.

**(c)** Likewise, the **fractional excretion of sodium (FENa)** is low (< 1%) in prerenal oliguria and high (> 3%) in renal failure. The FENa is determined as follows

$$\text{FENa} = \frac{\text{urine sodium} \times \text{serum creatinine}}{\text{urine creatinine} \times \text{serum sodium}} \times 100\%$$

**4. Polyuria** (excessive urine output) generally causes thirst and, therefore, is accompanied by **polydipsia** (excessive fluid intake). When free access to fluids is not possible, as with infants or the vomiting child, polyuria may contribute to dehydration and electrolyte disturbances.

**a. Causes** (Table 13-1; see also Ch 16 IV B 1). Polyuria most commonly is caused by disorders of renal concentrating ability or by diuretics, although it occasionally results from an abnormal desire for fluids (**psychogenic polydipsia**).

**b. Evaluation** of polyuria involves a **fluid deprivation test** under close supervision in the hospital. Serum osmolarity, urine osmolarity, and body weight are monitored.

**(1)** Failure to achieve an adequate increase in urine osmolarity indicates a concentrating defect (e.g., maximum urinary concentration should occur with a serum osmolality exceeding 300 or with an acute 3% weight loss).

**Table 13-1.** Causes of Polyuria

Central diabetes insipidus (ADH deficiency)
    Partial ADH deficiency
    Complete ADH deficiency
    Idiopathic diabetes insipidus
    Acquired diabetes insipidus
        Intracranial trauma or infection

Nephrogenic diabetes insipidus (ADH-resistant)
    Inherited nephrogenic diabetes insipidus
    Acquired nephrogenic diabetes insipidus
        Interstitial nephritis, chronic renal insufficiency, papillary necrosis
        Hypokalemia, sickle cell disease

Diuretic-induced polyuria
    Osmotic agents (glucose, mannitol)
    Volume expansion (intravenous fluids, resolution of acute renal failure)
    Diuretic agents (furosemide)

Abnormal fluid ingestion (psychogenic polydipsia)

ADH = antidiuretic hormone (vasopressin).

    **(2)** The defect can be further categorized as vasopressin-deficient or vasopressin-resistant by the response to administration of vasopressin [also called antidiuretic hormone (ADH)] or its analog, desmopressin (dDAVP).

## II. THE KIDNEY IN THE NEWBORN

### A. Developmental considerations

    **1. Nephrogenesis** begins early in the first trimester of pregnancy and continues actively until 36 weeks gestation. The very premature infant, therefore, will be born with far fewer than the one million nephrons that exist in each kidney of the infant born at term.

    **2.** The kidneys and genitourinary tract are the most common organ systems affected by **congenital anomalies,** although not all of these are significant.

    **3.** The fetal kidney excretes urine into the amniotic fluid at a brisk rate—up to 10 ml/kg/hr. **Fetal oliguria or anuria** results in **oligohydramnios,** which is associated with pulmonary hypoplasia, other internal abnormalities, and a characteristic facial appearance with low-set ears (**Potter syndrome**). The pulmonary hypoplasia may be incompatible with life.

    **4.** Significant intrauterine **urinary tract obstruction** may lead to abnormal and disorganized parenchymal development (**renal dysplasia**), and this may result in **renal insufficiency** even if the obstruction is relieved at birth.

### B. Renal function at birth.
Virtually every aspect of renal function has significant limitations at birth. Because of these limitations, all **drug use** in the neonate must be evaluated in terms of renal excretion and potential toxicity. The more **premature** an infant is, the more severe and prolonged the limitations are.

    **1. GFR.** At birth the GFR is low—about 5 ml/min, or 20–30 ml/1.73 m²/min. The GFR doubles by about 2 weeks of age; the increase depends on renal blood flow and its intrarenal distribution and on dietary protein load. The GFR reaches adult levels by age 2 years.

    **2. Serum creatinine.** Prior to the fifth day of life, creatinine levels reflect maternal levels and do not accurately indicate infant renal function.

    **3. Sodium handling.** The kidney in the newborn can neither excrete a sodium load adequately nor conserve sodium if deprived. The limited sodium conservation occurs in part because the distal nephron is relatively insensitive to aldosterone. This also explains the impaired secretion of **potassium** and **hydrogen** ions in the newborn.

    **4. Concentrating and diluting capacity.** Renal concentrating capacity is limited; the kidney in the newborn is able to concentrate urine to a level of about 600–700 mOsm/kg, or about half the normal adult value. Renal diluting capacity is unimpaired (50 mOsm/kg), although water loads are excreted more slowly because of the low GFR.

5. **Acid-base balance.** Decreases in bicarbonate reabsorption and hydrogen ion secretion combine to limit the kidney's ability to acidify the urine. As a result, the newborn frequently has a mild metabolic acidosis, with a serum bicarbonate of 20–22 mEq/L.

## C. Renal diseases in the newborn

1. **Acute renal failure** in the newborn is uncommon.
   a. **Etiology.** Acute renal failure generally is transient and due to severe perinatal insults such as asphyxia, sepsis, or cardiac failure. Other causes include nephrotoxic agents (e.g., radiocontrast agents, aminoglycosides) and renal vascular occlusion.
   b. **Diagnosis**
      (1) Most newborns with **oliguria** (urine flow less than 1 ml/kg/hr) do not have acute renal failure and respond to appropriate fluid challenge.
      (2) Any infant with suspected renal failure should be evaluated for **obstruction** using ultrasonography. Obstruction should be promptly relieved.
   c. **Therapy** for prolonged oliguric or anuric renal failure in the newborn may involve peritoneal dialysis to allow administration of the calories needed to prevent hypoglycemia and severe weight loss.

2. **Congenital renal abnormalities,** including **hypoplasia** (too little normal parenchyma) and **dysplasia** (disorganized parenchyma), generally do not cause renal failure in the newborn, although they may progress to end-stage renal disease later in childhood.

3. **Renal venous thrombosis** may occur as a consequence of hyperviscosity (e.g., from polycythemia or severe volume depletion). The infant with this condition generally presents with a flank mass and hematuria. Severe hypertension or acute renal failure is uncommon. Treatment is supportive. Long-term sequelae include diminished GFR, tubular dysfunction, and hypertension.

4. **Renal artery occlusion** generally is due to embolization from an umbilical artery catheter placed above the renal arteries. The infant presents with severe hypertension and signs of congestive heart failure. Therapy consists of antihypertensive medication to control the blood pressure.

## III. NEPHROTIC SYNDROME

### A. General considerations

1. **Definition.** Nephrotic syndrome is characterized by heavy proteinuria (urinary protein excretion exceeding 960 mg/m$^2$/day). This leads to hypoalbuminemia, edema, and hyperlipidemia. Nephrotic syndrome is not a single disease entity. It may accompany any glomerular disease.

2. **Pathogenesis.** Nephrotic syndrome develops when the glomerular basement membrane shows a marked, prolonged increase in permeability to plasma proteins. The underlying pathogenesis is unknown, but evidence suggests the importance of immune mechanisms.

### B. Minimal change disease (also called **lipoid nephrosis** and **nil lesion**) is so named because the histologic changes visible on electron microscopy are limited to effacement of epithelial foot processes.

1. **Incidence and etiology.** Although uncommon, minimal change disease accounts for 80% of all cases of nephrotic syndrome in children. It occurs at all ages but most commonly between age 2 and 5 years. The etiology is unknown.

2. **Clinical features and course**
   a. The affected child usually presents with edema, which may be generalized and severe. Fatigue, anorexia, abdominal pain, diarrhea, infection, and intravascular volume depletion may be present.
   b. Minimal change disease usually follows a relapsing course. Acute infections frequently trigger relapses, which may be detected promptly by urine testing with dipsticks.

3. **Diagnosis.** The typical patient with minimal change disease has normal renal function with no hematuria as well as normal blood pressure and serum complement levels, although exceptions are not uncommon.
   a. The best diagnostic indicator of minimal change disease, short of a renal biopsy, is the **response to steroid therapy**. A trial of steroid therapy should precede renal biopsy, therefore, if minimal change disease is suspected.

**b.** Table 13-2 lists other tests that are useful in establishing the diagnosis of nephrotic syndrome, in excluding other renal disease, and in monitoring for complications.

**4. Therapy**
   **a. Steroids. Prednisone** (2 mg/kg/day orally in 2 or 3 divided doses) is given for 4 weeks. Alternate-day therapy is then given (2 mg/kg as a single dose in the morning) to mimic endogenous glucocorticoid release and to minimize steroid side effects. The dose is slowly tapered over many weeks to prevent a rapid recurrence of proteinuria as well as to prevent untoward steroid withdrawal effects.
   **b. Alkylating agents.** A child with minimal change disease who fails to respond to steroids or who develops intolerable steroid toxicity may be treated successfully with either **cyclophosphamide** or **chlorambucil**. Because of their potentially serious side effects, these agents are used only when absolutely necessary.
   **c. Diuretics.** In the acute, edematous phase of minimal change disease, aggressive diuretic therapy may worsen the intravascular volume depletion. Diuretics do have a role in controlling the edema of chronic nephrotic states when intravascular volume depletion is not present.
   **d. Cyclosporine.** Recently, treatment with cyclosporine has been adopted. Although it appears to provide remission while being given, it does not provide long-term remission and, therefore, must be regarded as an expensive and potentially very toxic alternative to prednisone.
   **e. Supportive measures.** Edema is managed by restricting sodium but not fluid intake. Dietary protein intake of approximately 2 g/kg/day is optimal. Pneumococcal vaccine should be given, ideally when the child is in remission and not taking steroids. Because nephrotic syndrome is a hypercoagulable state, deep venipuncture as well as further volume depletion should be avoided.

**5. Prognosis.** The long-term outlook is good, as most cases of minimal change disease eventually remit permanently. The greatest concern is for steroid-related morbidity, especially growth retardation. Controversy surrounds the possibility that minimal change disease may rarely transform to another glomerulopathy, such as focal glomerulosclerosis.

**Table 13-2.** Tests Useful for Evaluating Nephrotic Syndrome

| Purpose | Test |
|---|---|
| Establish the presence of nephrotic syndrome | Timed urinary protein excretion<br>Total serum protein<br>Serum protein electrophoresis<br>Serum cholesterol and triglycerides |
| Exclude other renal disease* | Kidney function tests<br>    Blood urea nitrogen<br>    Serum creatinine<br>    Creatinine clearance<br>    Urinalysis (examine for cellular casts)<br>Serologic tests<br>    Complement component C3<br>    Total hemolytic complement ($CH_{50}$)<br>    Antinuclear antibodies<br>    Hepatitis B surface antigen<br>    Circulating immune complexes<br>Renal ultrasonography<br>Renal biopsy |
| Monitor for complications (including those related to steroid therapy) | Complete blood count<br>Appropriate cultures<br>Serum electrolytes<br>Bone densitometry (for steroid-induced demineralization)<br>Eye examinations (for steroid-induced cataracts) |

*Not all tests are necessary in all children.

**C. Other forms of nephrotic syndrome** (Table 13-3). The remaining 20% of cases of childhood nephrotic syndrome (i.e., those not associated with minimal change disease) occur with primary glomerulopathies, with systemic diseases, or secondary to toxic injuries. Accurate diagnosis is based on renal biopsy. Patients are less likely to be steroid-responsive and are more apt to progress to renal insufficiency than those with minimal change disease.

**IV. GLOMERULOPATHIES** are a heterogenous group of diseases involving the glomerulus, which vary greatly in etiology, presentation, course, and outcome. Most are immunologically mediated and are accompanied by varying degrees of hematuria, proteinuria, and azotemia. A large proportion of glomerulopathies are inflammatory and, thus, are referred to as **glomerulonephritis**.

**A. Postinfectious glomerulonephritis** may follow many viral, bacterial, fungal, and parasitic infections.

   **1. Acute poststreptococcal glomerulonephritis**
       **a. Pathogenesis.** This prototype of postinfectious glomerulonephritis is mediated by the inflammatory response to immune complex deposition.

**Table 13-3.** Representative Causes of Childhood Nephrotic Syndrome

**Primary nephrotic syndrome**
   Without glomerulonephritis
      Minimal change disease
      Focal segmental glomerulosclerosis
      Congenital nephrotic syndrome

   With glomerulonephritis
      Mesangial proliferative glomerulonephritis
      Membranoproliferative glomerulonephritis
      Membranous nephropathy
      Acute postinfectious glomerulonephritis

**Systemic diseases associated with nephrotic syndrome**
   Infections
      Viral (e.g., AIDS, hepatitis B, cytomegalovirus and Epstein-Barr virus
        infections)
      Bacterial (e.g., subacute bacterial endocarditis, shunt nephritis)
      Parasitic (e.g., malaria)

   Malignant diseases
      Lymphoma and leukemia
      Solid tumors (e.g., Wilms' tumor, carcinomas)

   Metabolic diseases
      Diabetes mellitus
      Hypothyroidism

   Inflammatory diseases
      Systemic lupus erythematosus
      Systemic vasculitis
      Henoch-Schönlein purpura

   Other disorders
      Sickle cell disease
      Renal vein thrombosis
      Hemolytic-uremic syndrome

**Exogenous agents associated with nephrotic syndrome**
      Allergens (e.g., pollens, venoms)
      Vaccines (e.g., DTP)
      Toxic agents (e.g., heavy metals, heroin)
      Medications (e.g., captopril, penicillamine)

AIDS = acquired immune deficiency syndrome; DTP = diphtheria and tetanus toxoids with pertussis.

**(1)** Glomerulonephritis usually follows infection with several specific types of streptococci, the so-called nephritogenic strains. There is a latent period of about 10 days (range, 1–4 weeks) between the streptococcal illness and the onset of glomerulonephritis.

**(2)** **Hypocomplementemia** (decreased levels of complement component C3) develops along with the nephritis; C3 levels return to normal within 8 weeks. (Other renal diseases with hypocomplementemia include membranoproliferative glomerulonephritis and glomerulonephritis that occurs in association with systemic lupus erythematosus, chronic infection, or inherited complement deficiencies.)

**b. Clinical features and course.** The presentation may vary from mild, asymptomatic microscopic hematuria to gross hematuria, nephrotic syndrome, or severe renal failure. The typical affected child has a brief period of brownish urine, a sediment showing red blood cell casts, and mild renal insufficiency with volume-dependent hypertension and edema. The interval of azotemia (increased BUN) is short, and complete recovery of renal function is the rule. Microscopic hematuria, however, may persist for several years.

**2. Other infections that may lead to glomerulonephritis** include:
   **a.** Bacterial (staphylococcal infection)
   **b.** Viral (hepatitis B, infectious mononucleosis)
   **c.** Fungal (histoplasmosis)
   **d.** Parasitic (toxoplasmosis, falciparum malaria)

**B. Mesangial proliferative glomerulonephritis** most frequently presents as recurrent or persistent hematuria or as frequently relapsing or steroid-resistant nephrotic syndrome. Histologically, the mesangium shows proliferation and, often, prominent immunoglobulin M (IgM) deposits. The course of this nephritis is variable: Some patients develop end-stage renal disease, whereas others recover completely.

**C. IgA nephropathy (Berger's disease)** is most commonly a focal glomerulonephritis, which is indistinguishable histologically from the nephritis of **Henoch-Schönlein purpura**.

**1. Clinical features.** IgA nephropathy usually presents as recurrent, brief episodes of gross hematuria accompanying upper respiratory illnesses. There may also be persistent microscopic hematuria.

**2. Therapy.** There is no effective therapy for this condition, although equivocal results have been yielded by alternate-day steroids, steroids plus azathioprine, and cyclosporine.

**3. Prognosis.** The outlook is good, although the child with associated nephrotic syndrome is at risk for developing renal insufficiency.

**D. Membranoproliferative glomerulonephritis** encompasses at least three types of chronic nephritis—**type I** (with subendothelial deposits), **type II** (with dense intramembranous deposits), and **type III** (with scattered deposits in the basement membrane)—any of which may present as either an acute or an indolent nephritis. Persistent or intermittent complement depletion may occur, particularly in type II.

**1. Clinical features and biopsy findings.** Membranoproliferative glomerulonephritis is commonly associated with azotemia, hypertension, or nephrotic syndrome.

**2. Therapy and prognosis.** Untreated membranoproliferative glomerulonephritis is generally a progressive disorder. Long-term stabilization of renal function may be achieved with prolonged alternate-day prednisone therapy.

**E. Membranous nephropathy** is uncommon in childhood, although it is the most common cause of nephrotic syndrome in adults.

**1. Pathogenesis.** Membranous nephropathy is the prototype of renal disease mediated by in situ immune complex formation (i.e., immune complexes form in the kidney and do not circulate in the blood). The condition may be idiopathic, it may occur in disorders characterized by chronic antigenemia (e.g., hepatitis B), or it may occur in association with other systemic disease (e.g., syphilis, systemic lupus erythematosus).

**2. Clinical features.** Children with membranous nephritis generally present with hematuria and proteinuria. Half of these children have nephrotic syndrome.

3. **Therapy and prognosis.** Therapy in children is supportive. Spontaneous long-term remissions are common and are sometimes permanent.

F. **Rapidly progressive (diffuse crescentic) glomerulonephritis** is very unusual in childhood. It may develop in the course of any form of glomerulopathy or in the absence of previously recognized renal disease.

   1. **Clinical features and biopsy findings.** This glomerulonephritis is characterized by the rapid decline of renal function (over weeks) and the presence of extensive glomerular epithelial crescent formation.

   2. **Therapy.** Aggressive therapy with large doses of corticosteroids, immunosuppressive agents, plasmapheresis, and anticoagulation sometimes is successful.

G. **Glomerulonephritis in Henoch-Schönlein (anaphylactoid) purpura** (see also Ch 8 V D 3 b). Renal involvement occurs in approximately half of the children with Henoch-Schönlein purpura.

   1. **Clinical features and biopsy findings**
      a. This syndrome of unknown etiology is characterized by small vessel vasculitis and by skin, joint, and gastrointestinal manifestations.
      b. Nephritis, ranging from microscopic hematuria to nephrotic syndrome or renal failure, may accompany the other findings or follow them by up to several weeks. Renal histology varies from focal to diffuse proliferative glomerulonephritis. IgA is regularly present.
      c. Hypertension, even in the absence of nephritis, occasionally may occur.

   2. **Therapy and prognosis.** There is no effective therapy for the nephritis. It generally resolves, although 5% of cases progress to chronic renal insufficiency. Nephrotic syndrome or acute renal failure at presentation is a worrisome prognostic feature.

H. **Renal involvement in systemic lupus erythematosus** (see also Ch 8 V C 1). Renal disease is a major concern in the management of childhood lupus.

   1. **Clinical features and biopsy findings**
      a. The extent of renal injury is variable, as reflected by urinary sediment and renal function, and the renal histology may show focal, diffuse proliferative, mesangial proliferative, membranous, or tubulointerstitial nephritis.
      b. The activity of the renal disease varies with the rest of the illness and may be monitored with serologic tests such as serum complement (C3) levels and anti–DNA antibody (Farr) titers.

   2. **Therapy** includes steroids and immunosuppressive agents.

I. **Sickle cell nephropathy** (see also Ch 14 III D 10)

   1. Renal involvement varying from a proliferative nephritis to focal glomerulosclerosis regularly occurs in sickle cell disease, with potentially serious renal insufficiency developing in adolescence or young adulthood.

   2. Children most commonly show a renal concentrating and acidifying defect. Microscopic or gross hematuria, the latter sometimes severe, may occur in children with sickle cell trait as well as in those with homozygous sickle cell disease.

J. **Diabetic nephropathy** [see also Ch 16 I A 1 f (3)] is the most common cause of end-stage renal disease in the United States. Because overt nephropathy is related to the duration of diabetes mellitus, it is not a common problem in childhood.

   1. **Clinical features.** The earliest clinical sign of nephropathy is asymptomatic microalbuminuria, although significant glomerular lesions may precede this marker.

   2. **Management.** Diabetic nephropathy appears to be related to and accelerated by chronic glomerular hyperfiltration and hypertension. Thus, pediatricians must be diligent in avoiding chronic hyperglycemia and in controlling hypertension in young patients with diabetes.

## V. URINARY TRACT INFECTION

A. **Incidence.** Urinary tract infection is common in infants and children. In newborns, it is twice as common in males, but in childhood, it is 10 times more common in females. About 5% of school-age girls develop a urinary tract infection, and 80% of these patients experience a recurrence.

**B. Localization.** A urinary tract infection is frequently classified as involvement of the renal parenchyma (**pyelonephritis**) or the bladder (**cystitis**). No laboratory study can accurately localize the infection, and localization usually is based on clinical findings. Unfortunately, the symptoms of a urinary tract infection in infants and young children frequently are nonspecific and vague. Most infections do not involve the renal parenchyma.

**C. Etiology and pathogenesis**

1. **Contamination by fecal flora.** In virtually all cases, a urinary tract infection results from fecal flora, especially coliform bacteria, ascending the urethra to the bladder. Factors important to the development of urinary tract infection include the ability of organisms to adhere to the urinary epithelium, surface immunoglobulins, completeness of bladder emptying, and urine pH. Pyelonephritis implies that organisms have ascended the ureters, as can occur in vesicoureteral reflux (retrograde flow of urine up the ureters from the bladder).

2. **Vesicoureteral reflux** is present in 35% of children with a urinary tract infection and is much less common in the general population. The relationship between vesicoureteral reflux and urinary tract infection is uncertain, but vesicoureteral reflux definitely increases the risk of pyelonephritis.
   a. In most cases, vesicoureteral reflux is due to a congenitally abnormal insertion of the ureter into the bladder wall. Mild vesicoureteral reflux may occur transiently with cystitis.
   b. **Renal scarring** is found in 50% of children with vesicoureteral reflux and infection. It is due to reflux of urine into the renal parenchyma (**intrarenal reflux**). In most cases, such scarring occurs before age 2 years, indicating the need for prompt diagnosis and treatment of urinary tract infection in infants. It is not known if vesicoureteral reflux, in the absence of infection or obstruction, can injure the kidney.

**D. Clinical features.** Recognizing urinary tract infection in children, particularly infants, may be difficult. The classic symptoms of cystitis (i.e., dysuria, urgency, frequency) often are absent, as are the flank pains and shaking chills associated with pyelonephritis in adults. Children with urinary tract infection may present with unexplained fever, failure to thrive, vague gastrointestinal and abdominal complaints, and enuresis.

**E. Diagnosis**

1. **Urine culture.** The diagnosis must be based on culture results, not on symptoms or urinalysis. Urine cultures should be obtained only in children in whom urinary tract infection is suspected, not in asymptomatic individuals. Reliable urine screening cultures are available in outpatient settings.
   a. **Definitive results.** A colony count of $10^5$ for a single organism generally is accepted as proof of infection.
   b. **Methods of urine collection**
      (1) **Clean-catch** samples can be 85% reliable.
      (2) Specimens obtained by **catheter or suprapubic aspiration** are more specific but cause discomfort and involve some risk.
   c. **Repeat culture** is required if symptoms do not improve within 48 hours of initiating antimicrobial therapy.
   d. **Follow-up culture** should be obtained at least 72 hours after completion of antimicrobial therapy.

2. **Imaging** is indicated for urinary tract infection in all children under age 2 years, in all boys, in girls with parenchymal infection, and in all children in whom localization of the infection is in doubt. Uncomplicated cystitis in school-age girls does not require radiologic evaluation if follow-up is assured.
   a. **Ultrasonography** should be performed to search for obstruction or urinary tract anomalies. It can be repeated serially to monitor renal growth.
   a. **Voiding cystourethrography** identifies vesicoureteral reflux and establishes the degree of reflux. The study is best performed after completion of therapy.

**F. Therapy**

1. **Uncomplicated cystitis.** Antimicrobial therapy is based on the results of urine culture and sensitivity testing. Generally, 10 days of therapy with amoxicillin or trimethoprim-sulfamethoxazole is effective and well tolerated. While short-course therapy is established effective therapy in adults, studies in children are equivocal and, therefore, such therapy is not recommended.

**2. Pyelonephritis**
  **a.** The same drugs used for cystitis yield antimicrobial urinary levels that are adequate to treat renal parenchymal infections. Often, however, the child with pyelonephritis is vomiting and severely ill. Furthermore, until the organism is identified, an aminoglycoside may be desirable, and hospitalization for initial parenteral antibiotic and fluid therapy is then indicated.
  **b.** An episode of pyelonephritis may be treated with 10–14 days of oral therapy. Recurrent episodes may require therapy for 4–6 weeks.

**3. Preventive therapy.** The child with vesicoureteral reflux, other urinary tract anomalies, or a recurrent urinary tract infection requires continuous antimicrobial therapy. A single daily low dose of nitrofurantoin is effective and well tolerated. Bacterial resistance seldom develops.

**G. Complications and prognosis.** Although urinary tract infection is frequently recurrent, the risk of progression to chronic renal insufficiency, even with pyelonephritis, is very low.

**1. Hypertension** is the most common long-term sequela of recurrent pyelonephritis.

**2. Renal scarring** also can result from pyelonephritis.
  **a.** Renal scarring is seen in infants and young children; it rarely develops in older children and adults. The progression of renal scars is an immunologically mediated process that is not understood.
  **b.** Renal scarring is frequently focal, and hypertrophy of normal renal tissue maintains normal overall function. It may also result in a peculiar renal outline, referred to as **pseudotumor formation**.

**3. Severe vesicoureteral reflux.** Most vesicoureteral reflux in childhood resolves spontaneously, but severe reflux may require surgery. Serial cystograms, preferably with radionuclides, are obtained every 18–24 months to monitor the resolution of vesicoureteral reflux. Antimicrobial prophylaxis should be continued as long as reflux is present.

## VI. HYPERTENSION

### A. Definition and incidence

**1. Definition.** Hypertension in childhood is defined as a blood pressure reading greater than the ninety-fifth percentile for age obtained on three separate occasions. Approximately 1% of the pediatric population and 3% of adolescents are hypertensive by this definition.

**2. Blood pressure norms** are available for boys and girls of different ages in the United States. These values show a progressive increase in blood pressure from infancy to adolescence. A "normal value" does not imply freedom from the long-term risk of cardiovascular disease and, therefore, is not necessarily a "healthy value."

### B. Etiology

**1. Primary hypertension** (also called **idiopathic** or **essential hypertension**) is by far the most common form of hypertension (as defined above) in children. As in adults, it probably is a heterogeneous group of disorders. The blood pressure elevation generally is mild to moderate and asymptomatic. If sustained for long periods, it is an important risk factor in the development of cardiovascular disease. Often, a strong family history of high blood pressure exists.

**2. Secondary hypertension**
  **a. Renal disease** is the most common cause of secondary hypertension. Virtually any renal disease, glomerular or interstitial, may be the cause. The hypertension may be transient or sustained and may be out of proportion in severity to the degree of renal insufficiency. Renal hypertension is due to salt and water retention with volume expansion or to a renin-mediated increase in vascular resistance.
  **b. Vascular causes** of hypertension (e.g., coarctation of the aorta, renal artery stenosis, renal artery occlusion), although uncommon, are important to identify since they may lead to severe, symptomatic hypertension and they may be curable. Anatomic vascular abnormalities are identified by angiography.
  **c. Endocrine causes** of hypertension are very uncommon and are conditions associated with

excess catecholamines or aldosterone. These include pheochromocytoma, primary or secondary aldosteronism, and congenital adrenal hyperplasia with 11-hydroxylase or 17-hydroxylase deficiency. Diagnosis is based on serum and urine concentrations of catecholamines and their metabolites, aldosterone, and—in the case of congenital adrenal hyperplasia—17-hydroxysteroids and 17-ketosteroids.

   **d. Neurologic disease** as a cause of hypertension often is hard to document. Increased intracranial pressure and the Guillain-Barré syndrome are well-recognized causes. Conditions such as cerebral palsy and seizure disorders are less definitely associated with hypertension. In the latter conditions, spasticity and hypertonicity may make accurate blood pressure determination difficult.

   **e. Miscellaneous causes**
   - **(1)** A variety of **medications** and **illicit drugs** may cause hypertension in some individuals. Table 13-4 lists agents frequently encountered in children and adolescents.
   - **(2)** Acute, significant **rises in serum calcium** may increase blood pressure. Children who are suddenly and completely immobilized may develop hypercalcemia and hypertension.
   - **(3)** Children who are placed in **traction** may develop hypertension independent of hypercalcemia.

**C. Diagnosis.** Most children with high blood pressure do not need an extensive or invasive evaluation.

**1. Basic evaluation**
   **a. History.** Significant items include previous growth and state of health, urinary tract symptoms or infections, medications, and family history of hypertension, stroke, or premature cardiovascular disease.

   **b. Physical examination**
   - **(1) Blood pressure readings** should be obtained when the heart rate is stable and repeated until values are consistent. Diastolic values are best expressed by both the phase 4 (muffling) and phase 5 (disappearance) Korotkoff sounds. Blood pressure readings should be obtained in all extremities, and **pulses** should be checked.
   - **(2) Auscultation** for murmurs and bruits and **funduscopic examination** of retinal vessels are important.

   **c. Laboratory studies** should include a urinalysis and measurement of serum electrolytes, BUN, and creatinine. Chest x-ray, electrocardiogram (ECG), or echocardiogram can exclude ventricular hypertrophy. Serum triglycerides, total cholesterol, and high-density lipoproteins are important indicators of additional risk for cardiovascular disease.

**2. Further evaluation for secondary hypertension** may be indicated by findings on the initial evaluation or by any of the following:
   **a. Very high blood pressure readings** (e.g., above 120/80 mm Hg in infants, 140/90 mm Hg in children, 160/100 mm Hg in adolescents)
   **b.** Any level of blood pressure that causes **symptoms** (e.g., headache, vomiting, signs of congestive heart failure)
   **c.** Hypertension that is **progressive**
   **d.** Hypertension that is **refractory to therapy**

**D. Therapy**

**1. Initial therapy** in mild hypertension should be nonpharmacologic, namely, reduction in salt intake and, if indicated, weight reduction and increased physical activity.

**Table 13-4.** Medications and Illicit Drugs That May Cause Hypertension

Adrenocorticotropic hormone (ACTH)
Corticosteroids (both glucocorticoids and mineralocorticoids)
Amphetamines
Birth control pills
Sympathomimetic agents (including phenylephrine eye drops in young children)
Phencyclidine (PCP, angel dust)

2. **Drug therapy** is given when the above measures do not suffice.
   a. **Approach.** Drugs should be chosen that can be taken infrequently and that will allow an active lifestyle including competitive sports. The lowest possible effective dose is determined by starting low and increasing the dose until the desired control has been attained or until side effects intervene.
   b. **Agents** used most often to treat childhood hypertension are shown in Table 13-5. Other agents, including newer β blockers, prazosin, minoxidil, clonidine, nifedipine, and captopril, are effective and well tolerated but are not officially approved for use in children.
3. **Therapy for secondary hypertension** involves eliminating the cause when possible as well as giving antihypertensive medication to stabilize the blood pressure and the patient. Surgery is indicated for coarctation of the aorta and renal artery stenosis. Balloon angioplasty is the optimal therapy for renal artery stenosis.

E. **Hypertensive emergencies.** When the blood pressure is severely elevated (e.g., 180/110 mm Hg), is producing symptoms, or is increasing rapidly, treatment must be given promptly (Table 13-6), and the child must be monitored closely.

## VII. FLUID AND ELECTROLYTE DISTURBANCES in children almost always are the result of gastrointestinal illness (e.g., diarrhea, vomiting) and involve some degree of dehydration. Most cases are mild and may be treated with oral fluids. When choosing among the many acceptable approaches to therapy, it is best to keep the approach as simple as possible.

A. **Maintenance water and electrolyte requirements** (Table 13-7) are the amounts required daily to maintain homeostasis in a person in a resting, basal state.

1. **Water.** Maintenance water requirements may be calculated as 1500 ml/m²/day for children weighing more than 1.5 kg. Maintenance water balances the following **natural losses**.
   a. **Insensible water loss.** Approximately 40% of maintenance water replaces evaporative, electrolyte-free water lost from the skin and lungs.

**Table 13-5.** Drugs Used to Treat Childhood Hypertension

| Drug | Dose | Frequency of Doses | Side Effects and Comments |
|---|---|---|---|
| **Thiazide diuretics** | | | |
| Chlorothiazide | 10 mg/kg | 1–2/day | May cause hypokalemia; ineffective with low GFR; no greater effect with higher doses; long-term antihypertensive effect is independent of volume depletion; useful adjunct to captopril therapy |
| Hydrochlorothiazide | 1 mg/kg | 1–2/day | |
| **Vasodilators** | | | |
| Hydralazine | 0.5–2.5 mg/kg | 3–4/day | Given with diuretic because of salt and water retention; may cause headache, flushing, tachycardia; maximum dose 300 mg/day |
| Minoxidil | 0.2–1.0 mg/kg | 2–3/day | Given only when refractory to other drugs; causes hypertrichosis |
| **β-Adrenergic antagonists** | | | |
| Propranolol | 1–3 mg/kg | 2–3/day | Not given to children with asthma |
| Metoprolol | 0.5–2.0 mg/kg | 2/day | $β_1$-Selective; not given to children with asthma |
| **ACE inhibitors** | | | |
| Captopril | 0.1–2.0 mg/kg | 3–4/day | May cause renal failure in renal artery stenosis; may cause proteinuria, hypokalemia |
| **Central sympatholytics** | | | |
| Methyldopa | 2.5–10.0 mg/kg | 3/day | Long pediatric experience but currently rarely used; drowsiness may preclude long-term use |

GFR = glomerular filtration rate; ACE = angiotensin-converting enzyme.

**Table 13-6.** Drugs Used to Treat Childhood Hypertensive Emergencies

| Drug | Dose | Side Effects and Comments |
|---|---|---|
| **Vasodilators** | | |
| Diazoxide | 3–5 mg/kg IV | Given within 15 seconds; dose is decreased in children on β blockers; causes tachycardia |
| Nitroprusside | 0.5–8.0 µg/kg/min IV | Must monitor thiocyanate levels for toxicity and follow anion gap |
| Hydralazine | 0.1–0.5 mg/kg IV | Given over 20 minutes; maximum dose 20 mg |
| **Calcium channel blockers** | | |
| Nifedipine | 0.2–0.6 mg/kg SL | Onset within 10 minutes; duration of action 1–6 hours |
| **α-Adrenergic antagonists** | | |
| Phentolamine | 1–5 mg/kg IV | Used for suspected pheochromocytoma; blood pressure may fall within minutes; severe hypotension may occur |

IV = intravenous; SL = sublingual.

      **b. Fecal loss.** About 5%–10% of maintenance water replaces fecal loss.
      **c. Urinary loss.** The remaining 50%–55% of maintenance water replaces urinary water loss. The amount of water lost in the urine is the amount necessary to excrete a basal renal solute load as urine that is neither concentrated nor diluted (i.e., with specific gravity of 1.010).

   **2. Electrolytes.** Maintenance electrolytes include sodium, potassium, and chloride; the daily requirements for these are shown in Table 13-7.

  **B. Dehydration states**

   **1. Etiologic considerations**
      **a.** Dehydration in the pediatric age-group generally is the result of **acute gastrointestinal illness,** in which losses from diarrhea, vomiting, or both are combined with inadequate oral fluid intake. The serum electrolyte concentrations in a child with dehydration reflect the magnitude and electrolyte composition of the intake and losses. Table 13-8 lists the approximate composition of gastrointestinal fluids. Table 13-9 shows the composition of oral fluids used to treat mild or early cases of gastrointestinal illness.
      **b.** The increased water requirements induced by various disease states may be exacerbated by such factors as fever, hyperventilation, ambient humidity, sweating, and increased metabolic rate.

   **2. Types of dehydration.** Although the classification of dehydration states by plasma osmolality is based on serum sodium levels, it is simplest to consider the water deficit and sodium deficit separately.
      **a. Isotonic dehydration.** Net sodium and water losses are proportionate. This form of dehydration is found in about 75% of children hospitalized for dehydration.
        **(1)** Serum sodium values are within the broad range of normal (130–150 mEq/L).
        **(2)** Although extracellular fluid (ECF) tonicity remains normal, gastrointestinal losses are unevenly hypotonic and there is a net loss of water from the intracellular fluid (ICF) as well.
      **b. Hypertonic dehydration.** Water is lost in excess of sodium.

**Table 13-7.** Daily Maintenance Requirements for Water and Electrolytes

| Substance | Requirement/24 hr |
|---|---|
| Water | 1500 ml/m$^2$* |
| Sodium | 2–3 mEq/kg |
| Potassium | 2–3 mEq/kg |
| Chloride | 2–3 mEq/kg |

*Amount of water is for patients weighing more than 1.5 kg.

**Table 13-8.** Approximate Composition of Gastrointestinal Fluids

| Fluid | Sodium (mEq/L) | Potassium (mEq/L) | Chloride (mEq/L) | Bicarbonate (mEq/L) |
|---|---|---|---|---|
| Gastric | 75 | 20 | 100 | 0 |
| Small intestinal | 135 | 15 | 100 | 30 |
| Large intestinal | 60 | 40 | 80 | 50 |
| Diarrhea (in infants) | 60 | 45 | 60 | 45 |

(1) **Hypernatremia** (serum sodium above 150 mEq/L) occurs in about 20% of cases of dehydration. With hypernatremia, the water loss is primarily from the ICF, and the ECF is relatively well preserved.

(2) **Signs.** The classic signs of dehydration (e.g., intravascular volume depletion, decreased skin turgor) frequently are absent. Instead, neurologic signs (e.g., irritability, lethargy, seizures) are prominent and the skin may feel doughy.

(3) **Associated abnormalities** include hyperglycemia, metabolic acidosis, and hypocalcemia.

c. **Hypotonic dehydration.** Sodium is lost in excess of water.

(1) **Hyponatremia** (serum sodium below 130 mEq/L) occurs in only about 5% of dehydrated children.

(2) **Signs**

(a) Because the losses are mainly from the ECF, the classic signs of dehydration and intravascular volume depletion (i.e., decreased skin turgor, decreased tearing, dry mucous membranes, sunken anterior fontanelle, tachycardia and orthostatic hypotension, low jugular venous pulsation) occur early.

(b) Neurologic signs, including seizures, may occur and are directly related to both the serum sodium concentration and the rapidity with which hyponatremia develops.

(3) **Associated abnormalities.** The various causes of hyponatremia (Table 13-10) must be considered.

3. **Degree of dehydration**

a. The extent of dehydration may be estimated from the change in body weight if the prior weight or growth charts are available. Acute weight loss may be assumed to equal water loss.

b. Reasonable clinical estimates of dehydration can be made on the basis of history and physical assessment: A loss of 5% generally correlates with subtle evidence of dehydration, a loss of 10% with obvious evidence, and a loss of 15% with signs of shock.

4. **Electrolyte deficits**

a. **Sodium deficit** occurs in all forms of dehydration, although the deficit is greatest in hyponatremic and smallest in hypernatremic states.

(1) **Isotonic dehydration.** The losses include uneven hypotonic losses, so that the net water deficit from the ICF approximates the loss from the ECF. Therefore, a 1-L deficit in a child with a normal serum sodium concentration consists of 0.5 L of ECF (sodium 140 mEq/L) and 0.5 L of ICF (sodium 5–10 mEq/L).

(2) **Hypertonic dehydration.** In hypernatremic states, the sodium deficit is smaller because losses from the ICF, where the sodium content is very low, comprise approximately three-fourths of the total loss.

**Table 13-9.** Composition of Oral Fluids Commonly Used to Treat Gastroenteritis

| | Carbohydrate (g/dl) | Sodium (mEq/L) | Potassium (mEq/L) |
|---|---|---|---|
| Pedialyte* | 2.5 | 45 | 20 |
| Gatorade | 4.6 | 23 | 3 |
| Kool-Aid | 10.5 | 3 | 0.1 |
| Ginger ale | 9.0 | 3.5 | 0.1 |
| Rehydralyte* | 2.5 | 75 | 20 |

*Oral rehydration solution.

**Table 13-10.** Causes of Hyponatremia

**Pseudohyponatremia**
  Hyperlipidemia
  Hyperproteinemia

**Dilutional hyponatremia**
  Hyperglycemia
  Congestive heart failure
  Nephrotic syndrome
  Liver disease
  Water intoxication
  SIADH
  Reset osmostat

**Depletional hyponatremia**
  Gastrointestinal loss
  Sweat loss
  Renal loss (adrenal insufficiency, chronic renal
    insufficiency, diuretics)

SIADH = syndrome of inappropriate antidiuretic hormone secretion.

    **(3) Hypotonic dehydration.** In hyponatremic states, ECF losses are accentuated, because the hypotonic ECF forces fluid to shift from the ECF into the ICF.
  **b. Potassium deficit** is difficult to estimate but generally approximates the sodium deficit found in isotonic states. The amount administered usually is limited by the concentration of potassium in intravenous fluids and should not exceed 40 mEq/L when infused into a peripheral vein.

**5. Treatment of dehydration**
  **a. Shock.** When signs of shock (e.g., hypotension, weak rapid pulse, poor peripheral perfusion, skin mottling) are present, intravascular volume should be reexpanded promptly without regard to electrolyte status. An isotonic volume expander such as 0.9% (normal) saline is given as 20 ml/kg over 30 minutes. Further fluid resuscitation is given as needed.
  **b. Isotonic dehydration.** Fluids that correct the deficit and provide daily maintenance requirements are given over 24 hours, with half of the total administered in the first 8 hours. Treatment of a 10% dehydrated child who weighs 10 kg and is 0.6 m² is as follows.
    **(1)** The child should receive 1 L of water for maintenance (1500 ml/m²) and 1 L of water for deficit replacement (10% of 10 kg). The child also should receive 20–30 mEq each of sodium and potassium for maintenance and 70 mEq each of these electrolytes for deficit replacement. (The sodium deficit represents the sodium concentration in the 0.5 L of deficit water estimated to come from the ECF. Again, the potassium deficit approximates the sodium deficit.)
    **(2)** Half of the total, or 1 L, of one-third normal saline in 5% dextrose should be given in the first 8 hours and the remainder given over the next 16 hours.
    **(3)** The child must be reevaluated at regular intervals, watching for sources of ongoing losses (e.g., continued diarrhea).
  **c. Hypertonic dehydration.** To avoid too rapid a reduction in sodium concentration, the deficit amounts should be given slowly and evenly over 48 hours, along with maintenance fluids.
  **d. Hypotonic dehydration**
    **(1)** The sodium required to convert a hyponatremic dehydrated state to an isonatremic one may be calculated using the formula

$$\text{required Na}^+ \text{ (mEq)} = 0.6 \times \text{body wt (kg)} \times [\text{desired Na}^+ \text{ (mEq/L)} - \text{observed Na}^+ \text{ (mEq/L)}]$$

    **(2)** The total sodium deficit should not be corrected completely because of the risk of neurologic damage, including **central pontine myelinolysis** (the osmotic demyelinization syndrome), which has been reported rarely in children.
      **(a)** Generally, a corrected serum sodium concentration of 125 mEq/L is reasonable.
      **(b)** When the initial serum sodium is very low (e.g., < 110 mEq/L), the correction should be more modest (e.g., correct to 115–120 mEq/L).

      **(c)** The correction may be made with 3% saline (1 ml = 0.5 mEq of sodium) given at a rate to increase serum sodium 1–2 mEq/L/hr.

    **(3)** Further correction of the dehydration may then proceed as with isotonic dehydration.

# VIII. ACID-BASE DISTURBANCES

## A. Normal acid-base homeostasis

1. Acid-base balance is maintained by the pulmonary excretion of carbon dioxide plus the renal excretion of excess hydrogen ions.

2. Acute changes in acid-base status are prevented by the body's buffer systems. The most important of these in the ECF is bicarbonate because it is plentiful, it can be conserved and generated by the kidney, and it links the lungs and kidneys by carbonic acid dissociation:

$$CO_2 + H_2O \rightleftharpoons H_2CO_3 \rightleftharpoons H^+ + HCO_3^-$$

3. The growing child excretes about 2–3 mEq of hydrogen ions per kilogram daily. Most of this net acid is derived from dietary protein. The kidney excretes net acid by acidifying the urine via the following mechanisms:
   a. Reclaiming all filtered bicarbonate
   b. Excreting urinary anions (e.g., phosphate), which combine with hydrogen ions to form titratable acid
   c. Producing ammonia, which may bind hydrogen ions to form ammonium ions

## B. Assessing acid-base status. Measuring a patient's serum electrolytes, blood pH, and blood gases provides the data for determining acid-base status.

1. **Serum electrolyte levels** provide the total carbon dioxide and permit calculation of the anion gap.
   a. The **total carbon dioxide** is almost identical to the serum bicarbonate plus small contributions of dissolved carbon dioxide and carbonic acid.
   b. The **anion gap** [serum sodium − (chloride + total carbon dioxide)] normally is less than 12 in older children and less than 17 in infants. A large anion gap means there is an excess of one or more unmeasured anions such as lactate or acetoacetate.

2. **Blood pH** indicates the net acid-base status and identifies **acidemia** (pH < 7.35) or **alkalemia** (pH > 7.45). The pH may be within the normal range in acid-base disorders if there is compensation for the primary disturbance or if there is a mixed disorder.

3. **Arterial blood gas analysis** provides the carbon dioxide partial pressure ($Pco_2$) that allows assessment of pulmonary ventilation. Analysis of blood gases also provides the amount of buffer base deficit or excess, which estimates the bicarbonate concentration.

## C. Acidosis results from any process that reduces the body's pH.

1. **Respiratory acidosis**
   a. **Causes.** Respiratory acidosis is caused by the accumulation of carbon dioxide as the result of pulmonary hypoventilation. It may occur with any cause of respiratory failure, including pulmonary disease, neuromuscular disease, and CNS depression.
   b. **Compensation.** The body attempts to compensate for respiratory acidosis by the renal conservation of bicarbonate and by increased excretion of hydrogen ion.
   c. **Therapy** is directed at restoring adequate ventilation. Alkalinizing agents should not be used.

2. **Metabolic acidosis**
   a. **Causes.** Metabolic acidosis is caused by the accumulation of net acid or the excessive loss of bicarbonate.
      (1) **Accumulation of net acid** occurs with ingestion of acid (e.g., salicylate intoxication, which also causes respiratory alkalosis by stimulating central hyperventilation), excess production of acid (e.g., lactic acidosis, diabetic ketoacidosis), or decreased excretion of acid (e.g., in renal failure). These forms of acidosis usually have a **wide anion gap**.
      (2) **Excess loss of bicarbonate** commonly occurs with diarrhea. It may also occur in renal disease, although renal failure affects all phases of urine acidification. Metabolic acidosis resulting from bicarbonate loss usually has a **normal anion gap** and is called **hyperchloremic metabolic acidosis**.

b. **Compensation.** The body's compensation for metabolic acidosis is increased respiratory minute ventilation (hyperventilation), leading to a reduction in $P_{CO_2}$ and returning pH toward normal. Maximum hyperventilation can lower the $P_{CO_2}$ to 12–15 mm Hg, which keeps the pH in the normal range with a bicarbonate concentration as low as 8 mmol/L.

c. **Renal tubular acidosis** is the term given to a heterogeneous group of disorders, all of which are characterized by hyperchloremic metabolic acidosis and tubular dysfunction but usually not by renal insufficiency. Renal tubular acidosis is classified broadly into three types. Table 13-11 lists representative causes for each type. Children with renal tubular acidosis may present with growth failure and with episodes of vomiting and dehydration.

(1) **Distal renal tubular acidosis (type I)** is characterized by failure of the distal nephron to secrete the 2–3 mEq/kg/day of dietary acid (hydrogen ion) necessary to maintain acid-base homeostasis. The urine cannot be maximally acidified and new bicarbonate cannot be generated. Chronic positive hydrogen ion imbalance results in buffering by bone. This leads to increased skeletal calcium resorption, hypercalciuria, and increased risk of nephrocalcinosis and stones. In most children, there is also a urinary bicarbonate leak, which has implications in determining the amount of therapy needed to correct the acidosis.

(2) **Proximal renal tubular acidosis (type II)** is characterized by decreased proximal tubular reabsorption of bicarbonate. A reduction in the normally variable renal threshold for bicarbonate causes a marked bicarbonate leak, which disappears when the serum bicarbonate falls below the threshold level (e.g., to 15 mmol/L). The defect may

**Table 13-11.** Types of Renal Tubular Acidosis in Children and Representative Causes

| Distal renal tubular acidosis (type I) | Proximal renal tubular acidosis (type II) |
|---|---|
| Isolated, primary | Isolated, primary |
|   Inherited |   Inherited |
|   Acquired |   Acquired |
| Associated with heritable disorders | Associated with carbonic anhydrase deficiency |
|   Sickle cell disease |   Inherited |
|   Marfan syndrome |   Acquired |
|   Wilson's disease |     Acetazolamide administration |
|   Ehlers-Danlos syndrome | Associated with Fanconi syndrome |
| Associated with renal disease |   Inherited |
|   Renal transplantation |     Cystinosis |
|   Obstructive uropathy |     Lowe syndrome |
|   Chronic pyelonephritis |     Tyrosinemia |
|   Acute tubular necrosis |     Galactosemia |
| Associated with other systemic disease |     Glycogen storage disease type I |
|   Systemic lupus erythematosus | Associated with renal disease |
|   Chronic active hepatitis |   Renal transplantation |
|   Malnutrition |   Nephrotic syndrome |
| Induced by drugs or poisons |   Medullary cystic disease |
|   Amphotericin B | Associated with other systemic disease |
|   Vitamin D |   Rubella syndrome |
|   Toluene |   Sjögren syndrome |
| |   Amyloidosis |
| |   Medullary cystic disease |
| | Induced by poisons |
| |   Heavy metals |
| |   Lindane |
| | **Type IV renal tubular acidosis** |
| |   Primary aldosterone deficiency |
| |   Hyporeninemic hypoaldosteronism |
| |   Mineralocorticoid-resistant hyperkalemia |
| |   Transient renal tubular acidosis in newborns |

be isolated or may occur with other proximal tubular abnormalities, such as glycosuria, aminoaciduria, or depressed phosphate reabsorption. Diffuse proximal tubular dysfunction is termed the **Fanconi syndrome**.

   (3) **Type IV renal tubular acidosis** includes a group of disorders, all of which are characterized by defects in distal tubular hydrogen ion and potassium secretion, leading to hyperchloremic metabolic acidosis and hyperkalemia.

   d. **Therapy**
      (1) **Renal tubular acidosis** is treated with alkalinizing agents. Doses of either bicarbonate or citrate must be sufficient to correct the acidosis completely. As much as 20 mEq/kg/day may be required to return the serum bicarbonate to a normal concentration. Adequate therapy restores normal growth in affected children.
      (2) **Metabolic acidosis other than renal tubular acidosis** sometimes is treated with alkalinizing agents, although such treatment is controversial.
         (a) In mild to moderate acidosis in which respiratory compensation has occurred and renal function is normal, therapy directed at the underlying cause of the acidosis is sufficient.
         (b) In severe acidosis (pH < 7.2), alkali therapy should be given to increase the serum bicarbonate concentration and to decrease the energy expended by compensatory respiratory effort. The amount of bicarbonate given should correct the pH to 7.2; it is essential to avoid fully correcting the base deficit, which places the patient at risk for **overshoot alkalosis**.

**D. Alkalosis** results from any process that increases the body's pH through either a reduction in $Pco_2$ or an increase in bicarbonate buffer base.

   1. **Respiratory alkalosis**
      a. **Causes.** Respiratory alkalosis is caused by the excessive loss of carbon dioxide as the result of hyperventilation, which is usually centrally mediated (e.g., salicylate intoxication, head injury, hysteria).
      b. **Compensation.** The body's attempt at renal compensation is through increased bicarbonate excretion.
      c. **Therapy** is directed at the cause of the hyperventilation.

   2. **Metabolic alkalosis**
      a. **Causes and compensation.** Metabolic alkalosis is caused by a loss of hydrogen ions or an increase in base.
         (1) The **most common cause** of metabolic alkalosis in children is the use of diuretics, which leads to volume contraction and potassium and chloride depletion. These in turn lead to increased bicarbonate reabsorption and aldosteronism with increased hydrogen ion secretion. Volume contraction with significant chloride and potassium loss due to recurrent vomiting is another common cause. A gain of base can be the result of excessive alkali administration.
         (2) **Less common causes** of metabolic alkalosis in children include Bartter syndrome, familial chloride diarrhea, chronic steroid administration, dietary chloride deficiency, chronic potassium depletion, and posthypercapneic states.
      b. **Therapy.** Metabolic alkalosis is treated by restoring intravascular volume and replacing potassium and chloride deficits. Correction of the underlying cause of the alkalosis (e.g., surgery for pyloric stenosis, discontinuing diuretic therapy) is essential. The use of acid to correct alkalosis through the infusion of ammonium chloride or dilute hydrochloric acid rarely is indicated and should be reserved for patients with severe alkalosis and those who cannot tolerate volume repletion.

## IX. RENAL FAILURE

   A. **Definition.** Renal failure occurs when the kidneys no longer meet the body's need to maintain water, electrolyte, and acid-base balance and to eliminate the end products of protein metabolism.

   1. Renal failure may be **acute or chronic**.

   2. Renal failure may be **oliguric or nonoliguric**.
      a. Renal failure involves a fall in GFR but not necessarily a fall in urine output. For example, if the normal GFR of 120 ml/min fell to 1 ml/min and tubular reabsorption was 0, 1440 ml of urine would still be excreted per day.

**b.** Just as renal failure is not always oliguric, oliguria does not always indicate renal failure. Differentiation is aided by history, physical examination, urine indices (see I C 3 b), and, if indicated, response to a fluid challenge.

**c.** Nonoliguric and oliguric renal failure are equally significant, but nonoliguric failure is easier to manage since fluid restriction need not be so severe and the patient can be given drugs, electrolytes, and calories.

## B. Acute renal failure

**1. Etiology and pathogenesis.** In childhood, acute renal failure frequently occurs as a component or complication of serious systemic illness (e.g., septic shock) or multiorgan injury (e.g., severe trauma). The pathogenesis is not completely understood but is multifactorial, involving hemodynamic, cellular, hormonal, and metabolic factors.

**a. Categories.** Acute renal failure is divided into three categories, based on the nature of the insult or disease.

**(1) Prerenal failure** occurs due to factors that decrease renal perfusion and impair the delivery of oxygen and energy substrate to the kidney. Prerenal factors include hypotension, severe hypertension, hypovolemia, hypoxemia, renal artery occlusion, decreased cardiac output, and hypoglycemia. Causes include dehydration, shock, septicemia, and heart failure.

**(2) Renal parenchymal failure.** Intrinsic renal parenchymal injury can affect glomerular function, tubular function, or both. Causes include all forms of glomerulonephritis, nephrotoxicity (e.g., from heavy metals, uric acid, myoglobin, or aminoglycoside antibiotics), and renal venous obstruction. Long-standing glomerular hyperfusion, as occurs with chronic hyperglycemia and excessive protein loads, may also cause renal parenchymal injury.

**(3) Postrenal failure** occurs due to factors that injure the kidney by obstructing urine flow. Causes include stones, Wilms' tumor, and congenital anomalies (e.g., obstructed ureteropelvic junction, posterior urethral valves).

**b. Acute tubular necrosis.** If prerenal, parenchymal, or postrenal insults are mild or promptly reversed, acute renal failure may not develop. If these factors are severe or prolonged, acute tubular necrosis will result.

**(1)** The renal failure that develops in acute tubular necrosis is generally transient, although chronic renal impairment and sequelae such as hypertension may result.

**(2)** If the insult is very severe, renal cortical necrosis may occur, with irreversible renal failure.

## 2. Complications

**a. Water retention** may lead to dilutional hyponatremia and possible neurologic effects ranging from lethargy to seizures or coma.

**b. Sodium retention** causes a compensatory expansion of the ECF, which can lead to edema, hypertension, or congestive heart failure.

**c. Renal ischemia** causes hyperreninemia, which can also lead to hypertension.

**d. Hyperkalemia** is a consequence of diminished filtration and failure of the distal nephron to secrete potassium. Hyperkalemia usually is not a serious problem unless there is a high potassium load (e.g., from tumor lysis syndrome) or until the GFR has fallen to less than 5 ml/min.

**e. Metabolic acidosis** develops from failure of renal acidification mechanisms and bicarbonate wasting.

**f. Uremic syndrome,** with anorexia, lethargy, and encephalopathy, results from the failure to excrete uremic toxins. These toxins remain poorly characterized.

## 3. Therapy

**a. Initial treatment** of acute renal failure is aimed at:

**(1)** Reversing or removing the underlying cause

**(2)** Minimizing the excretory work of the kidneys, especially reducing the nitrogen load by limiting protein intake and, if possible, drugs that are excreted by the kidneys

**(3)** Treating complications

**(4)** Providing adequate caloric intake

**b. Dialysis** is indicated when the above measures are inadequate prior to the spontaneous recovery of renal function. There is no specific BUN or creatinine level at which dialysis should be instituted.

**4. Recovery** from acute renal failure often involves a period of brisk urine output, the so-called **diuretic phase** or **recovery phase** of acute renal failure. Most often, this diuresis is appropriate and reflects excretion of water that accumulated in the earlier oliguric phase.

## C. Hemolytic-uremic syndrome

1. **Definition.** Hemolytic-uremic syndrome is an unusual acute nephropathy characterized by the triad of microangiopathic hemolytic anemia, thrombocytopenia, and acute renal failure. Although the kidney often is the only organ affected, other organs also may be involved, including the CNS, gastrointestinal tract, lungs, and myocardium. With systemic involvement, it is impossible to differentiate hemolytic-uremic syndrome from thrombotic thrombocytopenic purpura.

2. **Incidence.** Hemolytic-uremic syndrome may occur at any age. It is the most common cause of acquired acute renal failure in infants and children. Although it usually is sporadic, clusters of cases occur.

3. **Etiology and pathogenesis**
   a. Hemolytic-uremic syndrome generally is preceded by an infection, usually a gastrointestinal illness with diarrhea, although the syndrome has been reported as a sequela of virtually all types of viral and bacterial infections.
   b. The pathogenesis is believed to involve endothelial injury, leading to platelet aggregation and depletion. Platelet thrombi damage erythrocytes and lead to hemolysis. The vascular injury leads to renal ischemia and acute renal failure.

4. **Clinical features and course**
   a. The anemia and thrombocytopenia may be mild or profound. Renal insufficiency varies from mild, nonoliguric renal failure to severe oliguria lasting several days to many weeks. Progression to end-stage renal failure is uncommon.
   b. Long-term sequelae may include hypertension and varying degrees of renal insufficiency. Recurrences are uncommon but are seen in some individuals, even after renal transplantation.

5. **Therapy**
   a. The acute renal failure and hematologic problems are the targets of therapy. Transfusions (red cell, platelet, or both) may be required.
   b. Supportive treatment includes careful attention to nutrition.
   c. Dialysis may be needed when prolonged acute renal failure occurs.

## D. Chronic renal failure is a significant and irreversible reduction in GFR.

1. **Etiology.** Although any renal disorder, if severe enough, can lead to chronic renal failure, congenital nephropathies are the most common cause of chronic renal failure in childhood. Renal dysplasia, which may be a consequence of prenatal urinary tract obstruction, is the most common cause of progressive renal insufficiency in the first decade of life.

2. **Course.** Although chronic renal failure progresses at different rates in different individuals, the course in a particular patient may often be predicted accurately by plotting the reciprocal of the serum creatinine versus time. The result is usually a linear relationship that predicts the approximate time when replacement therapy will be needed.

3. **Complications and their management.** Besides the complications seen with acute renal failure, several additional problems occur with chronic renal failure.
   a. **Problems with nutrition and growth** are the most significant complications seen in children.
      (1) **Nutrition.** The goal of dietary management is to maximize caloric intake, reduce excretory solute load, and preserve residual renal function. The diet should be high in carbohydrates and fat, with limited protein (1.0–1.2 g/kg/day) and phosphorus intake.
      (2) **Growth.** Most children with chronic renal failure grow poorly due to a number of factors, including inadequate calories, acidosis, anemia, and renal osteodystrophy.
   b. **Renal osteodystrophy** results from several factors, including impaired vitamin D metabolism, decreased intestinal calcium absorption, phosphate retention (leading to hyperphosphatemia), secondary hyperparathyroidism, and metabolic acidosis. The combination of skeletal demineralization and hyperparathyroidism retards growth and leads to rickets.
      (1) Therapy with vitamin D metabolites [e.g., calcitriol (1,25-dihydroxyvitamin $D_3$) or dihydrotachysterol] prevents or heals the skeletal abnormalities but does not dramatically improve growth.

        **(2)** Calcium carbonate is given in doses that supply 500–1000 mg/m²/day of elemental calcium. This provides extra calcium for absorption and to act as a binder of dietary phosphate.

        **(3)** To prevent hyperphosphatemia, it often is necessary to limit phosphorus intake and to give phosphate binders. Either calcium carbonate or aluminum salts (50–100 mg/kg/day with meals) may be used.

    **c. Hyperkalemia.** Dietary potassium limitation usually is not needed until the GFR falls to very low levels (below 5 ml/min/1.73 m²). Potassium balance is maintained in chronic renal failure by increased excretion from remaining nephrons and significant intestinal potassium loss. A potassium-binding resin (e.g., sodium polystyrene sulfonate) may be given orally or rectally to remove potassium.

    **d. Anemia**

        **(1)** Normochromic, normocytic anemia is common in chronic renal failure for several reasons. Erythropoiesis is depressed because of low levels of erythropoietin and high levels of uremic toxins. Red blood cell survival is shortened. The uremic bleeding diathesis may result in gastrointestinal blood loss. Also, a nutritional folate or iron deficiency may exist.

        **(2)** Until recently, effective therapy was not available except for the careful use of blood transfusions. The availability of **recombinant erythropoietin,** however, has provided an effective, although very expensive, treatment for the anemia.

**E. End-stage renal disease.** When the progression of chronic renal failure is no longer adequately managed by medical means, replacement therapy is required, using hemodialysis, a peritoneal dialysis regimen, or transplantation.

    **1. Peritoneal dialysis.** Continuous ambulatory dialysis involves the placement of a permanent intraperitoneal (Tenckhoff) catheter. Peritoneal dialysis offers the advantage of technical simplicity and gives the child an increased feeling of well-being. Disadvantages include continued poor growth in the child and fatigue in the parents from the continuous nature of the therapy. Complications include infections around the catheter, peritoneal infections, and occlusion of the catheter.

    **2. Hemodialysis.** Chronic hemodialysis in children is performed at a dialysis center and generally requires three sessions per week, lasting 4–5 hours each. Besides the time and cost involved, disadvantages of hemodialysis include difficulty with vascular access, increased incidence of anemia, and side effects of dysequilibrium while on dialysis (i.e., headache, nausea, and muscle cramps). When children are switched from hemodialysis to peritoneal dialysis, they are more energetic and they (as well as their families) generally feel more independent.

    **3. Transplantation.** Renal transplantation is the therapy of choice for children with end-stage renal disease, since it provides the best opportunity for a reasonably normal life-style and for growth. Results are excellent and are better with transplants from living related donors than with cadaver transplants. Although renal transplantation may be carried out on infants, a child weighing at least 10 kg is at a lower risk for technical problems and infectious complications and may accept the kidney of an adult.

        **a.** Improvements in pretransplantation care include the judicious use of blood transfusions, particularly the use of donor-specific transfusions. Advances in immunosuppressive therapy include better recognition and treatment of rejection, the use of cyclosporine, and the more prudent use of corticosteroids, including alternate-day therapy.

        **b.** Post-transplantation growth acceleration ("catch-up growth") remains disappointing, particularly in older children and adolescents. Other problems that persist include:

            **(1)** The continued shortage of donor kidneys

            **(2)** Complications of immunosuppressive drug use, such as drug toxicity, susceptibility to infection, and a small, but definite, risk of malignancy

            **(3)** The absence of effective therapy for chronic rejection

**X. HEREDITARY RENAL DISEASES.** Most renal disease in childhood is not strictly heritable by dominant or recessive patterns. However, histocompatibility gene (HLA) associations occur with some conditions, including minimal change disease and membranoproliferative glomerulonephritis, making genetic predisposition likely. Some renal disorders are clearly heritable conditions. Several of the more common ones are considered in this section.

    **A. Hereditary nephritis (Alport syndrome)** is a progressive disorder with variable severity. Although it appears to be autosomal dominant, it commonly affects males more severely than females.

1. **Clinical features**
   a. The most common presentation in childhood is asymptomatic hematuria. Hypertension is also common. Renal insufficiency usually does not begin until the second decade.
   b. The nephropathy may occur alone or with auditory or visual problems. High-frequency sensorineural hearing loss occurs in one-third of the patients. Diverse eye problems, usually involving the lens, occur in 15% of patients.

2. **Diagnosis** is made by renal biopsy showing characteristic abnormalities, notably lamellation and thinning of the glomerular basement membrane, which is visible on electron microscopy.

3. **Therapy.** The only effective therapy is transplantation.

B. **Medullary cystic disease (nephronophthisis).** This serious and progressive disorder shows two distinct modes of inheritance that differ in age at presentation. Pathologically, both forms are characterized by small medullary cysts and tubular atrophy that progress to diffuse fibrosis and cystic enlargement.

1. **Clinical features**
   a. The **juvenile form** (also called **familial juvenile nephronophthisis**) is an autosomal recessive disorder that presents in the first decade as growth failure, polyuria, salt wasting, anemia, hypertension, and progressive renal failure. Renal biopsy must include deep medullary tissue to be diagnostic.
   b. The **adult form** is an autosomal dominant disorder that presents in adolescence or adulthood as similar symptoms with a similar course.

2. **Therapy.** There is no effective therapy. The disease does not recur in transplanted kidneys.

C. **Polycystic kidney disease.** Again, two types exist that differ in pattern of inheritance and age at onset.

1. **Infantile-type polycystic kidney disease** is an autosomal recessive disorder usually detected at birth.
   a. **Clinical features**
      (1) The infant presents with large kidneys and oliguria. (If the oliguria is present during intrauterine life, severe pulmonary hypoplasia may result and the condition may be incompatible with life.) Renal insufficiency is slowly progressive, although it varies in severity.
      (2) The condition is virtually always associated with hepatomegaly due to **congenital hepatic fibrosis,** which causes portal hypertension and secondary varices.
   b. **Therapy** for infantile polycystic disease includes both renal transplantation and some form of portosystemic vascular shunt.

2. **Adult-type polycystic kidney disease** is an autosomal dominant disorder that, despite its name, occasionally presents in childhood.
   a. **Clinical features**
      (1) Patients initially present with some combination of abdominal pain, flank mass, proteinuria, intermittent hematuria, hypertension, or urinary tract infection. Progressive renal failure develops later.
      (2) Adult polycystic disease is characterized by large cysts in both kidneys. Extrarenal cystic involvement of the liver, pancreas, or lungs is not unusual. Ten percent of patients have berry aneurysms.
   b. **Therapy.** Transplantation is the only effective treatment.

## XI. UROLOGIC PROBLEMS

A. **Renal trauma**

1. **Etiology.** Renal trauma in children is most commonly the result of a blunt blow to the abdomen or a deceleration injury (e.g., jumping from a height). Possible types of renal injury include contusions, cortical lacerations, calyceal lacerations, complete renal tears, and vascular pedicle injury.

2. **Clinical features.** The injury need not be severe or dramatic to result in the most common manifestation, hematuria. Other common symptoms are abdominal pain and tenderness, which may mimic an acute abdomen or renal colic. A flank mass may be present.

3. **Diagnosis.** Because the kidney with a cyst, tumor, or obstruction is more likely to bleed when injured, the kidneys should be imaged with ultrasonography and IVP. A nonfunctioning kidney suggests a vascular injury and should be investigated with arteriography.

4. **Therapy and prognosis**
   a. Therapy should be conservative except in cases with vascular avulsion or with uncontrolled, massive bleeding. Surgery is required in severe cases.
   b. Preservation of renal function in the injured kidney is likely.

5. **Complications** include delayed hemorrhage, urinoma, perinephric abscess, poor renal growth, obstruction due to clot or scar formation, and hypertension.

B. **Urolithiasis** during childhood is uncommon in the United States and consists mainly of renal stones. (In some parts of the world, bladder stones are more common.)

1. **Etiology** (Table 13-12). The occurrence of a stone in a child should prompt evaluation to determine the cause.

2. **Clinical features and diagnosis.** Signs and symptoms include hematuria and abdominal pain, which may be either vague or severe. The best diagnostic test is ultrasonography of the kidneys and pelvis.

3. **Therapy.** Maintenance therapy should be directed at prevention of further stones and close monitoring for their occurrence.
   a. High urinary flow rates are desirable in all causes of stones.
   b. In **hypercalciuria,** therapy is aimed at reducing urinary calcium with thiazides or dietary calcium restriction.
   c. Treatment of **cystinuria** (an autosomal recessive disorder with defective intestinal and renal transport of dibasic amino acids) involves urinary dilution and alkalinization and, occasionally, the use of penicillamine.

C. **Hypospadias** is the most common anomaly of the penis. There is a 10% risk of the defect in male siblings.

1. **Defect and associated anomalies**
   a. In hypospadias, the opening of the urethral meatus is on the ventral surface of the penis. Ventral curvature of the penis, known as **chordee,** usually is present.
   b. There is a 10%–15% risk of undescended testes with hypospadias. The risk of other anomalies of the urinary tract is not significant.

**Table 13-12.** Causes of Renal Calculi in Children

| Increased excretion of solute | Decreased excretion of solubilizing substances |
|---|---|
| Calcium | Citrate |
|   Idiopathic hypercalciuria |   Distal renal tubular acidosis |
|   Chronic furosemide therapy | Magnesium |
|   Distal renal tubular acidosis | Pyrophosphate |
|   Immobilization | |
|   Vitamin D excess | **Urinary stasis or decreased flow rate** |
|   Hyperparathyroidism |   Poor fluid intake |
| Oxalate |   Partial obstruction |
|   Primary oxaluria | |
|   Small bowel disease (increased oxalate absorption) | **Other disorders** |
|   Ethylene glycol (antifreeze) intoxication |   Chronic urinary tract infection |
|   Vitamin C excess |   Polycystic kidney disease |
| Cystine |   Medullary sponge kidney |
|   Cystinuria | |
| Uric acid | |
|   Cancer chemotherapy [e.g., for leukemia or lymphoma (tumor lysis syndrome)] | |
|   Lesch-Nyhan syndrome | |
|   Gout | |

**2. Clinical features.** Hypospadias has a spectrum of severity. In its most common form, hypospadias is of no clinical significance. When severe, it can be associated with ambiguous genitalia and serious voiding difficulty.

**3. Therapy,** when necessary, is surgical. When severe, hypospadias may require serial procedures to construct a urethra. Because the foreskin is used in these procedures, the newborn with hypospadias should not be circumcised.

**D. Epispadias and exstrophy of the bladder.** This sporadic and uncommon spectrum of embryologic anomalies results from faulty disappearance of the cloacal membrane.

**1. Epispadias**
   **a. Defect.** Epispadias in males is the opening of the urethra on the dorsal surface of the penis. In females, the most common counterpart is a bifid clitoris; a shortened urethra and bladder neck involvement also may occur in females.
   **b. Clinical features.** Epispadias in either sex may cause varying degrees of incontinence. When incontinence is present, a voiding cystourethrogram is indicated to evaluate reflux.
   **c. Therapy.** Surgery may be needed to reconstruct the urethra and bladder neck.

**2. Exstrophy**
   **a. Defect and associated clinical features.** Exstrophy is a serious anomaly in which the bladder extrudes through the abdominal wall. The kidneys and upper urinary tract usually are normal, but vesicoureteral reflux is common. When exstrophy is severe, there may be associated abnormalities of the pubic rami, the pelvic diaphragm, the vagina and uterus, the bowel and rectum, and the spinal cord.
   **b. Therapy.** Children with exstrophy require sophisticated care and extensive surgery. Immediate concerns include preventing infection and fluid and electrolyte disturbances.

**E. Cryptorchidism (undescended testes)** is present in 1% of 1-year-old males.

**1. Defect and associated clinical features**
   **a.** Failure of the testis to descend into the scrotum may be unilateral or bilateral. An **inguinal hernia** is often present. The true undescended testis must be differentiated from the **retractile testis** that results from an exaggerated cremasteric reflex.
   **b.** The undescended testis is susceptible to testicular torsion and trauma, and it has an increased potential for malignant degeneration in adulthood, regardless of whether it is corrected or remains undescended.

**2. Therapy.** Surgical treatment (**orchiopexy**) should be carried out before age 2 years to increase the chance for fertility.

**F. Testicular torsion** (i.e., twisting of the testis and spermatic cord, causing ischemia) is uncommon in childhood.

**1. Clinical features.** Although the child usually complains of scrotal pain and swelling, severe abdominal pain may be the initial symptom.

**2. Differential diagnosis** includes epididymitis, mumps orchitis, incarcerated inguinal hernia, and testicular tumors.

**3. Therapy.** Testicular torsion is a true surgical emergency, because delay leads to infarction and testicular necrosis.

**G. Urethral stenosis.** Stenosis of the urethral meatus in both sexes and urethral stenosis in the female are rare in children. True meatal stenosis occurs most commonly in the child with hypospadias.

**1. Clinical significance**
   **a.** These disorders are significant because they frequently are diagnosed incorrectly to explain a variety of urinary problems, such as recurrent urinary tract infections and enuresis.
   **b.** Because urethral stenosis is rare, females with recurrent urinary tract infections and enuresis should not be subjected to cytoscopy and urethral dilation.

**2. Therapy** is meatotomy and dilation, but these are rarely indicated.

### H. Neurogenic bladder

1. **Etiology.** Many neurologic conditions prevent adequate storage or elimination of urine from the bladder, but neurogenic bladder is most often the result of a spinal cord disorder, including meningomyelocele, trauma, and tumors.

2. **Clinical features.** Patients suffer from incontinence, regardless of whether the neurologic defect has caused spastic, flaccid, or uninhibited bladder emptying.

3. **Diagnosis.** Neurologic assessment must include attention to reflexes below the waist, including the anal and cremasteric reflexes. Cystometry and spinal cord imaging may be required.

4. **Therapy**
   a. Cholinergic agents may help to facilitate emptying the atonic bladder. Anticholinergic agents may help to inhibit uncontrolled or spastic bladder contractions.
   b. Repeated, regular bladder catheterization is the common approach in children with cord disorders who have sensory as well as motor deficits.
   c. Surgical procedures (urinary diversion, bladder enlargement, bladder neck reconstruction, antireflux surgery) are indicated in some children.

5. **Complications** of neurogenic bladder include recurrent or chronic urinary tract infection and obstruction. These, in turn, may lead to renal parenchymal damage.

## STUDY QUESTIONS

**Directions:** Each of the numbered items or incomplete statements in this section is followed by answers or by completions of the statement. Select the **one** lettered answer or completion that is **best** in each case.

1. Renal ultrasonography can provide useful information in the diagnosis of all of the following renal disorders EXCEPT

(A) Wilms' tumor
(B) severity of renal failure in acute tubular necrosis
(C) polycystic kidney disease
(D) ureteropelvic junction obstruction
(E) nephrocalcinosis

2. A 12-year-old girl has a physical examination so she can join the soccer team. A random urinalysis is normal except for 2 + protein on dipstick testing. The most reasonable next study would be

(A) BUN and serum creatinine measurements
(B) serum total protein and albumin measurements
(C) urine culture
(D) testing a 24-hour urine collection for total protein
(E) urinalysis of the first morning urine

3. Which of the following statements best characterizes the diagnosis of urinary tract infection in children?

(A) The presence of fever localizes the infection to the renal parenchyma
(B) The diagnosis is likely if there is pyuria with more than 10 white blood cells per high-power field
(C) The diagnosis is likely if a clean-catch specimen shows $10^5$ organisms of a single species
(D) Diagnosis is difficult because the typical causative organisms grow poorly in culture
(E) Vesicoureteral reflux localizes the infection to the lower urinary tract

4. Urinalysis may provide useful information about all of the following renal parameters EXCEPT

(A) renal phosphate handling
(B) renal protein loss
(C) renal concentrating capacity
(D) possible urinary tract infection
(E) possible glomerulonephritis

5. A 5-year-old, apparently healthy child has had three episodes of gross hematuria. All of the following laboratory procedures are indicated in the evaluation of this child EXCEPT

(A) examination of the urine for red cell morphology and casts
(B) renal and bladder ultrasonography
(C) prothrombin time, partial thromboplastin time, and platelet count
(D) urinary screening for hypercalciuria
(E) sulfosalicylic acid precipitation test for proteinuria

6. Most cases of childhood nephrotic syndrome occur in association with which of the following renal diseases?

(A) Acute postinfectious glomerulonephritis
(B) Diabetic nephropathy
(C) Membranoproliferative glomerulonephritis
(D) Membranous nephropathy
(E) Minimal change disease

7. A healthy, 14-year-old black girl experiences the sudden onset of gross hematuria, which persists for 2 days. All of the following are reasonable immediate steps in the evaluation of this patient EXCEPT

(A) hemoglobin electrophoresis to exclude hemoglobin S
(B) cytoscopy to establish the site of bleeding
(C) BUN and serum creatinine measurement
(D) urine culture
(E) renal ultrasonography to assess renal anatomy

1-B    4-A    7-B
2-E    5-C
3-C    6-E

8. A child receiving chemotherapy for T cell leukemia develops the tumor lysis syndrome with acute renal failure. All of the following laboratory results might be expected EXCEPT

(A) serum potassium 6.1 mEq/L (normal = 4–5 mEq/L)

(B) serum bicarbonate 29 mEq/L (normal = 24–26 mEq/L)

(C) serum sodium 130 mEq/L (normal = 138–142 mEq/L)

(D) serum phosphate 7.5 mEq/L (normal = 4–5 mEq/L)

(E) serum uric acid 11.2 mg/dl (normal = 3–6 mEq/L)

9. A 15-month-old girl has a history of poor oral fluid intake, occasional vomiting, rapid breathing, and decreased urine output. Physical examination reveals a pulse of 150/min, blood pressure of 120/80, and a respiratory rate of 60/min. There are bibasilar rales, and the liver is palpable 4 cm below the right costal margin. All of the following procedures might be helpful in evaluating the oliguria EXCEPT

(A) giving a fluid challenge with isotonic saline, 20 ml/kg

(B) determining the urine sodium concentration

(C) determining the BUN and serum creatinine levels

(D) giving a dose of intravenous furosemide

(E) calculating the fractional excretion of sodium

10. All of the following statements regarding the treatment of childhood urinary tract infections are true EXCEPT

(A) a 10-day course of either amoxicillin or trimethoprim-sulfamethoxazole is adequate for uncomplicated cystitis

(B) antibiotic prophylaxis should be used in children with vesicoureteral reflux

(C) short-course therapy is not accepted standard treatment for urinary tract infections in children

(D) treatment of pyelonephritis requires intravenous antibiotics to achieve adequate urinary antimicrobial levels

(E) follow-up cultures are indicated at least 72 hours after completing a course of therapy

11. All of the following statements regarding blood pressure in children are true EXCEPT

(A) blood pressure levels tend to increase with age throughout infancy and childhood

(B) family history is an important risk factor in the development of hypertension in childhood

(C) most cases of childhood hypertension have an identifiable cause

(D) to avoid blood pressure elevations due to anxiety, the reading should be obtained when the heart rate is stable and repeated until values are consistent

(E) initial therapy for children with hypertension includes exercise, weight loss, and salt restriction

8-B          11-C
9-A
10-D

**Directions:** Each group of items in this section consists of lettered options followed by a set of numbered items. For each item, select the **one** lettered option that is most closely associated with it. Each lettered option may be selected once, more than once, or not at all.

**Questions 12–15**

For each biopsy pattern, select the renal disease with which it is most likely to be associated.

(A) Minimal change disease
(B) Focal segmental glomerulosclerosis
(C) Henoch-Schönlein purpura
(D) Rapidly progressive glomerulonephritis
(E) Mesangial proliferative glomerulonephritis

12. Glomeruli have marked epithelial crescent formation

13. IgA is the primary immunoglobulin seen in glomeruli

14. IgM is the primary immmunoglobulin seen in glomeruli

15. The only histologic change is effacement of the epithelial foot processes

**Questions 16–19**

For each renal disorder, select the laboratory finding with which it is most likely to be associated.

(A) Hypocomplementemia
(B) Chronic hepatitis B antigenemia
(C) Microangiopathic anemia and thrombocytopenia
(D) Vesicoureteral reflux
(E) Elevated thyroxine and TSH levels

16. Hemolytic-uremic syndrome

17. Poststreptococcal glomerulonephritis

18. Recurrent pyelonephritis

19. Membranous nephropathy

12-D     15-A     18-D
13-C     16-C     19-B
14-E     17-A

## ANSWERS AND EXPLANATIONS

**1. The answer is B**  *[I B 5 a]*.
Ultrasonography offers no help in assessing renal function and, therefore, is not useful for diagnosing acute tubular necrosis. Wilms' tumor, polycystic kidney disease, ureteropelvic junction obstruction, and nephrocalcinosis all are associated with anatomic changes that are evident on ultrasonography, which is the imaging procedure of choice for delineating structural abnormalities.

**2. The answer is E**  *[I C 2 a (1)]*.
The most common cause of proteinuria in an otherwise healthy child or adolescent is postural proteinuria. This possibility may be investigated by obtaining a urine specimen after prolonged recumbency (e.g., after a night's sleep) and repeating the urinalysis. Persistent proteinuria would suggest the need for further evaluation, including a timed urine collection for measuring protein excretion. The serum proteins should not be low unless the proteinuria is in the nephrotic range. Urinary tract infection does not cause significant proteinuria and, thus, a urine culture would not be needed.

**3. The answer is C**  *[V E 1]*.
A colony count of $10^5$ for a single organism generally is accepted as proof of urinary tract infection. Although urine obtained for culture by suprapubic aspiration or catheterization is less likely to be contaminated, clean-catch specimens are very reliable in diagnosing urinary tract infection if collected properly. There is no practical, accurate way to localize the site of infection to the renal parenchyma or the lower urinary tract. The presence of fever or of vesicoureteral reflux is certainly not a differentiating symptom, as either may occur with cystitis. High fever, however, usually occurs only in pyelonephritis, and reflux definitely increases the risk of parenchymal involvement. Pyuria may occur in children without a urinary tract infection who have acute illnesses, especially those with fever and dehydration. Pyuria also may occur in any form of interstitial nephritis. Most urinary tract infections in children are caused by coliform bacteria, which grow regularly on standard culture media.

**4. The answer is A**  *[I B 1, 3 b (2)]*.
Urinalysis cannot estimate renal phosphate handling, which must be assessed by calculating the tubular reabsorption of phosphate. The presence of amorphous phosphates in the urine sediment is common and not abnormal. Renal concentrating capacity may be estimated by the urine specific gravity and protein loss by dipstick. Examination of the sediment may reveal pyuria or bacilluria (suggesting infection) or red cell casts (suggesting glomerulonephritis).

**5. The answer is C**  *[I C 1 a (1)]*.
Prothrombin time (PT), partial thromboplastin time (PTT), and platelet count are tests of the coagulation system. Hematuria rarely is the presenting sign of a bleeding diathesis, and so coagulation profiles are not necessary. Gross hematuria may occur in several forms of glomerulonephritis, including the mesangial proliferative form and immunoglobulin A (IgA) nephropathy. It also may occur in disorders affecting genitourinary tract structure, such as tumors, cysts, and stones. Thus, urinary sediment examinations are important, and urinary tract imaging is essential. The common association of recurrent macroscopic and persistent microscopic hematuria with hypercalciuria makes it important to screen for this condition with the urine calcium to creatinine ratio. Testing for proteinuria is important, because the combination of proteinuria and hematuria is likely to signify a serious renal disease. Sulfosalicylic acid precipitation gives a measure of the total urinary protein.

**6. The answer is E**  *[III B 1]*.
Nephrotic syndrome is not a single disease entity but, rather, a component of several glomerular diseases. It is characterized by heavy proteinuria leading to hypoalbuminemia, edema, and hyperlipidemia. Nephrotic syndrome develops when the glomerular basement membrane shows a marked, prolonged increase in permeability to plasma proteins. In children, 80% of cases of nephrotic syndrome occur in association with minimal change disease, a disease characterized by histologic changes that are limited to effacement of epithelial foot processes. The remaining 20% of cases of childhood nephrotic syndrome occur in association with primary glomerulopathies (e.g., acute postinfectious glomerulonephritis, membranoproliferative glomerulonephritis, membranous nephropathy), systemic diseases (e.g., diabetic nephropathy, sickle cell nephropathy), and toxic injuries.

**7. The answer is B**  *[I C 1 b]*.
Cystoscopy is an invasive procedure that has a role in the evaluation of persistent hematuria, although not immediately. More important to the initial evaluation of gross hematuria in this 14-year-old black girl

is to establish that there is normal renal function, infection-free urine, the absence of sickle cell trait, and the absence of major renal anomalies (e.g., cysts, stones, tumor). In this patient, hematuria associated with sickle cell trait is quite possible.

**8. The answer is B**  *[IX B 2]*.
The expected acid-base disturbance in acute renal failure is metabolic acidosis. The acidosis is the result of increased endogenous acid load, volume expansion, defective acid secretion, decreased excretion of titratable acid, and diminished ammonia production. Hyperkalemia, hyperphosphatemia, and hyperuricemia all are expected consequences of increased renal load and decreased renal excretion. The tumor lysis syndrome also increases the serum uric acid levels.

**9. The answer is A**  *[I C 3 b]*.
Despite the history of poor intake of oral fluid, this infant presents with signs of congestive heart failure and fluid overload. In view of these findings, a fluid challenge could be dangerous, and it is unlikely that she would respond. If the oliguria is the result of congestive heart failure and poor renal perfusion, the urine sodium concentration and fractional excretion of sodium should be low, the blood urea nitrogen (BUN) and serum creatinine should be normal or slightly elevated, and the child may respond well to furosemide.

**10. The answer is D**  *[V F 2]*.
Because antibiotics are eliminated through the kidneys, very high levels are achieved in renal parenchyma and parenteral administration is unnecessary to treat the infection. Intravenous antibiotics may be required initially, however, in the case of a severely ill and vomiting child with pyelonephritis. An episode of pyelonephritis usually requires 10–14 days of oral therapy. Uncomplicated cystitis usually requires a 10-day course of treatment. Continuous antimicrobial therapy is required for treatment of vesicoureteral reflux. Short-course therapy is not recommended for urinary tract infection in children. A follow-up culture should be obtained at least 72 hours after completion of antibiotic therapy.

**11. The answer is C**  *[VI B 1, D 1]*.
As in adults, hypertension in children typically has no identifiable cause and, thus, is classified as primary (idiopathic, essential) hypertension. Of those children with secondary hypertension, most have renal disease as the underlying cause. Evaluation of hypertension in children often reveals a family history of the condition. When measuring blood pressure, the readings should be obtained when the heart rate is stable and repeated until the values are consistent. Blood pressure levels tend to increase with age throughout infancy and childhood. Treatment of high blood pressure should begin with reduced salt intake, weight reduction (if indicated), and increased physical activity.

**12–15. The answers are: 12-D**  *[IV F]*, **13-C** *[IV G]*, **14-E** *[IV B]*, **15-A** *[III B]*.
Rapidly progressive glomerulonephritis may occur in association with several different glomerulopathies or as an idiopathic condition. Histologically, it shows extensive glomerular epithelial crescent formation.

The nephritis of Henoch-Schönlein purpura, indistinguishable histologically from IgA nephropathy, is usually a focal glomerulonephritis with deposition of IgA as the primary immunoglobulin.

In mesangial proliferative glomerulonephritis, besides the histologic finding for which the disease is named, there often are IgM deposits in the mesangium. The glomerular basement membrane and capillary endothelium are normal.

The only histologic change in minimal change disease is the effacement of epithelial foot processes, visible only on electron microscopy.

**16–19. The answers are: 16-C**  *[IX C 1]*, **17-A** *[IV A 1 a (2)]*, **18-D** *[V C 2]*, **19-B** *[IV E 1]*.
Hemolytic-uremic syndrome is characterized by the triad of microangiopathic hemolytic anemia, thrombocytopenia, and azotemia. Although these features may vary in severity, they generally all occur together.

Approximately 85% of cases of poststreptococcal glomerulonephritis show decreased serum levels of complement component C3. Levels return to normal within 8 weeks of the onset of disease.

Vesicoureteral reflux is present in about 35% of children with urinary tract infection and in a much higher percentage of those who develop pyelonephritis.

Although membranous nephropathy may be idiopathic, it often occurs in association with diseases characterized by chronic antigenemia. Hepatitis B is one such condition, and membranous nephritis has frequently been associated with the chronic form of this disease.

# 14
# Hematologic Diseases

Arnold J. Altman
John J. Quinn

## I. GENERAL PRINCIPLES

**A. Definition.** Hematologic disorders are those that produce either quantitative or qualitative defects in the cellular elements of the blood or in those soluble elements related to hemostasis. In evaluating hematologic data in the pediatric patient, it is important to recognize the normal developmental variations that are essential to proper interpretation of a particular blood response in infancy and childhood.

**B. Hematopoiesis**

1. **Prenatal hematopoiesis.** Hematopoietic tissue is derived from the mesenchymal layer of the embryo.
   a. The earliest evidence of hematopoiesis is seen in the blood islands of the **yolk sac** at about 2–3 weeks gestation. After the yolk sac becomes connected to the systemic circulation, stem cells migrate to the embryo proper and seed future sites of hematopoiesis.
   b. At 5–6 weeks gestation, hematopoiesis commences in the **liver,** which serves as the chief site of blood cell production until the sixth fetal month. The liver continues to produce hemic cells until 2 weeks after birth. The **spleen, lymph nodes,** and **thymus** are also sites of hematopoiesis during fetal life.
   c. Hematopoiesis commences in the **bone marrow** at about the fourth or fifth fetal month, and by the sixth month, the bone marrow becomes the chief focus of blood cell production.

2. **Postnatal hematopoiesis.** At birth, hematopoietic activity is present in most of the **bones,** especially the long bones. With progressive age, however, active marrow gradually recedes from the distal portions of the skeleton, so that by the age of 18 years, only the vertebrae, ribs, sternum, skull, and pelvis are active sites of blood production.

**C. Hematopoietic homeostasis.** Compared with most normal cells in the body, those in the peripheral blood have a relatively short life span—120 days for red blood cells, 10 days for platelets, and only 6–7 hours for neutrophils. Maintenance of adequate blood counts, therefore, requires continuous replenishment in massive quantities from the bone marrow. It has been estimated that the average adult must produce approximately 100–200 billion each of new red blood cells, neutrophils, and platelets daily to meet this demand.

1. **Requirements for hematopoiesis.** The following are major requirements for hematopoiesis:
   a. Pluripotential hematopoietic stem cells
   b. An inductive microenvironment
   c. Stimulatory factors for specific cell lines (e.g., erythropoietin, thrombopoietin)
   d. Nutrients (e.g., iron, vitamin $B_{12}$, folate, amino acids)

2. **Assessment of hematopoiesis.** In clinical practice, hematopoietic homeostasis is routinely assessed by **examination of the complete blood count and peripheral blood smear**. When quantitative abnormalities of any of the cellular elements are encountered, it is useful to distinguish between disorders of production and disorders of destruction. Daily production of red blood cells can be estimated by means of the **reticulocyte count,** while neutrophil and platelet production usually are evaluated by **examination of the bone marrow**.

## II. DISORDERS OF THE HEMATOPOIETIC STEM CELL

**A. Pancytopenia** is a reduction of red blood cells, white blood cells, and platelets. It is not a disease itself, but it may result from specific disease processes. The patient with pancytopenia may present with the pallor and lethargy of anemia, the infectious complications of neutropenia, or the hemorrhagic diathesis of thrombocytopenia. **Bone marrow examination** often is required to distinguish among bone marrow aplasia, bone marrow replacement (e.g., by leukemic cells), and peripheral autoimmune destruction (Evans syndrome).

**B. Bone marrow aplasia** severe enough to produce pancytopenia may be **congenital** or **acquired**. The distinction usually is not difficult because the congenital form is associated with characteristic phenotypic and cytogenetic abnormalities.

  **1. Constitutional aplastic anemia (Fanconi's anemia)**
  **a. Pathogenesis.** Fanconi's anemia is an autosomal recessive disorder; it is associated with chromosome fragility, which results in excessive breaks and recombinations. This abnormality is not limited to hematopoietic cells but is found in all cells of the body.
  **b. Clinical features.** Despite its congenital nature, Fanconi's anemia is not associated with significant anemia or thrombocytopenia until the affected child is 3–8 years of age.
    **(1)** There is a variety of **associated phenotypic abnormalities** that are of diagnostic value. Among these are abnormal skin pigmentation, retarded growth, renal abnormalities, and skeletal deformities (e.g., absent or hypoplastic thumbs, aplasia of the radii, aplasia of the first metacarpals).
    **(2)** **Other abnormal findings** include macrocytic red blood cell indices and an elevated fetal hemoglobin (Hb F) level. The bone marrow is hypoplastic.
  **c. Therapy** involves appropriate supportive care with red blood cell and platelet transfusions. Some patients respond to androgen therapy, but the effect often is transient. Bone marrow transplantation is the treatment of choice if a human leukocyte antigen (HLA)-matched donor is available.
  **d. Prognosis.** In the past, when the only treatment of Fanconi's anemia patients with pancytopenia was blood transfusions, only rare patients survived more than 4 years. For patients who respond to androgens or bone marrow transplantation, the outlook is more favorable.

  **2. Acquired aplastic anemia**
  **a. Etiology.** Acquired aplastic anemia may result from **exposure** to chemicals (e.g., benzene), drugs (e.g., chloramphenicol, sulfonamides), infectious agents (e.g., hepatitis virus), and ionizing radiation. In many instances, no clear-cut etiologic agent is identified, and the case is classified as **idiopathic**.
  **b. Clinical features.** The hypocellular marrow distinguishes acquired aplastic anemia from other forms of pancytopenia, such as leukemia and Evans syndrome, in which the marrow is not aplastic.
  **c. Therapy and prognosis.** Bone marrow transplantation is the treatment of choice. The prognosis of severe aplastic anemia is poor: 80% of patients die within 3 months of diagnosis unless a matched donor for a bone marrow transplant is available. Because exposure to sensitizing blood products compromises the success of the transplant, it is best to avoid transfusions (especially from family members) if transplantation is being considered.

## III. ANEMIA

**A. General considerations**

  **1. Definition.** Anemia is an abnormal decrease in the number of circulating red blood cells, in the hemoglobin concentration, and in the hematocrit. It is not a disease itself but is a symptom of another disorder.

  **2. Normal red blood cell values** in the pediatric years are listed in Table 14-1. It is important to consider the following developmental variations when evaluating an infant or child for anemia.
  **a. Hemoglobin level** and **hematocrit** are relatively high in the newborn; these values subsequently decline, reaching a nadir at about 7 weeks of age for the premature infant and at 2–3 months of age for the term infant. (This condition is the physiologic "anemia" of infancy.) Total hemoglobin concentration and hematocrit rise gradually during childhood, reaching adult values after puberty.

**Table 14-1.** Red Blood Cell Values in the Pediatric Years

| Age | Hemoglobin (g/dl) | | Hematocrit (%) | | Mean Corpuscular Volume (fl) | | Mean Corpuscular Hemoglobin (pg/cell) | |
|---|---|---|---|---|---|---|---|---|
| | Mean* | Lower Limit* | Mean | Lower Limit | Mean | Lower Limit | Mean | Lower Limit |
| 1–3 days (term infant) | 18.5 | 14.5 | 56 | 45 | 108 | 95 | 34 | 31 |
| 1 month | 14.0 | 10.0 | 43 | 31 | 104 | 85 | 34 | 28 |
| 2 months | 11.5 | 9.0 | 35 | 28 | 96 | 77 | 30 | 26 |
| 3–6 months | 11.5 | 9.5 | 35 | 29 | 91 | 74 | 30 | 25 |
| ½–2 years | 12.0 | 11.0 | 36 | 33 | 78 | 70 | 27 | 23 |
| 2–6 years | 12.5 | 11.5 | 37 | 34 | 81 | 75 | 27 | 24 |
| 6–12 years | 13.5 | 11.5 | 40 | 35 | 86 | 77 | 29 | 25 |
| 12–18 years Female | 14.0 | 12.0 | 41 | 36 | 90 | 78 | 30 | 25 |
| Male | 14.5 | 13.0 | 43 | 37 | 88 | 78 | 30 | 25 |

*Mean and lower limit of normal. Lower limit is 2 standard deviations below the mean. (Adapted from Dallman PR, Siimes MA: Percentile curves for hemoglobin and red cell volume in infancy and childhood. *J Pediatr* 94:26, 1979.)

    **b.** **Hb F** is the major hemoglobin of prenatal and early postnatal life. Hb F values decline postnatally; by 9–12 months of age, the Hb F values comprise less than 2% of the total hemoglobin concentration.

    **c.** **Mean corpuscular volume (MCV)** is relatively high during the neonatal period but declines during the latter part of infancy.

**3. Classification** (Table 14-2). In clinical practice, anemias are classified according to the **morphologic appearance** (i.e., color and size) of the red blood cells on the peripheral smear and according to the **MCV**. The suffix "chromic" refers to color, and the suffix "cytic" refers to size. The primary classifications are:

    **a.** **Hypochromic, microcytic** (small, pale red blood cells; a low MCV)

    **b.** **Macrocytic** (large red blood cells; a high MCV)

    **c.** **Normochromic, normocytic** (cells of normal size and shape; a normal MCV)

**B. Hypochromic, microcytic anemias**

  **1. General considerations**

    **a. Defect.** Hypochromic, microcytic red blood cells indicate impaired synthesis of the heme or globin components of hemoglobin.

      **(1)** **Defective heme synthesis** may be the result of iron deficiency, lead poisoning, chronic inflammatory disease, pyridoxine deficiency, or copper deficiency.

      **(2)** **Defective globin synthesis** is characteristic of the thalassemia syndromes.

    **b. Evaluation.** Laboratory studies that are useful in evaluating the hypochromic, microcytic anemias include determinations of serum iron levels, iron-binding capacity, and free erythrocyte protoporphyrin as well as quantitative measurements of the adult hemoglobin, Hb $A_2$, and Hb F levels.

  **2. Iron deficiency anemia** is by far the **most common cause of anemia in children**. Most cases result from inadequate intake of iron; however, loss of iron through hemorrhage must be considered in the differential diagnosis.

    **a. Pathogenesis**

      **(1)** **Nutritional iron deficiency** usually develops when rapid growth puts excessive demands on iron stores. This is seen mainly during:

        **(a)** **Infancy,** when iron stores at birth are inadequate due to low birth weight or when the diet is composed exclusively of milk or cereals with low iron content

        **(b)** **Adolescence,** when a rapid growth spurt often coincides with a diet of suboptimal iron content (this is a particular problem in girls, who also lose iron with menses)

      **(2)** **Iron deficiency resulting from blood loss** can occur prenatally, perinatally, or postnatally.

        **(a)** **Prenatal iron loss** can result from extrusion of fetal blood into the maternal circulation (fetomaternal transfusion) or into the circulation of a twin (twin-to-twin transfusion).

**Table 14-2.** Anemias of Infancy and Childhood

| Microcytic anemias | Normocytic anemias |
|---|---|
| Defects of heme synthesis | Hemolytic disorders |
|   Iron deficiency |   Disorders of the external milieu |
|     Nutritional |     Antibody-mediated |
|     Through blood loss (chronic) |     Microangiopathic |
|   Chronic inflammation |     Due to toxins |
|   Sideroblastic anemia |     Due to infectious agents |
|     Due to lead poisoning |     Due to hypersplenism |
|     Due to pyridoxine deficiency or dependency |   Disorders of the red blood cell membrane |
| Defects of globin synthesis |     Hereditary spherocytosis |
|   Classic thalassemias |     Hereditary elliptocytosis |
|   Thalassemic hemoglobinopathies |     Hereditary stomatocytosis |
|     Hemoglobin Lepore |     Paroxysmal nocturnal hemoglobinuria |
|     Hemoglobin E |   Hemoglobinopathies |
|     Hemoglobin Constant Spring |     Hemoglobin S |
| **Macrocytic anemias** |     Hemoglobin C |
| With megaloblastic bone marrow |     Unstable hemoglobins |
|   Vitamin $B_{12}$ deficiency |     Other hemoglobinopathies |
|   Folic acid deficiency |   Enzymopathies |
|   Hereditary orotic aciduria |     Disorders of the hexose monophosphate shunt (e.g., G6PD deficiency) |
| Without megaloblastic bone marrow |     Disorders of the Embden-Meyerhof pathway (e.g., PK deficiency) |
|   Liver disease | Hemorrhage (acute or subacute) |
|   Hypothyroidism | Hypoproduction disorders |
|   Bone marrow failure states |   Pure red blood cell aplasia |
|     Acquired aplastic anemia |     Transient erythroblastopenia of childhood |
|     Fanconi's anemia |     Drug-induced aplasia |
|     Diamond-Blackfan syndrome |     Chronic renal disease |
|     Myelodysplasia |   Pancytopenia |
| |     Acquired aplastic anemia |
| |     Fanconi's anemia |
| |     Bone marrow replacement (e.g., by leukemic cells) |

G6PD = glucose-6-phosphate dehydrogenase; PK = pyruvate kinase.

    **(b) Perinatal bleeding** may result from obstetric complications such as placental abruption or placenta previa.

    **(c) Postnatal blood loss** may be of an obvious cause (e.g., after surgery or due to trauma) or may be occult, as occurs in idiopathic pulmonary hemosiderosis, parasitic infestations, or inflammatory bowel disease.

  **b. Clinical features.** Iron deficiency is most commonly seen between 6 and 24 months of age. The typical patient is on a diet consisting almost exclusively of milk.

    **(1) Symptoms.** While mild iron deficiency is relatively asymptomatic, as it becomes more severe, the infant manifests irritability, anorexia, lethargy, and easy fatigability.

    **(2) Signs.** On physical examination, the milk-fed infant is fat, pale, and sallow; other findings include tachycardia and a systolic murmur. If the anemia is very severe (i.e., hemoglobin < 3 g/dl) or if the patient has complications that put added stress on the cardiovascular system, there may be signs of congestive heart failure (i.e., a gallop rhythm, cardiomegaly, distended neck veins, hepatomegaly, and rales).

  **c. Diagnosis**

    **(1)** Anemia may vary from very mild to very severe, depending on the degree and duration of iron deficiency. Small, pale red blood cells are evident on the peripheral smear, and this is reflected in the red blood cell indices; the reduction in MCV, mean corpuscular hemoglobin, and mean corpuscular hemoglobin concentration usually is proportional to the severity of the anemia.

    **(2)** The serum iron level is decreased, while the iron-binding capacity (the transferrin level) is increased and the percent of saturation is low (usually less than 20%). The serum ferritin level is decreased (which is a reflection of low iron stores in the bone marrow), and the level of free erythrocyte protoporphyrin is increased.

(3) Bone marrow examination usually is not clinically indicated to confirm the diagnosis. When performed, it demonstrates micronormoblastic hyperplasia of erythroid elements and decreased or absent stainable iron.

**d. Therapy**

(1) **Mild to moderate anemia** (i.e., hemoglobin > 3 g/dl without signs of cardiac decompensation) can be managed by administration of iron. This can be provided by the oral route at a dosage of 6 mg/kg/day of elemental iron. Therapy is continued for a period of 2–3 months after the hemoglobin level has returned to normal; this allows replenishment of tissue iron stores. Dietary counseling must be given simultaneously to provide the patient with adequate amounts of dietary iron. Parenteral administration of iron sometimes is employed when there is a gastrointestinal problem that would interfere with iron absorption or if there is concern about the reliability of administration.

(2) **Severe anemia.** Although infants can tolerate remarkable degrees of anemia, particularly if the decline in the hemoglobin concentration is gradual, patients with extremely severe anemia who have developed signs of cardiac decompensation should be transfused slowly with packed red blood cells until the clinical condition has stabilized.

**3. Anemia of chronic disease**

**a. Pathogenesis**

(1) The anemia of chronic disease is associated with a variety of disorders, including:

(a) Chronic inflammatory disease (e.g., Crohn's disease, juvenile rheumatoid arthritis)

(b) Chronic infection (e.g., tuberculosis)

(c) Malignancy

(2) Iron is not released from its storage sites in the macrophages; thus, it is unavailable for hemoglobin synthesis in developing erythroblasts.

(3) A modest decrease in the survival of red blood cells and a relatively limited erythropoietin response to the anemia also contribute to the development of anemia.

**b. Diagnosis**

(1) The anemia is mild in degree (i.e., hemoglobin concentration is 7–10 g/dl) with hypochromic, microcytic indices.

(2) As in iron deficiency anemia, the serum iron level is reduced. However, in contrast with iron deficiency anemia, the iron-binding capacity is reduced and the serum ferritin level is increased.

(3) Bone marrow examination shows micronormoblastic hyperplasia. There is an increase in storage iron, but a decrease in the number of iron-containing erythroblasts (sideroblasts).

**c. Therapy.** The anemia resolves when the underlying disease process is treated adequately. Therapy with medicinal iron is unnecessary unless concomitant iron deficiency is present.

**4. Sideroblastic anemia**

**a. Pathogenesis**

(1) Among the conditions that produce sideroblastic anemia in childhood are:

(a) Pyridoxine deficiency

(b) Pyridoxine dependency

(c) Lead poisoning

(2) Iron enters the erythroblast freely; however, due to a metabolic block, it cannot be incorporated into hemoglobin. Instead, it accumulates in the mitochondria, giving the cell a characteristic appearance (a ringed sideroblast) when stained for iron content.

**b. Diagnosis**

(1) All sideroblastic anemias are associated with hypochromic, microcytic indices. Stippled red blood cells may be found on the peripheral smear.

(2) The bone marrow shows micronormoblastic hyperplasia. Ringed sideroblasts and increased iron stores are evident when the cells are stained with Prussian blue.

**c. Therapy**

(1) A trial of pyridoxine (50–300 mg/day) should be instituted for several weeks.

(2) If the anemia is not responsive to the pyridoxine or related to a toxin that can be eliminated, treatment usually is not successful, and the patient may require support with red blood cell transfusions.

**5. Thalassemias**

  **a. Definition.** Thalassemias are hereditary hemolytic anemias characterized by decreased or absent synthesis of one or more globin subunits of the hemoglobin molecule. **α Thalassemia** results from reduced synthesis of α-globin chains, and **β thalassemia** results from reduced synthesis of β-globin chains.

  **b. Pathogenesis**

  **(1)** Among the mechanisms responsible for producing thalassemias are:

  **(a)** Gene deletion, which is the most common cause of α thalassemia

  **(b)** An abnormality in the transcription or processing of messenger RNA (mRNA), which occurs more frequently in β thalassemia

  **(c)** Thalassemic hemoglobinopathy, in which a structurally abnormal globin chain is produced in subnormal amounts (e.g., Hb Lepore, Hb E, Hb Constant Spring)

  **(2)** Excess unpaired globin chains are a hazard to the red blood cell because they produce insoluble tetramers that precipitate, causing membrane damage. This makes red cells susceptible to destruction within the reticuloendothelial system of the bone marrow (resulting in ineffective erythropoiesis) and within the reticuloendothelial system of the liver and the spleen (resulting in hemolytic anemia).

  **c. α Thalassemias** usually are the result of **gene deletion** (normally there are four α-globin genes per cell).

  **(1) Four genes deleted.** Failure to produce any α-globin chains results in an excess of γ-globin chains, which form tetramers. This hemoglobin variant is **Hb Bart's**. Hb Bart's has a high affinity for oxygen and does not release it to the tissues. The result is severe anemia, heart failure, hepatosplenomegaly, generalized edema, and death in utero due to hydrops fetalis.

  **(2) Three genes deleted (Hb H disease).** Sufficient α-globin is produced to allow the fetus to come to term, albeit with significant anemia and elevated levels of Hb Bart's. Anemia of moderate to extreme severity persists throughout life. The major postnatal hemoglobin is Hb H, which consists of tetramers of β chains.

  **(3) Two genes deleted (α thalassemia minor).** The patient experiences moderate hypochromic, microcytic anemia. α Thalassemia minor can be confused with mild to moderate iron deficiency.

  **(4) One gene deleted (silent carrier state).** The patient has a normal hematologic picture, including normal hemoglobin concentration, hematocrit, and red blood cell indices. The condition can be diagnosed only by quantitative measurement of globin chain synthesis or by gene analysis. A carrier can produce offspring with Hb H disease or α thalassemia minor.

  **d. β Thalassemias.** Since normally there are only two β-globin genes per cell, only two general types of β thalassemia are possible.

  **(1) Homozygous β thalassemia (β thalassemia major, Cooley's anemia).** Patients with this form of anemia usually are of Mediterranean background.

  **(a) Defect.** Molecular defects range from complete absence of β-globin synthesis (genotype $\beta^\circ/\beta^\circ$) to partial reduction in the gene product from the affected locus (genotype $\beta^+/\beta^+$).

  **(b) Clinical features and course.** Beginning in the middle of the first year of life, the infant develops a progressively **severe hemolytic anemia** associated with marked **hepatosplenomegaly**. If untreated, the hepatosplenomegaly becomes progressive and the infant develops anemia, failure to thrive, and **bone marrow hyperplasia**. The bone marrow hyperplasia produces characteristic features such as tower skull, frontal bossing, maxillary hypertrophy with prominent cheekbones, and overbite. Death usually occurs within the first few years of life due to congestive heart failure unless the patient is supported with blood transfusions.

  **(c) Diagnosis**

  **(i)** Despite the severity of anemia, there is reticulocytopenia, reflecting ineffective erythropoiesis. Peripheral blood smear shows marked hypochromia, microcytosis, anisocytosis, and poikilocytosis. The red blood cell indices are significantly reduced.

  **(ii)** On hemoglobin electrophoresis, Hb A is either markedly decreased or totally absent. Of the total hemoglobin concentration, 30%–90% is Hb F.

  **(d) Therapy.** The mainstay of treatment is **transfusion with packed red blood cells**. Splenectomy generally is considered when transfusional requirements exceed 250 ml/kg/yr.

(i) Even in the untransfused state, thalassemic patients develop iron overload due to hyperabsorption of dietary iron. The iron load becomes even greater with chronic transfusion therapy. When the bone marrow storage capacity for iron is exceeded, iron accumulates in parenchymal organs such as the liver, heart, pancreas, gonads, and skin, producing the complications of **hemochromatosis** ("bronzed diabetes"). Many patients succumb to congestive heart failure in their late teens and early twenties.

(ii) In an effort to prevent hemochromatosis, patients chronically on transfusion regimens are treated with chelating agents (e.g., desferoxamine), which promote iron removal from the body.

**(2) Heterozygous β thalassemia (β thalassemia minor)**

    **(a) Clinical features.** The growth and development of patients with this disorder are normal. The only abnormality is mild anemia (a hemoglobin level that is approximately 10 g/dl).

    **(b) Diagnosis**

        (i) Hypochromia, microcytosis, and anisocytosis are found disproportionately severe to the degree of anemia.

        (ii) Hemoglobin electrophoresis shows elevation of the Hb $A_2$ level and, sometimes, elevation of the Hb F level.

    **(c) Therapy.** No treatment is necessary. It is important, however, that β thalassemia minor is distinguished from iron deficiency to prevent inappropriate therapy with medicinal iron. Genetic counseling also is important.

## C. Macrocytic anemias

**1. General considerations**

    **a. Defect.** Macrocytic anemias are typified by large red blood cells (i.e., high MCV) in the peripheral blood. Some macrocytic anemias are associated with megaloblastic hematopoiesis, while others are not.

    **(1) Macrocytosis in association with megaloblastic hematopoiesis** indicates a **defect in DNA synthesis,** usually due to a deficiency of vitamin $B_{12}$, folate, or both. A much less common cause of megaloblastic anemia is **hereditary orotic aciduria,** a defect in nucleic acid processing.

    **(2) Macrocytosis in the absence of megaloblastic changes** is seen in **liver disease, hypothyroidism,** and **dysmyelopoietic states** (e.g., Diamond-Blackfan syndrome, Fanconi's anemia, preleukemia).

    **b. Evaluation**

    **(1) Macrocytic anemia with megaloblastic marrow** is characterized by the following hematologic and bone marrow findings.

        **(a)** Macroelliptocytes and hypersegmented neutrophils are evident on the peripheral smear.

        **(b)** The bone marrow is hypercellular with asynchrony between nuclear and cytoplasmic maturation. The nucleus remains relatively large with poor condensation of chromatin as the cytoplasm matures.

    **(2) Macrocytic anemia without megaloblastic marrow.** Since young red blood cells generally are larger than mature cells, significant reticulocytosis due to any cause also produces macrocytes in the peripheral smear and elevates the MCV.

**2. Folate deficiency**

    **a. Etiology**

    **(1) Dietary deficiency of folic acid** is unusual in developed countries. However, infants fed on boiled milk or goat's milk and children with severe anorexia may develop folic acid deficiencies.

    **(2) Impaired absorption of folate** is seen in malabsorptive states [e.g., regional enteritis (Crohn's disease), celiac disease] that affect the small bowel (primarily the jejunum). Patients usually have a history of weight loss, poor weight gain, irritability, lethargy, and abnormal stools.

    **(3) Increased demand for folate** is seen in conditions characterized by an increased cell turnover (e.g., pregnancy, chronic hemolysis, malignancy). Relative folate deficiency may develop if the diet does not provide adequate folate to meet these needs.

    **(4) Abnormal folate metabolism.** Certain anticonvulsant drugs (e.g., phenytoin and phenobarbital) interfere with folate metabolism.

    **b. Diagnosis** of folic acid deficiency is confirmed by the demonstration of a decreased folate level and by a hematologic response to a 50-$\mu$g test dose of folic acid.

    **c. Therapy.** The patient should receive 5–10 mg of folic acid orally daily until the anemia and megaloblastosis are corrected. Unless a true dietary deficiency exists, therapy should also be directed toward the underlying disease process.

  **3. Vitamin B$_{12}$ deficiency**

    **a. Etiology.** Dietary vitamin B$_{12}$ deficiency is rare in developed countries; the one exception occurs in the infant who is breast-fed by a mother who is a strict vegetarian. The usual cause of vitamin B$_{12}$ deficiency is a selective or generalized **absorptive problem**.

      **(1)** Vitamin B$_{12}$ is absorbed primarily in the terminal ileum; combination with a factor produced by the gastric parietal cells (**intrinsic factor**) is necessary for absorption to occur. Once absorbed into the bloodstream, vitamin B$_{12}$ is transported in the plasma by means of a specific transport protein (**transcobalamin II**).

      **(2)** Any condition that alters intrinsic factor production, interferes with intestinal absorption in the terminal ileum, or reduces transcobalamin II levels reduces the availability of vitamin B$_{12}$.

    **b. Clinical features.** Vitamin B$_{12}$ deficiency affects multiple tissues, including the gastrointestinal mucosa (exemplified by diarrhea and weight loss) and the nervous system (seen in subacute combined degeneration of the spinal cord).

    **c. Diagnosis** is confirmed by the demonstration of a subnormal serum level of vitamin B$_{12}$. The mechanism of malabsorption can be demonstrated by the **Schilling test**.

    **d. Therapy** for most forms of vitamin B$_{12}$ deficiency requires intramuscular injection of a loading dose (1000 $\mu$g) of the vitamin followed by monthly maintenance of intramuscular doses (100 $\mu$g).

**D. Normochromic, normocytic anemias**

  **1. General considerations.** Normochromic, normocytic anemias are a heterogeneous group of disorders. The distinction between those associated with shortened survival of red blood cells and those due to impaired production of red blood cells is facilitated by analysis of the reticulocyte count and analysis of the other cellular elements of the blood.

    **a.** A **low reticulocyte count** usually suggests bone marrow failure.

      **(1)** Anemia may be an isolated finding (pure red blood cell aplasia).

      **(2)** Anemia may occur in association with neutropenia and thrombocytopenia (pancytopenia).

    **b.** A **high reticulocyte count** with normal neutrophil and platelet counts is characteristic of a hemolytic or hemorrhagic disorder.

  **2. Pure red blood cell aplasia**

    **a. Congenital anemia (Diamond-Blackfan syndrome)** is transmitted in an autosomal recessive fashion. Although usually associated with macrocytosis, Diamond-Blackfan syndrome is discussed in this section to simplify comparison with other forms of red blood cell aplasia.

      **(1) Clinical features and diagnosis.** In many patients, anemia becomes apparent within the first few months of life, and most patients manifest anemia within the first year. In addition to anemia, patients with this condition have reticulocytopenia, macrocytic red blood cell indices, and elevated Hb F levels.

      **(2) Differential diagnosis.** The early appearance of anemia, the presence of neutropenia and thrombocytopenia, and a normal phenotypic expression differentiate Diamond-Blackfan syndrome from Fanconi's anemia, the other congenital anemia of childhood (see II B 1). The early presentation, macrocytosis, elevated Hb F level, and chronic course distinguish Diamond-Blackfan syndrome from transient erythroblastopenia of childhood.

      **(3) Therapy.** About 50% of patients with Diamond-Blackfan syndrome respond to corticosteroids; in some of these patients, red blood cell production can be maintained on remarkably low doses (e.g., 2.5–5.0 mg prednisone once or twice weekly). Other patients may require red blood cell transfusions to maintain hemoglobin at an adequate level.

    **b. Acquired anemia (transient erythroblastopenia of childhood)** is of unknown etiology but probably results from the prolonged effects of viral suppression of erythropoiesis.

      **(1) Clinical features and diagnosis.** Transient erythroblastopenia of childhood is seen somewhat later in infancy than is Diamond-Blackfan syndrome. The anemia, which sometimes can be very severe, is normochromic, normocytic. Aside from reticulocytopenia, there are no other abnormalities in the peripheral blood. The Hb F level is normal.

    **(2) Therapy.** Unless the anemia is severe enough to cause cardiac decompensation, no therapy is required. Most patients recover spontaneously with 2–4 weeks.

  **c. Other forms of acquired red blood cell aplasia**

    **(1) Disorders of the kidneys, liver,** and **thyroid gland** may result in hypoproliferation of the bone marrow.

    **(2) Hypoproliferative anemia** may follow **bacterial** and **viral infections**. The etiologic agent that is documented most often is **parvovirus**. Generally, the anemia is not severe unless the patient has an underlying hemolytic disorder; failure of the bone marrow to meet the increased red blood cell turnover in this case may lead to an **aplastic crisis**.

**3. Hemolytic anemias** are caused by either intrinsic defects of the red blood cell (**intracorpuscular**) or by factors extrinsic to the red blood cell (**extracorpuscular**). In general, intracorpuscular defects are hereditary, and extracorpuscular defects are acquired.

  **a. Hemolytic anemia associated with extracorpuscular defects.** The external milieu of the red blood cell consists of the plasma and the vascular endothelium. The presence of autoantibodies or isoantibodies, toxic chemicals, or infectious agents in the plasma may shorten red blood cell survival. Likewise, irregularities of the vascular endothelium (microangiopathic changes) may be damaging to the red blood cell.

  **b. Hemolytic anemia associated with intracorpuscular defects.** Intracorpuscular defects reflect abnormalities of the membrane, hemoglobin, or enzymes. With the exception of paroxysmal nocturnal hemoglobinuria, these disorders are hereditary.

    **(1) Membrane defects** include hereditary spherocytosis, hereditary elliptocytosis, hereditary stomatocytosis, and paroxysmal nocturnal hemoglobinuria.

    **(2) Hemoglobinopathies** result from a qualitative change in the structure of one of the globin chains. This can result in one or more of the following consequences:

      **(a)** No functional change

      **(b)** Alteration in electrical charge, which allows identification by hemoglobin electrophoresis

      **(c)** Alteration in solubility

        **(i)** Paracrystalline gel may form when hemoglobin is deoxygenated (e.g., Hb S).

        **(ii)** The hemoglobin may precipitate as Heinz bodies (e.g., unstable hemoglobins).

      **(d)** Alteration in oxygen affinity

        **(i)** High-affinity hemoglobins bind oxygen tightly and result in erythrocytosis.

        **(ii)** Low-affinity hemoglobins release oxygen easily and are associated with a physiologic anemia.

      **(e)** Alteration in ability to maintain heme iron in a reduced (i.e., $Fe^{2+}$) state

        **(i)** Methemoglobin (i.e., $Fe^{3+}$) forms.

        **(ii)** The patient appears mildly cyanotic.

    **(3) Enzymopathies** generally involve either the glycolytic (Embden-Meyerhof) pathway or the hexose monophosphate shunt.

      **(a)** The most common glycolytic enzyme involved is **pyruvate kinase (PK)**.

      **(b)** The most common hexose monophosphate shunt enzyme involved is **glucose-6-phosphate dehydrogenase (G6PD)**.

**4. Antibody-mediated hemolytic anemias**

  **a. General considerations**

    **(1) Major types**

      **(a) Autoimmune hemolytic anemias** are the result of antibodies generated by an individual's immune system against his own red blood cells.

      **(b) Isoimmune hemolytic anemias** result from antibodies produced by one individual against the red blood cells of another individual of the same species.

    **(2) Typical antibodies involved**

      **(a)** Antibodies of the **immunoglobulin G (IgG)** class, for the most part, are **warm-reactive** (i.e., they have maximal activity at 37° C).

        **(i)** These are **incomplete antibodies** in that they do not agglutinate red blood cells, although they coat the surface of the red blood cells. These antibodies fix early complement components but cannot activate the complement cascade through the entire hemolytic sequence.

      **(ii)** Hemolysis occurs extravascularly due to trapping of opsonized red blood cells by macrophages in the spleen and other reticuloendothelial organs.

      **(iii)** IgG antibodies are associated clinically with autoimmune diseases, lymphomas, and viral infections. Occasionally, no underlying etiology is demonstrable.

      **(iv)** They are identified by means of the direct Coombs' test.

   **(b)** Antibodies of the **IgM** class usually are **cold-reactive** (i.e., most have maximal activity at low temperatures).

      **(i)** These are **complete antibodies** in that they agglutinate red blood cells and activate the complement sequence through C9, causing lysis of red blood cells.

      **(ii)** Hemolysis occurs intravascularly.

      **(iii)** IgM antibodies are associated clinically with mycoplasma pneumonia, Epstein-Barr virus, and transfusion reactions.

   **(c)** **Donath-Landsteiner antibody**

      **(i)** Donath-Landsteiner antibody is of the **IgG** type, but it is exceptional in that it reacts best in the cold and can activate complement, causing hemolysis to occur intravascularly.

      **(ii)** Its clinical associations include syphilis and viral infections. It may also be idiopathic.

  **b. Autoimmune hemolytic anemias**

   **(1) Etiology.** Autoimmune hemolytic anemia may be idiopathic or the result of infectious agents, drugs, lymphoid neoplasms, or disorders of immune regulation (e.g., systemic lupus erythematosus, agammaglobulinemia).

   **(2) Therapy** depends on the etiology, clinical condition of the patient, and expected duration of the illness. As most cases of childhood autoimmune hemolytic anemia are idiopathic or postinfectious and self-limited, supportive care and judicious use of transfusions and corticosteroids are the therapies most commonly employed. Treatment modalities include:

      **(a)** Supportive care with bed rest and oxygen

      **(b)** Transfusion with packed red blood cells

      **(c)** Corticosteroids

      **(d)** Splenectomy

      **(e)** Immunosuppressive agents

  **c. Isoimmune hemolytic anemias** can be seen in hemolytic disease of the newborn [see Ch 5 V D 1 a (1)]. Hemolytic transfusion reactions are associated with isoimmune hemolytic anemias (e.g., the transfusion of type A blood into an individual with type B blood).

**5. Microangiopathic hemolytic anemias**

  **a. Defect and pathogenesis.** In these conditions, the red blood cells suffer mechanical damage due to irregularities in the vascular endothelium [e.g., in association with severe hypertension, chronic renal disease, artificial heart valves, hemolytic-uremic syndrome, giant hemangioma, or disseminated intravascular coagulation (DIC)]. The resulting hemolytic anemia occurs because of red blood cell fragmentation in the presence of small vessel disease.

  **b. Diagnosis** is supported by demonstration of red blood cell fragmentation on the peripheral smear in the form of burr cells, helmet cells, and other irregularly shaped red blood cells.

  **c. Therapy** involves supportive care and treatment of the underlying condition.

**6. Hereditary spherocytosis**

  **a. Defect.** Hereditary spherocytosis is an autosomal dominant type of hemolytic anemia associated with a **defect in spectrin,** the major supporting protein of the red blood cell membrane. The defect leads to a loss of membrane fragments and the formation of small, spherical red blood cells with a high volume to surface ratio (**microspherocytes**).

   **(1)** Microspherocytes have less deformability than normal red cells and, consequently, have difficulty in traversing small blood vessels.

   **(2)** The microspherocyte membrane is excessively permeable to sodium. This puts a metabolic strain on the cell because energy in the form of adenosine triphosphate (ATP) is required to pump excess sodium out of the red cell.

  **b. Pathogenesis.** The spleen plays a major role in the pathogenesis of hemolysis.

   **(1)** The spleen has the smallest vessels in the body; thus, the rigid microspherocytes are trapped in its microvasculature.

**(2)** Glucose and oxygen levels are very low in the sluggish splenic sinusoids; thus, the excess metabolic demands of the microspherocyte for ATP cannot be met.

**c. Clinical features**

**(1)** Hereditary spherocytosis may present in the newborn as jaundice, which is sometimes severe enough to require exchange transfusions.

**(2)** Infants and children may present with pallor or splenomegaly.

**(3)** Occasionally, patients may present with severe hypoproliferative anemia due to an aplastic crisis following a viral infection [see III D 2 c (2)].

**(4)** Teenagers and adults may develop gallstones and present with the symptoms of **cholecystitis**.

**d. Diagnosis**

**(1)** **Physical examination** usually is positive for pallor, icterus, and mild to moderate splenomegaly.

**(2)** **Laboratory findings**

**(a)** Mild anemia and reticulocytosis usually are present. During aplastic episodes, the anemia may become severe and the reticulocyte count declines.

**(b)** Diagnosis is confirmed by the demonstration of increased osmotic fragility.

**e. Therapy**

**(1)** **Supportive care** involves folic acid supplementation (to meet needs imposed by increased red blood cell turnover) and red blood cell transfusion (during aplastic crises).

**(2)** **Definitive therapy** is splenectomy, which alleviates anemia, reticulocytosis, and icterus; however, characteristic microspherocytes persist after splenectomy. Splenectomy should be postponed until the patient is 6 years of age to allow the full development of the immune system.

**7. Hereditary elliptocytosis**

**a. Defect.** Hereditary elliptocytosis is an abnormality involving the shape of red blood cells. It is characterized by varying degrees of red blood cell destruction and hemolytic anemia.

**b. Clinical features.** The clinical course is variable. Only 10%–15% of patients develop chronic hemolytic anemia (these patients usually have red cells with increased osmotic fragility). The newborn may present with icterus; peripheral smear shows bizarre fragmented forms of red blood cells as well as some characteristic oval-shaped cells. Later in life, the elliptocytes become more prominent.

**c. Therapy.** Asymptomatic patients require no treatment. Patients with chronic hemolysis require splenectomy when they are over 6 years of age.

**8. Hereditary stomatocytosis**

**a. Defect.** Stomatocytosis is a rare hereditary disorder. Characteristically, red blood cells have a central slit, or stoma, when seen on dried smear. The physiologic defect is a red cell membrane that is unusually permeable to sodium.

**b. Clinical features.** Most patients have mild symptoms associated with jaundice and occasional anemia.

**c. Therapy.** If the anemia is of sufficient severity to warrant treatment, splenectomy has been found to be palliative but not curative.

**9. Paroxysmal nocturnal hemoglobinuria**

**a. Defect.** Paroxysmal nocturnal hemoglobinuria is an uncommon, acquired membrane disorder characterized by red blood cells that are unusually sensitive to the action of hemolytic complement. Hemolysis is maximal during sleep when carbon dioxide partial pressure ($P_{CO_2}$) rises and pH falls, thereby activating the alternative pathway of complement activation.

**b. Clinical features.** The disorder is associated with attacks of hemoglobinuria, which usually—but not always—occur at night. The disorder often occurs in conjunction with hypoplastic anemia.

**c. Diagnosis** is confirmed by demonstrating increased lysis in an acidified serum test (**Ham test**) or in isotonic low ionic strength solutions (**sucrose-hemolysis test**).

**d. Therapy** is symptomatic. When the anemia is severe, patients may be transfused with packed red cells (which should be washed to remove complement prior to transfusion).

**10. Hb S disorders**

**a. Epidemiology.** This hemoglobinopathy is the most common cause of hemolytic anemia in the African-American population. It also is occasionally found in Greeks, Italians, Saudi Arabians, and Veddoids of southern India.

**b. Defect and pathogenesis**

(1) The molecular defect is due to an abnormal autosomal gene that substitutes valine for glutamic acid in the sixth position of the β-globin chain. This substitution results in an unusual solubility problem in the deoxygenated state. Under conditions of hypoxia, the hemoglobin aggregates into long polymers that align themselves into rigid paracrystalline gels (tactoids), which distort the red cell into a sickle shape.

(2) The clinical consequences of the solubility anomaly are:

(a) Shortened red blood cell survival (hemolytic anemia)

(b) Microvascular obstruction, which leads to tissue ischemia and infarction

**c. Heterozygous state (sickle cell trait).** About 10% of African-Americans are heterozygous for the Hb S gene. Both Hb A and Hb S exist in individuals with sickle cell trait; there is more Hb A than Hb S.

(1) **Clinical features.** Sickle cell trait usually is asymptomatic, unless the affected individual is subjected to hypoxemic stress. Otherwise, abnormalities may be limited to failure to concentrate urine, painless hematuria, or both.

(2) **Diagnosis.** Patients with sickle cell trait do not routinely manifest sickle cells on peripheral smear. Sickle cell trait may be diagnosed by hemoglobin electrophoresis or by solubility tests (e.g., precipitation with dithionate and phosphate, sodium metabisulfite slide test). It is important to detect the trait for purposes of genetic counseling.

(3) **Therapy.** No specific treatment is required; however, precautions to avoid hypoxemia associated with severe pneumonia, unpressurized flying, exercise at high altitudes, and general anesthesia are in order. Tourniquet surgery and deep hypothermia should be avoided.

**d. Homozygous state (sickle cell anemia)**

(1) **Clinical features**

(a) In the **asymptomatic period,** the high levels of Hb F during fetal life and during the first few months of postnatal life protect the patient.

(b) The **earliest clinical manifestation** may occur at 4–6 months of age, when the patient develops symmetrical painful swelling of the dorsal surfaces of the hands and feet (**hand-foot syndrome**). This is due to avascular necrosis of the bone marrow of the metacarpal and metatarsal bones. During this same period, the patient begins to develop progressive anemia with jaundice and splenomegaly.

(c) Two major **life-threatening problems relating to the spleen** affect infants.

(i) **Splenic sequestration crises.** The spleen may suddenly become engorged with red blood cells, trapping a significant portion of the blood volume. If not corrected rapidly, this can lead to hypovolemic shock and death.

(ii) **Overwhelming infection.** Despite its large size, in the early childhood years, the spleen does not efficiently perform its filtering function with respect to blood-borne microorganisms. Patients are very susceptible to overwhelming infection, particularly with encapsulated bacteria such as pneumococcus and *Hemophilus influenzae.*

(d) **Aplastic crises** can occur at any age when there is suppression of erythropoiesis in response to a viral infection [see III D 2 c (2)].

(e) **Vaso-occlusive episodes** can involve any tissue. Depending on the involved organ, a vaso-occlusive episode can produce abdominal pain, bone pain, cerebrovascular accident, pulmonary infarction, hepatopathy, or hematuria. These episodes often are precipitated by infection, dehydration, chilling, vascular stasis, or acidosis. Repeated vaso-occlusive episodes in the spleen lead to infarction and fibrosis of this organ; it gradually regresses in size and usually is no longer palpable after the age of 5 years.

(f) **Late manifestations.** By the time a patient reaches his late teens or early twenties, he is suffering the long-term consequences of chronic anemia, tissue hemosiderosis, and tissue infarction. Many succumb to progressive myocardial damage with congestive heart failure. Other long-term complications include gallstones, leg ulcers, renal damage, and aseptic necrosis of the long bones.

(2) **Therapy**

(a) **Infections**

(i) **Prevention.** Penicillin taken daily on a prophylactic basis has been demonstrated to reduce the incidence of overwhelming pneumococcal infection. Pneumococcal and *H. influenzae* vaccines also are useful in preventing infection.

      **(ii) Treatment.** A febrile episode that occurs suddenly must be considered sepsis until proven otherwise. Blood cultures should be obtained, and the patient should receive intravenous antibiotics against pneumococcus and *H. influenzae.*

    **(b) Vaso-occlusive episodes**

      **(i) Prevention** involves the avoidance of dehydration, hypoxia, chilling, and acidosis.

      **(ii) Treatment.** Analgesics should be given for pain. When a vital organ (the brain, liver, lung) is threatened or when the episode does not respond to hydration, transfusion with packed red blood cells may be necessary.

    **(c) Severe aplastic crises** should be treated by transfusion with packed red blood cells.

**11. Hemoglobin C disorder** is mild and usually detected only during examination for an unrelated medical condition.

    **a. Epidemiology.** This β-globin variant is found primarily in African-Americans. Approximately 3% of African-Americans are heterozygous for the Hb A and Hb C genes, and 1 in 10,000 is homozygous for Hb C.

    **b. Clinical features.** An Hb AC trait is asymptomatic, but target cells are found in the blood smear. Hb CC homozygotes have mild to moderate hemolytic anemia with target cells on the peripheral smear.

**12. Double heterozygous states.** A combination of Hb S and another abnormal hemoglobin or a combination of Hb S with a thalassemia gene produces a variety of clinical syndromes of varying severity.

    **a.** The **Hb SC heterozygote** tends to have a milder disease than the Hb SS homozygote; splenomegaly may be more prominent and pulmonary infarction a more common problem.

    **b.** The **Hb S–β thalassemia heterozygote** may have a clinical picture that is as severe as Hb SS disease; Hb S–α thalassemia, on the other hand, may be mild.

**13. Glucose-6-phosphate dehydrogenase (G6PD) deficiency** is the most common red blood cell metabolic disorder. It usually is transmitted in an X-linked recessive fashion.

    **a. Defects.** There are about 150 G6PD variants. The two prototypic forms are the A– variant and the Mediterranean variant.

      **(1)** The **A– variant** is found mainly in the African-American population and is associated with an isoenzyme that deteriorates rapidly (it has a half-life of 13 days).

      **(2)** The **Mediterranean variant** is found mainly in individuals of Greek and Italian descent and is associated with almost complete absence of enzyme activity, even in young cells, due to extreme instability (it has a half-life of several hours).

    **b. Pathogenesis**

      **(1)** G6PD-deficient cells do not generate an amount of reduced glutathione that is sufficient to protect the red blood cells from oxidant agents. Exposed sulfhydryl groups of hemoglobin are oxidized, predisposing the molecule to denaturation.

      **(2)** The heme and globin moieties dissociate, with the globin precipitating as Heinz bodies, which form disulfide bridges to the red cell membrane. The damaged red cells are then removed by the reticuloendothelial system; severely damaged cells may lyse intravascularly.

    **c. Clinical features**

      **(1)** The classic picture of G6PD deficiency is an **episodic hemolytic anemia** that usually is drug induced. However, it may also present as hemolysis precipitated by infection, neonatal jaundice, chronic nonspherocytic hemolytic anemia, or favism.

      **(2)** When patients with either the A − or the Mediterranean variant of G6PD deficiency are exposed to **oxidant drugs** (e.g., sulfonamides, salicylates, phenacetin), there is a lag period of 1–3 days, after which a brisk hemolytic process ensues. The subsequent course differs for the two variants, however.

        **(a)** Patients with the A − variant have self-limited hemolysis confined to the older red blood cell population. Recovery occurs as young red blood cells with enzyme activity sufficient to resist oxidant stress emerge from the bone marrow.

        **(b)** Patients with the Mediterranean variant have hemolysis that destroys most of their red blood cells and may require transfusions until the drug is eliminated from their bodies.

**d. Therapy**
  **(1)** Patients with variants of G6PD deficiency that are associated with acute acquired hemolysis should avoid drugs that initiate hemolysis.
  **(2)** Splenectomy does not benefit patients with G6PD deficiency.

**14. Pyruvate kinase (PK) deficiency** is clinically heterogeneous and is inherited in an autosomal recessive fashion.
  **a. Pathogenesis**
    **(1)** PK catalyzes the final step in the glycolytic pathway; the consequence of its deficiency is inadequate production of ATP. This puts metabolic stress on the red blood cells since ATP is required to energize the pump that maintains intracellular sodium and potassium ions at the proper levels; thus, PK-deficient cells lose potassium and gain sodium.
    **(2)** Reticulocytes, with their increased metabolic demands, are particularly vulnerable to destruction, especially in the sluggish splenic cords.
  **b. Clinical features**
    **(1)** The severity of hemolysis is variable; newborns may present with jaundice, chronic anemia, or splenomegaly.
    **(2)** Although the signs and symptoms of PK deficiency are the same as those of other chronic hemolytic anemias, due to selective destruction of reticulocytes, there may be an inappropriately low reticulocyte count in response to the anemia.
  **c. Therapy.** Splenectomy has proven beneficial in individuals with severe enzyme deficiency. Paradoxically, the reticulocyte count rises after splenectomy because the reticulocytes are then able to survive longer.

**IV. POLYCYTHEMIA (ERYTHROCYTOSIS)** refers to a greater than normal number of red blood cells in the blood. The term sometimes also implies a greater than normal number of leukocytes and platelets. Erythrocytosis is, perhaps, a more accurate term since it implies an increase in total concentration of red corpuscles, not an increase of leukocytes and platelets.

**A. Etiology.** Erythrocytosis may be caused by an increase in red blood cell mass (**absolute erythrocytosis**) or by a decrease in plasma volume, in which case the total number of circulating red corpuscles is unaffected, although their concentration is increased (**relative erythrocytosis**).

**B. Pathophysiology.** Abnormal elevation of hematocrit generally is considered to be a hematocrit of 55% and above. Cardiac work is increased by an excessively elevated hematocrit, which can increase blood viscosity, leading to diminished blood flow and decreased oxygen delivery to tissues.

**C. Relative erythrocytosis** is commonly associated with **dehydration**. Because an elevated hematocrit may reflect either an expansion of total red blood cell mass (absolute erythrocytosis) or a decrease in plasma volume (relative erythrocytosis), it is necessary that dehydration be ruled out before the high hematocrit is considered significant.

**D. Absolute erythrocytosis** may be due to a primary defect of the hematopoietic stem cell (**polycythemia vera**) or secondary to **elevated erythropoietin levels**.

  **1. Polycythemia vera,** in which leukocytes and platelets also are increased in number, is extremely rare in childhood.

  **2. Elevated erythropoietin levels,** leading to erythrocytosis, may be seen in the following clinical situations.
    **a. Hypoxia**
      **(1)** The most common cause of erythrocytosis in childhood is cyanotic cardiac disease. Pulmonary disease and high altitudes may also produce sufficient hypoxia to induce erythrocytosis.
      **(2)** Hemoglobins with a high affinity for oxygen do not release it readily to tissues. The consequent tissue hypoxia may be sufficient to induce an erythropoietin response, which can be diagnosed by demonstrating a $P_{50}$ (the partial pressure of oxygen at which half of the hemoglobin has oxygen bound to it) that is lower than normal.
    **b. Inappropriate erythropoietin production** by renal cysts, renal tumors, and some other tumors (e.g., cerebellar hemangioblastoma)

**V. LEUKOCYTE DISORDERS.** In most clinical settings, the status of the leukocyte population is assessed by measuring the total white blood cell count and the differential count. In evaluating these parameters, it is important to remember that for the first 4 years of life, there is a relative preponderance of lymphocytes.

**A. Disorders of leukocyte morphology**

1. **Chédiak-Higashi syndrome** is an autosomal recessive systemic disorder that is characterized by **giant cytoplasmic granular inclusions** in neutrophils.
   a. **Clinical features**
      (1) Recurrent, severe pyogenic infections
      (2) Partial albinism, photophobia, lymphadenopathy, and hepatosplenomegaly
      (3) A tendency to develop lymphoreticular malignancy
   b. **Diagnosis** is made by finding extremely large granules in peripheral blood neutrophils. Neutrophil movement also is impaired because of the large granules.
   c. **Therapy** involves antimicrobial treatment of the infections and blood or platelet transfusions for anemia.

2. **May-Hegglin anomaly** is a rare autosomal dominant disorder of leukocytes and platelets. **Döhle bodies** (large pale blue inclusions) are found in the cytoplasm of neutrophils, eosinophils, basophils, and monocytes. The disorder is characterized also by thrombocytopenia, giant platelets, and large platelet granules. Neutrophil function remains intact, but there may be platelet function abnormalities.

3. **Pelger-Hüet anomaly** is a common autosomal dominant trait that has no adverse effects on health. There is decreased nuclear segmentation of neutrophils, and neutrophil function is intact. Occasionally, Pelger-Hüet anomaly is seen as an acquired disorder (due to drugs, leukemia, infectious mononucleosis).

**B. Neutropenia**

1. **General considerations**
   a. **Definition.** Although the absolute neutrophil count (ANC) varies somewhat according to age and race, a value of 1500/mm$^3$ usually is considered the lower limit of normal. However, an increased propensity to infection is not seen until the ANC falls below 1000/mm$^3$. With an ANC of 500–1000/mm$^3$, patients are at higher risk for cutaneous and mucous membrane infections (e.g., furunculosis, gingivitis, mouth ulcers, perianal cellulitis). When the ANC is below 500/mm$^3$, the risk for severe visceral infections (including septicemia) increases proportionally to the lowering of the ANC.
   b. **Etiology and classification.** Neutropenia may occur in conjunction with anemia and thrombocytopenia as part of a generalized bone marrow dysfunction (e.g., aplastic anemia, malignancy) or as an isolated cytopenia. The discussion here is confined to isolated neutropenia. Isolated neutropenia may be the result of **either decreased production or increased destruction of neutrophils**. Determination of the etiology of neutropenia routinely requires bone marrow aspiration.

2. **Neutropenia due to decreased production of neutrophils**
   a. **Congenital or familial neutropenias.** A variety of chronic neutropenias, not all well-defined, appear to be of congenital origin or to follow a familial pattern. These vary in severity from benign disorders detected accidentally by routine blood count to disorders associated with frequent life-threatening infections. It is not always possible to predict prognosis based on ANC or bone marrow examination; instead, a combination of family history and clinical follow-up often is the best guide to patient management.
      (1) **Cyclic neutropenia**
         (a) **Clinical features.** Cyclic neutropenia is characterized by regular development of marked neutropenia, usually at 21-day intervals. Coincident with the neutropenia, the patient develops fever, oral ulcers, furunculosis, and other types of infection. Fatal infections are rare.
         (b) **Diagnosis.** Bone marrow changes are cyclic also but are out of phase with changes in the peripheral blood (i.e., myeloid hyperplasia is present at the time of maximal neutropenia). The defect is most likely to occur at the pluripotential stem cell level, resulting from failure or inhibition of the bone marrow. Red blood cell and platelet production also are affected but are not of clinical significance because of the longer half-lives of these cells.

**(2) Chronic benign neutropenia**

**(a) Clinical features.** This is a heterogeneous group of disorders, with variable inheritance patterns and morphologic features. Patients tend to have "nuisance" infections (i.e., mild furuncles, mouth ulcers) rather than life-threatening ones. The ANC usually is 300–1500/mm³.

**(b) Diagnosis.** The bone marrow often shows adequate numbers of myeloid precursors associated with an apparent arrest in development at any stage of maturation from promyelocyte to band form.

**(3) Severe congenital agranulocytosis** (congenital neutropenia; Kostmann's disease) is inherited through an autosomal recessive gene. The bone marrow shows maturation arrest at the promyelocyte or early myelocyte stage. Severe and often lethal pyogenic infections of the skin and respiratory tract occur, often beginning in the first month of life.

**(4) Neutropenia associated with metabolic or phenotypic abnormalities**

**(a) Metabolic diseases** associated with neutropenia include idiopathic hyperglycinemia, propionic acidemia, methylmalonic acidemia, and isovaleric acidemia. Patients with these diseases usually are quite ill with lethargy, vomiting, ketosis, and dehydration beginning in the neonatal period.

**(b) Cartilage-hair hypoplasia** is a variety of short-limbed dwarfism that is characterized by fine, silky hair, moderate neutropenia, and variable immunologic abnormalities.

**(5) Schwachman-Diamond syndrome** is characterized by metaphyseal chondrodysplasia, dwarfism, pancreatic exocrine insufficiency, and neutropenia. Patients may present early in life with diarrhea, failure to thrive, and recurrent sinopulmonary infections. Neither the neutropenia nor the dwarfism is amenable to therapy.

**(6) Neutropenia associated with immunologic disorders**

**(a)** Some cases of **congenital agammaglobulinemia** and **dysgammaglobulinemia** are associated with neutropenia, which may be transient, cyclic, or chronic.

**(b) Reticular dysgenesis** is a lethal disorder characterized by a selective failure of stem cells committed to myeloid and lymphoid development. There is deficiency of granulocytic and lymphocytic development, although erythroid and megakaryocytic elements are spared. The bone marrow is devoid of myeloid elements, and the thymus and spleen are devoid of lymphocytes.

**b. Neutropenia caused by infection.** Various bacterial and viral agents are associated with neutropenia in children. The mechanisms responsible for the neutropenia are ill-defined and probably include myelosuppression as well as increased peripheral utilization, sequestration, and margination.

**(1) Viruses** commonly causing neutropenia include influenza (A and B), hepatitis (A and B), respiratory syncytial, rubella, varicella, and Epstein-Barr viruses.

**(2) Bacterial infections** associated with neutropenia include typhoid, paratyphoid, brucellosis, and tularemia.

**c. Drugs and toxic agents**

**(1) Two patterns of drug-induced myelosuppression** are recognized.

**(a) Cytotoxic drugs,** such as methotrexate, cause regularly occurring, dose-dependent suppression of all marrow elements.

**(b) Idiosyncratic suppression** of neutrophil production can be caused by drugs such as sulfonamides, synthetic penicillins, antithyroid agents, and phenothiazines.

**(2) Heavy metals** and **benzene agents** also can suppress granulocytopoiesis.

**3. Neutropenia due to increased destruction of neutrophils**

**a. Immune-mediated neutropenia.** Antineutrophil antibodies may be self-produced (autoimmune) or transmitted to the patient from another individual (isoimmune).

**(1) Autoimmune neutropenia** may be idiopathic or occur secondary to drug sensitization, system disease (e.g., lupus), a neoplasm (e.g., lymphoma), or viral infection. Some patients respond to corticosteroid therapy.

**(2) Isoimmune neutropenia** results from the transfer of antineutrophil antibodies from the mother to the fetus. This may occur because the mother has been sensitized to an antigen on the fetal neutrophils or because the mother has an illness (e.g., lupus) that has induced an autoimmune process in her. When the neonatal neutropenia is severe, pyogenic infections of the skin, umbilical cord, respiratory tract, and bloodstream may develop. In most cases, the neutropenia resolves spontaneously when the maternal antibody is cleared from the infant's circulation.

**b. Drug-induced neutropenia.** In addition to their myelosuppressive effects, drugs may produce neutropenia by acting as haptens in immune neutropenia or by directly damaging circulating neutrophils. Neutropenia may resolve following the withdrawal of the offending drug or through the use of steroids.

**c. Splenic sequestration (hypersplenism).** Splenomegaly from any cause can lead to neutropenia due to trapping of the neutrophils. Red blood cells and platelets may be affected as well. Treatment of the underlying illness or splenectomy (if clinically indicated) usually resolves this form of neutropenia.

**C. Disorders of neutrophil function** (see Ch 8 II B 1)

**VI. HEMOSTASIS.** Normal hemostasis requires the integrity of three elements: **blood vessels, platelets,** and **soluble clotting factors** (Figure 14-1). Hemorrhage may result from deficiency or disorders of any of these elements.

**A. Hemorrhagic diathesis**

**1. Clinical features.** Indications of significant hemorrhagic diathesis include:
   **a.** Petechiae, purpura, or both
   **b.** Severe recurrent epistaxis (in the absence of an obvious local cause)
   **c.** Prolonged bleeding after dental extractions, surgical procedures, or major trauma
   **d.** Recurrent hemarthrosis

**2. Screening** the patient with a suspected hemorrhagic diathesis requires a battery of laboratory tests, including:
   **a.** A complete blood count
   **b.** The estimate of platelet number and assessment of platelet morphology on blood smear
   **c.** Partial thromboplastin time (PTT), which measures the integrity of the intrinsic and common pathways
   **d.** Prothrombin time (PT), which measures the integrity of the extrinsic and common pathways
   **e.** Measurement of bleeding time, which assesses vascular integrity and platelet function

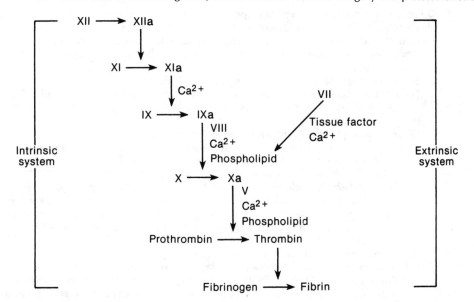

**Figure 14-1.** The coagulation cascade. The intrinsic pathway is initiated by activation of factor XII, whereas the extrinsic pathway is initiated by release of tissue factor and activation of factor VII. Both pathways converge with the activation of factor X. *a* = activated.

3. **General approach to management**

   a. Drugs that compromise platelet function (e.g., aspirin) must be avoided, as should deep venipunctures and intramuscular injections. The patient should be protected against trauma (especially to the head). Prolonged immobilization should be prevented.

   b. When the nature of the defect is identified, specific replacement measures should be employed.

   c. If the bleeding is life-threatening, fresh frozen plasma (10–20 ml/kg) can be used as a temporizing measure for defects in coagulation factors until a specific factor deficiency is identified.

B. **Disorders of blood vessels**

1. **Role of blood vessels in hemostasis.** Injury to a blood vessel elicits at least two responses that help to control bleeding.

   a. **Vasoconstriction** reduces blood flow through the injured vessel.

   b. **Subendothelial collagen** activates platelets and coagulation factors.

2. **Vascular abnormalities** leading to a bleeding diathesis include **vasculitis** as well as the following conditions.

   a. **Excessive capillary fragility** is seen in hereditary disorders of collagen synthesis (e.g., Ehlers-Danlos syndrome).

   b. **Hereditary hemorrhagic telangiectasia** is an autosomal dominant disorder. Vascular abnormalities occur throughout the body, especially on mucosal surfaces. Gastrointestinal bleeding may be severe. Iron deficiency anemia occurs invariably.

   c. **Vitamin C deficiency (scurvy)** results in impaired collagen synthesis. Walls of blood vessels are pliable due to the poor collagen support. Bleeding may also be due to qualitative platelet defects.

   d. **Henoch-Schönlein purpura** (see also Ch 8 V D 3 b) is a disease of children and young adults that is associated with a variety of clinical features, including arthritis, nephritis, urticaria, a characteristic purpuric rash involving the buttocks and lower extremities, and gastrointestinal pain.

C. **Disorders of platelets.** Platelet defects can be quantitative or qualitative. **Quantitative disorders** are detected by platelet estimate on a peripheral blood smear or platelet count. **Qualitative disorders** are detected by bleeding time or platelet aggregation studies.

1. **Quantitative disorders. Thrombocytopenia** is a decreased number of platelets (the normal platelet count is 150,000–350,000/mm$^3$); it is the most common cause of abnormal bleeding. The low platelet count may result from failure of production or from shortened survival. Platelet production is evaluated mainly by assessing the number of megakaryocytes in the bone marrow aspirate.

   a. **Thrombocytopenia due to decreased platelet production**

      (1) **Bone marrow failure** states associated with pancytopenia (see II and III C 1 a) are a cause of thrombocytopenia. Ineffective thrombopoiesis is associated with megaloblastic hematopoiesis.

      (2) **Amegakaryocytic thrombocytopenia** has a variable inheritance pattern, although when it is due to the **thrombocytopenia-absent radius (TAR) syndrome,** it is inherited as an autosomal recessive trait. The thrombocytopenia in TAR syndrome may be associated with renal disorders and congenital heart disease.

      (3) **Wiskott-Aldrich syndrome** (see also Table 8-3) has an X-linked recessive inheritance. Clinically, it is characterized by eczema, recurrent infections due to deficiencies in T cell and B cell immunity, and thrombocytopenia. The thrombocytopenia may be severe, and the bleeding often is aggravated by sepsis. Small platelets (**microthrombocytes**) are seen on peripheral smear.

   b. **Thrombocytopenia due to shortened survival**

      (1) **Immune-mediated thrombocytopenia** may be associated with **viral infection** or **drugs,** but most cases in childhood are **idiopathic.** The term **idiopathic thrombocytopenic purpura (ITP)** refers to a thrombocytopenia for which exogenous causes are not apparent. It seems that, in most patients, an autoimmune process increases platelet destruction. Opsonized platelets are trapped and destroyed in the reticuloendothelial system.

        **(a) Clinical features.** ITP may be seen after a mild viral illness or after an immunization. The onset usually is abrupt, with bleeding of the skin and mucous membranes. Bleeding is severe after trauma.

        **(b) Clinical course.** Severe internal hemorrhage is rare, despite a very low platelet count. In 80%–90% of cases, ITP resolves spontaneously within 1–6 months. However, some cases become relapsing or chronic. The mortality rate is less than 1%.

        **(c) Therapy.** Conservative management is advisable since the acute form of ITP observed in children resolves spontaneously in most cases. The use of corticosteroids is controversial, although some physicians advise a brief course early in acute, severe cases. Refractory cases may be treated with intravenous gamma globulin, splenectomy, or immunosuppressive agents.

    **(2) Hypersplenism** (see V B 3 c) is associated with thrombocytopenia as well as anemia and neutropenia.

    **(3) DIC** (see VI D 5) has also been associated with thrombocytopenia.

  **c. Thrombocytopenia in the newborn.** There are many causes of thrombocytopenia in the newborn. Among the most common are congenital infections (see the TORCH constellation in Chapter 7 II B), bacterial sepsis, immune-mediated causes, and DIC. In **immune-mediated thrombocytopenia** in the newborn, antibody is formed by the mother against antigen on her own platelets (autoimmune antibodies) or on the fetus' platelets (isoimmune antibodies). IgG antibodies cross the placenta and opsonize the infant's platelets. Platelets are trapped and destroyed within the infant's reticuloendothelial system.

    **(1) Autoimmune antibodies** are produced by women with ITP, lupus, and drug-induced thrombocytopenia. The mother is thrombocytopenic.

    **(2) Isoimmune antibodies** are produced by the mother whose fetus' platelets possess an antigen that her platelets lack. The mother's platelet count is normal.

**2. Qualitative platelet disorders (thrombocytopathies)** may be congenital or acquired. Thrombocytopathies are associated with platelets that, although sufficient in number, are dysfunctional in hemostasis.

  **a. Congenital causes of thrombocytopathies**

    **(1) Bernard-Soulier syndrome** is an inherited coagulation disorder characterized by mild thrombocytopenia, moderate to severe purpuric bleeding, and giant platelets on peripheral smear. There is an absence of the platelet membrane glycoprotein Ib, which is associated with the interaction between coagulation factor VIII and the platelet membrane that is required for normal platelet adhesion to collagen.

    **(2) Glanzmann's thrombasthenia** is an intrinsic platelet disorder characterized by deficiency of the platelet membarne glycoprotein IIb-IIIa complex. These platelets cannot absorb several cationic proteins or bind to each other. Thus, abnormalities are found in tests of platelet aggregation.

    **(3) Gray platelet syndrome** characteristically has a mild bleeding diathesis and a lack of alpha granules in blood platelets.

    **(4) Storage pool disease** is characterized by a deficient release reaction of blood platelets when they are physiologically stimulated. The platelets aggregate normally when stimulated by exogenous adenosine diphosphate (ADP) but do not release endogenous ADP in normal amounts. The number of dense granules in the platelets is below normal.

  **b. Acquired thrombocytopathies**

    **(1) Drug-induced** (specifically aspirin-induced) **thrombocytopathia** is the most common cause of platelet dysfunction. Aspirin inhibits the platelet release reaction. Normal amounts of the dense granule contents (e.g., ADP) are not released by platelets. The second wave of platelet aggregation is deficient.

    **(2) Myeloproliferative disorders** (disorders of bone marrow production) also are implicated in acquired platelet dysfunction.

**D. Disorders of soluble hemostatic factors**

  **1. Hemophilia A and von Willebrand's disease (factor VIII deficiency)**

    **a. General considerations.** Hemophilia A and von Willebrand's disease are the most common hereditary coagulation disorders.

      **(1)** These two diseases involve different regions of the factor VIII molecule and are associated with different functions of the molecule. The factor VIII molecule is a complex of two proteins: the factor VIII procoagulant protein (antihemophilic factor; **VIII:C**) and the factor VIII-related protein (the von Willebrand factor; **VIII:R**).

(2) Hemophilia A and von Willebrand's disease can be distinguished from each other by a number of clinical and laboratory features (Table 14-3).

**b. Hemophilia A**

(1) **Pathogenesis.** Hemophilia A results from a deficiency of VIII:C, which is the small molecular weight unit of the molecule (the large molecular weight unit is present in normal amounts). VIII:C acts as cofactor of the intrinsic pathway of coagulation. The defective gene is located on the X chromosome.

(2) **Clinical features.** The most characteristic features of hemophilia A are spontaneous or traumatic hemorrhages, which can be subcutaneous, intramuscular, or within joints (hemarthrosis).

(a) In infants, excessive bleeding may occur after circumcision, but it is usually not evident in the first year of life.

(b) Severely affected boys (i.e., those whose VIII:C activity is below 1%) show easy bruising and a propensity to hemarthrosis from the time they begin to walk.

(c) In later life, soft tissue, muscle, and joint bleeding dominate the clinical course; life-threatening internal hemorrhage may follow trauma.

(3) **Diagnosis.** The PTT is prolonged, indicating a deficiency in the intrinsic pathway. Factor VIII assay is required to confirm the diagnosis; a decrease in VIII:C activity with a normal level of VIII:R is diagnostic.

(4) **Therapy.** General supportive care is indicated for the hemorrhagic diathesis. Replacement therapy for severely affected patients is in the form of cryoprecipitate or factor VIII concentrate. Mildly or moderately affected patients may achieve adequate hemostatic levels of factor VIII following treatment with desmopressin (dDAVP), which releases the molecule from tissue stores.

**c. von Willebrand's disease**

(1) **Pathogenesis.** Transmission of the disease is variable. von Willebrand's disease results from a deficiency of VIII:C as well as VIII:R, which plays a central role in platelet adhesion.

(2) **Clinical features.** As is true with hemophilia A, the severity of von Willebrand's disease varies with the degree of deficiency of factor VIII. Usually, the bleeding is mild, with mucosal and cutaneous (platelet-type) bleeding most dominant. However, severe hemorrhage may occur following trauma.

(3) **Diagnosis.** There is prolonged bleeding time and prolonged PTT. Ristocetin-induced platelet aggregation is abnormal. VIII:R antigen measurement demonstrates deficiency.

(4) **Therapy.** Supportive measures are indicated for the hemorrhagic diathesis. Cryoprecipitates are preferred in replacement therapy, because factor VIII concentrate lacks sufficient VIII:R multimers to correct platelet dysfunction. Mildly or moderately affected patients may be treated with desmopressin for mild bleeding episodes.

**2. Hemophilia B (factor IX deficiency; Christmas disease)** is inherited as an X-linked recessive disorder.

**a. Clinical features.** Hemophilia B has a bleeding diasthesis similar to that of hemophilia A (i.e., deep-muscle hematomas, hemarthrosis, significant bleeding after trauma or surgery).

**b. Diagnosis.** The PTT is prolonged. The activity of factor IX is decreased.

**c. Therapy.** General supportive measures are indicated for the bleeding diathesis. Replacement therapy is with prothrombin complex concentrate (which is a mixture of coagulation factors II, VII, IX, and X).

**Table 14-3.** Clinical and Laboratory Features of Hemophilia A and von Willebrand's Disease

|  | **Hemophilia A** | **von Willebrand's Disease** |
|---|---|---|
| **Molecular defect** | VIII:C | VIII:C; VIII:R |
| **Mode of inheritance** | X-linked recessive | Autosomal dominant |
| **PTT** | Prolonged | Prolonged |
| **Bleeding time** | Normal | Prolonged |
| **Ristocetin cofactor** | Normal | Decreased |
| **Bleeding diathesis** | Deep muscle hematomas; hemarthroses | Mucous membranes |

PTT = partial thromboplastin time.

3. **Vitamin K deficiency.** Coagulation factors II, VII, IX, and X (which are synthesized in the liver) as well as the antithrombotic factors protein C and protein S are dependent on vitamin K. When the vitamin is deficient, normal coagulation does not occur.
   a. **Etiology**
      (1) Vitamin K deficiency can occur in **malabsorption states** and other gastrointestinal disorders. **Drugs** (e.g., coumarin) that are vitamin K antagonists can interfere with metabolism of the vitamin.
      (2) **Hemorrhagic disease of the newborn** can occur in neonates if the now routine administration of vitamin K at birth is omitted.
   b. **Therapy.** Nutritional disorders and malabsorption states respond to parenteral administration of vitamin K. Fresh frozen plasma or the prothrombin complex concentrate is indicated for severe bleeding.

4. **Liver disease.** All of the coagulation factors, with the exception of factor VIII, may be deficient in liver disease. In addition, hepatic clearance of activated clotting factors may be impaired. Thus, both PTT and PT are prolonged. Fresh frozen plasma is indicated in therapy (prothrombin complex concentrates are to be avoided because activated factors may produce intravascular coagulation).

5. **Disseminated intravascular coagulation (DIC)**
   a. **Etiology.** DIC occurs secondary to other disease processes.
   b. **Pathogenesis.** Intravascular activation of the coagulation cascade leads to fibrin deposition in the small blood vessels, tissue ischemia, release of tissue thromboplastin, consumption of labile clotting factors (i.e., platelets, factors II, V, and VIII, and fibrinogen), and activation of the fibrinolytic system.
      (1) **Damage to the vascular endothelium** occurs in renal disease, sepsis, and in patients with giant hemangioma.
      (2) **Introduction of thromboplastic substances into the circulation** occurs in acute promyelocytic leukemia.
      (3) **Impairment of clearance of activated clotting factors** occurs in liver disease.
   c. **Clinical features**
      (1) The bleeding diathesis is diffuse. There is oozing from venipuncture sites and around indwelling catheters; gastrointestinal and pulmonary bleeding as well as hematuria occur; bleeding occurs from traumatized sites.
      (2) Thrombotic lesions affect the extremities, skin, kidney, and brain.
   d. **Diagnosis.** The PTT and PT are prolonged. There is thrombocytopenia and hypofibrinogenemia. The levels of fibrin degradation products are elevated. Microangiopathic erythrocyte morphology is apparent on blood smear.
   e. **Therapy.** The primary disease process should be treated. Supportive measures are indicated for the bleeding diathesis. If bleeding persists or if thromboses are present, heparinization with replacement of platelets and clotting factors (i.e., fresh frozen plasma) should be considered.

## STUDY QUESTIONS

**Directions:** Each of the numbered items or incomplete statements in this section is followed by answers or by completions of the statement. Select the **one** lettered answer or completion that is **best** in each case.

1. All of the following conditions are characterized by hypochromic, microcytic red cells EXCEPT

(A) iron deficiency anemia
(B) α thalassemia major
(C) β thalassemia minor
(D) G6PD deficiency
(E) anemia of chronic disease

2. Which of the following statements regarding the anemia of chronic disease is true?

(A) MCV is elevated
(B) Serum iron level is elevated
(C) Serum iron-binding capacity is elevated
(D) Marrow iron stores are increased
(E) Iron therapy is required to raise hemoglobin level

3. Hemolytic-uremic syndrome is a disorder of which of the following?

(A) The red cell membrane
(B) The vascular endothelium
(C) Hemoglobin
(D) The glycolytic pathway
(E) Immune regulation

4. Which of the following hemolytic anemias is NOT associated with an intracorpuscular defect?

(A) Hereditary spherocytosis
(B) Sickle cell anemia
(C) Autoimmune hemolytic anemia
(D) G6PD deficiency

5. All of the following disorders are associated with prolonged bleeding time EXCEPT

(A) hemophilia A
(B) von Willebrand's disease
(C) aspirin-induced thrombocytopathia
(D) Bernard-Soulier syndrome
(E) ITP

6. Patients with DIC present with all of the following hematologic abnormalities EXCEPT

(A) thrombocytopenia
(B) microangiopathic blood smear
(C) hypofibrinogenemia
(D) prolonged PTT
(E) low levels of fibrin degradation products

7. Which of the following is NOT a characteristic of Fanconi's anemia?

(A) Hematologic abnormalities in infancy
(B) Pancytopenia
(C) Skeletal anomalies
(D) Chromosome fragility

8. A 7-year-old patient with known hereditary spherocytosis presents with pallor, low-grade fever, and splenomegaly. Blood counts are as follows: hemoglobin 3 g/dl, reticulocyte count 2%, white blood cell count 8000/mm³, and platelet count 200,000/mm³. The most likely diagnosis is

(A) acute splenic sequestration crisis
(B) aplastic crisis
(C) hemolytic crisis
(D) acute leukemia
(E) superimposed iron deficiency

---

1-D     4-C     7-A
2-D     5-A     8-B
3-B     6-E

**Directions:** Each item below contains four suggested answers of which **one or more** is correct. Choose the answer

    **A**  if **1, 2, and 3** are correct
    **B**  if **1 and 3** are correct
    **C**  if **2 and 4** are correct
    **D**  if **4** is correct
    **E**  if **1, 2, 3, and 4** are correct

9. Further hematologic evaluation is indicated for

(1) a full-term newborn with a hemoglobin level of 12 g/dl
(2) a 2-month-old infant with a hemoglobin level of 10 g/dl
(3) a 2-year-old child with a MCV of 100
(4) a full-term newborn with a MCV of 105

10. Clinical characteristics of sickle cell anemia include

(1) onset of significant anemia within the first 2 months of life
(2) hand-foot syndrome
(3) splenomegaly throughout life
(4) splenic hypofunction

11. Studies indicated in the evaluation of a patient with neutropenia include

(1) bone marrow aspiration
(2) nitroblue tetrazolium test
(3) antineutrophil antibodies
(4) leukocyte alkaline phosphatase

9-B
10-C
11-B

## ANSWERS AND EXPLANATIONS

**1. The answer is D** *[III D 3 b (3) (b)].*
In glucose-6-phosphate dehydrogenase (G6PD) deficiency, an enzymopathy, the red blood cell morphology is normochromic, normocytic. In other anemias listed in the question, failure of hemoglobin production due to lack of iron (iron deficiency), unavailability of iron (anemia of chronic disease), or defective globin chain production (thalassemias) leads to production of hypochromic, microcytic red blood cells.

**2. The answer is D** *[III B 3].*
The anemia of chronic disease is a hypochromic, microcytic anemia [i.e., anemia characterized by a low mean corpuscular volume (MCV)], which is associated with failure to release iron from marrow storage sites. Both serum iron and iron-binding capacity are low, but marrow iron stores are increased. The anemia improves when the underlying illness is treated and usually does not respond to iron therapy.

**3. The answer is B** *[III D 5 a].*
Hemolytic-uremic syndrome is a microangiopathic hemolytic anemia resulting from mechanical damage to the red cells suffered due to irregularities in the renal vascular endothelium. This results in the characteristic red cell fragmentation on the peripheral smear, seen as burr cells, helmet cells, and other irregularly shaped red cells.

**4. The answer is C** *[III D 3 a, 4 b].*
Autoimmune hemolytic anemia results from an abnormality outside the red cell (i.e., the presence of antibody). Thus, it is an extracorpuscular defect. Hereditary spherocytosis is a disorder of the red cell membrane. Sickle cell anemia and G6PD deficiency are disorders of hemoglobin and a constituent enzyme of the red cell, respectively.

**5. The answer is A** *[VI D 1 b (3)].*
Prolonged bleeding time usually reflects abnormalities of platelet number, platelet function, vessel wall, or von Willebrand factor (which mediates platelet adhesion and aggregation). In classic hemophilia (hemophilia A), the only abnormality is in the procoagulant piece of the factor VIII molecule, which plays no role in platelet aggregation or adhesion. On the other hand, in von Willebrand's disease, the entire factor VIII molecule is deficient, including the portion that interacts with platelets. Bernard-Soulier syndrome results from a defect in a platelet membrane receptor molecule that is associated with platelet adhesion. In idiopathic thrombocytopenic purpura (ITP), it appears that an autoimmune process causes increased platelet destruction. Aspirin inhibits platelet release.

**6. The answer is E** *[VI D 5 d].*
In disseminated intravascular coagulation (DIC), activation of the coagulation system results in depletion of platelets as well as certain labile coagulation proteins (i.e., factors II, V, and VIII and fibrinogen). In addition, fibrin strands formed within the microvasculature can damage red blood cell membranes, resulting in microangiopathic morphologic abnormalities, such as helmet cells and burr cells on blood smear. The levels of fibrin degradation products are elevated in DIC.

**7. The answer is A** *[II B 1 b].*
Although Fanconi's anemia is a congenital disorder, the hematologic abnormalities associated with it usually do not appear until the patient is 3–8 years of age. Fanconi's anemia is an autosomal recessive disorder of bone marrow, which may be severe enough to produce pancytopenia. The genetic defect is chromosome fragility, resulting in excessive breaks and recombinations. Among the many phenotypic abnormalities are skeletal anomalies and retarded growth.

**8. The answer is B** *[III D 6 c, d].*
Temporary suppression of erythropoiesis (as suggested in this patient by the inappropriately low reticulocyte count) can occur in conjunction with even a mild infectious process. In the patient with a hemolytic disorder, even a few days of reticulocytopenia can produce a profound decline in the hemoglobin level. The enlarged spleen represents the consequences of chronic hemolysis and possible early congestive heart failure; acute splenic sequestration crisis is characteristic of sickle cell anemia, not hereditary spherocytosis. Acute hemolytic crisis is characteristic of G6PD deficiency. Acute leukemia is unlikely in view of the normal white blood cell and platelet counts. Superimposed iron deficiency is a possible diagnosis, but it is unlikely in a 7-year-old child unless there is a concomitant hemorrhage.

**9. The answer is B (1, 3)** *[Table 14-1].*
The normal full-term newborn is relatively polycythemic, with an average hemoglobin concentration of 18 g/dl; by 2 months of age, the physiologic "anemia" of the newborn is apparent and a hemoglobin concentration of 10 g/dl would be considered normal. The red blood cells of the normal full-term newborn are relatively macrocytic, but the MCV declines rapidly thereafter. A high MCV in a 2-year-old child is distinctly abnormal.

**10. The answer is C (2, 4)** *[III D 10 d (1)].*
Significant levels of fetal hemoglobin (Hb F) are present at birth and persist throughout the first few months of life; thus, β-chain abnormalities (e.g., Hb S) do not become clinically significant until later in the first year of life. The earliest clinical manifestation of sickle cell anemia occurs at 4–6 months of age, when the infant develops symmetrical painful swelling of the dorsal surfaces of the hands and feet (hand-foot syndrome). Because of recurrent episodes of infarction, the spleen usually shrinks to a fibrotic nubbin by the time the patient is 5 years old.

**11. The answer is B (1, 3)** *[V B 2 a, 3 a].*
Bone marrow aspiration is useful to assess production and maturation of granulocytes and to rule out bone marrow aplasia or replacement. Antineutrophil antibodies are useful in diagnosing autoimmune neutropenias. The nitroblue tetrazolium test is used for the diagnosis of chronic granulomatous disease, a disorder of neutrophil function that is not associated with neutropenia. Leukocyte alkaline phosphatase is used to distinguish between the neutrophilia of inflammatory disease and that of chronic granulocytic leukemia.

# 15
# Oncologic Diseases

John J. Quinn
Arnold J. Altman

## I. GENERAL PRINCIPLES OF ONCOLOGIC DISEASES IN CHILDREN

**A. Incidence.** Approximately 1 in 600 children between the ages of 1 and 15 years develop cancer, making it the second most common cause of death, after injuries, in this age-group.

**B. Types**

1. **Common types of cancer in children** (Table 15-1). Leukemia and solid tumors represent the majority of childhood neoplasms. The solid tumors are of diverse types and, in contrast to adult cancers, are predominantly of nonepithelial origin and are responsive to chemotherapeutic agents.

2. **Uncommon types of cancer in children.** Typical adult-type carcinomas (e.g., lung, colon, breast) are rare during childhood.

**C. Predisposing factors.** Most childhood malignancies are of unknown etiology and occur in otherwise healthy children. Certain children, however, are at an increased risk for cancer because of their constitutional makeup or because of exposure to cancer-causing agents.

1. **Genetic factors.** Conditions that predispose children to malignancy are listed below.
   a. **Genetic mutations**
      (1) **Hereditary acquisition** of these mutations may occur. Wilms' tumor and retinoblastoma are embryonal cancers of the kidney and eye, respectively. Up to 40% of retinoblastomas and 20% of Wilms' tumors are hereditary. These tumors have variable penetrance. They occur in young children and often are bilateral.
         (a) Wilms' tumor and retinoblastoma are postulated to evolve in two distinct steps, or **hits,** which produce genetic abnormalities that result in tumor formation:
            (i) **Prezygotic (germline) inheritance** of the first mutation
            (ii) **Postzygotic (somatic) mutation,** which induces malignancy in the tissue rendered susceptible by the first mutation
         (b) Each of the two mutations may inactivate or delete one of the two alleles of a regulatory gene carried on homologous chromosomes. If the affected alleles regulate or suppress an oncogene, their loss may result in uncontrolled expression of the oncogene and excessive growth of tissue under its influence.
         (c) Both alleles must be inactivated for tumors to develop. Tumors only form in individuals homozygous for defects at them, therefore these sites of inactivation or mutation are termed **recessive oncogenes**. They may actually contain anti-oncogenes, which—if inactivated on both homologous chromosomes—permit expression of otherwise suppressed oncogenes.
      (2) **Sporadic acquisition** is more common than hereditary acquisition. Spontaneously occurring retinoblastoma and Wilms' tumor comprise 60% and 80% of cases, respectively. Two steps (hits) also have been postulated for their induction.
         (a) Occasionally, the first step occurs in the germ cells of the affected individual, and the mutation can be passed on to the progeny of this individual.
         (b) More frequently, both steps or mutations occur postzygotically. Their limitation to somatic tissue precludes their inheritance.
      (3) **Germline and somatic mutations** typically are not associated with detectable karyotypic abnormalities. When these abnormalities do occur, they can be detected in all of the patient's cells if one of the steps was germline or in only the tumor cells if both steps were somatic.

**Table 15-1.** Types of Childhood Cancer

| Cancer | Incidence | |
| --- | --- | --- |
| | **White Children (%)** | **African-American Children (%)** |
| Leukemia | 30.9 | 24.3 |
| Central nervous system | 18.3 | 21.6 |
| Lymphoma including Hodgkin's | 13.8 | 11.3 |
| Neuroblastoma | 6.8 | 5.4 |
| Soft tissue sarcoma | 6.2 | 8.6 |
| Wilms' tumor | 5.7 | 8.1 |
| Bone | 4.7 | 3.6 |
| Eye | 2.5 | 4.1 |
| Germ cell | 2.4 | 4.1 |
| Liver | 1.3 | . . . |
| Other | 7.4 | 8.9 |

    **(4) Chromosome abnormalities**
        **(a)** In both sporadic and hereditary cases of retinoblastoma, abnormalities localized to the long arm of chromosome 13 have been detected. This region is thought to contain the retinoblastoma gene. Tumor formation occurs only in cells homozygous for abnormalities in this region of the chromosome. Cells susceptible to tumor formation have already received a first hit on one number 13 chromosome. They become tumor cells when they are rendered homozygous for the abnormality on chromosome 13 by development of a second hit on the other number 13 chromosome, a process that results in loss of constitutional heterozygosity for genetic information at this location.
        **(b)** In a few sporadic cases of Wilms' tumor associated with aniridia and genitourinary tract abnormalities, there has been deletion of genetic material from the short arm of chromosome 11.
  **b. Defects in DNA repair** cause increased chromosome fragility, which predisposes to malignancy. The following are examples.
    **(1) Fanconi's anemia.** Patients with this constitutional aplastic anemia often have short stature, renal and skeletal abnormalities, and a propensity to develop leukemia.
    **(2) Bloom syndrome.** Leukemias, lymphomas, and carcinomas occur in high frequency in these individuals with sun-sensitive facial telangiectasia, short stature, and immunodeficiency.
    **(3) Ataxia-telangiectasia.** Lymphoid malignancies are common in these patients with widespread telangiectasia, cerebellar dysfunction, and immunodeficiency.
  **c. Immunodeficiencies.** Children born with congenital immunodeficiencies have a 100-fold increased risk of malignancy, particularly of the lymphoid system. In addition to Bloom syndrome and ataxia-telangiectasia, the congenital disorders include the following.
    **(1) Wiskott-Aldrich syndrome** is an X-linked disorder characterized by progressive T cell dysfunction, eczema, thrombocytopenia, and a propensity to develop lymphomas.
    **(2) Common variable immunodeficiency** predisposes affected individuals to stomach cancer and lymphomas, both of which do not usually manifest until adulthood.
    **(3) X-linked lymphoproliferative syndrome** in males results in severe infections with the Epstein-Barr virus, which, if the acute infection does not end fatally, induces lymphoma formation.
  **d. Abnormalities of chromosome number.** Patients with trisomy 21 (Down syndrome) have an incidence of acute leukemia that is 15 times greater than that of the normal population.
  **e. Neurocutaneous disorders.** Neurofibromatosis is a dominantly inherited disorder characterized by neurofibromas, cutaneous pigmented lesions (café-au-lait spots), bony abnormalities, and a tendency to develop malignancy in the neurofibromas and in other tissues, which may result in acute leukemia, neuroblastoma, or soft tissue sarcoma (see also Ch 17 VIII A).
**2. Infections.** Two viruses that infect cells of the immune system have been associated with malignancy.
  **a. Epstein-Barr virus** has as its target the human B cell, which it renders capable of continuous

cell division. If the patient is unable to mount an effective immune response that limits the B cell proliferation, one of the continuously dividing B cells may undergo a specific chromosome change that transforms it into a malignant cell.

    **(1)** This sequence is seen with endemic **Burkitt's lymphoma** and with lymphomas similar to Burkitt's that develop in patients who have been immunosuppressed by chemotherapeutic agents or other factors.

    **(2)** The specific chromosome abnormality consists of translocation of a portion of the long arm of chromosome 8, which contains the c-*myc* oncogene, onto the area of another chromosome (14, 2, or 22) that controls immunoglobulin chain synthesis, a specific B cell function.

  **b.** **Human immunodeficiency virus (HIV),** a retrovirus, has as its target the human helper T cell, which plays a critical role in modulating immune function.

    **(1)** Viral destruction of helper T cells may lead to **acquired immune deficiency syndrome (AIDS),** which is characterized by an increased susceptibility to opportunistic infections and malignancies (see Ch 8 II E). Children most often develop AIDS perinatally from an HIV-infected mother or from transfusions.

    **(2)** Pediatric patients with AIDS are susceptible to lymphoid malignancies such as **Burkitt's lymphoma,** but, to date, few children have developed **Kaposi's sarcoma**.

  **3.** **Environmental factors.** Although many environmental carcinogens and toxic exposures are associated with the development of cancer in adults, childhood cancers caused by environmental factors and toxic exposures are probably rare.

  **a.** One known risk factor for childhood cancer is prior treatment of malignancy in a child (i.e., with chemotherapeutic agents, ionizing radiation, or both). For example, leukemias and lymphomas have developed in children who have been treated for Hodgkin's disease with combined chemoradiotherapy, bone cancers have developed in children who have been heavily irradiated, and brain tumors have developed in children given cranial irradiation.

  **b.** Epidemiologic studies suggest possible links between in utero cannabis exposure and the development of acute nonlymphocytic leukemia (ANLL). A link between exposure to electromagnetic radiation from power lines and the development of acute lymphocytic leukemia (ALL) has also been suggested.

## D. Clinical features

  **1.** **Constitutional symptoms.** Fever, night sweats, and unintended weight loss of greater than 10% are nonspecific symptoms that are often associated with advanced cases of childhood cancer.

  **2.** **Abdominal masses.** The intra-abdominal tissues are the most common sites of solid tumor formation. Frequently, a visible or palpable mass is detected whose location is determined by the tissue from which it arises. Pain may be present, especially if the mass suddenly enlarges due to bleeding within it.

    **a.** **More common tumors**

      **(1)** **Wilms' tumor** arises from the kidneys.

      **(2)** **Neuroblastoma** arises from sympathetic neural tissue located in either the adrenal medulla or in the paraspinal ganglia.

    **b.** **Less common tumors**

      **(1)** **Rhabdomyosarcoma** arises from the abundant mesenchyme of the abdomen and pelvis.

      **(2)** **Hodgkin's disease** and **non-Hodgkin's lymphoma** develop in intra-abdominal lymphoid tissue.

      **(3)** **Hepatoblastoma** and **hepatocellular carcinoma** occur in the liver.

      **(4)** **Germ cell tumors** originate in the ovaries.

      **(5)** **Leukemic infiltration** and **metastases** may cause enlargement of the liver, spleen, and intra-abdominal lymph nodes.

  **3.** **Intrathoracic masses**

    **a.** **Mediastinal masses** are the most common type of intrathoracic mass. The type of tumor that causes the mediastinal enlargement determines the location of the mass within the mediastinum. Large masses may cause wheezing and hypoxia from severe airway compression, which is a medical emergency. Dysphagia and hoarseness can develop from compression of the esophagus and the recurrent laryngeal nerve, respectively.

    **(1) Anterior mediastinal masses** usually are due to thymic involvement in non-Hodgkin's lymphoma or ALL (see II B) but can also be due to a malignant thymoma or a germ cell tumor.

    **(2) Middle mediastinal masses** suggest Hodgkin's disease or metastatic involvement of leukemia, non-Hodgkin's lymphoma, or neuroblastoma.

    **(3) Posterior mediastinal masses** usually are neural tumors, such as neuroblastoma or, in patients with neurofibromatosis, neurofibrosarcoma.

  **b. Intrapulmonary lesions** are less common than mediastinal masses and are metastatic in nature. Nodular pulmonary metastases develop in Wilms' tumor, soft tissue sarcomas, bone cancers, germ cell tumors, hepatoblastomas, and Hodgkin's disease. Neuroblastoma is the only solid tumor in which pulmonary metastases are rare.

**4. Lymph node enlargement** (lymphadenopathy) usually is the response to an infectious or inflammatory stimulus. However, it can also be due to the proliferation of neoplastic cells within the lymph node.

  **a. Suppuration** strongly suggests an acute bacterial infection. Other findings, such as degree of hardness, matting, or tenderness, cannot reliably distinguish benign from neoplastic adenopathy.

  **b. Rapidly enlarging nodes or nodes in the supraclavicular region** should increase the suspicion of malignancy.

    **(1)** Leukemias, Hodgkin's disease, non-Hodgkin's lymphoma, and metastatic solid tumors can all cause nodal enlargement.

    **(2)** Metastases from abdominal tumors often enlarge the left supraclavicular nodes.

    **(3)** Metastases from thoracic tumors often enlarge the right supraclavicular nodes.

**5. Bone pain.** Expansion of the marrow cavity or destruction of cortical bone by leukemic cells or by a metastatic tumor can cause considerable pain.

  **a.** If the long bones of the lower extremities are involved, a limp or difficulty in walking may develop.

  **b.** If the skull is involved, proptosis or palpable nodules may develop.

  **c.** Neuroblastoma and the primary bone cancers (i.e., Ewing's sarcoma, osteogenic sarcoma) are most likely to produce bone metastases. Primary bone cancers and histiocytosis X can also produce pain at their site of origin.

**6. Soft tissue masses.** Rhabdomyosarcomas often arise on the trunk or extremities and produce palpable tumors. Bone tumors that break through the cortex and infiltrate the soft tissues can also produce palpable tumors.

**7. Intracranial lesions.** Any space-occupying lesion can produce signs and symptoms of increased intracranial pressure (e.g., papilledema, ocular palsies, headaches, vomiting).

  **a.** Numerous primary intracranial malignancies usually arise below the tentorium.

  **b.** Discrete metastatic lesions from solid tumors also occur and are more often supratentorial.

  **c.** CNS involvement occurs in acute leukemia and takes the form of diffuse meningeal infiltration, which also causes increased intracranial pressure.

**8. Bone marrow failure**

  **a. Diffuse replacement** of the normal marrow elements characterizes the acute leukemias and results in anemia, thrombocytopenia, and a paucity of mature and functional leukocytes, especially neutrophils (see II A 3 a).

  **b. Less extensive infiltration** (e.g., as occurs with solid tumor metastases) may result in anemia and leukoerythroblastic changes on peripheral smear, consisting of teardrop-shaped, fragmented, and nucleated red blood cells and a shift in the granulocyte series to the left, down to and including the myeloblast stage. Tumor cells often are cohesive, and clumps of primitive cells in the marrow resulting from solid tumor metastases are termed **syncytia**.

**E. Staging.** Current classification systems employ numerical staging; advanced disease is indicated by high numbers and usually is associated with a poor prognosis. Staging systems only apply to solid tumors with a propensity to disseminate and do not apply to the leukemias, which always are disseminated at the time of diagnosis.

**1. Stage I** tumors are truly **localized** to their organ of origin and, if treated by surgery, must be totally resected with no microscopic or gross disease remaining.

2. **Stages II and III** refer to **more advanced localized** disease than stage I tumors, for which surgical resection does not result in complete tumor removal. Patients with stage II tumors generally have less residual disease following surgery than patients with stage III tumors. For malignancies primary to the lymph nodes, the meaning of stage II and III designations is somewhat different and indicates the degree of spread within the lymphoid system.

3. **Stage IV** is indicative of **disseminated** disease with hematogenous metastases or spread to distant nodes in tumors that are not primary to the lymph nodes.

F. **Therapeutic strategies.** Childhood cancers are among the most curable human malignancies. To achieve a cure, therapy often involves multiple disciplines working in concert.

1. **Surgery.** Total or partial removal (**debulking**) of solid tumors contributes greatly to the cure of disease. Very large tumors that cannot be removed at initial surgery sometimes can be rendered operable after their size has been decreased by radiotherapy, chemotherapy, or both.

2. **Radiotherapy.** The ionizing radiation beam can be directed at specific tumor locations. Radiotherapy plays an important role in the following situations:
   a. Destruction of localized residual tumor that cannot be surgically removed
   b. Reduction in the size of large tumors to render them operable
   c. Palliative and curative therapy of discrete metastatic foci
   d. Eradication of leukemic cells in sanctuary sites (see II A 3 d)
   e. Local control of selected malignancies of lymphoid, osseous, and mesenchymal origin for which surgery is not indicated

3. **Chemotherapy.** Many different antineoplastic drugs have been developed during the last 4 decades, and their use is based on the following principles.
   a. **Chemotherapy interferes with cell growth and division.**
   b. **Chemotherapy produces adverse effects on normal as well as malignant cells.**
      (1) Normal cells that are most likely to be affected are rapidly dividing, particularly those of the bone marrow, gastrointestinal tract, and hair follicles. However, many types of cells and many diverse organs may be affected by the toxicity of a specific chemotherapeutic agent.
      (2) The toxic effect of some agents is dose-related and may be avoided by not exceeding a certain dose.
      (3) Drugs with dissimilar toxicities often can be used in combination to enhance a malignant cell kill without enhancing the toxicity to normal cells. Even when the toxicity of two or more agents is additive, they often can be used in combination if the toxicity is reversible and if the patient receives appropriate supportive care during the period of drug-induced toxicity. This ability to use drugs in combination has greatly enhanced the curative role of chemotherapy.
   c. **Chemotherapy is most likely to effect a cure for any malignancy when the tumor cell burden is small.** Chemotherapy, however, can be curative in any of the following situations.
      (1) **Primary therapy for disseminated malignancy.** In this situation, there is no opportunity to control the disseminated disease locally with either surgery or radiotherapy. The leukemias are the principle examples of systemic malignant diseases that are treated primarily with chemotherapy. Metastatic solid tumors also require chemotherapy for control but often are not as responsive as the leukemias.
      (2) **Reduction in bulk disease.** Large solid tumors that cannot be managed initially with surgery, radiotherapy, or both can sometimes be successfully treated by these means if their size is first reduced by chemotherapy.
      (3) **Destruction of micrometastases.** Patients with nonmetastatic solid tumors for which local surgery, radiotherapy, or both appear completely adequate often have recurrences at distant sites. They are thought to have clinically inapparent spread (**micrometastases**), which, in the absence of systemic therapy, produces gross metastatic disease. These patients—with their small tumor burdens—respond very well to adjuvant chemotherapeutic regimens designed to destroy micrometastases.

4. **Bone marrow transplantation.** Some disseminated malignancies that are not cured by standard doses of chemotherapy and radiotherapy, particularly leukemias, may be cured by high doses if the irreversible toxicity of the therapy can be avoided. Toxicity to bone marrow is the limiting factor in many treatment regimens. If marrow destruction by high therapeutic doses

can be circumvented by transplantation of new marrow, then potentially curative doses of chemotherapy and radiotherapy can be administered. The following types of marrow transplants can be performed.

**a. Types**

**(1)** In **syngeneic transplants,** the donor and recipient are identical twins and, thus, are genetically identical. This is a rare occurrence.

**(2)** In **allogeneic transplants,** the donor and recipient are not identical twins.

**(a)** Donors usually are related to the recipient. Most commonly they are siblings, but occasionally they can be other family members. Although there is no genetic identity between the donor and recipient, there must be histocompatibility [human leukocyte antigen (HLA) matching]. If there is not, either the new marrow will be rejected or, frequently, the T cells in the donated marrow will mount an immune response against the body of the recipient, which manifests as **graft-versus-host disease (GVHD).** A related HLA-matched family member can be found for, at most, 1 in 3 individuals who require an allogeneic transplant. Less commonly, donors unrelated to the recipient can be identified. Because of the tremendous diversity of HLA antigens, it is more difficult to find an HLA match between two unrelated individuals. Searches for an unrelated donor require access to databases that have information on the HLA types of large numbers of potential donors.

**(b)** Even with histocompatibility between the donor and recipient of an allogeneic transplant, there is still a significant risk of GVHD. This can be particularly severe when the donor is not related to the recipient.

**(3)** In **autologous transplants,** the patient is the donor.

**(a)** For these transplants, the patient's marrow must be collected and stored prior to administering the marrow-ablative doses of therapy.

**(b)** There is no risk of GVHD with autologous transplants, but there is a risk of reinfusing malignant cells with the normal marrow cells. Techniques are currently being developed to "purge" the marrow in vitro of malignant cells prior to its return to the patient. Most commonly used are monoclonal antibodies directed against tumor-associated antigens or chemotherapeutic agents.

**b. GVHD**

**(1) Clinical features**

**(a)** GVHD produces mild to severe lesions in the skin, gastrointestinal tract, and liver.

**(b)** Profound immunodeficiency develops in patients with severe forms of GVHD, and they often die of complicating infections.

**(2) Prevention**

**(a)** Prevention of GVHD may be possible with post-transplant administration of immunosuppressive agents (e.g., methotrexate, cyclosporine) and use of techniques that remove the T cell mediators of GVHD from the marrow prior to its infusion into the recipient. These latter techniques often dramatically decrease the incidence and severity of GVHD but may be associated with an increased risk of rejection of the transplanted marrow and with relapse of the malignancy.

**(b)** Intensive post-transplant immunosuppression or T cell depletion could also extend the scope of bone marrow transplantation to include non–HLA-identical individuals as donors. This is an especially important consideration, since an HLA-identical family member donor cannot be identified for many patients in need of transplants.

## II. THE LEUKEMIAS

**A. General considerations.** Collectively, these hematologic malignancies account for the greatest percentage of cases of childhood cancer—that is, 31% of all neoplastic disease in white children and 24% in African-American children.

**1. Classification.** Leukemias are classified on the basis of leukemic cell morphology into **lymphocytic leukemias,** which are proliferations of cells of lymphoid lineage, and **nonlymphocytic leukemias,** which are proliferations of cells of granulocyte, monocyte, erythrocyte, or platelet lineage. They are also classified on the basis of their natural history in the prechemotherapy era.

**a. Acute leukemias** constitute 97% of all childhood leukemias. If untreated, they are rapidly fatal within weeks to a few months of the diagnosis, but with treatment, they often are curable. The malignant cells, which are very immature in appearance and function, are termed **blasts**.

(1) **Acute lymphocytic leukemia (ALL)** is also termed **acute lymphoblastic leukemia** due to the distinguishing characteristic of the presence of large numbers of lymphoblasts in the bone marrow. ALL is the most common pediatric neoplasm and accounts for 80% of all childhood acute leukemia.

(2) **Acute nonlymphocytic leukemia (ANLL)** accounts for the remaining 20% of cases of acute leukemia in children.

b. **Chronic leukemias** comprise 3% of childhood leukemias; even without treatment, patients can survive for many months to years. Unfortunately, the chronic leukemias evolve into forms of acute leukemia that cannot be cured by available chemotherapy. All chronic leukemias in children are of nonlymphocytic lineage. The leukemic cells are more mature and functional than the blasts of acute leukemias.

2. **Epidemiology.** In addition to children with syndromes associated with abnormalities of chromosome number or stability or with immunodeficiency states (see I C 1 b–d), the following individuals are at increased risk for leukemia.

a. **Identical twins** have a 20% risk of leukemia if one twin develops it during the first 5 years of life.

b. **Children with solid tumors** (e.g., Hodgkin's disease, Wilms' tumor) who have undergone intense treatment may develop leukemia as a secondary malignancy.

c. **Children with congenital marrow failure** states, such as **Schwachman-Diamond syndrome** (exocrine pancreatic insufficiency and neutropenia) and **Diamond-Blackfan syndrome** (congenital red cell aplasia), have an increased risk of leukemia.

d. **African-American children** appear to have an increased incidence of ANLL and a decreased incidence of ALL.

3. **Clinical features**

a. **Bone marrow failure.** Replacement of the normal hematopoietic elements by the leukemic cell population results in decreased production of red blood cells, normal white blood cells, and platelets. As a consequence, presenting clinical features of leukemia are similar to those of aplastic anemia. Signs and symptoms of marrow failure often predominate in the child with newly diagnosed leukemia, and most of these children will have one or more of the following symptoms.

(1) **Anemia** that accompanies bone marrow failure is surprisingly well tolerated considering its degree of severity. It develops slowly, unless there is superimposed hemorrhage from thrombocytopenia. It does, however, produce:
(a) Pallor
(b) Irritability
(c) Decreased activity

(2) **Hemorrhagic diathesis**
(a) Bleeding due to thrombocytopenia is common but usually superficial. It manifests as:
(i) Petechiae and ecchymoses in the skin
(ii) Mucosal bleeding, such as epistaxis or melena
(b) If there is associated disseminated intravascular coagulation (DIC) or extreme leukocytosis [see II A 5 a (4)], occasionally there may be severe and life-threatening bleeding, such as in the CNS.

(3) **Infection** due to a paucity of functional white blood cells, especially granulocytes, may be present.
(a) Fever is the usual manifestation of infection.
(b) Localized signs of infection, such as rales with pneumonia or pus formation in an abscess, may not be apparent in these granulocytopenic patients.
(c) Infection often quickly disseminates and produces bacteremia and sepsis.

b. **Reticuloendothelial system filtration**
(1) **Lymphadenopathy** is common, especially in ALL, and may be so massive as to resemble that in the lymphomas.
(2) **Hepatosplenomegaly** also may be present. Both the liver and the spleen can be minimally to massively enlarged.

c. **Bone pain** (see I D 5)

**d. Involvement of sanctuary sites.** Sanctuary sites are rarely involved at the time of diagnosis but may be involved with the recurrence of disease. These sites are the:

**(1) CNS,** where involvement manifests as diffuse meningeal infiltration with signs of increased intracranial pressure (see I D 7 c)

**(2) Testes,** one or both of which may be involved, with infiltration producing enlargement that is out of proportion to the child's sexual development

**4. Laboratory findings**

**a. Peripheral blood.** A normal complete blood count does not preclude a diagnosis of leukemia, but abnormalities frequently are present.

**(1) Anemia** is present in most patients and is normochromic and normocytic, with a low reticulocyte index indicative of decreased marrow production of red blood cells.

**(2) Thrombocytopenia** also is very common. If the platelet count is less than 20,000/mm$^3$, as is often the case, there usually are hemorrhagic manifestations. Anemia, thrombocytopenia, or both are present in 90% of patients.

**(3) Neutropenia** often is present. Even if the patient has a high total white blood cell count, few of the cells are mature neutrophils. The following distribution of white blood cells is seen:

**(a)** Low ($<$ 5000/mm$^3$) in one-third of patients

**(b)** Normal (5000–20,000/mm$^3$) in one-third of patients

**(c)** High ($>$ 20,000/mm$^3$) in one-third of patients

**(4) Blast cells** are commonly seen on peripheral smear, especially if the white blood cell count is normal or high.

**b. Bone marrow** shows extensive replacement of the normal elements by leukemic cells. Even if there are blasts in peripheral blood, a diagnosis of leukemia should always be confirmed by bone marrow examination.

**5. Therapy**

**a. Supportive care.** Treatment of any complications in the child with newly diagnosed leukemia is essential and lifesaving.

**(1) Transfusional support** often is necessary. Blood products often are irradiated prior to transfusion to destroy any donor lymphocytes that could mount a graft-versus-host reaction in the immunocompromised leukemia patient.

**(a)** Packed red blood cells are used to correct significant anemia.

**(b)** Platelet concentrates are used for severe thrombocytopenia.

**(c)** Granulocytes rarely are needed. Their use is controversial, but they may play a role in the management of granulocytopenic patients with infections that do not respond to antibiotics.

**(2) Treatment of infection** is essential. Patients usually are granulocytopenic. If they become febrile, appropriate cultures (blood, urine, sites of local infection) should be obtained promptly and intravenous administration of broad-spectrum antibiotics begun immediately thereafter. A chest x-ray also should be obtained to look for infiltrates.

**(3) Metabolic support** is necessary in patients with large malignant cell burdens as represented by a high white blood cell count or significant organ infiltration. These patients are likely to develop a tumor lysis syndrome characterized by one or more of the following metabolic abnormalities.

**(a) Hyperuricemia** may develop from a breakdown of purines released by dying leukemic cells. The uric acid can precipitate in the renal tubules and cause renal failure. This may be prevented by:

**(i)** Vigorous hydration to promote uric acid excretion

**(ii)** Alkalinization of the urine to increase uric acid solubility

**(iii)** Administration of allopurinol, a xanthine oxidase inhibitor, to block uric acid formation

**(b) Hyperkalemia** also may develop and cause serious cardiac arrhythmias if not corrected.

**(c) Hyperphosphatemia** also develops, which can cause a reciprocal fall in serum calcium, which may result in:

**(i)** Tetany

**(ii)** Potentiation of the effect of hyperkalemia on the heart

**(iii)** Precipitation of calcium phosphate in the renal tubules

**(4) Treatment of hyperviscosity.** White blood cell counts greater than 100,000/mm$^3$, especially in patients with ANLL, can cause significant hyperviscosity. The white blood cell count may be lowered by exchange transfusions or leukopheresis. Without treatment, the hyperviscosity may interfere with blood flow to the:

    **(a)** CNS, causing hemorrhagic infarction

    **(b)** Lungs, causing hypoxemia

  **(5) Treatment of compressive symptoms.** Large collections of malignant cells in the anterior mediastinum may produce an obstructing mass, resulting in compressive symptoms such as hypoxemia from airway compromise and obstruction of the superior vena cava, producing a syndrome consisting of facial plethora, venous distension, and increased intracranial pressure. If the mass and the compressive symptoms do not decrease with the institution of chemotherapy, radiotherapy to the mass may be effective.

  **b. Antileukemic therapy** is administered in distinct phases with distinct objectives.

    **(1) Remission induction.** This initial phase lasts at least 4 weeks, during which maximal cytoreduction is achieved. If successful, at the conclusion of remission induction, bone marrow should demonstrate normal hematopoiesis and contain less than 5% blasts, complete blood count values should return to normal, and abnormal physical findings due to leukemia should be gone.

    **(2) Consolidation** aims to:

      **(a)** Kill additional leukemic cells with further systemic therapy

      **(b)** Prevent leukemic relapse within the CNS by therapy specifically directed toward the CNS

    **(3) Maintenance** is the longest phase of therapy. Its objectives are to:

      **(a)** Continue the remissions achieved in the previous phases

      **(b)** Produce whatever additional cytoreduction is necessary to cure the leukemia

    **(4) Discontinuation of antileukemic therapy** is possible for patients who remain in remission throughout their prescribed course of maintenance therapy. During this phase, most patients continue in an indefinite remission and are cured of their leukemia. A minority of patients develop relapse (recurrence) in either bone marrow or extramedullary sites, such as the CNS or testes.

## B. Acute lymphocytic leukemia (ALL)

  **1. Epidemiology.** ALL is the most common type of childhood leukemia. It is more common in white children than in African-American children and more common in males than in females (1.2–1.3 times). ALL is associated with a peak incidence in the 3- to 5-year-old age-group for white children only.

  **2. Classification**

    **a. Morphologic classification** of ALL is based on the following features.

      **(1) Appearance of the leukemic lymphoblasts.** According to the French-American-British (FAB) classification, leukemic lymphoblasts subdivide into three categories.

        **(a) L1 lymphoblasts** are small, with scant cytoplasm and absent or inconspicuous nucleoli. They are by far the most common type of cells in children with ALL.

        **(b) L2 lymphoblasts** are larger, with more abundant cytoplasm and one or more prominent nucleoli. They are much less common than L1 cells and are sometimes mistaken for myeloblasts.

        **(c) L3 lymphoblasts** are large, with deeply basophilic and vacuolated cytoplasm and prominent nucleoli. They are rare and usually indicative of the equally rare B cell ALL.

      **(2) Enzymatic evaluation.** Terminal deoxynucleotidyl transferase (TdT) is a unique DNA polymerase that is found in almost all lymphoblasts but only rarely in ANLL blasts.

      **(3) Histochemical evaluation** shows:

        **(a)** Absence of enzymes characteristic of ANLL blasts

        **(b)** In many cases, block-like accumulations of glycogen on periodic acid-Schiff (PAS) stain

    **b. Immunologic classification** (Figure 15-1) considers ALL to be a heterogeneous group of malignancies comprised of immature lymphoid cells arrested at various stages of development. On the basis of immunophenotype, ALL is divided into the following subtypes.

      **(1) Non-T, non-B cell ALL** accounts for 80% of all cases. Cells from patients with this type of ALL are lymphoid precursors that, under normal circumstances, would have differentiated into mature B cells capable of synthesizing a distinct immunoglobulin molecule or mature T cells capable of synthesizing a T cell antigen receptor. Often, the malignant leukemic cells have begun to rearrange their immunoglobulin chain genes

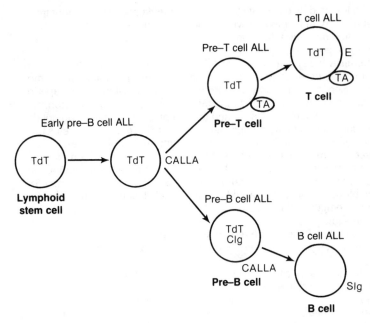

**Figure 15-1.** Scheme of B cell and T cell development and types of acute lymphocytic leukemia (*ALL*) that result from blocks at various stages of development. Current terminology considers both common acute lymphocytic leukemia antigen (*CALLA*)-negative and CALLA-positive early pre–B cell ALL and pre–B cell ALL as forms of non-T, non-B cell ALL. The exact precursor cell that gives rise to the T cell lineage is not known definitively and may not be the cell depicted in this scheme. *TdT* = terminal deoxynucleotidyl transferase; *TA* = thymic antigen; *E* = sheep red cell receptor; *CIg* = cytoplasmic immunoglobulin; *SIg* = surface immunoglobulin.

and their T cell receptor genes but not to the point where they can synthesize a functional gene product that indicates a commitment to the B cell or T cell lineage. Thus, these cells may be blocked at very early stages of their development. These cells are clonal in origin; in a given patient, they all demonstrate the same pattern of gene rearrangement. Non-T, non-B cell ALL is considered a **malignancy of B cell precursors,** because rearrangement of immunoglobulin chain genes is more common and more advanced than rearrangement of T cell antigen receptor genes and because the cells express early B cell differentiation antigens. Non-T, non-B cell ALL is **subdivided based on reactivity with the common acute lymphocytic leukemia antigen (CALLA)** into the following subtypes.

(a) **CALLA-negative early pre–B cell ALL** is less common than CALLA-positive ALL and consists of early pre–B cells that are not yet able to synthesize CALLA or cytoplasmic immunoglobulin.

(b) **CALLA-positive ALL** is more common than CALLA-negative ALL and may be one of the following.

  (i) **Early pre–B cell CALLA-positive ALL** consists of cells that synthesize CALLA but not cytoplasmic immunoglobulin; this is the most common subtype in children with ALL.

  (ii) **Pre–B cell ALL** consists of cells that usually continue to synthesize CALLA and have matured to the point where they synthesize cytoplasmic immunoglobulin consisting of only heavy chains, all of which are identical in the cells of any given patient.

(2) **B cell ALL** accounts for 1% of cases and is characterized by cells that lack TdT activity and often no longer express CALLA. These cells synthesize complete immunoglobulin molecules, which are expressed on their surface. The cells from any given patient all synthesize the same molecule consisting of one specific light chain and one specific heavy chain. This is the most mature form of ALL of B cell lineage and the only form of ALL in which the cells have a distinct appearance (L3) in the FAB classification.

(3) **T cell ALL** accounts for the remaining 19% of cases of ALL. The malignant cells show evidence of T cell lineage by expression of T cell antigens on their surface and by more advanced and definitive rearrangement of the genes for the T cell receptor. T cell ALL is subdivided into:

(a) Sheep red blood cell receptor-negative or so-called **pre–T cell ALL**

(b) Sheep red blood cell receptor-positive or **typical T cell ALL**

3. **Prognosis.** Presenting clinical and laboratory features for each patient with newly diagnosed ALL determine the probability that the child will remain in remission when treated with current

antileukemic therapy. Certain factors (e.g., age, sex, leukemic cell burden as reflected by white blood cell count or organ infiltration, morphology, immunophenotype) are used to determine prognosis. The Childrens Cancer Group assigns patients a good, intermediate, or poor prognosis based on the following features.

**a. Good prognosis patients** have an 80% or greater chance of cure. Features of these patients include:

  **(1)** Age between 2 and 10 years
  **(2)** White cell count less than 10,000/mm$^3$
  **(3)** Absence of L3 cells
  **(4)** Absence of lymphomatous features [see II B 3 c (3)]
  **(5)** Platelet count greater than 100,000/mm$^3$, if male

**b. Intermediate prognosis patients** have a 50% or greater chance of cure. Patients in this group include:

  **(1)** Males age 2–10 years with good prognostic features, whose platelet count is less than 100,000/mm$^3$
  **(2)** Children age 1–2 years without lymphomatous features or L3 morphology, whose white cell count is less than 50,000/mm$^3$
  **(3)** Children age 2–10 years without lymphomatous features or L3 morphology, whose white cell count is 10,000–50,000/mm$^3$

**c. Poor prognosis patients** have less than a 50% chance of cure. Patients in this group include:

  **(1)** Children age 1–10 years with a white cell count greater than 50,000/mm$^3$ but no lymphomatous features
  **(2)** Children older than 10 years, regardless of white cell count or the presence of lymphomatous features
  **(3)** Children with lymphomatous features ("leukemia/lymphoma syndrome") as defined by a combination of:
    **(a)** One or more of the following clinical features:
      **(i)** Massive splenomegaly
      **(ii)** Anterior mediastinal mass
      **(iii)** Massive lymphadenopathy
    **(b)** One or more of the following laboratory features:
      **(i)** Hemoglobin greater than 10 g/dl
      **(ii)** White cell count greater than 50,000/mm$^3$
      **(iii)** Blasts with T cell phenotype
  **(4)** Children younger than 1 year, in whom ALL often is associated with high white cell count, massive organomegaly, CALLA-negativity, and translocations involving chromosome 11 at a site where the C-*ets-1* proto-oncogene is located
  **(5)** Children with B cell ALL with L3 cells

**d. Other prognostic features**

  **(1)** Within any given category, there are other factors that may determine prognosis.
    **(a)** Factors that worsen the prognosis for any type of ALL include inadequate therapy, male sex, and CNS leukemia at diagnosis.
    **(b)** Factors that worsen the prognosis for non-T, non-B cell ALL include CALLA negativity, cytoplasmic immunoglobulin (pre–B cell ALL), and fewer than 53 chromosomes within the leukemic cells. Pseudodiploidy due to the presence of a chromosome translocation within the leukemic cells is strongly associated with a poor prognosis. These translocations include:
      **(i)** t(9;22)—the Philadelphia chromosome—which is seen in various types of non-T, non-B cell ALL
      **(ii)** t(4;11), which is seen in some cases of early pre–B cell ALL
      **(iii)** t(1;19), which is seen in some cases of pre–B cell ALL
      **(iv)** t(11;14), which is seen in some cases of T cell ALL
      **(v)** t(8;14), which is seen in most cases of B cell ALL with L3 morphology
  **(2)** Morphology impacts on prognosis. Children whose blasts have a predominantly L1 morphology have a better prognosis than those with blasts with L2 morphology. L3 morphology, because of its association with the B cell immunophenotype, carries a poor prognosis.
  **(3)** Immunophenotype links certain prognostic features.
    **(a)** T cell ALL usually carries a poor prognosis and is associated with such features as:
      **(i)** Male sex

 **(ii)** A high white cell count
 **(iii)** Lymphomatous features
 **(iv)** Predilection for CNS involvement
 **(b)** CALLA-positive non-T, non-B cell ALL of the early pre–B cell type (cytoplasmic immunoglobulin negative) often carries a good prognosis and is associated with such features as:
 **(i)** Occurrence during the 3- to 5-year-old age peak
 **(ii)** Association with a low or normal white cell count

4. **Therapy**
 a. **Remission induction** is successful in over 95% of children. At least three drugs—prednisone, vincristine, and ʟ-asparaginase—are employed; other drugs sometimes are added to regimens for patients with an intermediate or poor prognosis.
 b. **Consolidation** consists of continued systemic therapy, which may be very intense for poor prognosis patients. Intrathecal therapy with methotrexate, sometimes in conjunction with cranial irradiation, is given for CNS prophylaxis. Radiotherapy adds to the toxicity of CNS therapy and is reserved primarily for high-risk patients. It may cause:
 **(1)** Learning disabilities, especially in young children
 **(2)** Transient somnolence syndrome
 **(3)** Fatal leukoencephalopathy (rare)
 **(4)** Brain tumors (rare)
 c. **Maintenance therapy** often consists of periodic "reinduction" pulses of prednisone and vincristine as well as:
 **(1)** Daily oral 6-mercaptopurine and weekly oral methotrexate for low-risk patients
 **(2)** More intensive multiagent therapy for intermediate- and poor-risk patients

5. **Outcome**
 a. **Continuous complete remission** is the most common outcome for children with ALL and is especially likely in those with a good prognosis.
 b. **Relapses** still occur in 30%–40% of patients. Up to 75% of relapses occur while initial chemotherapy is still being administered. Relapse can occur in the:
 **(1)** Bone marrow, which is the most common site of recurrence
 **(2)** CNS, which was the most common site of recurrence prior to CNS prophylaxis
 **(3)** Testes, which are becoming the most common site of extramedullary relapse
 c. **Salvage chemotherapy** sometimes can retrieve children with:
 **(1)** Isolated extramedullary relapses in the CNS or testes
 **(2)** Bone marrow relapses that occur later than 6 months after elective discontinuation of therapy
 d. **Current chemotherapy** regimens frequently produce additional remissions in children with bone marrow relapses on chemotherapy or within 6 months of its discontinuation, but they are rarely curative. Most of these patients will ultimately die of their ALL unless they can be retrieved by bone marrow transplantation. At least one-third of children with relapsed ALL who can undergo allogeneic transplantation from an HLA-matched relative are cured of their otherwise fatal disease. Results with other types of bone marrow transplants (unrelated HLA-matched, autologous) are not as good.

C. **Acute nonlymphocytic leukemia (ANLL)**

1. **Epidemiology.** ANLL accounts for 20% of all childhood leukemia. It is more common in males than in females and more common in African-American children than in white children. ANLL is not associated with an early childhood peak.

2. **Classification.** The FAB classification employs morphologic and histochemical information to subdivide ANLL into the following subtypes.
 a. **M1 (myeloblastic leukemia without maturation).** The cells have abundant cytoplasm and prominent nucleoli and resemble L2 lymphoblasts. However, they are TdT negative, and they are positive for one or more of the following histochemical stains:
 **(1)** Peroxidase
 **(2)** Sudan black B
 **(3)** Chloroacetate esterase
 b. **M2 (myeloblastic leukemia with differentiation).** The cells have the same histochemical features as M1 cells but also have readily discernible azurophilic granules, which may coalesce into Auer rods.

    **c. M3 (promyelocytic leukemia).** The abundant azurophilic granules in the cells may serve as a source of procoagulant material, which causes DIC and can greatly increase the severity of the bleeding tendency present at initial diagnosis.

    **d. M4 (myelomonocytic leukemia).** Some of the cells have myeloblastic features by morphology and histochemistry, others have monocytic features and stain for nonspecific esterase, and still others have features of both lineages. M4 with eosinophilia is a distinct subtype associated with:

        **(1)** Abnormalities of chromosome 16

        **(2)** Propensity for meningeal involvement

        **(3)** Good response to chemotherapy

    **e. M5 (monoblastic leukemia)** is characterized by nonspecific esterase-positive cells, propensity for gum and CNS involvement, and association with DIC.

    **f. M6 (erythroleukemia).** The malignant cells are predominantly megaloblastic erythroid precursors, but myeloblasts are also present.

    **g. M7 (megakaryoblastic leukemia),** unlike M1 through M6, cannot be defined by morphologic features alone. Its diagnosis requires one or both of the following:

        **(1)** Detection of platelet peroxidase by electron microscopy

        **(2)** Detection of platelet-specific proteins by immunologic techniques

**3. Therapy**

    **a. Remission induction** generally requires more intensive chemotherapy than that administered for ALL. Most regimens employ at least an anthracycline and cytosine arabinoside (ara-C). Myelosuppression is severe, and good supportive care is essential. Remission is achieved in 80% of children.

    **b. After remission induction,** the following options are available:

        **(1)** Further chemotherapy consisting of:

            **(a)** Consolidation therapy with intensive systemic therapy and prophylactic therapy to the CNS

            **(b)** Maintenance therapy, which is a component of some, but not all, regimens

        **(2)** Bone marrow transplantation (allogeneic if the patient has an HLA-matched donor, autologous if the patient does not)

**4. Prognosis**

    **a.** The best chemotherapeutic regimens are curative for slightly less than half of the patients.

    **b.** The best allogeneic bone marrow transplantation regimens are curative for up to two-thirds of the patients.

    **c.** Since some relapsed patients can be salvaged by allogeneic bone marrow transplantation, the best initial regimen is still under study for patients with HLA-matched donors.

## D. Chronic myelogenous leukemia (CML)

**1. Classification.** Two types of CML occur during childhood.

    **a. Adult CML,** which is twice as common as juvenile CML, is a clonal myeloproliferative disorder arising from a neoplastically transformed stem cell. The neoplastic cells almost invariably contain the Philadelphia chromosome t(9;22). This translocation results in fusion of the c-*abl* oncogene on chromosome 9 to the breakpoint cluster region (*bcr*) of chromosome 22. The hybrid c-*abl/bcr* region transcribes a novel tyrosine kinase, which may promote the replicative advantage enjoyed by the neoplastic clone.

    **b. Juvenile CML** is a form of myelomonocytic leukemia, which is characterized by a proliferation of cells of monocyte and granulocyte origin. It is not a variant of adult CML, and its cells do not contain the Philadelphia chromosome.

**2. Clinical features**

    **a. Adult CML**

        **(1) Symptoms.** Adult CML occurs in older children and teenagers who present with:

            **(a)** Lassitude and weight loss from hypermetabolism

            **(b)** Bone pain

            **(c)** Increasing abdominal girth from massive splenomegaly

        **(2) Characteristic laboratory findings** include:

            **(a)** Extreme hyperleukocytosis characterized by:

               **(i)** A white cell count greater than 100,000/mm$^3$

               **(ii)** A predominance of more mature granulocytes on peripheral smear

               **(iii)** Eosinophilia and basophilia

            **(b)** Normal to increased platelet count
            **(c)** Mild anemia
            **(d)** Extreme myeloid hyperplasia in the bone marrow
            **(e)** The Philadelphia chromosome

    **b. Juvenile CML**
        **(1) Symptoms.** Juvenile CML occurs predominantly in children less than 5 years old and in males, who present with:
            **(a)** Suppurative lymphadenopathy
            **(b)** Moderate hepatosplenomegaly
            **(c)** Desquamative, erythematous rash
            **(d)** Purpura
            **(e)** Pulmonary infiltrates
        **(2) Characteristic laboratory findings** include:
            **(a)** Anemia with characteristics of fetal erythropoiesis
            **(b)** Thrombocytopenia
            **(c)** Moderate hyperleukocytosis characterized by:
                **(i)** A mean white cell count of $60,000/mm^3$
                **(ii)** An increase in monocytes and granulocytes in the peripheral blood
            **(d)** An increase in monocytes and granulocytes and a decrease in megakaryocytes in the bone marrow

  **3. Prognosis**
    **a. Adult CML** has a median survival of more than 2 years and can be subdivided into the following phases.
        **(1)** During **chronic CML,** the disease manifestations can be well controlled by chemotherapy.
        **(2)** During **accelerated CML,** clinical and laboratory findings show marked deterioration and patient responsiveness to therapy diminishes.
        **(3)** During **blastic CML,** which is of short duration, the disease acquires the features of a fatal acute leukemia. Blast crisis can be:
            **(a) Myeloid,** which is more common than lymphoid and usually is unresponsive to further therapy
            **(b) Lymphoid,** which usually is briefly responsive to therapy
    **b. Juvenile CML** is more rapidly fatal, with a median survival of 9 months.

  **4. Therapy**
    **a. Chemotherapy** is not curative of either type of childhood CML.
    **b. Bone marrow transplantation** has been curative of both adult and juvenile CML. For patients with adult CML, bone marrow transplantation is much more efficacious if it is done during the chronic phase.
    **c. Interferon** has been shown to decrease the proliferation of the Philadelphia chromosome–positive cells in adult CML. In some patients, there has been a transient decrease or disappearance of Philadelphia chromosome–positive cells from the bone marrow.

## III. NON-HODGKIN'S LYMPHOMAS are a heterogeneous group of diseases characterized by neoplastic proliferations of immature lymphoid cells, which, unlike the malignant lymphoid cells of ALL, accumulate primarily outside the bone marrow.

  **A. Epidemiology.** Non-Hodgkin's lymphomas comprise approximately 6% of all childhood cancers. They occur predominantly in older children and teenagers and have a strong predilection for males.

    **1. Childhood non-Hodgkin's lymphomas** differ from many adult cases in that they are:
      **a.** Predominantly extranodal in presentation
      **b.** As likely to be T cell lymphomas as B cell lymphomas
      **c.** Highly aggressive
      **d.** Rarely of nodular histology

    **2. Burkitt's lymphoma** occurs in an endemic form in Africa, where it presents as a mass in the jaw or abdomen. Induction of the B cell lymphoma in Africa has been linked to a prior Epstein-Barr virus infection occurring in a young child who has been immunosuppressed by malaria or another infection (see I C 2 a). Burkitt's lymphoma and other closely related forms of B cell lymphoma also develop in children immunosuppressed by HIV infection.

**B. Classification**

1. **Morphology.** Almost all cases are diffuse lymphomas and are classified as highly aggressive. The following types occur.

   a. In **lymphoblastic non-Hodgkin's lymphoma,** the cells resemble the L1 and L2 cells seen in the usual cases of childhood ALL.

   b. In **nonlymphoblastic non-Hodgkin's lymphoma,** the cells resemble transformed cells of the germinal center and may be:

      (1) Small noncleaved or Burkitt's type cells resembling L3 cells

      (2) Large transformed lymphoid cells, which, because of their size, have erroneously been called histiocytes

2. **Immunology**

   a. T cell origin is demonstrated in almost half of the cases. The cells generally have a lymphoblastic morphology and contain TdT.

   b. B cell origin is demonstrated in most other cases. The cells are nonlymphoblastic and lack TdT activity.

   c. Non-T, non-B cell origin is uncommon.

   d. True histiocytic or nonlymphoid origin is rare.

**C. Clinical features.** All childhood non-Hodgkin's lymphomas are rapidly growing, and thus, symptom duration is short.

1. **Anterior mediastinal masses,** sometimes associated with pleural effusions, are the most common presentation of T cell, or lymphoblastic, lymphomas. They can produce:

   a. Respiratory distress from airway compromise

   b. Superior vena cava syndrome [see II A 5 a (5)]

2. **Abdominal masses** are the most common presentation of B cell, or nonlymphoblastic, lymphomas. They can cause:

   a. Abdominal enlargement from a rapidly growing tumor, sometimes producing pain, ascites, and urinary tract obstruction

   b. Intestinal obstruction, by serving as the lead point for an intussusception

3. **Peripheral lymph node enlargement** can be seen with any type of childhood non-Hodgkin's lymphoma.

4. **Less common presentations** include:

   a. Obstructing nasopharyngeal tumor

   b. Bone tumor

   c. Skin tumor

**D. Staging.** Various systems are employed for different types of childhood non-Hodgkin's lymphoma. They all distinguish:

1. **Local disease** of limited bulk, often confined to one side of the diaphragm and carrying a good prognosis

2. **Extensive disease** within the mediastinum or abdomen

3. **Hematogenous dissemination,** especially to the bone marrow and meninges

**E. Therapy**

1. **Extensive surgical debulking** (i.e., removal of at least 90% of the tumor) improves survival for abdominal lymphomas.

2. **Systemic chemotherapy** is needed in all cases to shrink the local tumor and to prevent dissemination to the bone marrow or to a leukemic phase. The intensity and duration of therapy depends on the type of lymphoma and on the stage of the disease.

3. **CNS prophylaxis** in some form is required in most patients.

4. **Radiotherapy** is indicated in treatment sites where there is:

   a. Life-threatening obstruction that does not respond to chemotherapy

   b. Bulk tumor for which chemotherapy alone is judged inadequate

**F. Prognosis.** With appropriate management of the metabolic consequences of rapid cell turnover [see II A 5 a (3)] and with the institution of therapy, a favorable outcome often is achieved. Without therapy, rapid and widespread dissemination occurs.

    **1. T cell lymphomas** spread to the bone marrow and meninges and then closely resemble T cell ALL.

    **2. B cell lymphomas** of Burkitt's type spread to the bone marrow and meninges and closely resemble B cell (L3) ALL.

## IV. HODGKIN'S DISEASE in children behaves similarly to the disease in adults.

**A. Epidemiology.** Hodgkin's disease accounts for 4% of all childhood cancer. It occurs in older children and teenagers and has a slight female predominance.

**B. Clinical features**

    **1. Localized adenopathy,** especially in the cervical region, is the most common presenting symptom.

    **2. Systemic symptoms** occur in up to 30% of children and consist of:
        **a.** Temperature exceeding 38° C
        **b.** Drenching night sweats
        **c.** Weight loss in excess of 10% of body weight in 6 months

**C. Classification** based on histopathology divides Hodgkin's disease into:

    **1. Lymphocyte predominance,** with many lymphocytes and a few Reed-Sternberg cells

    **2. Mixed cellularity,** in which there are more Reed-Sternberg cells admixed with a heterogeneous population of reactive cells

    **3. Lymphocyte depletion,** with many Reed-Sternberg cells and a few reactive cells

    **4. Nodular sclerosis,** in which dense fibrotic bands separate islands of reactive cells and Reed-Sternberg cell variants called **lacunar cells**

**D. Staging.** Approximate stage can be assigned by a combination of clinical and laboratory tests, but definitive staging often requires exploratory laparotomy with splenectomy, which is indicated if precise staging is needed to determine the type of therapy to be employed. Four stages are defined; however, for any given stage, patients are further subdivided into "A" or "B" depending on the absence (A) or presence (B) of systemic symptoms.

    **1. Stage I.** Disease is confined to one group of nodes.

    **2. Stage II.** Disease is present in more than one group of nodes but is limited to one side of the diaphragm. Approximately 60% of children have localized (stage I or II) disease.

    **3. Stage III.** Disease involves nodes on both sides of the diaphragm with the spleen considered a node.

    **4. Stage IV.** There is hematogenous spread to the liver, bone marrow, lungs, or other non-nodal sites.

**E. Therapy and prognosis.** Prognosis is good and varies from a 90% cure of stage I disease to a 50% cure of stage IV disease.

    **1. Radiotherapy** to involved nodes plus the next node group to which spread could occur is often used for localized disease. For patients treated with radiotherapy alone, chemotherapy can sometimes be used as successful salvage therapy for relapse.

    **2. Combination chemotherapy** is indicated for all stage IV and many stage III patients and for patients with localized but bulky disease, such as a large mediastinal mass. Chemotherapy often is given in conjunction with radiotherapy.

    **3. Late effects of therapy** are numerous. Most serious are:
        **a.** Secondary malignancies (e.g., ANLL, non-Hodgkin's lymphoma) in patients treated with combined radiotherapy and procarbazine-containing chemotherapy regimens

**b.** Thyroid gland dysfunction (hypothyroidism, benign and malignant tumors) following neck irradiation
**c.** Growth disturbances following irradiation
**d.** Sterility

**V. NEUROBLASTOMA** is a malignancy of neural crest cells, which, in the course of their normal development, give rise to the paraspinal sympathetic ganglia and the adrenal medulla.

**A. Epidemiology.** Its 7% incidence makes neuroblastoma the second most common solid tumor of childhood. Only brain tumors are more common. Neuroblastoma occurs predominantly in infants and preschool children, with over half of the patients younger than 2 years old and one-third younger than 1 year. There is a slight male predominance.

**B. Clinical features** are extremely variable and reflect the widespread distribution of neural crest tissue.

**1. Primary sites**
**a. Abdominal tumors** are the most common presentation, accounting for 70% of the cases; half arise from extra-adrenal tissue and half from the adrenal medulla. Presenting features are:
**(1)** Abdominal mass, which often displaces the kidneys anterolaterally and inferiorly
**(2)** Abdominal pain
**(3)** Systemic hypertension, if there is compression of the renal vasculature
**b. Thoracic tumors** are the next most common presentation and are located in the posterior mediastinum. Presenting features are:
**(1)** Respiratory distress
**(2)** Incidental finding on a chest x-ray that was obtained for unrelated symptoms
**c. Head and neck tumors** present as palpable tumors sometimes with **Horner syndrome,** which consists of:
**(1)** Miosis
**(2)** Ptosis
**(3)** Enophthalmos
**(4)** Anhidrosis
**(5)** Heterochromia of the iris on the affected side
**d. Epidural tumors** arise from the posterior growth in dumbbell fashion of abdominal or thoracic tumors. They grow through the neural foramina into the epidural space, where they compress the spinal cord, producing back pain and symptoms of cord compression. Patients with this presentation require rapid evaluation with imaging studies to define the epidural component of the tumor and then therapy to prevent cord ischemia and its neurologic sequelae.

**2. Metastases** are common at diagnosis and often cause the symptoms that lead to the diagnosis of neuroblastoma.
**a. Nonspecific symptoms** of metastatic disease include:
**(1)** Weight loss
**(2)** Fever
**b. Specific symptoms** of metastatic disease include:
**(1)** Bone marrow failure (see I D 8)
**(2)** Cortical bone pain, resulting in a limp if present in the lower extremity
**(3)** Orbit problems, resulting in:
**(a)** Proptosis
**(b)** Periorbital ecchymoses
**(4)** Liver infiltration, causing hepatomegaly
**(5)** Distant lymph node enlargement (see I D 4)
**(6)** Skin infiltration, causing palpable subcutaneous nodules

**3. Remote effects** occasionally are seen.
**a.** Watery diarrhea may occur in patients with differentiated tumors, which secrete vasoactive intestinal peptide.
**b.** Acute myoclonic encephalopathy is a rare manifestation associated with an excellent prognosis. Patients present with:
**(1)** Opsoclonus (rapid eye movements)
**(2)** Myoclonus
**(3)** Truncal ataxia

**C. Staging** generally follows the pattern described in I E, with the following exceptions.

1. **Stage II** tumors must not be large enough to cross the midline.

2. **Stage III** tumors cross the midline.

3. **Stage IVS** tumors are small primary tumors that occur in young infants with metastases limited to the skin, liver, and bone marrow but not to cortical bone.

**D. Tumor markers** are extremely useful in evaluating children with neuroblastoma.

1. **Urinary markers.** Catecholamines are elaborated by most tumors and are useful for diagnosis, for following response to therapy, and for detection of recurrence. Particularly useful markers whose urinary excretion can be measured include:
   **a.** Vanillylmandelic acid (VMA)
   **b.** Homovanillic acid (HVA)

2. **Serum markers.** Elevation of the following serum markers often is associated with a poor prognosis:
   **a.** Neuron-specific enolase
   **b.** Ferritin
   **c.** Lactic dehydrogenase

3. **Oncogene marker.** Amplification of the N-*myc* oncogene within the tumor cells also is associated with a poor prognosis.

**E. Therapy**

1. **Surgery** alone often suffices for stage I and stage II patients.

2. **Spontaneous regression without any therapy** is common in stage IVS infants. Surgical removal of the small primary tumor is indicated to prevent late local recurrence.

3. **Chemotherapy** often can produce dramatic tumor regression in stage III and IV disease, but it is infrequently curative even when combined with radiotherapy and surgical debulking.

4. **Autologous and allogeneic bone marrow transplantation** is being explored for stage III and stage IV patients who have a poor prognosis.

**F. Prognosis** depends on the following factors.

1. **Age.** Infants less than 1 year old have the best prognosis.

2. **Stage**
   **a.** Stage I and stage II patients and stage IVS infants have a good prognosis.
   **b.** Most stage III and stage IV patients have a poor prognosis.

3. **Histopathology** may be an important feature. The degree of differentiation of the tumor cells and the pattern of their growth may, in selected cases, influence prognosis.

4. **Tumor markers** (see V D)

**VI. WILMS' TUMOR.** Neoplastic embryonal renal cells of the metanephros give rise to this kidney tumor, which is composed of an admixture of cells (blastemal, epithelial, and stromal) in varying proportions. The epithelial cells form tubules.

**A. Epidemiology.** Wilms' tumor accounts for 6% of all childhood cancers. It is predominantly a tumor of the first 5 years of life, with an approximately equal incidence throughout each of those 5 years. There is an equal occurrence in males and females.

**B. Clinical features**

1. **Abdominal mass** is by far the most common presentation. On imaging studies, the mass characteristically occurs within the kidneys and displaces and distorts the renal collecting system.

2. **Abdominal pain,** especially with hemorrhage into the tumor, is characteristic. There may be associated fever and anemia.

3. **Hematuria** is not common but, when present, is more often microscopic than gross.

4. **Hypertension** occurs in approximately one-fourth of all patients and may be related to elaboration of renin by tumor cells or, less frequently, to compression of the renal vasculature by the tumor.

    5. **Genetic factors** (see I C 1)

    6. **Associated abnormalities** that occur in a few patients include:
      **a.** Hemihypertrophy
      **b.** Genitourinary tract abnormalities
      **c.** Mental retardation
      **d.** Aniridia
        **(1)** Children with sporadic (as opposed to hereditary) aniridia are at increased risk for development of Wilms' tumor. In many of these children, a deletion of the short arm of chromosome 11 can be demonstrated.
        **(2)** Children with both sporadic aniridia and the chromosome deletion (11p13) have an almost 50% chance of developing Wilms' tumor.
        **(3)** Children with sporadic aniridia, chromosome deletion, and Wilms' tumor may also have mental retardation and genitourinary tract abnormalities, including ambiguous genitalia in affected males.

**C. Staging** is similar to that for other solid tumors (see I E). An additional stage, **stage V,** designates those 5% of patients with tumor in both kidneys. Most patients have relatively localized disease; only 10%–15% of patients have distant metastases at diagnosis.

**D. Diagnosis**

    1. **Appropriate imaging studies** are used to define the site of origin within the kidneys and to evaluate the contralateral kidney for tumor.

    2. **Search for distant metastases** is undertaken. Sites may include:
      **a.** Lungs
      **b.** Liver
      **c.** Bone (in patients with an unfavorable histology)
      **d.** Brain (in patients with an unfavorable histology)

**E. Therapy.** Dramatic advances in survival have occurred with the use of combined modality therapy.

    1. **Surgery** involves removal of the primary tumor, lymph nodes, and selected metastases.

    2. **Radiotherapy** involves treatment of residual local disease and selected metastatic foci.

    3. **Chemotherapy** varies in duration and intensity, depending on the patient's stage and histology.
      **a.** Actinomycin D and vincristine are used to treat all stages of disease.
      **b.** Additional agents, including doxorubicin, are used to treat patients with a poor prognosis.

**F. Prognosis.** Patients with localized disease and a favorable histology have a greater than 90% chance of survival. Poor prognosis patients have a less than 50% chance of survival.

    1. **Stage**
      **a.** Patients with distant metastases (stage IV) do least well.
      **b.** Stage V patients often do well with individualized management of their bilateral tumors.

    2. **Histopathology**
      **a.** Ninety percent of patients have a favorable histology, and most, in absence of distant metastases, do very well.
      **b.** Ten percent have unfavorable histologies and often do poorly, even if their disease is localized. They usually have:
        **(1)** Anaplastic Wilms' tumor
        **(2)** Sarcomatous Wilms' tumor

## VII. SOFT TISSUE SARCOMAS are tumors of primitive mesenchyme.

**A. Rhabdomyosarcoma** arises from the embryonal mesenchyme from which skeletal muscle originates.

    1. **Pathology.** Rhabdomyosarcoma can be divided into two pathologic categories.
      **a. Tumors of favorable histology** occur in 80% of affected children and are predominantly embryonal.
      **b. Tumors of unfavorable histology** occur in the remaining 20% of affected children and are of various subtypes.

2. **Clinical features.** Rhabdomyosarcoma is heterogeneous in presentation. The following are common sites of occurrence.
    a. **Head and neck** (38%)
        (1) **Orbit tumors** have a rapid onset of symptoms due to their confinement by the bony orbit. They present as:
            (a) Exophthalmos
            (b) Ptosis
            (c) Eyelid swelling
        (2) **Nasopharyngeal and middle ear tumors** are associated with:
            (a) Discharge
            (b) Polypoid mass
            (c) Airway obstruction
            (d) Chronic otitis media
            (e) Spread to the adjacent meninges, causing increased intracranial pressure and cranial nerve palsies
        (3) **Neck tumors** cause:
            (a) Mass
            (b) Pain
            (c) Cervical and brachial plexus palsy
    b. **Genitourinary tract** (21%)
        (1) **Bladder and prostate tumors** cause:
            (a) Urinary obstruction
            (b) Hematuria
        (2) **Vaginal and uterine tumors** cause:
            (a) Vaginal bleeding
            (b) Polypoid tumor with glistening membrane (sarcoma botryoides, or "cluster of grapes") extruding from the vaginal orifice
    c. **Extremity tumors** (18%) present as solid masses on the upper or lower extremities.
    d. **Miscellaneous presentations** occur with a mass or obstructing lesion in the following locations:
        (1) Trunk
        (2) Retroperitoneum
        (3) Paratesticular region
        (4) Perianal region
        (5) Gastrointestinal and biliary tracts

3. **Therapy**
    a. **Surgery**
        (1) Complete excision is indicated for those locations where disfigurement will not result.
        (2) If disfigurement would result, either chemotherapy, radiotherapy, or both are used as alternatives to surgery or to shrink the tumor to permit easier removal.
    b. **Radiotherapy** is used for local tumors and metastases.
    c. **Chemotherapy** is used as an adjuvant to other therapy and for local and metastatic tumors. The intensity of therapy depends on the location, stage, and histology of the tumor.
    d. **Irradiation of adjacent meninges** is indicated for patients with head and neck tumors with a propensity for meningeal spread. **Intrathecal chemotherapy** is sometimes administered to these patients as well. Appropriate therapy to the meninges has eliminated them as a frequent site of recurrence in children with tumors adjacent to them.

4. **Prognosis** has dramatically improved over the years by judicious use of all therapeutic modalities.
    a. Children with primary tumors of the orbit have an **excellent** (90%) survival rate without need for disfiguring surgery.
    b. Children with primary tumors of the genitourinary tract often are spared extensive pelvic surgery and still enjoy a **good** survival rate (as high as 75%).
    c. **Poor** prognosis is still seen with:
        (1) Extremity tumors
        (2) Retroperitoneal tumors
        (3) Metastatic disease

**B. Rare soft tissue sarcomas**

1. **Fibrosarcomas** often arise in the distal portion of the extremities. They are more commonly seen in young children for whom the prognosis is excellent with surgical treatment alone.

2. **Liposarcomas** also are more common in young children and carry an excellent prognosis, provided that total surgical excision is possible.

3. **Synovial sarcomas** most commonly develop around the knee joint.

4. **Primitive neuroectodermal tumors** arise from peripheral nerves. These tumors have a characteristic translocation, t(11;22), and often present as masses on the chest or extremities. Unlike other rare soft tissue sarcomas, primitive neuroectodermal tumors have a greater metastatic potential and require aggressive systemic chemotherapy.

**VIII. BONE TUMORS.** Primary malignant bone tumors account for 4% of childhood cancer. Two highly malignant tumors predominate: Ewing's sarcoma and osteogenic sarcoma.

A. **Ewing's sarcoma** is an undifferentiated sarcoma of uncertain histogenesis, which arises primarily in bone. A possible neurogenic origin has been suggested for the highly undifferentiated Ewing's sarcoma cells because these cells have a t(11;22), which is the same translocation that is found in the cells from primitive neuroectodermal tumors of the peripheral nervous system (see VII B 4). Occasional cases of Ewing's sarcoma arise in the soft tissues of the extremities and paravertebral region rather than in bone and are referred to as **extraosseous** Ewing's sarcoma.

1. **Epidemiology.** Ewing's sarcoma is seen primarily in adolescents and is 1.5 times more common in males than females. It is rarely seen in African-Americans.

2. **Clinical features**
    a. Pain and localized swelling are the most common presenting complaints.
    b. Sometimes there are systemic manifestations, including:
        (1) Fever
        (2) Leukocytosis
        (3) Elevated erythrocyte sedimentation rate
    c. Any bone can be affected. Likely sites are:
        (1) Mid- to proximal femur and pelvic bones
        (2) Other long bones, the ribs, and the scapula

3. **Diagnosis**
    a. X-rays characteristically show a destructive lesion possibly associated with periosteal elevation or a soft tissue mass.
    b. Metastases should be suspected, especially to the lungs and to other bones.

4. **Therapy**
    a. **Radiotherapy** is the usual mode of treatment of the primary tumor.
    b. **Chemotherapy**—which consists of cyclophosphamide and doxorubicin, as well as other agents—plays an important role in:
        (1) Reduction of primary tumor bulk
        (2) Prevention of metastases
        (3) Treatment of patients with metastases at diagnosis

5. **Prognosis**
    a. The prognosis is very good for patients with distal extremity nonmetastatic tumors treated with chemotherapy and radiotherapy.
    b. The prognosis is poor for patients with:
        (1) Metastatic disease at diagnosis
        (2) Tumors of the pelvic bones
        (3) Tumors in the proximal femur

B. **Osteogenic sarcoma** is a malignant tumor of the bone-producing mesenchyme.

1. **Epidemiology.** Osteogenic sarcoma is the most common primary malignant bone tumor seen in pediatric patients. It is seen mainly in adolescents and is twice as common in males as compared with females.

2. **Clinical features**
    a. Pain and swelling are common.
    b. Systemic manifestations are rare.
    c. Half of all cases occur in the proximity of the knee joint.
    d. The most common tumor sites in decreasing order of frequency are:
        (1) Distal femur

(2) Proximal tibia
(3) Proximal humerus
(4) Proximal femur
e. Metastases are primarily to the lungs.
f. Radiographic findings include:
(1) Destructive lesions
(2) Periosteal reaction, with a characteristic radial "sunburst" as the tumor breaks through the cortex and new bone spicules are produced

3. **Therapy**
a. **Surgery** plays an important role.
(1) Various limb salvage surgical procedures that limit resection to the tumor-bearing portion of the bone often are performed.
(2) Amputation is performed when limb salvage is not possible.
b. **Chemotherapy** also is of great importance and clearly improves disease-free survival. Particularly effective agents include:
(1) High-dose methotrexate, which must be given with citrovorum factor rescue
(2) Doxorubicin
(3) Cisplatin

4. **Prognosis.** With aggressive adjuvant chemotherapy, survival is improved to greater than 50%. Aggressive treatment of metastatic disease is indicated, as some patients can be salvaged with aggressive chemotherapy and surgical resection of pulmonary metastases.

## IX. BRAIN TUMORS. 
Collectively, brain tumors are the second most common form of childhood cancer, accounting for 20% of the total. They are of diverse types, each with unique characteristics, locations, and growth rates.

A. **Special problems in management of pediatric brain tumors**

1. The blood-brain barrier limits the delivery of chemotherapy by the systemic route.

2. The developing brain of infants and young children is vulnerable to the toxicity of therapeutic modalities (e.g., radiotherapy).

3. The proximity of some tumors to important areas of brain function precludes their extensive surgical resection.

4. There is a tendency for the tumors to spread within rather than outside the neuraxis.

B. **Classification**

1. **Location.** Two-thirds of brain tumors arise below and one-third arise above the tentorium.

2. **Histology.** Most brain tumors fall into two distinct groups.
a. **Tumors of astrocytic origin**
(1) **High-grade astrocytomas** arise primarily above the tentorium and present as:
(a) Focal neurologic deficits
(b) Signs of increased intracranial pressure (see I D 7)
(c) Focal seizures
(2) **Low-grade astrocytomas** arise primarily below the tentorium in the cerebellum, where they present as:
(a) Signs of increased intracranial pressure
(b) Signs of cerebellar dysfunction (e.g., ataxia, nystagmus)
(3) **Brain stem gliomas** present as:
(a) Multiple cranial nerve palsies
(b) Ataxia
(c) Long tract signs
b. **Tumors of neuroepithelial origin**
(1) **Medulloblastoma** is the most common malignant brain tumor in children and characteristically presents as a cerebellar tumor causing:
(a) Signs of increased intracranial pressure
(b) Cerebellar dysfunction

        **(c)** Propensity for rapid spread throughout the neuraxis by the cerebrospinal fluid (CSF) pathways, which is more common in young children and carries a poor prognosis

    **(2) Primitive neuroectodermal tumors** are much less common than medulloblastomas and are highly malignant. They present as cerebral masses with symptoms similar to cerebral astrocytomas.

## C. Therapy

1. **Surgery** plays an important role in the management of tumors whose location permits resection.
   a. Resectable tumors include cerebellar and cerebral tumors.
   b. Brain stem gliomas generally are not resectable, and their location often makes even biopsy hazardous.

2. **Radiotherapy** plays a major role in the management of tumors in all locations and is indicated for most tumors except for completely resected low-grade astrocytomas.
   a. Unfortunately, the doses delivered often are associated with significant toxicity, which is especially severe in young children and includes:
      (1) Learning disabilities
      (2) Growth failure
      (3) Primary hypothyroidism when the neck is in the radiation field
   b. For tumors that tend to spread throughout the neuraxis (e.g., medulloblastomas), the whole neuraxis (cranium and spine) must be irradiated.

3. **Chemotherapy** is a relatively recent addition to the armamentarium and has shown promise in:
   a. Prolonging survival of patients with high-grade astrocytomas
   b. Increasing the cure rate of select patients with medulloblastomas

## D. Prognosis

1. The prognosis is **excellent** for completely resected low-grade cerebellar astrocytomas.

2. The prognosis is **good** for many medulloblastomas, particularly if they:
   a. Occur in children older than age 4 years
   b. Are relatively small in size
   c. Have not spread

3. The prognosis is **poor** for:
   a. Brain stem gliomas
   b. Medulloblastomas that occur in young children, are large in size, and spread into the CSF and to distant sites in the neuraxis

# X. LIVER TUMORS

**A. Epidemiology.** Liver tumors account for only 1% of childhood cancer. However, they are the most common epithelial malignancy of childhood.

**B. Clinical features.** Liver tumors present as a mass, primarily in the right upper quadrant. They often elaborate α-fetoprotein (AFP), which is a tumor marker useful for diagnosis, for following response to therapy, and for detection of recurrence. Two types of tumors occur.

1. **Hepatoblastoma,** the most common type, occurs in infants and young children.
   a. It often is associated with thrombocytosis and metastasizes primarily to the lung.
   b. It has an outcome that depends on whether it can be completely resected.
   c. Hepatoblastoma that is not resectable sometimes may be sufficiently reduced in size by chemotherapeutic agents (e.g., doxorubicin and cisplatin) to permit curative resection.

2. **Hepatocellular carcinoma,** which is less common than hepatoblastoma, is seen in older children and teenagers.
   a. It often is multifocal and is less curable than hepatoblastoma.
   b. Hepatocellular carcinoma may be related to a preceding hepatitis B infection, just as in adults.

**XI. GERM CELL TUMORS** arise from precursors of egg and sperm cells.

   A. **Common sites of origin** include the **gonads** (testes, ovaries) and **ectopic sites** (sacrococcyx, anterior mediastinum).

   B. **Histologies** represent the degree to which the cells remain pluripotent and undifferentiated.

   1. Multipotential cells form embryonal carcinoma.

   2. Cells with embryonic or somatic differentiation form teratomas, which may be benign or malignant.

   3. Cells with extraembryonic differentiation form:
      a. Yolk sac or endodermal sinus tumors
      b. Trophoblastic tumors or choriocarcinomas

   4. Cells with a commitment to pure germ cell differentiation form:
      a. Seminomas in males (rare in children)
      b. Dysgerminomas in females

   C. **Diagnostic markers**

   1. **AFP** is produced by embryonal carcinomas and endodermal sinus tumors.

   2. **Human chorionic gonadotropin (HCG)** is produced by embryonal carcinomas and choriocarcinomas.

   D. **Clinical features**

   1. **Testicular tumors** present as painless intrascrotal swelling and always require radical orchiectomy with high ligation of the spermatic cord. Additional therapy and prognosis depend on:
      a. Age, with most infants less than 2 years old having an excellent prognosis with surgery alone
      b. Stage
      c. Histology
      d. Metastatic potential for spread to the retroperitoneal nodes and lungs via the lymphatics and blood, respectively

   2. **Ovarian tumors** commonly present as abdominal or pelvic masses. They may sometimes produce severe pain of acute onset that results from torsion of the tumor. Uncommon presentations include precocious puberty or virilism. Therapy includes:
      a. **Complete surgical resection**
      b. **Chemotherapy** for patients with the most common histology, endodermal sinus tumor, and for selected other histologies
      c. **Radiotherapy** for dysgerminomas

   3. **Sacrococcygeal germ cell tumors** are the most common germ cell tumors and the most common solid tumor in newborns.
      a. These tumors usually are benign when diagnosed in the first 2 months of life.
      b. Such tumors in older infants and children often are malignant and associated with a poor prognosis.

   4. **Mediastinal teratomas** are benign in 80% of cases. They are most likely to be malignant and carry a poor prognosis in older adolescents.

**XII. HISTIOCYTOSIS X** refers to a heterogeneous group of disorders that are characterized by proliferation of histiocytes. The wide range of clinical presentations has made classification confusing and suggests a spectrum of diseases—possibly associated with abnormalities of immune regulation—ranging from benign and indolent processes to highly aggressive processes. Whether the aggressive forms of the disease are true malignancies remains unanswered.

   A. **Histology.** The proliferating histiocytes are dendritic cells. These weakly phagocytic cells are components of the bone marrow–derived mononuclear phagocytic system from which circulating monocytes and phagocytic tissue macrophages also arise. These dendritic cells are called **Langerhans cells**.

   1. Langerhans cells primarily are located in the epidermis to which they migrated from the bone marrow.

    **2.** These cells serve as antigen-presenting cells.

    **3.** On electron microscopy, Langerhans cells contain an identifying structure called the **Birbeck granule**.

  **B. Etiology.** Although the etiology is unknown, an abnormality of immune regulation has been suggested because many cases are associated with dysmorphic changes in the thymus.

  **C. Clinical features**

    **1. Eosinophilic granuloma** is a benign and self-limited disease. It is uncommon in infants. Eosinophilic granuloma usually is limited to a single bone lesion that is painful and located in the femur or skull.

    **2. Hand-Schüller-Christian disease** is a more chronic and extensive disease. It also is uncommon in infants. Hand-Schüller-Christian disease commonly involves the bone and skin. It occasionally presents as a classic triad of:
      **a.** Skeletal lesions
      **b.** Diabetes insipidus
      **c.** Exophthalmos

    **3. Letterer-Siwe disease** is an acute disease that often terminates in fatal sepsis. It occurs in infants.
      **a.** Letterer-Siwe disease involves the skin, liver, spleen, lymph nodes, bone marrow, and lungs.
      **b.** Bone lesions are less striking than in the other forms of histiocytosis X.
      **c.** A poor outcome is heralded by dysfunction of one or more of the following: lungs, liver, and bone marrow.

**XIII. RETINOBLASTOMA** is a rare congenital malignancy that arises from neural tissue within the retina.

  **A. Genetic factors** (see I C 1 a)

  **B. Clinical features**

    **1.** Usually there is an abnormal white pupil, or **"cat's eye,"** and strabismus sometimes is present.

    **2.** Most tumors are localized to the globe at diagnosis. Metastases occur late and spread to the:
      **a.** Meninges via the optic nerve
      **b.** Bone marrow and cortical bone via the blood

  **C. Therapy** is highly specialized. The goal is to cure and to preserve useful vision whenever possible.

    **1. Surgical enucleation** is indicated for:
      **a.** Most cases of unilateral disease
      **b.** The most severely involved eye in bilateral cases

    **2. Radiotherapy** is indicated to:
      **a.** Treat any residual orbital disease
      **b.** Manage the remaining eye in bilateral cases along with other physical modalities (e.g., laser therapy, cryotherapy)

    **3. Chemotherapy** is employed in select cases as:
      **a.** An adjuvant
      **b.** A palliative for the few patients with disseminated disease

  **D. Prognosis**

    **1.** The prognosis is **excellent** for those cases that are limited to the eyes.

    **2.** There is a **poor** prognosis with dissemination.

## STUDY QUESTIONS

**Directions:** Each of the numbered items or incomplete statements in this section is followed by answers or by completions of the statement. Select the **one** lettered answer or completion that is **best** in each case.

1. Which of the following conditions has a better prognosis if it occurs in a child less than 1 year old?

(A) Neuroblastoma
(B) ALL
(C) Medulloblastoma
(D) Histiocytosis X
(E) Juvenile CML

2. Graft-versus-host disease is best avoided by

(A) caring for recipients in a germ-free environment
(B) purging B cells from the bone marrow prior to infusion
(C) making sure donors and recipients are HLA matched
(D) performing transplantation while the patient is in remission
(E) limiting transplantation to patients older than 10 years of age

3. Which of the following immunophenotypes is most common in children with ALL?

(A) B cell ALL
(B) T cell ALL
(C) Pre–T cell ALL
(D) CALLA-positive non-T, non-B cell ALL
(E) CALLA-negative non-T, non-B cell ALL

4. Radiotherapy plays a role in the treatment of pediatric cancer in each of the following situations EXCEPT

(A) palliation of symptoms from discrete metastatic foci
(B) eradication of local residual disease for stage I surgically resected tumors
(C) destruction of malignant cells prior to bone marrow transplantation
(D) prevention of meningeal leukemia in children with ALL
(E) treatment of localized Hodgkin's disease

5. Which of the following conditions is NOT associated with chromosome abnormalities?

(A) Eosinophilic granuloma
(B) Retinoblastoma
(C) Adult CML
(D) Burkitt's lymphoma

6. Which of the following statements about pediatric brain tumors is FALSE?

(A) They can arise above or below the tentorium
(B) They usually spread beyond the neuraxis
(C) Their response to radiotherapy is good
(D) Medulloblastoma is the most common brain tumor in children

7. An 11-year-old boy with hemophilia develops a large left supraclavicular mass that grows over a 3-week period. He has received many transfusions in the past but does not have a factor VIII inhibitor. The mass does not regress with factor VIII therapy. The most likely diagnosis is

(A) non-Hodgkin's lymphoma
(B) metastatic neuroblastoma
(C) Kaposi's sarcoma
(D) ANLL
(E) hemorrhage into the tissues of the supraclavicular region

8. A 2-year-old boy presents with a large left-sided abdominal mass, which, on intravenous pyelogram, appears to arise within the left kidney and to distort and displace the collecting system. On chest x-ray, multiple pulmonary nodules are present. The most likely diagnosis is

(A) neuroblastoma
(B) Wilms' tumor
(C) non-Hodgkin's lymphoma
(D) rhabdomyosarcoma
(E) hepatoblastoma

| | | |
|---|---|---|
| 1-A | 4-B | 7-A |
| 2-C | 5-A | 8-B |
| 3-D | 6-B | |

9. A 15-year-old boy presents with a large anterior mediastinal mass. Laboratory findings include a white cell count of 180,000/mm³, with 97% blasts on differential; the blasts are positive for terminal deoxynucleotidyl transferase (TdT). The most likely diagnosis is

(A) juvenile CML
(B) adult CML
(C) T cell non-Hodgkin's lymphoma
(D) ANLL
(E) T cell ALL

**Questions 10–12**

An 8-year-old girl presents with fever, numerous bruises over her entire body, and pain in both legs. Physical examination reveals pallor, a soft midsystolic murmur, the spleen at 2 cm below the left costal margin, and ecchymoses and petechiae on the face, trunk, and extremities. Findings on complete blood count include a hemoglobin of 6.3 g/dl, white cell count of 2800/mm³ (10% neutrophils, 1% bands, 2% monocytes, 87% lymphocytes), and platelet count of 29,000/mm³.

10. Which of the following would be the most appropriate initial diagnostic test?

(A) Heterophile antibody
(B) Bone marrow aspiration
(C) Sedimentation rate
(D) Skeletal survey
(E) Liver and spleen scan

11. If the patient's bone marrow were replaced by CALLA-positive lymphoblasts with L1 morphology, her risk of relapse would be

(A) high
(B) intermediate
(C) low
(D) undetermined

12. If the patient were to become febrile to 39.5° C, appropriate responses would include all of the following EXCEPT to

(A) administer aspirin for the fever
(B) obtain a blood culture
(C) obtain a chest x-ray
(D) obtain a urine culture
(E) start intravenous broad-spectrum antibiotics

**Directions:** Each item below contains four suggested answers of which **one or more** is correct. Choose the answer

|   |   |
|---|---|
| A | if **1, 2, and 3** are correct |
| B | if **1 and 3** are correct |
| C | if **2 and 4** are correct |
| D | if **4** is correct |
| E | if **1, 2, 3, and 4** are correct |

13. Features that are associated with a good prognosis for a patient with ALL include

(1) CALLA-positive non-T, non-B cell blasts
(2) a white cell count of 57,000/mm³
(3) an age of 7 years
(4) a large mediastinal mass

14. True statements regarding Wilms' tumor include which of the following?

(1) Metastasis to bone marrow is common
(2) Adjuvant chemotherapy is required for cure
(3) Patients have elevated levels of homovanillic acid
(4) Cure often is possible if the tumor histology is favorable

---

9-E       12-A
10-B     13-B
11-C     14-C

**Directions:** The group of questions below consists of lettered choices followed by several numbered items. For each numbered item select the **one** lettered choice with which it is **most** closely associated. Each lettered choice may be used once, more than once, or not at all.

**Questions 15–18**

For each presentation, choose the disease with which it is most likely to be associated.

(A) Neuroblastoma
(B) Wilms' tumor
(C) Rhabdomyosarcoma
(D) Acute promyelocytic leukemia
(E) Histiocytosis X

15. Development of a right flank mass in a 2-year-old boy with aniridia

16. Intracranial hemorrhage from severe thrombocytopenia and hypofibrinogenemia

17. Protrusion of "cluster of grapes" from the vagina

18. Diabetes insipidus

15-B      18-E
16-D
17-C

# ANSWERS AND EXPLANATIONS

**1. The answer is A** *[V F 1]*.
Age less than 1 year old is a favorable prognostic indicator in neuroblastoma. Histiocytosis X in an infant is much more likely to present as Letterer-Siwe disease, which often has a fatal outcome. Infants with acute lymphocytic leukemia (ALL) do particularly poorly, and children with medulloblastoma who are less than 4 years old do not do as well as older children. Children with juvenile chronic myelogenous leukemia (CML) do poorly at any age.

**2. The answer is C** *[I F 4]*.
Without human leukocyte antigen (HLA) matching, severe graft-versus-host disease (GVHD) is almost certain. Purging transplants of T cell mediators may also prevent GVHD, but purging them of B cells would have no effect. Caring for recipients in a germ-free environment may decrease the incidence of infection and, in at least aplastic anemia patients, of GVHD, but this is not nearly as important as matching at the major histocompatibility loci. Remission status does not influence GVHD occurrence. GVHD increases in both incidence and severity with increasing patient age. Therefore, children older than 10 years of age would be expected to have a higher rather than lower incidence of GVHD.

**3. The answer is D** *[II B 2 b (1) (b) (ii)]*.
Non-T, non-B cell ALL accounts for 80% of all cases of ALL in children. Non-T, non-B cell ALL is divided into common acute lymphocytic leukemia antigen (CALLA)-positive and CALLA-negative ALL subtypes. CALLA-positive non-T, non-B cell ALL is three to four times more common than its CALLA-negative counterpart, which has an incidence similar to both types of T cell ALL. T cell ALL is subdivided into pre–T cell ALL (sheep red cell receptor-negative) and typical T cell ALL (sheep red cell receptor-positive). B cell ALL is rare, accounting for 1% of cases of ALL in children.

**4. The answer is B** *[I E 1]*.
Surgically resected tumors classified as stage I have no need for local radiotherapy, as they can be totally resected with no microscopic or gross disease left behind. Radiotherapy can be very useful in relieving pain and the compressive symptoms from metastases. Total body irradiation plays an important role in the cytoreduction that precedes transplantation. Cranial irradiation is an important component of the central nervous system (CNS) prophylaxis regimen for ALL patients who have a poor prognosis. Radiotherapy plays a definitive role in the treatment of patients with localized Hodgkin's disease.

**5. The answer is A** *[XII B, C]*.
Eosinophilic granuloma is a form of histiocytosis X—a group of disorders of unknown etiology characterized by proliferation of histiocytes. Eosinophilic granuloma has not been associated with any chromosome abnormalities. Adult CML, which is twice as common as juvenile CML, is a clonal myeloproliferative disorder arising from a neoplastically transformed stem cell. These neoplastic cells almost invariably contain the Philadelphia chromosome t(9;22). In both sporadic and hereditary retinoblastoma, abnormalities localized to the long arm of chromosome 13 have been detected. The specific chromosome abnormality in Burkitt's lymphoma consists of a translocation of a portion of the long arm of chromosome 8, which contains the c-*myc* oncogene, onto the area of another chromosome (14, 4, or 22) that controls immunoglobulin synthesis.

**6. The answer is B** *[IX A 4]*.
Collectively, brain tumors are the second most common form of childhood cancer, accounting for 20% of the total, with medulloblastoma being the most common type. While brain tumors can arise above or below the tentorium, most arise below the tentorium. There is a tendency for brain tumors to spread within rather than outside the neuraxis. Radiotherapy plays a major role in the management of tumors in all locations and is indicated for most tumors except for completely resected low-grade astrocytomas.

**7. The answer is A** *[I C 2 b; III A–C]*.
The boy described in this case study is at high risk for developing a human immunodeficiency virus (HIV) infection and may, as a consequence, develop an acquired immune deficiency syndrome (AIDS)-associated, aggressive B cell lymphoma. Kaposi's sarcoma occurs less commonly than lymphoma in pediatric patients with AIDS. Metastatic neuroblastoma can present in this fashion, but the boy's age and hemophilia make this unlikely. Acute nonlymphocytic leukemia (ANLL) usually does not produce this degree of adenopathy and would be unusual in a hemophiliac. Hemorrhage always is a possible diagnosis in a child with hemophilia, but failure of the mass to respond to appropriate treatment and absence of an inhibitor interfering with response to treatment make this very unlikely.

**8. The answer is B** *[VI B, D].*
The classic x-ray appearance of Wilms' tumor is an abdominal mass that occurs within the kidney, distorting and replacing the renal collecting system; metastases to the lungs are noted on chest x-ray. Neuroblastoma arises above the kidney and displaces it anterolaterally and inferiorly and rarely metastasizes to the lungs. B cell non-Hodgkin's lymphomas often arise in the abdomen but not from the kidney, and they do not produce nodular pulmonary metastases. Rhabdomyosarcomas may arise in the retroperitoneum but are much rarer than Wilms' tumor and are extrarenal. They do spread to the lungs. Hepatoblastomas most commonly arise in the right rather than left lobe of the liver and produce right-sided masses. They should not distort the intrarenal architecture. They do, however, metastasize to the lungs.

**9. The answer is E** *[II B 2 a (2)].*
A teenage boy with a high white blood cell count ALL most likely has T cell disease. Both the presence of the mediastinal mass and the terminal deoxynucleotidyl transferase (TdT) in the blasts are much more suggestive of T cell ALL than of ANLL; TdT is found in almost all lymphoblasts of patients with ALL, whereas it is rare in ANLL. CML of either the adult or juvenile type would be unlikely because of the predominance of blasts in the blood, and juvenile CML would also be unlikely due to the patient's age. The presence of many circulating blasts indicates a leukemia rather than a lymphoma.

**10–12. The answers are: 10-B** *[I D 8 a; II A 3 a–c, 4 b]*, **11-C** *[II B 3 a]*, **12-A** *[II A 3 a (2)].*
This child's presentation is typical of ALL. She has signs and symptoms of anemia and thrombocytopenia as well as bone pain and splenomegaly, and her complete blood count values indicate pancytopenia. In this situation, bone marrow aspiration is the most appropriate test to see whether the bone marrow can produce adequate numbers of blood cells and, if not, whether the marrow is aplastic or replaced by malignant cells. A heterophile antibody would be useful only if infectious mononucleosis were a strong possibility. Splenomegaly, immune thrombocytopenia, and hemolytic anemia can be seen with mononucleosis, but leukopenia and bone pain would not be expected to occur with a typical Epstein-Barr virus infection. The sedimentation rate is not a specific enough test to be useful in this patient and would not provide a diagnosis. Skeletal survey may show leukemic lines, but their presence or absence cannot substitute for bone marrow examination, which is much more definitive and provides material for diagnosis of the specific type of leukemia. Liver and spleen scan would show splenic enlargement but would not provide a specific diagnosis.

A low white cell count, age of 8 years, and L1 morphology of lymphoblasts all are typical of low-risk ALL in a girl. If the patient were a boy, a platelet count of less than 100,000/mm$^3$ would increase the risk to intermediate. There are no high-risk features in this patient, such as high white cell count, age less than 1 year, massive splenomegaly or other lymphomatous features, or L3 morphology of the lymphoblasts.

Aspirin should not be used as an antipyrectic in a thrombocytopenic patient, since salicylates interfere with platelet function and would worsen the bleeding tendency. Prompt institution of intravenous broad-spectrum antibiotics, however, is mandatory in the febrile, neutropenic patient. Blood and urine cultures should be obtained prior to initiating antibiotic therapy. A chest x-ray also should be performed to detect any infiltrates. Administration of antipyretics is not contraindicated after the appropriate tests have been rapidly performed and after antibiotic therapy has begun.

**13. The answer is B (1, 3)** *[II B 3].*
Factors used to determine the prognosis of ALL in children include age, sex, leukemia cell burden, organ infiltration, morphology, and immunophenotype. Most patients with a good prognosis have non-T, non-B cell ALL that is CALLA-positive. They are further characterized by a white cell count less than 10,000/mm$^3$ and an age of 2–10 years. A poor prognosis is associated with age less than 1 year, a white cell count greater than 50,000/mm$^3$, a mediastinal mass, massive lymphadenopathy and splenomegaly, age over 10 years, blasts with a T cell phenotype or mature B cell (surface immunoglobulin-positive) phenotype, and hemoglobin greater than 10 g/dl.

**14. The answer is C (2, 4)** *[VI E, F].*
Most patients with favorable histologic types of Wilms' tumor are cured. To accomplish cure, chemotherapy is required even in the absence of metastases. Metastases are most commonly to the lung, whereas bone marrow is rarely, if ever, involved. Homovanillic acid (HVA) is produced by neuroblastoma and not by Wilms' tumor.

**15–18. The answers are: 15-B** *[VI B 6 d]*, **16-D** *[II A 3 a (2) (b), C 2 c]*, **17-C** *[VII A 2 b (2) (b)]*, **18-E** *[XII C 2 b].*
Children with sporadic aniridia have an increased risk for Wilms' tumor. Many of these children also will

have deletion of a portion of the short arm of chromosome 11, and this further increases their risk for Wilms' tumor.

Acute promyelocytic leukemia usually is associated with disseminated intravascular coagulation (DIC) from triggering of the coagulation cascade by the primary granules released by dying promyelocytes. This can be associated with severe consumptive thrombocytopenia and depletion of coagulation factors (e.g., fibrinogen, factor VIII). Patients may die quickly of bleeding complications (e.g., intracranial hemorrhage) unless their DIC is promptly recognized and treatment of the hemorrhagic diathesis promptly instituted.

Vaginal rhabdomyosarcoma characteristically presents as a glistening membranous polypoid tumor that extrudes from the vaginal orifice. Its appearance resembles a cluster of grapes.

Patients with the Hand-Schüller-Christian disease form of histiocytosis X may have infiltration of the posterior pituitary gland, which causes decreased antidiuretic hormone production. As a consequence, these patients develop diabetes insipidus.

# 16
# Endocrine and
# Metabolic Disorders
Susan K. Ratzan

## I. DISORDERS OF CARBOHYDRATE METABOLISM

**A. Diabetes mellitus** is a heterogeneous group of disorders characterized by hyperglycemia and abnormal energy metabolism, which is due to absent or diminished insulin secretion or action at the cellular level. **Insulin-dependent diabetes mellitus (IDDM), type I,** is the most common endocrine-metabolic disease in childhood, occurring in 1 in 500 children and adolescents. **Noninsulin-dependent diabetes mellitus (NIDDM), type II,** also occurs in childhood, but is much less frequently diagnosed because of its milder or absent symptoms. Diabetes mellitus may be associated with other diseases or syndromes, such as cystic fibrosis, Prader-Willi syndrome, and Werner syndrome. A rare, usually transient form of IDDM may be seen in the newborn.

**1. IDDM**

    **a. Etiology.** Although the precise etiology of IDDM is unknown, the pathologic process that ultimately results in the loss of insulin secretion by the beta cells in the islets of Langerhans has been related to genetic, autoimmune, and environmental factors.

        **(1) Genetic factors**

            **(a)** There is an increased frequency of certain histocompatibility antigens [i.e., human leukocyte antigens (HLAs) DR3 and DR4] among individuals with IDDM. When both DR3 and DR4 are inherited, the relative risk of developing IDDM is additive.

            **(b)** There is an increased incidence of IDDM among first-degree relatives; 2%–5% of siblings and offspring will develop IDDM. Concordance for identical twins is 40%–50%.

        **(2) Autoimmune factors.** Evidence for an autoimmune basis for the disease consists of the presence of circulating islet cell antibodies in the serum of over 85% of individuals with recent-onset IDDM and the increased appearance of the other autoimmune diseases (e.g., Hashimoto's thyroiditis, Addison's disease, celiac disease) in children with IDDM.

        **(3) Environmental factors.** The role of environmental factors in the pathogenesis of IDDM is less well understood. Although viruses have long been suspected to play a role, it is unlikely that a single virus is directly responsible for the development of the disease in all cases.

    **b. Pathophysiology**

        **(1)** When 90% of the functioning beta cells have been destroyed, loss of insulin secretion becomes clinically significant. With the loss of insulin, the major anabolic hormone, a catabolic state develops, which is characterized by **decreased glucose utilization and increased glucose production** via gluconeogenesis and glycogenolysis, leading to **hyperglycemia.** In the state of insulin deficiency, levels of counter-regulatory hormones (i.e., glucagon, epinephrine, growth hormone, and cortisol) are elevated. These hormones stimulate lipolysis, fatty acid release, and ketoacid production.

        **(2)** When the blood glucose concentration is persistently above the renal threshold for glucose reabsorption (i.e., 180 mg/dl), the resultant **glucosuria** causes an osmotic diuresis with increased urine output and increased fluid intake. Ketones are produced in abundant amounts when insulin deficiency is severe. If insulin treatment is not initiated, **diabetic ketoacidosis** ensues. This deranged metabolic state is characterized by hyperglycemia, metabolic acidosis (ketoacidosis), dehydration, and lethargy, which may progress to coma and death.

    **c. Clinical features.** Although IDDM may present at any age, the most common time is in early adolescence. Typically, the child develops frequent urination (**polyuria**) and increased thirst (**polydipsia**). Symptoms may wax and wane for a period of days or weeks but eventually become constant. Nocturia or enuresis may occur. If the disease is not discovered, significant **weight loss** may result, and with increasing insulin deficiency, the odor of ketones on the breath may be noted. Nausea, abdominal pain, and vomiting are symptoms of **diabetic ketoacidosis** and result in severe **dehydration**.

    **d. Diagnosis** of IDDM in a child with polyuria, polydipsia, and glucosuria who is otherwise well rests on **documentation of hyperglycemia.**

        **(1)** A **random blood glucose level** greater than 200 mg/dl, which is verified on a repeat test, is sufficient to make the diagnosis of IDDM.

        **(2)** Early in the course of the disease, glucosuria and hyperglycemia may be transient. In this situation, a **fasting and 2-hour postmeal blood glucose** measurement may be helpful in making the diagnosis, if the fasting glucose level is higher than 140 mg/dl and the 2-hour glucose level is higher than 200 mg/dl. The presence of islet cell antibodies in the serum, increased levels of glycosylated hemoglobin, a family history of IDDM, or all three features may increase suspicion of developing IDDM. However, absence of these features does not rule out IDDM.

        **(3)** A standard oral glucose tolerance test is not indicated if fasting hyperglycemia is present or if a random or 2-hour postmeal glucose level is higher than 200 mg/dl.

    **e. Therapy.** The immediate goal of treatment is to **restore fluid and electrolyte losses,** either orally or intravenously, depending on the severity of the illness, and to **reverse the catabolic state** by replacing insulin.

        **(1) Insulin replacement**

            **(a) Dosage.** The usual insulin-dependent child or adolescent requires 0.75–1.0 U/kg of insulin daily when the diabetes is fully developed. However, early in the course of the disease, the requirement may be less than 0.5 U/kg/day, especially during the "honeymoon," or remission, phase of IDDM. For this reason, the initial dose should be tailored to the estimated degree of insulin deficiency and calculated for the child's weight (i.e., a ketonuric child or one who initially presented with ketoacidosis should be given 0.5 U/kg/day after the ketoacidosis is cleared).

                **(i)** The total daily dose is divided between short-acting regular insulin and intermediate-acting [isophane insulin suspension (NPH) or Lente] insulin in 1:3 proportion. It is conventional to give two-thirds of the daily dose before breakfast and one-third before the evening meal.

                **(ii)** Recently, many physicians have begun to treat all children with a split-dose regimen from the onset of the disease in an attempt to maintain better 24-hour blood glucose control.

                **(iii)** More intensive insulin replacement plans consist of multiple (3–4) doses of regular insulin before meals supplemented with intermediate-acting insulin once or twice daily.

            **(b) Source.** Most children with IDDM now receive human insulin as opposed to insulin derived from animal sources (beef/pork or pork). Human insulin is less immunogenic than animal-source insulin. However, the advantages of the lower titer of insulin antibodies remain to be proven.

        **(2) Diet.** The principles of sound nutritional practices are the basis for diet and meal-planning for children with IDDM.

            **(a)** A meal plan that promotes normal growth and weight gain, that incorporates the prudent recommendations of the American Heart Association concerning fat intake, and that encourages high-fiber foods is appropriate. The American Diabetes Association Exchange Diet incorporates these healthful practices and provides consistency in type and distribution of calories throughout the day while allowing flexibility of food choices.

            **(b)** Since food intake must match the time course of insulin absorption, meals and snacks must be roughly equivalent in calories from day to day and must be eaten on time. During and following periods of heavy exercise, increased food intake may be required to avoid hypoglycemia.

        **(3) Exercise.** Children with IDDM should be encouraged to exercise regularly. Since strenuous exercise may result in hypoglycemia due to increased noninsulin-dependent uptake of glucose, physical education classes are best scheduled after meals or extra food should be eaten before exercise. There should be no restrictions on individual or organized athletic programs because of IDDM.

**(4) Patient education.** Children with IDDM and their families should be taught the principles of home management by trained diabetes educators. This training should be individualized and include the pathophysiology of diabetes in lay language, the techniques of insulin injection and home blood glucose monitoring, the recognition and treatment of hypoglycemia and hyperglycemia, the significance of ketonuria, and the management of diabetes during intercurrent illness. Eventually, the child and family should learn how to make minor insulin dose changes. Education is an ongoing process, and periodic reinforcement of home management is important as the child grows older and more independent of his family.

**(5) Psychological support and counseling.** The diagnosis of IDDM arouses strong emotional responses in the child and in family members, including grief, anger, guilt, resentment, and fear. Although these responses are normal, adjustment to the disease is facilitated by open discussion of these emotions.

**(6) Medical follow-up.** Regular follow-up visits every 3–4 months to a pediatrician with expertise in diabetes or to a regional pediatric diabetes program are indicated.

  **(a)** The glycosylated hemoglobin level should be measured as an objective index of blood glucose control over the preceding 2 months, and lipid levels should be measured periodically.

  **(b)** Because of the increased risk of autoimmune thyroid disease in children with IDDM, periodic assessment of thyroid function, including thyroxine level, $T_3$ resin uptake, thyroid-stimulating hormone (TSH) levels, and thyroid autoantibody determination, should be carried out (see III A 2).

  **(c)** Although long-term complications of diabetes are rare in children, blood pressure measurement and funduscopic examination should be performed during each visit.

  **(d)** For adolescents who have had diabetes for more than 5 years, a more rigorous examination for retinopathy, nephropathy, and neuropathy should be carried out.

**f. Complications** of IDDM may be divided into **immediate complications,** which include hypoglycemia and diabetic ketoacidosis, and **late complications,** which are those generally associated with a long duration of IDDM.

**(1) Hypoglycemia (insulin reaction)**

  **(a) Symptoms** of hypoglycemia may be related to sympathetic discharge (e.g., sweating, tremulousness, hunger) and should be readily recognizable by the child or family. More severe symptoms (e.g., lethargy, bizarre behavior, slurred speech, unconsciousness, seizures) are caused by glucose deprivation to the central nervous system (CNS). This may occur in combination with sympathetic symptoms or alone.

  **(b) Therapy** should be aimed at raising the blood glucose level above 100 mg/dl. The child should consume 4 oz of calorie-containing drink or food if she is able to swallow. When neuroglycopenic symptoms occur, the child needs assistance in treatment of the hypoglycemia episode. If the child is unconscious or having seizures, 1 mg of glucagon should be injected intramuscularly.

**(2) Diabetic ketoacidosis** is caused by relative or absolute insulin deficiency, which results in **hyperglycemia** and **metabolic acidosis with respiratory compensation**. This condition of accelerated catabolism is abetted by increased levels of glucagon, epinephrine, growth hormone (GH), and cortisol, which accelerate the rate of lipolysis and ketoacid production. The most common cause of diabetic ketoacidosis in a known diabetic is **omission of insulin doses**. The condition may be triggered by intercurrent illness, which may be associated with some degree of insulin resistance.

  **(a) Symptoms** are polyuria, polydipsia, fatigue, headache, dry mouth, nausea, abdominal pain, and vomiting. Lethargy may progress to obtundation and coma.

  **(b) Physical findings** include tachycardia and hyperpnea (Kussmaul's respiration), the respiratory compensation for metabolic acidosis; hypotension indicates marked dehydration and intravascular volume depletion. The child appears acutely ill, anxious, and dehydrated. The abdomen is mildly tender but without rebound or localized tenderness. Bowel sounds may be diminished. Physical examination must rule out intercurrent illness or infection.

  **(c) Laboratory studies** should include a complete blood count and determination of electrolyte, glucose, blood urea nitrogen (BUN), and creatinine levels and, in more severe illness, arterial blood gas determination.

(i) The hemoglobin and hematocrit usually are increased because of hemoconcentration. The white cell count may show marked leukocytosis (> 20,000), with a predominance of neutrophils and immature forms as a result of the metabolic stress.

(ii) The serum sodium level usually is low or normal. A low serum sodium level may be caused by dilution from the osmotic effect of marked hyperglycemia (i.e., a glucose level > 700 mg/dl) or "pseudohyponatremia," an artifact of measurement if the patient's serum is lipemic.

(iii) The serum potassium level usually is normal or high and does not reflect total body potassium depletion. A low serum potassium level (< 3.5 mEq/L) indicates profound potassium depletion and potential for life-threatening hypokalemia during the early course of treatment of diabetic ketoacidosis.

(iv) The bicarbonate level is low, ranging from 2 to 19 mEq/L, depending on the severity and duration of the illness.

(v) The BUN level may be considerably elevated on the basis of prerenal azotemia; the serum creatinine level is normal or minimally elevated.

(vi) Arterial blood gases indicate metabolic acidosis with respiratory compensation; pH typically is 6.9–7.3. Oxygen partial pressure ($Po_2$) is greater than 95 mm Hg (normal); carbon dioxide partial pressure ($Pco_2$) is less than 30 mm Hg (low) as the patient blows off carbon dioxide in an attempt to buffer the metabolic acid.

(d) **Therapy** should be carried out in an intensive care unit with frequent monitoring of the vital signs, neurologic status, and fluid input and output. If the patient is not alert, a nasogastric tube should be placed to empty stomach contents and prevent aspiration.

(i) The first aim of therapy is to replace fluids and electrolytes and to reexpand the vascular volume. The latter may be accomplished by an infusion of 10–20 ml/kg of normal saline over 2 hours.

(ii) The next consideration is insulin replacement. For all patients except those with mild diabetic ketoacidosis (i.e., a bicarbonate level > 15 mEq/L), continuous infusion of intravenous regular (crystalline) insulin is the most easily controlled and predictable. A priming intravenous dose of 0.1 U/kg of regular insulin is immediately followed by 0.1 U/kg/hr of regular insulin.

(iii) After the initial bolus of normal saline has been infused, half normal saline at a rate of one and one-half to twice the maintenance rate usually is adequate to begin to replace deficits. To this solution, 5%–10% dextrose should be added to maintain the blood glucose level between 200 and 300 mg/dl.

(iv) Vigorous replacement of potassium, using 40 mEq/L of potassium chloride should begin as soon as urine output is established and the serum potassium level is less than 5 mEq/L.

(v) Correction of the acidosis with bicarbonate is controversial. Rapid infusion of bicarbonate is contraindicated because it may cause deterioration of neurologic function and depression of cerebrospinal fluid (CSF) pH. In severe diabetic ketoacidosis (pH < 7.10), bicarbonate may be given over a period of 4 hours for partial correction of the acidosis.

(e) **Complications of diabetic ketoacidosis** include hypoglycemia, hypokalemia, and cerebral edema, which, although rare, is frequently fatal. A worsening mental status, confusion, unequal pupils, decerebrate posture, or seizures indicate cerebral edema. Early recognition and aggressive treatment to decrease intracranial pressure are associated with an improved outcome.

(3) **Late complications of IDDM.** There is increasing evidence that the long-term complications of diabetes have a metabolic basis. Proving the relationship of blood glucose control to complications of diabetes is an area of active research investigation.

(a) Complications associated with a long duration (i.e., > 10 years) of IDDM include **microvascular disease** of the eye (**retinopathy**), the kidney (**nephropathy**), and the nerves (**neuropathy**). These problems may be seen in the older adolescent patient.

(b) The other major category of late complications is **large vessel atherosclerotic complications,** leading to premature myocardial infarction and stroke.

g. **Future directions of research in IDDM** include development of an implantable insulin pump, islet cell and whole pancreas transplantation, immunotherapy for diabetes prevention, and an improved understanding of the genetic and environmental factors in IDDM.

2. **NIDDM** occurs in children and adolescents, but because it is **usually asymptomatic,** it is infrequently diagnosed. In some families, NIDDM appears to be inherited as an autosomal dominant trait.
   a. **Etiology.** NIDDM is caused by insulin deficiency that is more modest than that in IDDM and occasionally by resistance to insulin action, with normal or increased insulin secretion but decreased insulin receptors.
   b. **Therapy** consists of **maintenance of normal body weight.** Insulin treatment is indicated if there is fasting hyperglycemia (i.e., a glucose concentration > 140 mg/dl). Oral hypoglycemic agents generally are not used in children and adolescents.

B. **Hypoglycemia.** A variety of conditions and disease states may disrupt glucose homeostasis and result in hypoglycemia. Certain causes of hypoglycemia are more common at some ages than at others. This knowledge provides a useful way of approaching and understanding hypoglycemia in infancy and childhood.

   1. **Glucose homeostasis.** Blood glucose is the major energy source for all tissues, and maintenance of normal glucose homeostasis is critical for efficient energy metabolism. Glucose homeostasis depends on the interplay of endocrine and metabolic or enzymatic processes that control glucose uptake and utilization as well as on glucose production during periods of feeding and fasting to assure a continuous supply.
      a. Blood glucose in the fetus is dependent on transplacental passage of maternal glucose and substrate reserves. At birth, the newborn is abruptly cut off from the maternal supply of glucose and is dependent on oral intake of calories and his own endocrine and metabolic function for maintenance of normal glucose levels.
      b. During the adjustment to extrauterine life, blood glucose levels are somewhat lower without apparent ill effects. Premature infants and infants with a low birth weight have slightly lower blood glucose levels than full-term infants.
      c. There is disagreement over the definition of hypoglycemia in infants and children and whether low blood glucose level is "normal" for premature infants. Thus, it is prudent to initiate therapy for any infant with a blood glucose below 40 mg/dl and to monitor closely any infant with a blood glucose of 40–50 mg/dl.

   2. **Hypoglycemia in the newborn** has a varied presentation. Newborn symptoms may include jitteriness, pallor, cyanosis, apnea, a poor sucking reflex, hypotonia, and seizures.
      a. **Transient hypoglycemia** is a relatively mild form of hypoglycemia occurring in newborns known to be at risk for hypoglycemia in the first 24–48 hours of life.
         (1) **Etiology.** High-risk groups include premature infants, infants who are small for gestational age, infants of diabetic mothers, and infants with perinatal asphyxia.
         (2) **Clinical features and diagnosis.** Hypoglycemia may be asymptomatic, detected only on routine screening, or symptomatic.
         (3) **Therapy.** Whereas asymptomatic hypoglycemia can be managed by the institution of feedings, symptomatic hypoglycemia should be treated with intravenous glucose infusion.
         (4) **Prognosis** for these infants is excellent.
      b. **Severe or recurrent hypoglycemia.** If the newborn requires continuous intravenous glucose for more than 48 hours, a single blood sample drawn at the time of hypoglycemia should be analyzed for: glucose, insulin, GH, cortisol, thyroid hormone, and TSH. The glucose response to glucagon injection may also be helpful, which is noted 15 and 30 minutes after an intramuscular injection of 0.03 mg/kg (up to 1.0 mg).
         (1) **Hyperinsulinism**
            (a) **Etiology and pathogenesis.** The etiology of hyperinsulinism is unclear. Rarely is there a discrete area of hyperplasia or an islet cell adenoma. Nesidioblastosis, a disorganized scattering of beta cells outside the islets of Langerhans, has been described frequently in the surgically removed pancreas. However, its significance in the pathogenesis of hyperinsulinism is in question.
            (b) **Clinical features and diagnosis.** Infants with hyperinsulinism are normal or above normal in weight. Insulin levels at the time of hypoglycemia are inappropriately elevated, usually higher than 12 μU/ml when the glucose level is less than 40 mg/dl.

(c) **Therapy.** These infants require large amounts of intravenous glucose. Treatment with oral diazoxide 10–15 mg/kg in 3 divided doses may ameliorate symptoms. Recently, some children have been treated with an injectable analogue of somatostatin, which inhibits insulin release. Children who cannot be managed medically require near-total (90%–95%) pancreatectomy.

(d) **Prognosis** for normal neurologic development is guarded. It does appear to correlate with the severity and duration of recurrent hypoglycemia. Thus, appropriate monitoring and aggressive treatment to normalize the blood glucose level are indicated.

(2) **Congenital hypopituitarism**

(a) **Clinical features.** Affected infants are of normal birth weight and may have associated midline defects, such as optic nerve hypoplasia and absence of the septum pellucidum (septo-optic dysplasia), and microphallus. They also have prolonged neonatal jaundice.

(b) **Diagnosis.** At the time of hypoglycemia, GH and cortisol levels are inappropriately low. Infants may also have low $T_4$ with normal TSH levels. Hypoglycemia resolves with replacement of thyroid hormone, steroids, and GH; however, deficiency of vasopressin (diabetes insipidus) may be unmasked after replacement therapy with thyroid hormone and cortisol.

(c) **Therapy.** Diabetes insipidus may be treated with a diluted solution of desmopressin (dDAVP) given 1μg intranasally every 12 hours. Untreated congenital hypopituitarism is frequently fatal in the newborn period. Replacement therapy is lifesaving.

(d) **Prognosis** for neurologic development is uncertain. Neurologic development may be impaired by associated CNS malformation.

3. **Hypoglycemia in infants and children.** Hypoglycemia beyond the neonatal period is quite rare. Hyperinsulinism, GH deficiency, hypocortisolism secondary to **adrenocorticotropic hormone (ACTH) deficiency,** and primary adrenal insufficiency (**Addison's disease**) may present as symptomatic hypoglycemia. Certain hepatic enzyme deficiencies, which result in impaired glycogenolysis or gluconeogenesis, may present during infancy as profound metabolic acidosis, ketonuria, and hypoglycemia. These deficiencies include glycogen storage disease types I, III, and IV; hereditary fructose intolerance; fructose 1,6-diphosphatase deficiency; and galactosemia. The presence of marked hepatomegaly with failure to thrive and hypotonia should suggest one of these defects; the actual diagnosis may require liver biopsy for assay of the specific enzyme. In children age 1–4 years, the most common cause of hypoglycemia is ketotic hypoglycemia.

a. **Ketotic hypoglycemia.** The typical child with this form of hypoglycemia is a toddler who has had one or more episodes of early morning lethargy, pallor, and sweating, with or without a seizure. The blood glucose level during an episode is lower than 40 mg/dl. Large amounts of ketones are present in the urine. The child is otherwise well. Episodes are associated with a decreased intake of food due to intercurrent illness.

(1) **Etiology.** Ketotic hypoglycemia appears to be due to a diminished tolerance for normal fasting. At the point of hypoglycemia, infusion of alanine (the major gluconeogenic substrate) results in prompt elevation of the blood glucose level, implying normal gluconeogenic mechanisms. GH and cortisol levels are high, and insulin levels are appropriately low. Glucose response to injected glucagon is minimal. This has been postulated to be an exaggeration of the limited ability of children to tolerate prolonged fasting compared to adults, perhaps related to smaller muscle mass, which limits substrate availability.

(2) **Diagnosis** is best made by monitoring blood glucose throughout a 24-hour fast. If the blood glucose level falls below 40 mg/dl, additional blood for insulin, glucose, cortisol, and GH measurement is obtained as well as urine for ketone bodies. The fast should be terminated when the blood glucose level is below 40 mg/dl with a glucagon tolerance test (i.e., glucagon is administered intramuscularly at 0.03 mg/kg, up to 1.0 mg, with the blood glucose level checked at 15 and 30 minutes).

(3) **Therapy** is avoidance of fasting by eating small meals frequently, up to six times daily. Monitoring urine for ketone bodies during intercurrent illness may be helpful in alerting to symptoms of hypoglycemia. Symptoms generally disappear after the age of 6–8 years.

    **b. Hyperinsulinism.** In the older child and adolescent, hyperinsulinism may present as erratic episodes of unpredictable or bizarre behavior, loss of consciousness, or seizures.

        **(1) Etiology.** As opposed to the neonate or young infant with hyperinsulinism due to a diffuse functional process, in the older child, a functioning islet cell adenoma may be found.

        **(2) Diagnosis** may be reached by monitoring the blood glucose level on a 24-hour fast. The child usually becomes hypoglycemic in 6–12 hours. Ketone bodies are not present in the urine, and the glucose response to glucagon is brisk. Insulin levels are inappropriately and sometimes markedly elevated during hypoglycemia.

        **(3) Therapy.** The tumor may be localized by arteriography. Surgical excision is curative.

    **c. Nonhypoglycemia.** Occasionally, parents relate concern about hypoglycemia as a cause of hyperactivity, inattentiveness at school, headache, and low energy. If clinical suspicion is low, documentation of the blood glucose level when symptoms are present may persuade parents that hypoglycemia is not present. If parental concern is great, a 24-hour fast documents normal fasting ability. There is little substantiation that reactive hypoglycemia is a defined entity in children. Oral glucose tolerance testing is not helpful in the evaluation of children with hypoglycemia.

**II. HYPERLIPIDEMIC DISORDERS.** Identification of hypercholesterolemia as a major risk factor for the development of coronary heart disease has focused attention on the diagnosis and treatment of lipid abnormalities. Recent evidence demonstrates that lowering the serum cholesterol level in adults reduces the risk for subsequent coronary morbidity. This information, as well as the recognition that atherosclerotic lesions can be identified in children and adolescents, has prompted a more aggressive approach to the diagnosis and treatment of hyperlipidemia in children.

    **A. General considerations**

        **1. Normal lipoprotein metabolism.** Cholesterol and triglyceride are transported in blood in particles called lipoproteins. There are **four major classes of lipoproteins,** which are classified according to density and electrophoretic mobility.

        **a. Chylomicrons** are large, triglyceride-rich particles produced in the intestine by dietary fat and cleared by the action of lipoprotein lipase.

        **b. Very low-density lipoproteins (VLDLs)** are rich in triglyceride and are synthesized in the liver and catabolized to low-density lipoproteins.

        **c. Low-density lipoproteins (LDLs)** are rich in cholesterol. LDLs must bind to specific LDL receptors to be taken into cells and degraded.

        **d. High-density lipoproteins (HDLs)** contain cholesterol and are synthesized from chylomicrons and VLDLs directly in the liver and intestine. A high HDL cholesterol level conveys low risk of coronary heart disease.

        **2. Identification of individuals with hyperlipidemia** depends on the measurement of fasting total cholesterol, triglyceride, and HDL cholesterol levels. Elevated LDL cholesterol and low HDL cholesterol are associated with increased cardiovascular risk. LDL cholesterol may be calculated as

$$\text{LDL cholesterol} = \text{total cholesterol} - \left( \text{HDL cholesterol} + \frac{\text{triglyceride}}{5} \right)$$

        **a.** The definition of normal lipid levels depends on the reference population and the amount of saturated fat and cholesterol in the diet. In children in the United States, the mean and ninety-fifth percentile for total cholesterol are 160 and 200 mg/dl, respectively, and the mean and ninety-fifth percentile for triglyceride are 75 and 120 mg/dl, respectively.

        **b.** Although triglyceride levels rise slowly with age, cholesterol levels are relatively constant throughout childhood and adolescence, and the differences between the sexes are not of practical significance.

        **3. Screening children for hyperlipidemia.** Because of increased interest in preventive medicine and proven cardiac benefit of reducing serum cholesterol in adults, there has been increasing interest in identifying children at risk. Although mass screening programs for hyperlipidemia in children have not been instituted, it is advisable to screen all children with a family history of hyperlipidemia or premature heart disease. For children with milder elevation of total cholesterol levels (200–250 mg/dl), a low-cholesterol, low-fat diet and identification of and counseling about reducing other risk factors (e.g., smoking, hypertension, obesity) are recommended.

**B. Primary hyperlipidemias.** Primary disorders of lipid metabolism are a heterogeneous group of genetically determined diseases. The expression of the diseases may be affected by diet, obesity, diabetes, or other environmental factors. Certain types of primary hyperlipidemias predispose affected individuals to premature atherosclerosis and others to pancreatitis or neurologic sequelae, usually in adulthood. Although five separate subtypes (i.e., subtypes I, II, III, IV, and V) were described in the past, it is more useful clinically to separate the hyperlipidemias by which fraction, or fractions, are elevated.

1. **Familial hypercholesterolemia.** Marked elevation of total and LDL cholesterol levels with normal triglyceride levels is the **most common genetic hyperlipidemia in childhood**. It is inherited as an autosomal codominant trait and occurs in about 1 in 500 individuals.

   a. **Pathogenesis**
      (1) The **heterozygous form** is associated with a total cholesterol level usually higher than 300 mg/dl and a high risk of coronary heart disease by the age of 30–40 years. These individuals have approximately a 50% reduction in LDL receptor activity.
      (2) The **homozygous form** is associated with a total cholesterol level of 600–1000 mg/dl. In this rare condition, myocardial infarction in the first decade of life and death by the age of 20 years is common. This disorder is caused by a total deficiency of LDL receptors, which prevent uptake and catabolism of LDL cholesterol.

   b. **Therapy**
      (1) Treatment of the **heterozygous form** of familial hypercholesterolemia in children consists of a **strict diet** low in cholesterol and total fat and an increased polyunsaturated-to-saturated fat ratio. Adherence to the diet may result in a 10%–15% reduction in the LDL cholesterol level. If the cholesterol remains above 300 mg/dl, the addition of cholestyramine or colestipol (bile acid–binding resins that remove cholesterol from the enterohepatic circulation) is safe and efficacious. Lovastatin, a new drug that inhibits cholesterol biosynthesis, has shown promising results in adults. There is little or no experience with other lipid-lowering drugs in children, and, therefore, they are not recommended.
      (2) The **homozygous form** of familial hypercholesterolemia is **very resistant to treatment** since there is virtually a total absence of LDL receptors in affected patients. Some lowering of the cholesterol level may be achieved by repeated exchange transfusion, portocaval shunting, or liver transplantation.

2. **Familial combined hyperlipidemia (elevated cholesterol and triglycerides).** This combination is more common than previously recognized in children and appears to be dominantly inherited. Adults have premature coronary artery disease and peripheral vascular disease.

3. **Mild to moderate hypertriglyceridemia.** This pattern of hyperlipidemia also is rarely found in children. In adults, it has been associated with obesity, glucose intolerance, and hyperuricemia, and it may be aggravated by alcohol ingestion and some drugs.

4. **Severe hypertriglyceridemia.** In children and adolescents, elevation of fasting triglyceride levels over 1000 mg/dl may be caused by familial deficiency of lipoprotein lipase, which results in hyperchylomicronemia. This may result in recurrent pancreatitis, hepatosplenomegaly, and eruptive xanthomas. Treatment consists of severe restriction of dietary fat. Severe hypertriglyceridemia secondary to elevation of both chylomicron and VLDL levels is rare in children.

**C. Secondary hyperlipidemia.** Hypercholesterolemia may be secondary to hypothyroidism, nephrotic syndrome, diabetes, and liver disease, or it may be induced by a diet high in saturated fat and cholesterol. Elevated triglyceride levels may be present in poorly controlled diabetes, obesity, glycogen storage disease, and renal failure, or it may be secondary to use of certain drugs (e.g., oral contraceptives, thiazide diuretics, β blockers). In each of these instances, treatment is directed at the primary disease process, or the offending medication is removed.

## III. DISORDERS OF THE THYROID GLAND

**A. General considerations.** A good understanding of thyroid physiology and the assessment of thyroid function in children is necessary to recognize, diagnose, and treat thyroid disorders.

1. **Thyroid function.** Thyroid hormone is critical for normal postnatal somatic growth and neurologic development in infants and children.
   a. Thyroid hormone is essential for normal maturation of the CNS in children. Deficiency of thyroid hormone in the first 2 years of life may result in severe psychomotor retardation.

   **b.** Thyroid hormone is also necessary for normal skeletal growth and maturation in growing children. In both children and adults, it plays a major role in oxidative metabolism and heat production.

**2. Thyroid metabolism**
   **a. Synthesis. Iodide** absorbed from the intestine is trapped in the thyroid gland and is organically bound to **tyrosine** residues of thyroglobulin. Iodination of tyrosine forms **monoiodotyrosine (MIT)** and **diiodotyrosine (DIT),** which condense to form **thyroxine ($T_4$)** and **triiodothyronine ($T_3$).**
   **b. Feedback control.** Thyroid hormone synthesis is controlled by a negative feedback loop involving the CNS at the level of the hypothalamus and pituitary gland.
      **(1)** Low levels of circulating thyroid hormones stimulate hypothalamic release of **thyrotropin-releasing hormone (TRH),** which then stimulates production of **TSH** in the pituitary gland. TSH stimulates increased production of $T_4$ and $T_3$ by the thyroid gland.
      **(2) Circulation.** $T_4$ and $T_3$ circulate in plasma bound to thyroid-binding proteins—thyroxine-binding globulin (TBG) and thyroxine-binding prealbumin (TBPA). Protein-bound $T_4$ and $T_3$ account for over 99% of circulating thyroid hormones. The free (i.e., not protein-bound) $T_4$ and $T_3$ are the metabolically active forms of the hormone.

**3. Assessment of thyroid function** involves measurement of thyroid hormones and testing of thyroid responsiveness. The most commonly used tests are the following.
   **a. Radioimmunoassay** is used to measure the serum concentration of several hormones.
      **(1)** $T_4$ as measured by radioimmunoassay may be affected by processes that increase either fraction of $T_4$. For example, estrogen treatment stimulates production of TBG, thereby increasing the total $T_4$ by raising the $T_4$ bound to TBG. The free $T_4$ is normal, and the patient is, therefore, clinically euthyroid (i.e., the thyroid gland functions normally). Measurement of free $T_4$ is possible but usually not necessary for appropriate diagnosis.
      **(2)** $T_3$ as measured by radioimmunoassay is particularly useful in diagnosing hyperthyroidism.
      **(3) TBG** may be measured directly by radioimmunoassay.
      **(4) TSH** measurement by radioimmunoassay is valuable in the diagnosis of primary hypothyroidism (elevated TSH). In newer more sensitive assays, very low levels of circulating TSH can be distinguished from normal levels and may be supportive of a diagnosis of hyperthyroidism.
   **b. Thyroid gland imaging**
      **(1) Technetium 99m ($^{99m}$Tc) scanning** of the thyroid is the most commonly used thyroid imaging technique used in children.
         **(a)** $^{99m}$Tc is most useful for identification of areas of **decreased uptake of the radionuclide ("cold" nodules)** and for localization of ectopic thyroid tissue or absence of thyroid tissue.
         **(b)** $^{99m}$Tc is trapped only by the thyroid and has a half-life of only 6 hours; thus, it is not a great risk to the child.
      **(2) Ultrasonography** of the thyroid gland may be used for characterization of cystic lesions.
   **c.** $T_3$ **resin uptake** is a widely used test that is an indirect measure of the patient's thyroid-binding protein and, as such, is helpful in interpreting the effect of increased or decreased binding protein on the measurement of total $T_4$ (the test does not measure the patient's $T_3$). Radioactive $T_3$ is added to the patient's serum along with an insoluble binder of $T_3$, such as resin. Radioactive $T_3$ binds to unoccupied binding sites on the patient's binding proteins, and the remaining radioactive $T_3$ subsequently is bound to the resin added to the sample.
      **(1)** If the total $T_4$ is high because of an elevated protein-bound fraction (e.g., due to pregnancy or oral contraceptives), the $T_3$ resin uptake will be low.
      **(2)** Conversely, if the $T_4$ is low because of a low protein-bound fraction (e.g., due to congenital deficiency of TBG), the $T_3$ resin uptake will be high.
      **(3)** In hyperthyroidism, the $T_4$ (total $T_4$) and $T_3$ resin uptake are high. In hypothyroidism, the $T_4$ and $T_3$ resin uptake are low.
   **d. Free thyroxine index** is an estimate of free $T_4$, taking into account the patient's level of thyroid hormone-binding protein as measured by $T_3$ resin uptake. This test is a calculation, not a direct measurement, based on the total $T_4$ and $T_3$ uptake.
   **e. TRH stimulation test** measures the TSH response to an intravenous injection of TRH. Samples for TSH are measured before and every 15 minutes up to 1 hour after TRH injection.
      **(1)** Because of negative feedback suppression of $T_4$ on the pituitary thyrotroph, the TSH response to TRH is suppressed even in subtle hyperthyroidism.

**(2)** In hypothyroidism, the TSH response to TRH is increased. The test for hypothyroidism is more difficult to interpret than that for hyperthyroidism.

**f. Thyroid receptor antibody tests** measure a heterogeneous group of immunoglobulins that bind to the TSH receptor on thyroid cells and stimulate thyroid growth and function.

**(1)** Two types of tests have been recently developed.

**(a)** One measures **thyroid-stimulating immunoglobulins (TSI)**.

**(b)** The other test measures **thyrotropin-binding inhibition immunoglobulin (TBII)**.

**(2)** The presence of TBII and TSI correlates with disease activity in hyperthyroidism (Graves' disease) in childhood, and their measurement may be useful in predicting the likelihood of clinical remission.

**g. Radioactive iodine uptake** rarely is performed in children as a diagnostic test due to the high levels of radiation exposure. Iodine 123 ($^{123}$I) is preferred over $^{131}$I because of its shorter half-life and lower radiation dose.

**B. Hypothyroidism** may occur at birth (**congenital hypothyroidism**) or at any time during childhood or adolescence (**juvenile hypothyroidism**). Because of the importance of thyroid hormone for normal brain growth and development in the first 2 years of life, the clinical considerations are different for infants than for older children and adolescents.

**1. Congenital hypothyroidism,** unlike most thyroid diseases, affects males and females equally.

**a. Etiology**

**(1) Developmental thyroid defect** (thyroid agenesis or dysgenesis) is the primary cause of congenital hypothyroidism.

**(2) Defective biosynthesis of thyroid hormone** (frequently resulting in goiter) also may cause the disorder.

**(3) Transient congenital hypothyroidism** may occur as a result of transplacental passage of maternally ingested goitrogens (e.g., iodide expectorants, antithyroid drugs or maternal antithyroid antibodies).

**b. Clinical features.** Because thyroid hormone does not appear to be necessary for fetal growth, infants with congenital hypothyroidism are normal in size. The severity of symptoms and physical findings correlates with the degree of hypothyroidism.

**(1) Symptoms.** Although a newborn rarely may have some physical features of hypothyroidism in the first week of life, usually it is not apparent. Often the first symptom is **prolonged neonatal jaundice.** Other symptoms that develop in the first 1–2 months of life are feeding problems, lethargy, and constipation.

**(2) Physical findings** are coarse facies with large, open fontanelles; large, protruding tongue; hoarse cry; umbilical hernia; cool, dry, mottled skin; hypotonia; and delayed development.

**(3) Severe manifestations.** Severe congenital hypothyroidism is characterized by short limbs, epiphyseal dysgenesis, impaired physical growth and development, and mental retardation.

**c. Diagnosis**

**(1)** The diagnosis of congenital hypothyroidism is made by documenting decreased serum concentrations of total $T_4$, decreased $T_3$ resin uptake, and elevated serum concentrations of TSH.

**(2)** Assessment of skeletal age (e.g., by knee x-ray) may show retardation of skeletal maturation to less than 36 weeks gestation, suggesting intrauterine hypothyroidism.

**(3)** A $^{99m}$Tc thyroid scan prior to initiating therapy may be helpful in ascertaining the etiology of congenital hypothyroidism, which may have prognostic and genetic implications.

**(a)** Absence of $^{99m}$Tc uptake indicates thyroid agenesis.

**(b)** Increased $^{99m}$Tc uptake in a normally positioned gland implies an enzymatic defect in thyroid hormone production.

**(c)** An ectopic gland is demonstrated by abnormal localization of $^{99m}$Tc uptake.

**d. Therapy**

**(1)** Thyroid hormone replacement, using synthetic L-thyroxine as a single daily oral dose, should be instituted after confirming blood tests are drawn. The dosage for infants is approximately 10 μg/kg. As the child grows, the dosage is adjusted to maintain the serum $T_4$ in the high-normal range (10–14 μg/dl).

**(2) Follow-up.** Growth and neurologic development are evaluated at regular follow-up visits every 2–3 months in the first 2 years, with somewhat less frequent follow-up visits after 2 years of age.

    **e. Prognosis.** When the diagnosis of congenital hypothyroidism is delayed beyond 3 months of age, a high proportion of children suffer **permanent neurologic impairment**.

    **f. Screening.** Since congenital hypothyroidism is a relatively common problem (occurring in 1 in 4000 births) and because it was expected that early recognition, before clinical suspicion was aroused, might prevent neurologic sequelae, techniques for mass screening for hypothyroidism were developed in the 1970s. Neonatal screening for hypothyroidism has become widely applied. The results from follow-up of children diagnosed through neonatal screening by 1 month of age indicate that neurologic function and intelligence are normal when compared to those of their siblings. Screening also enables genetic counseling for families of children with less common familial forms of congenital hypothyroidism (i.e., dyshormonogenesis).

**2. Juvenile (acquired) hypothyroidism.** When symptoms appear after the first year of life, hypothyroidism is presumed to be acquired. Juvenile hypothyroidism is more common in girls than in boys, as are most thyroid diseases.

    **a. Etiology**

        **(1)** The most common cause of juvenile hypothyroidism is **autoimmune destruction** of the thyroid secondary to chronic lymphocytic thyroiditis (Hashimoto's thyroiditis).

        **(2)** Other causes include ectopic thyroid dysgenesis, goitrogens (e.g., iodide cough syrup, antithyroid drugs), and surgical or radioactive iodine ablation for treatment of hyperthyroidism.

    **b. Clinical features**

        **(1) Symptoms.** Slow linear growth is the hallmark of hypothyroidism in childhood. Puberty usually is delayed although occasionally may be paradoxically precocious. Other symptoms include cold intolerance, small appetite, lethargy, and constipation. School performance usually is not impaired, and behavior problems are rare.

        **(2) Physical findings.** Affected children may have coarse, puffy facies with a flattened nasal bridge; immature body proportions; stocky habitus; paucity of speech and spontaneous movement; dull, dry, thin hair; and rough, dry skin with a pale, waxy hue. Deep tendon reflexes show delayed relaxation time ("hung" reflexes).

    **c. Diagnosis**

        **(1)** The diagnosis is made on the basis of documentation of decreased serum concentrations of total $T_4$, decreased $T_3$ resin uptake, and elevated serum concentrations of TSH.

        **(2)** Skeletal maturation may be markedly delayed and indicates the duration of hypothyroidism.

        **(3)** The presence of circulating thyroid autoantibodies implies an autoimmune basis for the disease.

        **(4)** A $^{99m}$Tc thyroid scan is not indicated unless there are irregularities in thyroid consistency on palpation. In that case, a scan looking for a thyroid nodule would be appropriate.

    **d. Therapy**

        **(1)** Thyroid hormone replacement therapy is begun with synthetic L-thyroxine, approximately 3–5 μg/kg as a single daily oral dose. The adequacy of replacement can be judged by measurement of serum $T_4$ and TSH, which should be in the normal range.

        **(2)** Transient deterioration of school performance and behavior as the child adjusts to newfound energy levels is common.

    **e. Prognosis**

        **(1)** Unless hypothyroidism develops around the time of puberty when skeletal maturation is nearly complete, the prognosis for catch-up growth is good. However, there is some evidence that some children may not reach their genetic potential for growth. Other signs and symptoms resolve completely.

        **(2)** Children with autoimmune hypothyroidism are at increased risk for other associated autoimmune diseases, such as diabetes mellitus and adrenal insufficiency (Schmidt syndrome). Children with Down syndrome have an increased incidence of hypothyroidism and hyperthyroidism.

## C. Hyperthyroidism

**1. Etiology**

    **a. Graves' disease** (thyrotoxicosis), or hyperthyroidism secondary to diffuse thyroid hyperplasia (diffuse toxic goiter), is the most common cause of hyperthyroidism. It is an autoimmune thyroid disorder in which enlargement and hyperfunction of the thyroid gland may be stimulated by circulating immunoglobulins, particularly abnormal immunoglobulin G (IgG), a thyroid-stimulating immunoglobulin that binds to thyrotropin receptors on thyroid cells. The increased levels of free $T_4$ suppress TSH to undetectable levels. Thus, thyroid hyperfunction is not TSH dependent.

**b. Neonatal Graves' disease.** Neonatal hyperthyroidism is thought to be caused by transplacental passage of thyroid-stimulating immunoglobulins (i.e., IgG).

**c. Other etiologies** for hyperthyroidism in children are rare but include hyperfunctioning "hot" thyroid nodule and acute suppurative thyroiditis.

**2. Epidemiology.** Girls are more commonly affected than boys (in a ratio of 4:1), and there often is a family history of Graves' disease or Hashimoto's thyroiditis. The usual age at presentation is adolescence; it is unusual before age 5 years.

**3. Clinical features**

**a. Symptoms.** The onset of symptoms is insidious, and emotional lability, increased appetite, heat intolerance, weight loss, frequent loose stools, deterioration of behavior and school performance, and poor sleeping are the most common symptoms. Weakness and inability to participate in sports sometimes are noted.

**b. Physical findings.** On physical examination, the child appears fidgety, flushed, and warm. Marked tachycardia, fever, diaphoresis, nausea, and vomiting indicate **thyroid storm,** which is a sudden exacerbation of symptoms.

(1) Proptosis and widened palpebral fissures may be present.

(2) The thyroid gland usually is diffusely enlarged, smooth, firm but not hard, and nontender.

(3) The precordium is hyperactive, and resting tachycardia and widened pulse pressure are present.

(4) The skin is velvety smooth, warm, flushed, and moist.

(5) A fine tremor of outstretched fingers may be seen. Proximal muscle weakness may be present.

**c. Graves' ophthalmopathy** is caused by lymphocytic infiltration of the conjunctiva, extraocular eye muscles, and retrobulbar soft tissue and may cause redness and edema of the conjunctiva, decreased mobility of the eye, and proptosis. Its course may not follow that of hyperthyroidism. Most of the 60% of children who have some evidence of ophthalmopathy experience mild symptoms; in only a few of the patients is the involvement severe or progressive.

**d. Neonatal Graves' disease**

(1) Some infants born to women with Graves' disease exhibit jitteriness, stare, hyperactivity, increased appetite, and poor weight gain.

(2) Tachycardia is present, and thyromegaly may be detectable.

(3) Thyroid hormone levels are elevated above the normal range for the newborn, and TSH is suppressed.

**4. Diagnosis**

**a.** Hyperthyroidism is diagnosed by documentation of increased serum concentrations of total $T_4$ and total $T_3$, increased $T_3$ resin uptake, and low or suppressed levels of TSH. If $T_4$ levels are borderline, absence of the TSH response to TRH injection indicates autonomous thyroid hyperfunction.

**b.** $^{131}$I uptake is helpful if thyroid enlargement is not present. Increased $T_4$ with low $^{131}$I uptake may point to surreptitious overdosing with thyroid hormone.

**5. Therapy**

**a. Medications**

(1) Initial treatment consists of antithyroid medication, either **propylthiouracil [PTU]** (300–600 mg/day) or **methimazole** (30–60 mg/day) in three divided doses. PTU offers the advantage of blocking the peripheral conversion of $T_4$ to $T_3$. The addition of propranolol (10–20 mg four times daily) may give symptomatic relief until preformed thyroid hormone is discharged from the thyroid and thyroid hormone levels begin to fall, usually in 2–4 weeks.

(a) About 5% of patients experience side effects (e.g., skin rash, arthralgias, drug-induced hepatitis) while on antithyroid medication.

(b) Less common, but more serious, is the occasional occurrence of **agranulocytosis.** If the child develops high fever, sore throat, or oral ulceration, a white blood cell count should be obtained. Agranulocytosis usually is reversible, but alternative therapy for hyperthyroidism must be selected.

**(2)** About 40%–50% of children with Graves' disease go into a natural remission and may be taken off antithyroid medication after 12–24 months of treatment.

**(3)** Recurrent hyperthyroidism, long-standing disease, and a large thyroid gland indicate continuing disease activity. More recently, the continuing presence of circulating TBII and TSI predicts continued disease activity.

**b. Surgery**

**(1) Subtotal thyroidectomy** usually is selected for recurrent hyperthyroidism after a course of medical treatment or if the patient is noncompliant with medical therapy.

**(2) Complications** include postoperative hypoparathyroidism and recurrent laryngeal nerve damage in 1%–5% of patients. Most children require thyroid hormone replacement after surgery.

**c. Radioactive iodine.** Although ablation of thyroid tissue by radioactive iodine has traditionally been reserved for adults, it has been used regularly in some centers as the preferred treatment for children with no untoward effects on subsequent fertility or fetal wastage.

**(1)** The risk for immediate and long-term complications is low.

**(2)** The choice of surgery versus radioactive iodine should probably be left to the patient and family after a thorough discussion of both forms of therapy.

**(3)** As with surgery, most children eventually require thyroxine replacement for hypothyroidism after receiving radioactive iodine.

**d. Therapy for thyroid storm.** The extremely hypermetabolic state of thyroid storm requires immediate hospitalization and treatment with iodide, PTU, β blockers, and supportive care as well as treatment of any other intercurrent illness that may have triggered the episode.

**e. Therapy for neonatal Graves' disease.** Therapy with PTU (5–10 mg/kg every 6 hours) is instituted. Propranolol and iodide solution may be added in very symptomatic infants. Initially, infants should be monitored closely for signs of congestive heart failure. Neonatal Graves' disease usually resolves over the first several months of life.

**D. Thyroiditis** (i.e., inflammation of the thyroid gland) may be chronic, subacute, or acute. Each type has a distinct clinical presentation, course, and treatment.

**1. Chronic lymphocytic thyroiditis (CLT)** is commonly referred to as **Hashimoto's thyroiditis** and is the most common thyroid condition in childhood and adolescence. Girls are affected more than twice as often as boys.

**a. Clinical features**

**(1) Asymptomatic thyroid enlargement (goiter)** is the most common presenting complaint or physical finding. The thyroid gland is diffusely enlarged, and the surface may feel pebbly. With long duration, the gland becomes hard and nodular.

**(2)** Although most children are euthyroid, a few may be **hypothyroid** and very rarely some may have symptoms of **thyrotoxicosis (Hashitoxicosis)**. Distinguishing Hashimoto's thyroiditis from Graves' disease may be difficult, since elements of both diseases may coexist.

**b. Diagnosis** is made on the basis of physical findings and laboratory data.

**(1)** The most significant laboratory test supporting the diagnosis is the presence of high titers of thyroid autoantibodies in the serum. Antithyroglobulin and antimicrosomal antibodies are the most commonly found.

**(2)** Measurement of serum concentrations of $T_4$ and TSH may be normal, or $T_4$ levels may be normal with elevated TSH (**"compensated" hypothyroidism**), or $T_4$ levels may be decreased with elevated TSH (hypothyroidism).

**(3)** Thyroid scanning is not indicated unless a nodule is suspected. Needle biopsy rarely is done in children.

**c. Therapy** with L-thyroxine is reserved for those children with evidence of hypothyroidism, either decreased serum concentrations of $T_4$ or normal $T_4$ with elevated TSH. The disease may resolve completely with or without treatment in up to 50% of children with Hashimoto's thyroiditis. In some children, thyroid function continues to deteriorate and permanent hypothyroidism results.

**2. Subacute thyroiditis** is a rare nonsuppurative inflammatory disease of the thyroid, which is thought to have a viral etiology, although a specific virus is not identified in most cases.

**a. Clinical features**

**(1)** Typically, the child complains of sore throat and pain in the area of the thyroid gland. Pain may be referred to the angle of the jaw or the ear and is worse on movement of the neck.

**(2)** Symptoms of systemic illness (e.g., fever, malaise) are frequent. Examination reveals a tender, swollen thyroid gland.

**b. Diagnosis**

**(1)** In the early stages of the disease, serum $T_4$ concentrations may be moderately elevated and TSH levels suppressed, presumably secondary to discharge of preformed thyroid hormone from the gland. Thyroid uptake of radionuclide is very low. Symptoms of hyperthyroidism usually are mild and do not require treatment.

**(2)** Leukocytosis and elevated erythrocyte sedimentation rate are usual in the systemic phase of the illness.

**(3)** In the latter stages of the disease (2–6 months), hypothyroidism is common but ultimately resolves in almost all cases.

**c. Therapy** is symptomatic. Aspirin and nonsteroidal anti-inflammatory drugs to relieve pain and tenderness are sufficient in milder cases. Occasionally steroids are required for more severe cases.

**3. Acute thyroiditis** is a term usually reserved for acute bacterial infection of the thyroid, which may be suppurative or nonsuppurative. The most common causative organisms are *Staphylococcus aureus, Streptococcus hemolyticus,* and pneumococcus.

**a. Clinical features.** The child presents with an acute toxic febrile illness with marked tenderness in the area of the thyroid that is exacerbated by extension of the neck. The thyroid is extremely tender to palpation, and there may be increased warmth and erythema of the overlying skin.

**b. Diagnosis**

**(1)** Laboratory studies show leukocytosis with a left shift and an elevated erythrocyte sedimentation rate. Unlike subacute thyroiditis, serum levels of $T_4$ and TSH are normal, as is the 24-hour uptake of radioactive iodine.

**(2)** Ultrasonography may identify an abscess.

**(3)** Needle aspiration for culture identifies the bacterial organism.

**c. Therapy** with high-dose parenteral antibiotics is begun immediately. An abscess requires surgical drainage.

**d. Prognosis.** Complete recovery with normal thyroid function is the rule.

**E. Thyroid nodules** are rare in children. Although the etiology is uncertain, there is a high incidence of palpable nodules found in children who received irradiation to the neck area while they were infants.

**1. Pathology.** Thyroid nodules in children may be solitary nodules, which usually are benign (e.g., benign adenoma, cysts, lymphocytic thyroiditis) but may be malignant.

**a.** The most common type of thyroid carcinoma is **well-differentiated follicular carcinoma**.

**b.** An unusual and highly malignant, sometimes familial, form of thyroid cancer is **medullary thyroid carcinoma**. Medullary thyroid carcinoma is associated with **multiple endocrine adenomatosis type II (MEA II),** which includes pheochromocytoma and parathyroid hyperplasia or adenoma (see V B 1, 2).

**2. Diagnosis**

**a.** The patient history should include symptoms of hypothyroidism and hyperthyroidism, previous head or neck irradiation, and family history of thyroid or other endocrine disease.

**b.** Laboratory evaluation includes serum concentration testing of $T_4$, $T_3$ resin uptake, TSH, and thyroid antibodies.

**c.** The presence of a palpable mass in the thyroid is the major indication for performing a thyroid scan. As many as 30%–40% of isolated **"cold" nodules** (decreased radioisotope uptake) prove to be thyroid carcinoma in children. Most of the remaining nodules are benign adenomas or cystic lesions.

**d.** Fine needle aspiration under local anesthesia is useful for differentiating benign from malignant lesions.

**e.** Occult medullary thyroid carcinoma or precancerous C cell hyperplasia of the thyroid can be detected by calcium or pentagastrin infusion. A positive calcitonin response to the stimulation test is an indication for total thyroidectomy.

**3. Therapy**

**a. Benign nodules.** A nodule may be presumed to be benign if there is no predisposing condition or clinical characteristics of malignancy and the fine needle biopsy is negative for malignant cells. In this case, observation of the patient while on thyroid hormone suppression is indicated.

**b. Malignant nodules** require surgical removal. Hemithyroidectomy or subtotal thyroidectomy with lymph node excision is sufficient for well-differentiated unilateral carcinoma and usually affords an excellent prognosis. Total thyroidectomy is performed for medullary thyroid carcinoma. Postoperative drug therapy with L-thyroxine is used to suppress TSH.

**c. Metastatic thyroid cancer** is treated with radioiodine ablation.

## IV. DISORDERS OF THE PITUITARY GLAND.

The pituitary gland is a complex structure that has two distinct portions—the anterior and posterior lobes–with different embryonic origins and separate hormonal functions.

**A. Disorders of the anterior lobe.** The anterior lobe of the pituitary gland (also called the **adenohypophysis**) is derived from a diverticulum of the primitive oral cavity. Hypothalamic polypeptides reach the anterior lobe through the median eminence and the portal vasculature of the pituitary gland. The hormones produced in the anterior lobe are **GH, TSH, ACTH,** gonadotropins [i.e., **luteinizing hormone (LH)** and **follicle-stimulating hormone (FSH)**], and **prolactin**. Children are more likely to have a deficiency than an excess of pituitary hormones. Hypersecretory pituitary adenomas, which are very rare in children, usually are prolactin- or GH-secreting adenomas.

**1. GH disorders**

**a. Normal GH function**

**(1)** GH is an anabolic polypeptide hormone that stimulates growth of all tissues. Its most striking effect is on the lengthening of long bones. Its action on long bone growth appears to be mediated through another polypeptide hormone, **insulin-like growth factor 1 (IGF-1),** which is generated in the liver and other tissues.

**(2)** GH release from the anterior lobe is stimulated by the hypothalamic peptide, **growth hormone releasing factor (GRF),** and is inhibited by **somatostatin.**

**(3)** Other substances and factors play a role in GH release, and many form the basis of testing for abnormalities of GH secretion, including sleep, exercise, hypoglycemia, amino acids (e.g., arginine), β blockers, sex hormones, and other drugs (e.g., L-dopa, clonidine).

**b. GH deficiency** is associated with a variety of clinical conditions and syndromes, either as an isolated deficiency or in combination with other pituitary hormone deficiencies (**panhypopituitarism**).

**(1) Clinical features**

**(a) Congenital hypopituitarism**—a rare form of GH deficiency—may be familial and frequently is fatal if not diagnosed in the neonatal period. In these infants, profound hypoglycemia, prolonged jaundice, and low levels of cortisol, GH, and thyroid hormone require immediate treatment. When this syndrome is associated with optic nerve hypoplasia (blindness) and absence of the septum pellucidum, it is called **septo-optic dysplasia**.

**(b) Secondary GH deficiency.** GH deficiency may be secondary to **CNS tumors** (e.g., craniopharyngioma, glioma, pinealoma), **trauma, surgery** involving the hypothalamus or pituitary gland, **irradiation,** or malignant (histiocytosis) or infectious **infiltration**.

**(c) Idiopathic GH deficiency** accounts for most cases of GH deficiency. Usually, the defect is in the hypothalamus, resulting in deficient GRF stimulation of pituitary somatotrophs.

**(i)** Since GH does not appear to be necessary for fetal growth, affected newborns are of normal size. Growth velocity slows after 6–12 months of age, so that by age 2 years, height is below the fifth percentile.

**(ii)** Male infants may have microphallus secondary to intrauterine gonadotropin deficiency.

**(iii)** Symptomatic hypoglycemia may occur in the newborn period.

**(iv)** Older children with idiopathic GH deficiency have very short stature with growth velocities of less than 5 cm/yr. They may have mild truncal adiposity, frontal bossing, a flat nasal bridge, and a high-pitched voice. Skeletal maturation is significantly delayed.

**(2) Diagnosis.** Because GH is secreted in sporadic bursts, with the major surge coming after sleep onset (stages 3 and 4), GH levels are low throughout most of the day. To differentiate the normal low basal GH level from disease states associated with absent or diminished GH secretion, GH **provocative tests** have been developed.

        **(a)** GH levels greater than 10 ng/ml after exercise, insulin-induced hypoglycemia, and arginine infusion as well as L-dopa, glucagon, and clonidine administration are considered evidence of normal GH secretory capacity.

        **(b)** Peak levels of 7–10 ng/ml are intermediate and may indicate partial GH deficiency or a neurosecretory defect and must be interpreted in the clinical context.

        **(c)** Levels less than 7 ng/ml on two separate provocative tests indicate classic GH deficiency. Children with normal or intermediate GH response to provocative testing may have a neurosecretory defect. In these children, a trial of GH therapy may be warranted.

     **(3) Therapy.** Prior to 1985, human GH extracted from human cadaver pituitary glands was used for treatment of GH-deficient children. In 1986, human recombinant GH became widely available and is currently the only GH approved for human use in the United States.

        **(a)** GH is given by subcutaneous injection daily or every other day. In young infants with hypoglycemia, daily injections are necessary.

        **(b)** With a theoretically unlimited supply of GH, new uses for GH in the treatment of short stature from other etiologies are being explored. Girls with Turner syndrome have shown encouraging preliminary results as have some children with idiopathic short stature.

  **c. GH-secreting adenomas** cause acromegaly in the postadolescent child with fused epiphyses. In the younger child, it causes pituitary gigantism.

     **(1) Clinical features** include increased perspiration, headache, acral enlargement, and visual impairment. Carbohydrate intolerance, galactorrhea, joint pain, and delayed puberty also may be present.

     **(2) Diagnosis**

        **(a)** Elevation of GH levels may be variable, but integrated 24-hour GH secretion is increased as reflected in a significant increase in IGF-1 levels.

        **(b)** GH levels are not suppressible by glucose ingestion, as they are in normal individuals.

     **(3) Therapy.** Neurosurgical excision of the adenoma relieves progression of symptoms. Drug therapy with bromocriptine may ameliorate symptoms of GH excess but is not curative.

**2. TSH deficiency.** Isolated TSH deficiency is exceedingly rare. However, TSH deficiency in combination with other pituitary hormone deficiencies is common.

  **a. Hypothyroidism secondary to TSH deficiency** tends to be more subtle in its clinical manifestation than primary hypothyroidism. Therefore, all children who are being evaluated for GH deficiency should have evaluation of $T_4$, $T_3$ resin uptake, and TSH levels.

  **b. GH therapy** may induce or unmask TSH deficiency. Consequently, children on GH therapy should have yearly screening for secondary hypothyroidism. Treatment consists of thyroid hormone replacement as in primary hypothyroidism.

**3. ACTH deficiency** as an isolated defect has been reported. More commonly, ACTH deficiency occurs along with deficiency of other pituitary hormones.

  **a. Clinical features** are secondary to hypocortisolism and include hypoglycemia, fatigue, and poor tolerance of intercurrent illness.

  **b. Diagnosis** is based on failure to increase cortisol levels after insulin-induced hypoglycemia (on an insulin tolerance test).

**4. Gonadotropin deficiency**

  **a. Clinical features.** Gonadotropin (LH and FSH) deficiency presents in infancy as microphallus in the male. Hypogonadotropic hypogonadism becomes evident later, as the child's pubertal development falls significantly behind the expected age range for puberty.

  **b. Diagnosis**

     **(1)** Gonadotropin deficiency may occur as an isolated defect, as part of a recognizable syndrome [e.g., Kallmann syndrome (anosmia and hypogonadism), Prader-Willi syndrome (characterized by hypotonia, obesity, short stature, mental retardation), and anorexia nervosa] or within the context of multiple pituitary hormone deficiencies.

     **(2)** There is no specific test that clearly separates hypogonadotropic hypogonadism from constitutional delayed puberty.

**5. Prolactin-secreting adenomas** may be very small (microadenoma) or large, creating primarily neurologic symptoms.

**a. Clinical features** related to high prolactin levels include galactorrhea and delayed or arrested pubertal development.

**b. Therapy.** Surgical excision is curative. If this is not possible, medical treatment with bromocriptine may ameliorate symptoms.

**B. Disorders of the posterior lobe.** The posterior lobe of the pituitary gland (also called the **neurohypophysis**) develops—along with the pituitary stalk—as a downgrowth of neural tissue from the area of the third ventricle. Neural fibers connect the neurohypophysis with hypothalamic nuclei, the site of synthesis of **arginine vasopressin** [antidiuretic hormone (ADH)] and **oxytocin,** which, together, comprise a neuroendocrine unit.

**1. ADH disorders**

**a. Normal ADH function.** ADH is an octapeptide that has an antidiuretic effect on the collecting ducts in the kidney. This allows water to be reabsorbed and concentrated urine to be excreted, allowing the tonicity of body fluids to remain constant during periods of reduced water intake. ADH secretion is stimulated by hypovolemia through baroreceptors in the carotid sinus, by hyperosmolality through osmoreceptors in the hypothalamus, by the upright position, and by stress and anxiety.

    **(1)** Through an active process, sodium and chloride are removed from the glomerular filtrate in the ascending limb of the loop of Henle, which is impermeable to water. Therefore, urine delivered to the distal convoluted tubule is dilute.

    **(2)** In the presence of ADH, the collecting duct becomes permeable to water and water is passively reabsorbed into the hypertonic interstitium, concentrating urine to an osmolality greater than 1000 mOsm/L and reducing urine volume.

**b. Diabetes insipidus** is a condition marked by the inability to concentrate urine appropriately despite a normal countercurrent osmotic gradient in the kidney. With loss of ADH secretion, 24-hour urine output may reach 5–10 L/day. Urine osmolality remains low (about 100 mOsm/L).

    **(1) Etiology.** Diabetes insipidus may occur as an isolated idiopathic defect, or it may be accompanied by anterior pituitary hormone deficiency (as in septo-optic dysplasia). It may occur after head trauma, after surgical interruption of the pituitary stalk (e.g., for craniopharyngioma), and with tumors and infections of the CNS. There is a rare familial form of diabetes insipidus.

    **(2) Clinical features.** The patient has polyuria and polydipsia even when water-deprived. Frequently, the onset of symptoms of excessive thirst and urination is abrupt. The child prefers cold water to other fluids. Caloric intake diminishes, and growth and weight gain may fall off. Neurologic and visual complaints may be present if diabetes insipidus is secondary to a tumor.

    **(3) Diagnosis.** If the child's first morning urine is dilute (specific gravity of less than 1.015), a **water deprivation test** must be done. After a water load of 20 ml/kg is given in the morning, the child should not be given anything by mouth until the test is ended. Meticulous hourly measurements of weight and urine output are recorded.

        **(a)** Urine specific gravity and osmolality are measured on each sample. Serum sodium and osmolality are measured hourly after 4 hours.

        **(b)** The test is terminated when 3%–5% of body weight is lost or when the serum osmolality rises to 300 mOsm/L or more and urine osmolality remains constant and dilute (< 250 mOsm/L) over a 2-hour period. Hemoconcentration may result in a high-normal serum sodium level.

        **(c)** At the end of the test, a long-acting analogue of ADH, dDAVP, 5–10 μg, is given intranasally, and the child may drink. A further rise in urine osmolality by 100 mOsm/L or more indicates ADH-deficient diabetes insipidus.

        **(d)** Documentation of responsiveness to ADH is important in differentiating ADH-deficient diabetes insipidus from nephrogenic diabetes insipidus and other renal diseases associated with decreased concentrating ability (e.g., renal tubular acidosis, sickle cell disease, and other types of chronic renal disease) [see also Ch 13 I C 4].

    **(4) Therapy** with dDAVP intranasally every 12–24 hours provides relief of symptoms of polyuria and polydipsia.

**c. Nephrogenic diabetes insipidus** is a rare X-linked recessive disease of renal unresponsiveness to ADH. Male infants are severely affected.

    **(1) Clinical features** include polyuria, failure to thrive, and bouts of hyperpyrexia and vomiting, leading to severe hypernatremic dehydration in infancy.

    (2) **Diagnosis.** Failure to respond to ADH at the end of the water deprivation test in the absence of other renal disease suggests the diagnosis of nephrogenic diabetes insipidus (see also Ch 13 I C 4).

    (3) **Therapy** consists of provision of ample fluids at all times, including during the course of intercurrent illness. Thiazide diuretics, by promoting sodium diuresis and volume contraction, provide some relief of symptoms.

  **d. Thirst and osmotic regulation abnormalities.** Children with these abnormalities usually have significant CNS disease.

    (1) **Clinical features and diagnosis.** The serum sodium level is chronically elevated without symptoms of thirst, while urine remains dilute. With water deprivation and induction of more severe hyperosmolality, ADH may be secreted.

    (2) **Therapy** with dDAVP allows urine concentration with normal serum sodium. Care must be taken by the patient to avoid excess fluids and hyponatremia while taking dDAVP.

  **e. Psychogenic water drinking.** This disorder of compulsive water drinking is rare in children.

    (1) The history of other neurotic behaviors, gradual onset of symptoms, failure to get up at night to drink and urinate, and the finding of low normal serum sodium levels and osmolality with dilute urine may suggest this diagnosis.

    (2) The ability to concentrate urine on a water deprivation test may be less than normal because of "washout" of the renal concentration gradient. However, urine osmolality eventually rises while serum osmolality and sodium remain in the normal range.

  **f. Syndrome of inappropriate antidiuretic hormone (SIADH)**

    (1) **Clinical features.** SIADH causes expansion of the vascular volume and hyponatremia, which may lead to lethargy, confusion, and seizures. In children, SIADH is occasionally associated with pulmonary and CNS disease (e.g., pneumonia, bacterial meningitis). It also is associated with some chemotherapeutic agents (e.g., vincristine, cyclophosphamide).

    (2) **Therapy** involves fluid restriction. Symptomatic hyponatremia is treated with infusion of 3% sodium chloride solution.

**2. Oxytocin disorders.** Oxytocin is an octapeptide that differs from ADH by two amino acids, which results in marked reduction in antidiuretic properties. Its major function is in promoting uterine contraction and milk ejection. Deficiency of oxytocin is not associated with a recognized pediatric clinical problem.

## V. DISORDERS OF THE ADRENAL GLAND

**A. Disorders of the adrenal cortex.** The products of adrenocortical steroidogenesis are glucocorticoids, mineralocorticoids, and sex steroids. **Cortisol,** the major glucocorticoid, is stimulated by pituitary ACTH under a negative feedback loop. **Aldosterone,** the principal mineralocorticoid, is controlled by the renin-angiotensin system. The major sex steroids are **androgens.** Inherited deficiency of various enzymes involved in cortisol and aldosterone synthesis leads to a group of diseases called **congenital adrenal hyperplasia.** Autonomous hyperfunctioning of the adrenal cortex leads to **hypercortisolism** or **Cushing's disease,** and decreased adrenocortical secretion may be caused by primary adrenal insufficiency (**Addison's disease**) or a lack of ACTH stimulation (**secondary adrenal insufficiency**).

**1. Congenital adrenal hyperplasia (adrenogenital syndrome).** The clinical characteristics of congenital adrenal hyperplasia depend on which enzyme in the pathway of cortisol synthesis is deficient. Even for a specific enzyme, variability exists in the severity of disease expression and timing of onset of symptoms. It is helpful to review the pathways of adrenal steroidogenesis (Figure 16-1) to appreciate better the consequences of an enzyme defect on decreased synthesis of cortisol or aldosterone, increased ACTH production, and overproduction of precursors that are shunted to androgens. The two most common defects are 21-hydroxylase deficiency and 11-hydroxylase deficiency.

  **a. 21-Hydroxylase deficiency** accounts for 90% of cases of congenital adrenal hyperplasia and occurs in several forms. These disorders are inherited as autosomal recessive traits. The gene is HLA-linked on the short arm of chromosome 6.

    (1) **Classic salt-wasting 21-hydroxylase deficiency** is a severe deficiency resulting in decreased cortisol and aldosterone secretion, increased ACTH, and increased precursor

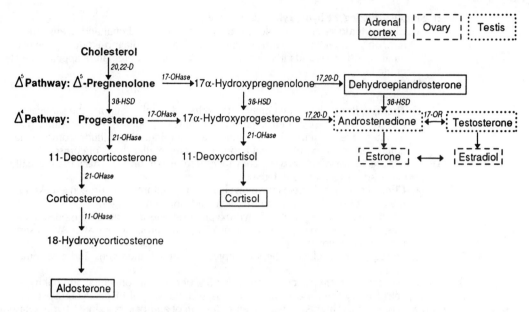

**Figure 16-1.** Summary of steroidogenesis in the adrenal cortex, ovary, and testis. *20,22-D* = 20,22-desmolase; *17,20-D* = 17,20-desmolase; *17-OHase* = 17-hydroxylase; *21-OHase* = 21-hydroxylase; *11-OHase* = 11-hydroxylase; *3β-HSD* = 3β-hydroxysteroid dehydrogenase/isomerase system; *17-OR* = 17-oxidoreductase. (Reprinted from Bullock J: Endocrine physiology. In *NMS Physiology,* 2nd edition. Baltimore, Williams & Wilkins, 1991, p 365.)

of the 21-hydroxylase step, **17-hydroxyprogesterone**. 17-Hydroxyprogesterone is metabolized to adrenal androgens, namely dihydroepiandrosterone (DHEA) and androstenedione. There is a one in four recurrence rate in siblings of children with classic salt-wasting 21-hydroxylase deficiency.

**(a) Clinical features**

    **(i)** Female infants are born with ambiguous genitalia. Clitoromegaly and labioscrotal fusion may lead to erroneous male sex assignment. Because there is normal ovarian development, internal genital structures are female. Male infants have no genital abnormalities.

    **(ii)** Symptoms of salt-wasting, vomiting, dehydration, and shock develop in the first 2–4 weeks of life. Infants are hyponatremic, hyperkalemic, acidotic, and often hypoglycemic.

**(b) Diagnosis** rests on measurement of markedly elevated levels of 17-hydroxyprogesterone in the serum. HLA family studies have shown that all affected siblings share the same HLA type. Thus, after the birth of an affected infant, HLA typing of amniotic fluid cells, as well as measurement of elevated 17-hydroxyprogesterone in amniotic fluid, permit prenatal diagnosis in subsequent pregnancies.

**(c) Therapy** consists of:

    **(i)** Cortisol replacement (20–25 mg/m²/day of oral hydrocortisone divided and given every 8 hours) to suppress ACTH and overproduction of androgens

    **(ii)** Mineralocorticoid (fludrocortisone 0.1 mg/day) adjusted to suppress the plasma renin level

    **(iii)** Surgical correction of female genital abnormalities

**(d) Follow-up.** These children must be monitored closely for linear growth and sexual development.

    **(i) Undertreatment,** indicated by elevated 17-hydroxyprogesterone, androstenedione, and renin levels and by accelerated advancement of skeletal maturation, leads to excessive growth, premature sexual hair growth and virilization of male and female children, and ultimately to premature epiphyseal fusion and adult short stature.

    **(ii) Overtreatment** with cortisol suppresses growth and may cause symptoms of hypercortisolism.

  **(2) Simple virilizing 21-hydroxylase deficiency**

   **(a) Clinical features** are due solely to overproduction of adrenal androgens. Therefore, only female infants with ambiguous genitalia are diagnosed during the neonatal period. Boys and girls have excessive growth and premature appearance of pubic hair.

   **(b) Diagnosis** is based on the measurement of elevated 17-hydroxyprogesterone in serum.

   **(c) Therapy.** Principles of treatment with cortisol and follow-up are the same as for salt-wasters. Some children, even without clinical symptoms of salt-wasting, have elevated levels of renin. The addition of a mineralocorticoid (fludrocortisone) facilitates suppression of adrenal androgens with smaller doses of cortisol.

  **(3) Nonclassic 21-hydroxylase deficiency (acquired or late-onset).** This variant usually occurs in adolescent or adult females.

   **(a) Clinical features.** Patients develop signs and symptoms of androgen excess (i.e., menstrual irregularities, hirsutism, acne, advanced bone age).

   **(b) Diagnosis.** Basal levels of 17-hydroxyprogesterone may be only modestly elevated. However, the excessive rise of 17-hydroxyprogesterone after ACTH stimulation is diagnostic.

   **(c) Therapy** with a glucocorticoid suppresses adrenal androgens and ameliorates symptoms.

 **b. 11-Hydroxylase deficiency** accounts for about 5% of cases of congenital adrenal hyperplasia. Lack of 11-hydroxylase results in decreased conversion of 11-deoxycortisol to cortisol, with precursors shunted toward overproduction of androgens, as in 21-hydroxylase deficiency. 11-Hydroxylase also is necessary for conversion of deoxycorticosterone to corticosterone in the aldosterone pathway.

  **(1) Clinical features.** Overproduction of deoxycorticosterone, which itself has mineralocorticoid activity, results in hypertension and hypokalemia in most of these patients.

  **(2) Diagnosis** is based on the measurement of increased 11-deoxycortisol and deoxycorticosterone in serum or their tetrahydrometabolites in the urine. Serum androstenedione and testosterone also are elevated, and renin and aldosterone are suppressed. In the milder nonclassic form, the biochemical abnormalities are expressed after ACTH stimulation.

 **c. Other defects.** Other, extremely rare, forms of congenital adrenal hyperplasia may be caused by deficiencies of **cholesterol desmolase, 3β-hydroxysteroid dehydrogenase,** and **17-hydroxylase.** A nonclassic form of 3β-hydroxysteroid dehydrogenase may present clinically in prepubertal or pubertal females as precocious adrenarche or excessive virilization. Treatment strategies are the same as for 21-hydroxylase deficiency.

**2. Primary adrenal insufficiency** may be congenital or acquired and results in decreased cortisol secretion alone or with diminished aldosterone.

 **a. Etiology**

  **(1)** Primary adrenal insufficiency in the newborn may be due to adrenal hypoplasia, familial unresponsiveness to ACTH, adrenal hemorrhage, or overwhelming sepsis **(Waterhouse-Friderichsen syndrome).**

  **(2)** In older children and adolescents, **autoimmune adrenal insufficiency** may occur alone or in association with another autoimmune endocrinopathy (e.g., thyroiditis, IDDM). Tuberculosis and fungal destruction of the adrenal gland are rare.

  **(3) Adrenoleukodystrophy** is a group of X-linked recessive inherited disorders of long-chain fatty acid metabolism, resulting in progressive neurologic deterioration and adrenal insufficiency.

  **(4)** Adrenal insufficiency may occur after withdrawal of pharmacologic steroid therapy as a result of **suppression of pituitary ACTH.**

 **b. Clinical features**

  **(1) Symptoms** include weakness, nausea, vomiting, weight loss, and salt-craving.

  **(2) Physical findings** include postural hypotension and increased pigmentation, especially over joints and on scar tissue, lips, nipples, and the buccal mucosa.

  **(3) Adrenal crisis** is characterized by fever, vomiting, dehydration, and shock that may be triggered by intercurrent illness, surgery, or trauma.

 **c. Diagnosis.** The characteristic electrolyte abnormalities are hyponatremia, hyperkalemia, and mild metabolic acidosis. The serum cortisol level is low (< 5 μg/dl) and fails to rise after acute injection of ACTH (cosyntropin at 250 μg intravenously). If the acute ACTH stimulation test is abnormal, a prolonged ACTH stimulation test (3–5 days) is necessary to rule out an atrophic adrenal gland secondary to chronic ACTH deficiency (**secondary adrenal insufficiency**).

**d. Therapy**

   **(1) Treatment of adrenal crisis.** Diagnostic studies should not delay treatment of this life-threatening illness. Rehydration and correction of electrolyte abnormalities are needed immediately.

   **(a)** Large quantities of 5% dextrose in normal saline are given, along with acute administration of intravenous glucocorticoid in stress doses (hydrocortisone at 100–200 mg/m$^2$/day divided and given every 4 hours).

   **(b)** Treatment with equivalent amounts of dexamethasone instead of hydrocortisone permits ACTH testing to be carried out while treatment is initiated, since dexamethasone does not interfere with measurement of cortisol after ACTH stimulation.

   **(2) Long-term treatment** of adrenal insufficiency consists of maintenance doses of oral glucocorticoid (hydrocortisone at 20 mg/m$^2$/day) and mineralocorticoid (fludrocortisone at 0.1 mg/day). The glucocorticoid dosage must be increased during significant intercurrent illness, trauma, or surgery to prevent acute adrenal insufficiency.

**3. Cushing syndrome** is a group of signs and symptoms that develop as a result of excessive cortisol, either due to endogenous overproduction of cortisol or exogenous treatment with pharmacologic doses of cortisol for other illnesses.

**a. Etiology**

   **(1) Bilateral adrenal hyperplasia (Cushing's disease)** is the most common etiology in children older than age 7 years. This is now generally believed to be due to chronic oversecretion of ACTH by a **pituitary tumor**. In many instances, the tumor is a microadenoma.

   **(2) Adrenal tumors** also may cause Cushing syndrome. Most adrenal tumors are adenomas, although in younger children and infants the possibility of malignant adrenal carcinoma is greater. Although most adrenal tumors are virilizing, rare feminizing adrenal tumors have been reported.

**b. Clinical features.** The classic manifestations of Cushing syndrome in childhood are slow growth, truncal obesity, rounded "moon" facies, buffalo hump, purple striae, and acne. Hypertension and muscle weakness are common.

**c. Diagnosis.** Initial laboratory studies document the presence of increased cortisol secretion. Elevated serum cortisol levels and absence of the normal diurnal variation are difficult to interpret in the stressed or hospitalized child.

   **(1)** A **24-hour urine test** for free cortisol is the most discriminating test. Failure to suppress the morning serum cortisol level to less than 5 μg/dl after receiving 0.3 mg/m$^2$ of dexamethasone at 11 P.M. the night before (the **overnight dexamethasone suppression test**) is supportive of possible Cushing syndrome.

   **(2)** A **prolonged dexamethasone suppression test** is needed to differentiate Cushing's disease (bilateral adrenal hyperplasia due to pituitary adenoma) from Cushing syndrome due to adrenal tumor, if both the 24-hour urine free-cortisol test and the overnight suppression test are positive. Low-dose oral dexamethasone (1.2 mg/m$^2$/day divided and given every 6 hours for 2 days) is followed by a high dose (4.8 mg/m$^2$/day for 2 days), with monitoring of serum cortisol and 24-hour urine free-cortisol levels.

   **(a)** If serum and urine cortisol levels are suppressed to less than 50% of the baseline on the first 2 days, Cushing syndrome is not present.

   **(b)** Failure to suppress levels on the first 2 days (low-dose dexamethasone) but suppression on the last 2 days indicates bilateral adrenal hyperplasia due to pituitary adenoma.

   **(c)** Failure to suppress levels on high-dose dexamethasone indicates adrenal tumor.

   **(3)** A **computed tomography (CT) scan** of the pituitary and adrenal areas also is warranted.

**d. Therapy**

   **(1)** Bilateral adrenal hyperplasia usually is treated by surgical excision of the pituitary adenoma. Transsphenoidal microsurgery is the treatment of choice for microadenomas. Some children have been treated with pituitary irradiation.

   **(2)** Adrenal tumors are treated by surgical excision. Chemotherapy for malignant metastatic disease may be palliative.

**(3)** In all cases when surgery is performed, perioperative steroid coverage must be provided to prevent possible adrenal insufficiency.

**B. Disorders of the adrenal medulla.** The adrenal medulla is composed of chromaffin cells derived from neural crest tissue. The adrenal medulla produces catecholamines (**epinephrine** and **norepinephrine**) in response to sympathetic nervous system stimulation. Catecholamines exert widespread metabolic effects on glycogenolysis, lipolysis, and gluconeogenesis as well as effects on the cardiovascular system. The physiologic effects on vasodilation and cardiac muscle contractility are mediated through α- and β-adrenergic receptors on target cell surfaces. The major clinical problems arising from the adrenal medulla are tumors (see Chapter 15 V for discussion of neuroblastoma).

1. **Pheochromocytoma** is a rare tumor of chromaffin tissue. The most common site of occurrence is the adrenal medulla, but the tumor also may occur in extra-adrenal sites in the chest and abdomen. Most tumors in childhood are benign. Morbidity and mortality result from the effects of overproduction of catecholamines. Pheochromocytoma may occur as an isolated tumor or in association with MEA types II and III (see V B 2 b, c).
   a. **Clinical features.** Hypertension usually is sustained but may be paroxysmal. Headache, vomiting, pallor, and sweating are prominent. Hypertensive encephalopathy may be life threatening.
   b. **Diagnosis** is based on finding elevated levels of epinephrine, norepinephrine, or their metabolites (e.g., metanephrine, normetanephrine) and 3-methoxy-4-hydroxymandelic acid (VMA) in a 24-hour urine sample.
      **(1) Imaging studies.** An attempt to localize the tumor by noninvasive measures first should be made using abdominal ultrasonography and CT or magnetic resonance imaging (MRI) scanning. Tumors in the thorax may be identified on chest x-ray or chest CT. $^{123}$I-metaiodobenzylguanidine scintigraphy is helpful in imaging the adrenal medulla as well as extra-adrenal chromaffin tissue.
      **(2) Invasive procedures** (e.g., venography for blood sampling for catecholamines, selective arteriography) may precipitate a hypertensive crisis and should be performed only after α-adrenergic blockade.
   c. **Therapy** for pheochromocytoma is surgical excision.
      **(1)** Careful attention must be given to perioperative control of hypertension and other symptoms. Preoperative medication consists of the long-acting α blocker phenoxybenzamine sometimes combined with a β blocker. Intraoperatively, acute exacerbations of hypertension are treated with the short-acting α blocker phentolamine. The peripheral vasodilator nitroprusside may also be used.
      **(2)** Hypotension due to reduced vascular volume after the tumor is removed is managed with aggressive fluid replacement.
      **(3)** Glucocorticoids must be given if bilateral adrenalectomy is done.
   d. **Follow-up.** Postoperative levels of urinary catecholamines and metabolites should be normal. Persistent symptoms and elevated levels indicate residual tumor. Tumors may recur many years after initial successful treatment.

2. **Multiple endocrine adenomatosis (MEA) syndromes** are a group of familial disorders involving hyperplasia or neoplasia of a variety of endocrine tissues. Symptoms are related to the specific hormone that is secreted.
   a. **MEA I.** Tumors of the anterior lobe of the pituitary gland, the pancreatic islet cells, and the parathyroid glands may occur.
      **(1)** Nonfunctioning pituitary tumors may cause hypopituitarism. Hyperfunctioning pituitary tumors may cause acromegaly or gigantism, hyperprolactinemic syndromes, or Cushing's disease.
      **(2)** Islet cell tumors may cause hypoglycemia (with secretion of insulin), intractable peptic ulcers (with secretion of gastrin), or hyperglycemia (with secretion of glucagon).
      **(3)** Hyperparathyroidism from hyperplasia or parathyroid tumor causes hypercalcemia.
   b. **MEA II.** This cluster includes pheochromocytoma, parathyroid hyperplasia, and medullary thyroid carcinoma (see III E 1 b).
   c. **MEA III.** This syndrome consists of multiple mucosal neuromas of the lips, eyelids, and tongue; marfanoid body habitus; and skeletal abnormalities, with medullary thyroid carcinoma and pheochromocytoma.

## VI. DISORDERS OF THE GONADS

**A. Disorders of sexual differentiation of the newborn.** The diagnosis and management of clinical problems related to abnormal differentiation of the newborn require an understanding of the process of normal sexual differentiation of male and female infants.

1. **Normal sexual differentiation.** The human embryonic gonad is undifferentiated prior to 45–50 days gestation. The internal sexual ducts consist of both male (**wolffian**) and female (**müllerian**) structures at this early stage. Thereafter, sexual differentiation proceeds along distinctly different paths dictated by the genetic and hormonal factors in the male and female fetus.

    a. **Male differentiation.** The male genotype is 46,XY.

        **(1)** Determinants on the Y chromosome direct the synthesis of **testis-determining factor (TDF)**. In the presence of TDF, the undifferentiated gonad differentiates as a testis; in the absence of TDF, the undifferentiated gonad differentiates as an ovary.

        **(2)** The fetal testes secrete **testosterone** from **Leydig cells** under the direction of human chorionic gonadotropin (HCG) and fetal pituitary gonadotropin.

            **(a)** High local concentrations of fetal testosterone stabilize wolffian structures, which develop into the vas deferens, epididymis, and seminal vesicles.

            **(b)** Testosterone is converted to **dihydrotestosterone (DHT)** by the action of 5α-reductase. DHT is necessary for differentiation of the external genitalia into the scrotum, phallus, and phallic urethra, which is complete by 12–14 weeks gestation.

            **(c)** The fetal testes also contain **Sertoli cells,** which secrete antimüllerian factor (AMF), causing regression of müllerian ducts in the male fetus by 8 weeks gestation.

    b. **Female differentiation.** The female genotype is 46,XX. Female differentiation occurs in the absence of testicular determining factors (i.e., Y chromosome, TDF, testosterone, DHT, and AMF).

        **(1)** In the absence of a Y chromosome and TDF, the undifferentiated gonad develops as an ovary.

        **(2)** In the absence of AMF, müllerian ducts develop into the fallopian tubes, uterus, and upper one-third of the vagina.

        **(3)** In the absence of testosterone and DHT, the wolffian ducts degenerate and the external genitalia differentiate as the clitoris, labia majora and minora, and separate urethral and vaginal openings.

2. **Abnormal sexual differentiation** results in a newborn who appears sexually ambiguous, neither completely male nor completely female.

    a. **Male pseudohermaphroditism** refers to infants who are genetic 46,XY males (with testes) but who appear to have signs of incomplete masculinization, including hypospadias, a small phallus, and a poorly developed scrotum with or without descended testes. Male pseudohermaphroditism can be caused by a variety of endocrine disorders involving testosterone synthesis, metabolism, or action at the cellular level.

        **(1)** **Defects in testosterone synthesis and metabolism** are very rare and may be caused by one of five enzyme deficiencies inherited as autosomal recessive traits. The first three result in defects in cortisol synthesis as well and, therefore, are classified as forms of **congenital adrenal hyperplasia** (see V A 1).

            **(a)** **Cholesterol desmolase deficiency** results in severe salt-wasting. Profound deficiency in mineralocorticoid, glucocorticoid, and androgen results in death in infancy in spite of adrenal steroid replacement.

            **(b)** **3β-Hydroxysteroid dehydrogenase deficiency.** Males are incompletely virilized because of deficient testosterone synthesis. Females may be mildly virilized. Diagnosis rests on measurement of elevated serum DHEA and 17-hydroxypregnenolone.

            **(c)** **17-Hydroxylase deficiency.** Because this defect results in increased deoxycorticosterone, a weak mineralocorticoid, hypokalemia and hypertension may be present. Males have ambiguous genitalia because of the inability to produce sex steroids. Females have normal sexual differentiation but fail to develop secondary sex characteristics at puberty.

**(d) 17-Oxidoreductase deficiency** prevents conversion of androstenedione to testosterone. Diagnosis may be made in infancy by finding an increased ratio of androstenedione to testosterone after stimulation wth HCG.

**(e) 17,20-Desmolase deficiency** is an extremely rare cause of male pseudohermaphroditism that results from the inability to convert progestogens to androgens. The defect can be demonstrated by an abnormal ratio of progestogens and androgens in the basal state and after HCG stimulation.

**(2) Defects in androgen action**

**(a) 5α-Reductase deficiency** impairs conversion of testosterone to DHT.

(i) Males are born with ambiguous genitalia because DHT is necessary for masculinization of the male external genitalia. Some of these infants are assigned a female sex because of the minimal virilization apparent at birth.

(ii) At puberty, testosterone-dependent pubertal changes take place, such as clitoral enlargement and descent of inguinal testes into the rugated labioscrotal folds. Muscle mass increases, and the voice deepens. In one isolated community, a large number of affected children were raised as females. Some of these individuals changed to a male gender role after puberty.

(iii) The diagnosis of a 5α-reductase deficiency may be made in childhood by finding an increased ratio of testosterone to DHT after HCG stimulation.

**(b) Androgen resistance syndromes (testicular feminization syndrome).** In the normal male newborn, testosterone levels are significantly elevated for the first several months. **Inappropriately elevated neonatal testosterone with high LH** might indicate androgen resistance due to a receptor defect or failure of normal negative feedback suppression. The pattern of normal to high testosterone with high LH is well documented in postpubertal individuals with androgen resistance.

(i) In **complete androgen resistance,** an XY male infant with testes appears as an unambiguous female because of complete resistance to androgen action at the cellular level. The first clue to this disorder may be the discovery of testes in inguinal hernia sacs in early childhood. Some children may present as adolescent females with primary amenorrhea. Because the undescended testes produce AMF in utero, the vagina is a shallow, blind-ending pouch. If the testes are not removed before the time of puberty, normal female breasts develop from the increased conversion of testosterone to estrogen by the testes.

(ii) In **partial androgen resistance,** the affected XY individual has ambiguous genitalia. The diagnosis of partial androgen resistance is difficult to make in the newborn with an XY karyotype. Since it is inherited as an X-linked recessive trait, the infant's mother must be a carrier and half of her siblings would be expected to be female carriers or affected males. Therefore, a family history of infertile or cryptorchid relatives is suggestive.

**b. Female pseudohermaphroditism** refers to infants who are genetic 46,XX females (with ovaries) but who appear masculinized at birth. Exposure of the female XX infant to increased androgen during the critical period of 8–12 weeks gestation causes a variable degree of labioscrotal fusion, formation of a urogenital sinus, and clitoral enlargement. Exposure after the twelfth week cannot cause labioscrotal fusion, but it can induce clitoral enlargement. Some infants appear to be cryptorchid males at birth.

**(1) Congenital adrenal hyperplasia.** Defects that cause female pseudohermaphroditism are 21-hydroxylase deficiency, 11-hydroxylase deficiency, and 3β-hydroxysteroid dehydrogenase deficiency.

**(2) Maternal androgen or progestin exposure.** With increasing awareness of the effects of medication and other drugs on the developing fetus, exogenous ingestion of androgenic substances is a rare cause of female pseudohermaphroditism. Occasionally, a virilizing tumor or disease during pregnancy in the mother may cause this syndrome. A detailed history of the pregnancy, including drugs taken and medical illness, should be obtained.

**c. Abnormal gonadal differentiation**

**(1) True hermaphroditism** occurs when there is both ovarian and testicular tissue present in the gonads. In approximately 80% of cases, the karyotype is 46,XX, and in the remainder it is 46,XY or mosaicism. The exact etiology is unknown.

**(a) Clinical features.** Usually there is significant masculinization and, consequently, most true hermaphrodites are raised as males. Gynecomastia and cyclic hematuria from uterine bleeding may occur.

**(b) Diagnosis.** True hermaphroditism may be strongly suspected in an infant with ambiguous genitalia, an XX karyotype, and normal serum 17-hydroxyprogesterone levels, ruling out 21-hydroxylase deficiency. The final diagnosis rests with surgical exploration and demonstration of gonads containing both ovarian and testicular tissue.

**(2) Mixed gonadal dysgenesis** involves a karyotype of 45X/46XY.

**(a) Clinical features.** There is a spectrum of appearance of the external genitalia from completely male to completely female.

**(i)** The gonads may appear as streak ovaries to dysgenetic testes and are often asymmetric. The more testicular tissue that is present, the greater is the likelihood of wolffian duct development on the side of that gonad.

**(ii)** Because of the 45X cell line, some somatic features of Turner syndrome may be present (e.g., short stature, webbed neck, congenital heart disease).

**(b) Diagnosis** is made by karyotyping.

**d. Other defects in external genital development** include hypospadias and microphallus.

**(1) Hypospadias** of varying degrees of severity may occur alone or with other birth defects, especially of the genitourinary system (see also Ch 13 XI C).

**(2) Microphallus** describes males with abnormally small but well-differentiated genitalia. Standards are available for assessing stretched penile length from infancy through adulthood. Genital growth in males is dependent on fetal pituitary gonadotropin stimulation of the fetal testis.

**(a) Etiology.** Microphallus may indicate postnatal hypogonadotropic hypogonadism, as in Kallmann syndrome, or may present as part of congenital hypopituitarism.

**(b) Therapy** with testosterone (25–50 mg every 3 weeks for 3 months) may demonstrate responsiveness to testosterone and has a positive cosmetic effect, without significantly advancing skeletal maturation.

**3. Management of the child with ambiguous genitalia**

**a. Complete diagnostic evaluation** should be undertaken as soon as possible after the birth of a child with ambiguous genitalia. Parents should be encouraged to delay naming and announcing the child's sex until diagnostic workup is complete. A careful family and pregnancy history and physical examination are the basis for further testing.

**(1) Physical examination.** The size of the phallus, position of the urethra, palpable gonads (usually testes), and other dysmorphic or asymmetric features should be noted.

**(2) Laboratory studies** initially include chromosome analysis and evaluation of electrolyte, testosterone, LH, FSH, and 17-hydroxyprogesterone levels. Radiographic dye study of the urogenital sinus often is helpful to delineate the presence of a vagina and cervix, and occasionally fallopian tubes may be seen. Pelvic ultrasonography may demonstrate the presence of ovaries and a uterus.

**(a) If the karyotype is 46,XX** and the 17-hydroxyprogesterone level is elevated, the most likely diagnosis is 21-hydroxylase deficiency. If the 17-hydroxyprogesterone level is normal, true hermaphroditism is likely. Measurement of 11-deoxycortisol and DHEA levels rules out the remote possibility of 11-hydroxylase deficiency or 3β-hydroxysteroid dehydrogenase deficiency.

**(b) If the karyotype is 46,XY,** measurement of gonadal and adrenal steroids before and after ACTH and HCG stimulation identifies rare forms of congenital adrenal hyperplasia and defects in testosterone synthesis and metabolism.

**(i)** Infants must be monitored closely for evidence of salt-wasting and glucocorticoid deficiency while awaiting diagnostic test results.

**(ii)** Diagnosis of partial androgen resistance depends on a family history compatible with X-linked recessive inheritance. High neonatal testosterone levels with elevated LH levels are suggestive of androgen resistance.

**b. Gender assignment.** It is important to arrive at the most specific diagnosis possible for a variety of therapeutic and management considerations.

**(1)** Even markedly **masculinized females with 21-hydroxylase deficiency** should be raised as female, since they have reproductive potential with adequate medical management of their disease and cosmetic repair of the external genitalia.

**(2)** For **46,XY males with ambiguous genitalia,** gender assignment should be based on consideration of the possibility of normal adult sexual function as a male. This generally depends on the size of the phallus and the surgeon's estimation of surgical correctability of the hypospadias.

        **(a)** Dysgenetic testes and ovotestes should be removed because of their potential for malignant transformation.

        **(b)** Gonads that do not agree with gender assignment should be removed to avoid the possibility of undesirable hormonal influences at puberty.

    **c. Therapy**

        **(1)** Appropriate hormonal replacement at the usual age of puberty should be provided.

        **(2)** Genetic and sexual counseling for families and for children is an important aspect of medical care.

        **(3)** In general, full but sensitive disclosure of all test results in an age-appropriate manner leads to successful psychosexual adjustment in adulthood.

**B. Disorders of puberty.** Normal pubertal development occurs as the period of transition from sexual immaturity to the sexually mature adult state (see Ch 4 II C 2; Tables 4-1–4-3; Figures 4-2, 4-3). During this time, secondary sex characteristics are acquired and reproductive capacity is attained due to the secretion of gonadal steroids under the direction of gonadotropin-releasing hormone (Gn-RH) and pituitary gonadotropins (i.e., FSH and LH). Deficiencies or defects in the functioning of these secretions may result in abnormal pubertal development.

    **1. Delayed puberty**

      **a. Female delayed puberty.** By definition, the absence of secondary sex characteristics at age 14 years is considered delayed. Normal secondary sex characteristics but absence of menarche by age 16 years also is considered delayed (**primary amenorrhea**).

        **(1) Constitutional delay of puberty** is less commonly diagnosed in girls than in boys.

            **(a) Etiology.** Constitutional delay of puberty is a designation reserved for otherwise healthy children (see VIII B 1). Delayed puberty may be secondary to a variety of endocrine and systemic diseases, such as hypothyroidism, sickle cell anemia, rheumatoid arthritis, inflammatory bowel disease, chronic renal failure, and others.

            **(b) Clinical features.** Girls with constitutional delay of puberty frequently are short but growing at normal prepubertal growth velocities. Bone age often is significantly delayed; however, there is no evidence of other endocrine or systemic disease. There is frequently a strong history of delayed puberty or menarche in adult family members. Late but otherwise normal puberty occurs.

        **(2) Primary ovarian failure.** Girls with primary ovarian failure develop castrate levels of gonadotropins by the usual age of puberty (10–12 years) because of lack of feedback of gonadal steroids on the pituitary gland.

            **(a) Turner syndrome** is the most common cause of primary ovarian failure (see Ch 7 IV C 1).

            **(b) Prepubertal surgical removal or irradiation** of the ovaries for treatment of cancer also may cause primary ovarian failure.

            **(c) Autoimmune ovarian failure** may occur in association with other autoimmune diseases, adrenal insufficiency, thyroiditis, hypoparathyroidism, and IDDM.

        **(3) Hypogonadotropic hypogonadism** may be difficult to distinguish from delayed puberty because, in each situation, gonadotropin levels are low and the response to Gn-RH stimulation is also minimal. This disorder often is part of other recognizable syndromes.

            **(a) Kallmann syndrome** involves anosmia with hypogonadotropic hypogonadism.

            **(b) Hypopituitarism** may include gonadotropin deficiency as one of several deficient pituitary hormones.

            **(c) Hypothalamic and pituitary tumors** such as adenoma, microadenoma (especially one secreting prolactin), craniopharyngioma, and pinealoma may be associated with hypogonadotropic hypogonadism.

            **(d) Anorexia nervosa** may cause delayed puberty or, in older adolescents, secondary amenorrhea due to gonadotropin deficiency.

            **(e) Prader-Willi syndrome** is characterized by short stature, obesity, mental retardation, and hypogonadotropic hypogonadism [see Ch 7 IV D 1 d (2)].

      **b. Male delayed puberty.** The earliest sign of puberty in males is testicular enlargement. Absence of any evidence of puberty by age 14 years is considered delayed.

        **(1) Constitutional delay of puberty** is the most common cause of delayed puberty in boys. Frequently these boys are short (at or below the fifth percentile) but growing at a low to normal prepubertal growth velocity. The bone age is significantly delayed. The physical examination is normal except for sexual immaturity. There usually is a family history of delayed pubertal development.

**(2) Primary testicular failure.** In boys with primary testicular failure, gonadotropin levels are elevated in the castrate range by the usual age of puberty because of the lack of testosterone feedback on the pituitary gland.

    **(a) Congenital bilateral anorchia ("vanishing testes" syndrome).** Boys with this syndrome have normal male sexual differentiation with apparent cryptorchidism. However, no testes are found on surgical exploration, and there is no testosterone response to HCG stimulation. Since there are normal male external genitalia and there are no müllerian remnants internally, it is presumed that testes must have been present in early fetal life and subsequently "vanished."

    **(b) Chemotherapy, irradiation, surgical excision, trauma, and infection** in the prepubertal boy may result in testicular failure.

    **(c)** Primary testicular failure also may be associated with the normal onset of puberty. In **Klinefelter syndrome** (see also Ch 7 IV C 2), a common cause of testicular failure, puberty begins at the usual age and secondary sex characteristics are acquired. However, these boys have small, firm testes and often have gynecomastia.

**(3) Hypogonadotropic hypogonadism.** As in females, isolated hypogonadotropic hypogonadism in males may occur alone or as part of a recognizable disease (e.g., Kallmann syndrome, hypopituitarism, CNS tumors, Prader-Willi syndrome).

  **c. Diagnosis**

    **(1)** A careful **history** and **physical examination** should be taken, including height and weight, Tanner staging of pubertal development (see Tables 4-1–4-3), smell testing, and presence of dysmorphic features or signs of other endocrine or systemic disease.

    **(2) Laboratory studies** include an evaluation of bone as well as FSH, LH, prolactin, $T_4$, TSH, and testosterone or estrogen levels. To rule out systemic disease, complete blood count, erythrocyte sedimentation rate, electroyte, and BUN evaluations may be helpful. Depending on the clinical situation, CT or MRI scan of the head and testing of other pituitary hormones may be indicated.

  **d. Therapy**

    **(1)** Treatment with appropriate sex steroid replacement for adolescents with a permanent cause of delayed puberty (either primary gonadal failure or hypogonadotropic hypogonadism) should be instituted at the usual age of puberty. Since sex steroids promote epiphyseal fusion while stimulating linear growth, this effect must be taken into consideration when treating children with short stature, especially due to GH deficiency. In children with eunuchoid proportions, epiphyseal fusion is desirable.

    **(2)** For adolescents with constitutional delay of puberty, smaller doses of the appropriate sex steroid may be used for a short course of treatment (3–6 months). This will initiate some development of secondary sex characteristics and be psychologically beneficial while not promoting premature epiphyseal fusion and loss of adult height.

**2. Precocious puberty.** Sexual development is considered to be precocious if there are any secondary sex characteristics present in girls before age 7½ years and in boys before age 9 years. True **central (gonadotropin-dependent) precocious puberty** appears to be more common in girls than in boys. In girls, there rarely is underlying CNS disease, and it is, therefore, considered "idiopathic." There is a significant incidence of CNS pathology, especially tumors, in males with central precocious puberty.

  **a. Premature thelarche** refers to the frequent finding of **isolated breast development** in very young girls. The usual age of onset is 12–24 months.

    **(1) Etiology.** It has been postulated that premature thelarche is due to small transient bursts of estrogen from the prepubertal ovary or from increased sensitivity to low levels of estrogen in some prepubertal girls.

    **(2) Clinical features.** Gonadotropins and serum estrogen levels are in the prepubertal range. Linear growth acceleration and advanced skeletal maturation are not present. Breast development does not progress, and no other signs of puberty develop.

    **(3) Diagnosis.** This nonprogressive, benign condition can be distinguished from true precocious puberty by the normal growth rate and bone age associated with premature thelarche.

  **b. Premature adrenarche** describes the **early appearance of sexual hair** (i.e., before age 8 years in girls and age 9 years in boys).

    **(1) Etiology.** This benign condition is believed to be due to early maturation of adrenal androgen secretion (adrenarche) in some children.

    **(2) Clinical features.** Levels of adrenal androgens are normal for pubertal stage but elevated for chronologic age. Bone age may be slightly, but not usually significantly, advanced.

    **(3) Diagnosis.** Children with premature adrenarche must be evaluated for other causes of increased androgen production, such as congenital adrenal hyperplasia due to 21-hydroxylase, 11-hydroxylase, or 3β-hydroxysteroid dehydrogenase deficiency or adrenal tumor. In children with evidence of significant androgen effect (e.g., advanced bone age, growth acceleration, acne), measurement of adrenal steroids and androgens before and after ACTH will identify those with congenital adrenal hyperplasia.

  **c. Precocious isosexual puberty** may be divided into two types—gonadotropin-dependent and gonadotropin-independent. This distinction has etiologic and therapeutic considerations.

    **(1) Gonadotropin-dependent precocious puberty (GDPP)** may be considered normal puberty beginning at an abnormally early age.

      **(a) Etiology.** GDPP may be idiopathic (as it is in most girls) or secondary to structural or functional disturbance in the CNS where the onset of puberty originates. However, a variety of diseases of the CNS have been associated with GDPP, including tumors (e.g., glioma, pinealoma, hamartoma), hydrocephalus, head injury, congenital malformation, and infection.

      **(b) Clinical features** are progressive development of secondary sex characteristics, beginning in girls before age 7½ years and in boys before age 9, accompanied by a growth spurt, causing the child's height to cross isobars on the growth curve. If the GDPP is secondary to another problem in the CNS, a history of neurologic disease or abnormal neurologic findings on physical examination may be present. Because sex steroids stimulate growth while promoting epiphyseal fusion, precocious puberty causes premature closure of the epiphyses and adult short stature. Behavior problems related to early sexual development and tall stature in childhood are relatively common.

      **(c) Diagnosis** is based on evidence of growth acceleration, significantly advanced bone age, and pubertal levels of gonadotropins and estrogen or testosterone. Because of the episodic secretion of gonadotropins and sex steroids early in GDPP, random daytime measurements may be low. A pubertal pattern of elevated gonadotropins after an intravenous infusion of Gn-RH is indicative of GDPP.

      **(d) Therapy.** Although treatment with injections of medroxyprogesterone acetate had been used for years to suppress menses and diminish secondary sex characteristics, this therapy did not prevent premature epiphyseal fusion and adult short stature. Recently, some long-acting analogues of Gn-RH have been discovered that inhibit gonadotropin release. These have been used in clinical trials for the treatment of children with GDPP with promising results, both in decreasing secondary sexual development and in slowing growth and skeletal maturation.

    **(2) Gonadotropin-independent precocious puberty (GIPP)** is a rare cause of precocious sexual development. Examples of GIPP are McCune-Albright syndrome (polyostotic fibrous dysplasia of bone), some cases of familial precocious puberty in males (testitoxicosis), and Leydig cell tumors and hyperplasia. Gonadotropins are low, and there is no increase in gonadotropins after Gn-RH infusion. GIPP does not respond to treatment with analogues of Gn-RH.

    **(3) Ectopic HCG production** by neoplasms may stimulate Leydig cell growth and hypersecretion of testosterone with the clinical presentation of precocious puberty in males. Tumors include hepatoblastoma, pinealoma, and retroperitoneal carcinoma. High LH levels (due to cross-reaction with HCG in radioimmunoassay) and low FSH levels are a clue to ectopic HCG production.

    **(4) Hypothyroidism** paradoxically may be associated with sexual precocity. Both gonadotropins and prolactin are elevated. Galactorrhea may be present. Unlike the case in other forms of precocious puberty, growth is arrested in hypothyroidism and bone age is delayed. Treatment of hypothyroidism may stop progression of sexual development.

**VII. DISORDERS OF CALCIUM METABOLISM.** Calcium and phosphorus homeostasis is maintained by having adequate nutritional intake of calcium, phosphorus, and vitamin D and a normally mineralized skeleton, the major reservoir of these minerals. The serum calcium and phosphorus are finely regulated by the action of **parathyroid hormone (PTH),** which acts on the bone and kidneys to raise the serum levels of calcium and lower the levels of phosphorus. Abnormalities of vitamin D and PTH may have profound effects on the serum levels of calcium and phosphorus and on the skeleton.

**A. Disorders of the parathyroid glands**

    **1. Primary hyperparathyroidism** is rare in childhood. The disorder may be isolated or occur as part of MEA I or II (see V B 2). Increased PTH levels cause increased mobilization of calcium and phosphorus from bone. The effect of increased PTH on the kidneys is decreased tubular reabsorption of phosphorus. Thus, the serum levels of calcium are elevated (**hypercalcemia**) and the phosphorus levels are low.

        **a. Clinical features**

            **(1)** Symptoms are related to hypercalcemia and include nausea, vomiting, constipation, lethargy, confusion, and weakness.

            **(2)** Hypertension and renal colic secondary to kidney stones are common.

        **b. Diagnosis**

            **(1) Laboratory studies** show elevated serum levels of calcium (total and ionized), low levels of phosphorus, increased alkaline phosphatase, and low tubular reabsorption of phosphorus (less than 80%). PTH levels are elevated relative to the elevated serum calcium. PTH secretion is autonomous.

            **(2) Radiographs** of bone show subperiosteal bone resorption that is especially evident in the clavicles.

        **c. Therapy** involves excision of the tumor if an adenoma is found and subtotal parathyroidectomy for hyperplasia.

    **2. Secondary hyperparathyroidism.** Diseases that cause **hypocalcemia** stimulate PTH to be released. The elevated PTH then restores the serum calcium to normal, but not elevated, levels but at the expense of having low phosphorus levels.

        **a. Etiology.** Conditions that are associated with secondary hyperparathyroidism are chronic renal disease, liver disease, and lack of vitamin D. In each of these situations, the initiating event is related to lack of intake, absorption, or metabolism of vitamin D, which leads to the hypocalcemic stimulus for PTH secretion.

        **b. Diagnosis and therapy.** The radiographic manifestation is rickets, and treatment is provision of adequate vitamin D.

    **3. Hypoparathyroidism**

        **a. Idiopathic hypoparathyroidism** may present in the neonatal period or at any time during childhood. The etiology may be autoimmune.

            **(1) Clinical features.** Symptoms are caused by low serum levels of calcium and include seizures, tetany, numbness of the face and extremities, and carpopedal spasm. Associated diseases may be thyroiditis, diabetes, adrenal insufficiency, and mucocutaneous candidiasis.

            **(2) Diagnosis.** At the time when serum calcium levels are low and phosphorus levels are high, the PTH levels are inappropriately low, indicating lack of PTH response to the hypocalcemia signal.

        **b. Pseudohypoparathyroidism** also presents as symptomatic hypocalcemia, but PTH levels are very high, indicating PTH unresponsiveness due to a receptor or postreceptor defect. Patients with pseudohypoparathyroidism have distinctive skeletal and facial characteristics, including short stature, round facies, a short thick neck, and short metacarpals. Mental retardation is common.

        **c. Therapy**

            **(1) Vitamin D** is the treatment for idiopathic hypoparathyroidism and pseudohypoparathyroidism.

                **(a)** Since low levels of PTH inhibit 1,25-hydroxylation of vitamin D in the kidneys, PTH deficiency is associated with a deficit of 1,25-dihydroxyvitamin $D_3$ (calcitriol), the most active metabolite of vitamin D. Treatment with 1,25-dihydroxyvitamin $D_3$ overcomes the deficit and also stimulates increased calcium absorption in the intestine.

                **(b)** Other forms of vitamin D, such as 25-hydroxyvitamin $D_3$ (calcidiol) and vitamin $D_3$ (cholecalciferol), also are effective but are required in larger doses. Because of the longer half-life of vitamin $D_3$, however, toxicity (hypercalcemia) is more serious.

(2) **Oral calcium supplementation** may speed the restoration of normal calcium levels. These children should have serum calcium and phosphorus levels monitored frequently to avoid hypercalcemia and potential nephrocalcinosis and renal damage.

4. **Neonatal hypocalcemia**
   a. **Early hypocalcemia** (serum calcium levels < 7 mg/dl) in the first 24–48 hours of life usually is associated with prematurity.
      (1) Immaturity of the parathyroid response to the normal fall in serum calcium levels after birth is believed to be the cause.
      (2) Clinical conditions associated with hypocalcemia in the first 2 days of life are birth asphyxia and maternal diabetes.
      (3) Hypocalcemia may be treated with oral calcium supplementation or intravenous calcium infusion for seizures.
   b. **Late hypocalcemic tetany** may occur in the first few weeks of life in infants receiving high-phosphate diets (i.e., cow's milk). Increased phosphate intake precipitates hypocalcemia and, therefore, is not recommended.
   c. **Idiopathic hypoparathyroidism** may present in the neonatal period with hypocalcemic seizures.

## B. Rickets

1. **General features of rickets**
   a. **Defect.** Rickets is characterized by bone lesions that are caused by **failure of osteoid,** the growing cellular matrix of bone, **to become mineralized.** The undermineralized bone is less rigid and the growing, remodeling bone bends and twists abnormally.
   b. **Clinical features**
      (1) Characteristic physical findings are bowing of the legs, thickening of the costochondral junction (rachitic rosary), knobby prominence of the wrists and knees, and growth failure. In infants, craniotabes (thinning of the skull bones) and fractures are common.
      (2) The radiographic manifestations are readily visible in views of the wrists and knees, with widening of the space between the end of the metaphysis and the epiphysis. The ends of the metaphysis are cupped, widened, and irregular or frayed.

2. **Variants of rickets** may be caused by vitamin D deficiency secondary to decreased intake, decreased absorption or decreased metabolism of vitamin D, or by lack of adequate calcium and phosphorus for normal bone mineralization caused by either deficient mineral intake or increased losses by the kidneys.
   a. **Nutritional rickets.** Lack of vitamin D in the diet results in decreased calcium absorption in the intestine. Hypocalcemia stimulates PTH secretion, which then causes increased reabsorption of calcium from bone and decreased renal reabsorption of phosphorus.
      (1) **Etiology.** Despite fortification of many foods with vitamin D to provide the minimum requirement of 400 IU daily, nutritional rickets still occurs in individuals with low vitamin D intake, such as food faddists. Often other aggravating factors are present besides decreased vitamin D intake, such as decreased exposure to the sun due to dark skin pigmentation, overcrowded inner city living conditions, and the winter season.
      (2) **Clinical features.** In classic nutritional rickets, the serum calcium level is low (or it may be normalized by the secondarily high PTH), the phosphorus level is low, and the alkaline phosphatase level is high because of active bone resorption from secondary hyperparathyroidism.
      (3) **Therapy** with 5000–10,000 units/day of vitamin D for several weeks, followed by provision of 400 IU/day in the diet, is curative.
   b. **Rickets associated with abnormal metabolism of vitamin D**
      (1) **Vitamin D–dependent rickets,** an autosomal recessive disease, is thought to be due to absence of the renal enzyme $1\alpha$-hydroxylase, which converts 25-hydroxyvitamin $D_3$ to the active metabolite 1,25-dihydroxyvitamin $D_3$.
         (a) **Clinical features.** Vitamin D–dependent rickets presents in the same way as nutritional rickets. The serum calcium level is low (or normal), the phosphorus level is low, and PTH is elevated. Usually 25-hydroxyvitamin $D_3$ levels are normal, while 1,25-dihydroxyvitamin $D_3$ levels are low.
         (b) **Therapy** with physiologic doses of 1,25-dihydroxyvitamin $D_3$ is curative.

(2) **Chronic renal disease.** One of the factors leading to **renal osteodystrophy**—the complex of osteopenia, osteitis fibrosis, and rickets associated with chronic renal failure—is decreased activity of 1α-hydroxylase in the kidneys. Therefore, treatment of renal osteodystrophy includes 1,25-dihydroxyvitamin $D_3$.

(3) **Chronic liver disease,** such as biliary atresia and other cholestatic diseases, may result in rickets from decreased intestinal absorption of vitamin D, a fat-soluble vitamin, or from decreased 25-hydroxylation in the liver itself. The treatment of choice is 25-hydroxyvitamin $D_3$ or 1,25-dihydroxyvitamin $D_3$.

(4) **Chronic anticonvulsant therapy.** Phenobarbital and phenytoin cause increased metabolism of calcidiol and may be associated with rickets. Usually other nutritional and environmental factors also are present in children with seizure disorders who present with clinical rickets. Increased demand for vitamin D can be satisfied by increasing the daily intake to 1000–2000 IU/day for children on chronic anticonvulsant therapy whose exposure to sunlight and nutritional intake is marginal.

c. **Rickets due to mineral deficiency**

(1) **X-linked hypophosphatemia (familial hypophosphatemia).** The primary defect in this inheritable form of rickets is a renal tubular defect resulting in phosphate "wasting." The serum calcium level is normal, the phosphorus level is low, and the alkaline phosphatase level is elevated. The 25-hydroxyvitamin $D_3$ level is normal, but the 1,25-dihydroxyvitamin $D_3$ level is low or normal, which is inappropriate given the hypophosphatemic stimulus for increasing 1α-hydroxylase activity. This may imply a defect in vitamin D metabolism as an additional etiologic factor.

(a) **Clinical features.** Biochemical abnormalities and radiographic signs of rickets are evident in the first few months of life. Subsequently, these children have severe rickets and short stature.

(b) **Therapy** consists of oral phosphate to replace renal losses and 1,25-dihydroxyvitamin $D_3$. Care must be taken to avoid vitamin D intoxication with hypercalciuria, nephrocalcinosis, and hypercalcemia.

(2) **Rickets of prematurity (metabolic bone disease of the premature infant).** Infants born prematurely have decreased bone mineralization compared to full-term infants because they do not benefit from the major skeletal accretion of calcium and phosphorus occurring in utero during the last trimester.

(a) **Clinical features.** Human milk and standard infant formulas that provide adequate calcium and phosphorus for the full-term infant are not adequate for the needs of the premature infant, as evidenced by the occurrence of severe osteopenia and rickets, resulting in fractures, in some premature infants. In these infants, serum calcium level is normal, and phosphorus level is low. 1,25-Dihydroxyvitamin $D_3$ levels are elevated, probably because of the hypophosphatemic stimulus.

(b) **Therapy.** Fortifying human milk or formulas with additional calcium and phosphorus results in improvement in bone mineralization and healing of fractures and rickets.

VIII. **APPROACH TO THE PEDIATRIC PATIENT WITH SHORT STATURE.** This section discusses the general approach to the evaluation of the child or adolescent with short stature. Many of the specific endocrine disorders that may result in short stature are described in detail elsewhere in this chapter.

A. **Growth assessment**

1. **Growth charts.** Assessment of growth in childhood begins with accurate and serial measurements that are plotted on the appropriate growth chart. The most widely accepted charts for children in the United States are those compiled by the United States National Center for Health Statistics.

2. **History.** Information that may have a bearing on the child's growth is gathered from talking with the child and his caregivers, usually the parents.

   a. Birth history, review of past growth and medical records, and a careful review of symptoms referable to each organ system must be obtained.

   b. Behavior problems and school performance should be noted.

   c. Growth records kept by the parents, school, and doctors' offices are helpful. If such records are not available, indirect information about growth may be ascertained by asking about frequency of shoe and clothing size changes and height relative to siblings and peers.

   **d.** Information about genetic potential for height may be gathered by recording the heights of parents, siblings, and other relatives. A family history of other medical problems also is relevant.

   **e.** The child should be questioned sensitively about the impact of short stature on his relationships with peers, participation in sports, and other social activities. Parents' perceptions also should be noted in these matters.

**3. Physical examination.** The following aspects should receive special attention during a physical examination.

   **a. Height**

   **(1) Recumbent length** is plotted for children from birth to 24 months of age. **Standing heights** are plotted for children 2–18 years of age. A **stadiometer** or other measuring device fixed to the wall measures height most accurately.

   **(2)** In addition to height, **arm span** and **upper-to-lower body segment ratio** should be measured.

   **b. General appearance and activity.** Dysmorphic features in a pattern suggestive of a specific syndrome, obesity, and general appropriateness of behavior to the examiner and family members should be noted.

   **c. Skin** is examined for abnormal pigmentation or cyanosis, and the skin and hair texture are noted for possible clues to hypothyroidism.

   **d. Head, ears, and eyes** are examined for midline defects (e.g., clefts) and for ocular or dental anomalies. Visual field examination is performed. Funduscopy is performed to look for optic nerve abnormalities, which might indicate increased intracranial pressure or an underlying CNS disease causing GH deficiency.

   **e. Neck.** The thyroid is palpated to determine its size, consistency, and the presence of nodules.

   **f. Chest and heart** are examined for evidence of chronic cardiopulmonary disease or heart murmur.

   **g. Abdomen.** Tenderness or bloating may indicate chronic gastrointestinal disease, such as celiac disease or inflammatory bowel disease.

   **h. Genitalia.** Anomalies of the genitalia, such as undescended testes and hypospadias in males and clitoromegaly and labial fusion in females, should be noted. Stretched penile length and testicular size should be recorded. Tanner staging for breast and pubic hair development in girls and genital and pubic hair development in boys should be documented.

   **i. Extremities.** Abnormalities of digits, joints, and body proportions should be noted and compared to published norms for age and sex.

   **j. Neurologic examination** is performed to rule out underlying CNS disease, especially any tumor that might cause GH deficiency.

**B. Short stature** generally can be ascribed to several broad categories of medical problems. On the basis of previous growth and medical records and the current medical, family, and social history and physical examination, the laboratory evaluation focuses on a relatively small number of tests of both diagnostic and prognostic significance. Broad diagnostic categories will be discussed in the order of those most frequently found among children presenting to an endocrinologist with the complaint of short stature.

**1. Constitutional delay of growth and development** is a more common diagnosis among boys referred for short stature than among girls, perhaps because of greater social value placed on height for boys than for girls.

   **a. Growth assessment**

   **(1)** These children grow at or below the fifth percentile at normal growth velocities, which results in a curve that is parallel to the fifth percentile.

   **(2)** Puberty is delayed and generally reflects significantly delayed skeletal maturation. Because these children fail to enter puberty at the usual age, their short stature and sexual immaturity are accentuated at this time when compared to those of normally developing peers.

   **(3)** Family members usually are of average height, but there often is a family history of short stature in childhood and delayed puberty in other family members.

   **b. Diagnosis.** Minimal diagnostic tests are indicated, including thyroid studies, complete blood count, erythrocyte sedimentation rate, electrolytes, BUN, and bone age assessment. These children have no findings suggestive of other endocrine or chronic systemic disease, and the normal growth velocity argues against such diagnoses.

  **c. Counseling.** These children and their families should be counseled about this pattern of growth and development as a variant of normal conditions and reassured about their potential for normal height, usually in the range expected for their families.

  **d. Therapy.** In many instances, reassurance that no significant endocrine disease exists and that normal growth and puberty with reasonable adult stature are expected is all that is required. Treatment with the anabolic steroid oxandrolone is controversial but appears to be helpful in some boys, mostly for the psychological benefit of modestly increasing muscle mass and growth velocity. There is no convincing evidence that final adult stature is either augmented or reduced by this treatment. Because of the illicit use of anabolic steroids by many athletes, oxandrolone is no longer available in the United States for treatment of short stature. For boys and girls with no signs of puberty by age 14 years and with a diagnosis of constitutional delay of growth and development, a short course (4–6 months) of the appropriate sex steroid may be helpful.

**2. Familial (genetic) short stature**

 **a. Growth assessment**

  **(1)** These children establish growth curves at or below the fifth percentile by age 2–3 years. They are otherwise completely healthy, with a normal physical examination. Bone age in these children is normal. Therefore, puberty occurs at the usual age and, thus, limits potential for growth late into adolescence.

  **(2)** Short stature usually is found in at least one parent. However, since the inheritance of height is complex, occasionally short stature may be present only in more distant relatives.

 **b. Diagnosis.** The same minimal diagnostic evaluation may be performed in these children as for those with apparent constitutional delay of growth to rule out subtle thyroid dysfunction or chronic disease.

 **c. Counseling.** Because puberty occurs at the expected time, these children seem to be at less of a disadvantage socially and emotionally compared to those with constitutional delay, despite the fact that their potential for adult height in the normal range is less.

**3. GH deficiency** (see also IV A 1 b). Fewer than 5% of children referred to endocrinologists for short stature have GH deficiency.

 **a. Growth assessment.** Children with classic GH deficiency grow at subnormal growth velocities (< 5 cm/yr) and have significant retardation of skeletal maturation. Therefore, evaluation with GH testing should be reserved for children who satisfy those criteria.

  **(1)** A history of birth asphyxia or neonatal hypoglycemia, or physical findings of microphallus or midline defects, is strongly suggestive of idiopathic GH deficiency.

  **(2)** GH deficiency secondary to a hypothalamic or pituitary tumor usually is associated with other neurologic or visual complaints and findings. In an older child with more recent onset of subnormal growth, the index of suspicion for tumor should be high.

 **b. Diagnosis.** After establishing that current growth velocity is less than 5 cm/yr and that thyroid function is normal and other systemic disease is unlikely, GH testing should be carried out. Evaluation for other pituitary hormone deficiencies also should be performed.

 **c. Therapy**

  **(1)** For children deemed GH-deficient, biosynthetic human GH (0.03–0.05 mg/kg) is given by subcutaneous injection every day. Accelerated growth velocity on GH treatment results in some catch-up growth in most children.

  **(2)** If puberty is delayed beyond age 14 years, the addition of sex steroids may be considered, both to augment the growth response to GH and to stimulate secondary sexual development. In children who have permanent gonadotropin deficiency, sex steroids may need to be replaced indefinitely as physiologically as possible.

  **(3)** Treatment with cortisol, thyroid hormone, and vasopressin (ADH) may be needed, depending on the degree of hypopituitarism.

  **(4)** Although some GH-deficient children release GH when stimulated by GRF, treatment with GRF currently is not an available alternative to GH therapy except in the research setting.

**4. Primary hypothyroidism** (see also III B) causes marked growth failure, with growth velocity less than 5 cm/year, and marked retardation of skeletal maturation. Because primary hypothyroidism is easily treatable, almost all children with short stature should have $T_4$, $T_3$ resin uptake, and TSH levels measured, even in the absence of obvious symptoms, to rule out any degree of hypothyroidism.

5. **Cushing's disease** [see also V A 3 a (1)] is a very rare cause of short stature in children. However, **hypercortisolism** (from either exogenous treatment with pharmacologic doses of steroids or endogenous oversecretion) may have a profound growth-suppressing effect. Usually other features of Cushing syndrome are evident.

6. **Primordial growth failure** has been used to describe a large diverse group of children who have normal endocrine function but who have inherent limitations on skeletal growth.
   a. **Etiology.** The cause of short stature in these children usually is easily identified on the basis of abnormal body proportions (skeletal dysplasias), dysmorphic features (chromosome abnormalities), and other characteristics of the history or physical examination (e.g., Prader-Willi syndrome, Noonan syndrome, intrauterine growth retardation).
   b. **Diagnosis.** Special attention should be given to the evaluation of **girls with short stature**. While a short girl with all of the physical stigmata of Turner syndrome may be easily identified, the features may be quite subtle in some girls. Therefore, girls with short stature and delayed puberty should have gonadotropins and chromosomes measured. Elevated gonadotropins indicating primary ovarian failure and chromosome abnormalities are diagnostic of Turner syndrome (see Ch 7 IV C 1).
   c. **Therapy.** Although children with primordial growth failure are not thought to have classic GH deficiency, the response to GH treatment in these children is being explored.

7. **Chronic systemic disease.** The impact of chronic systemic disease on growth is well known.
   a. **Types of diseases**
      (1) Cyanotic congenital heart disease, poorly controlled diabetes mellitus, and severe rheumatoid arthritis have a deleterious effect on growth, probably related to a combination of nutritional deficits and increased metabolic demands created by the disease process.
      (2) Some chronic diseases may have minimal symptoms and yet have a significant effect on growth. The two best known categories of chronic diseases that may present first as short stature are gastrointestinal diseases, specifically inflammatory bowel disease (Crohn's disease) and celiac disease, and renal disease associated with renal tubular acidosis or uremia.
   b. **Diagnosis.** Screening studies that may be helpful are complete blood count, erythrocyte sedimentation rate, serum electrolytes, and BUN. In some children where there is no explanation for growth failure, additional diagnostic tests for gastrointestinal disease are performed.

8. **Psychosocial deprivation.** In some children, a hostile, abusive, or neglectful environment appears to result in functional GH deficiency.
   a. **Clinical features.** Children with psychosocial deprivation characteristically show bizarre behavior, including hoarding food, gorging, drinking from puddles and toilet bowls, immature speech, disturbed sleep-wake cycles, and diminished perception of pain. Clinically, they resemble children with GH deficiency, with marked retardation of bone age and delayed puberty.
   b. **Diagnosis.** If GH testing is done while the children remain in the hostile environment, it usually shows a blunted response. When taken out of that environment, the children show catch-up growth, and testing reverts to normal.

C. **Tall stature.** Occasionally children appear to be growing too rapidly. Children who are growing above the ninety-fifth percentile should be examined carefully for signs of precocious puberty or adrenal androgen excess.

1. Most children have **familial tall stature**. Occasionally, early adolescent girls with familial tall stature may request treatment to reduce adult stature. High-dose estrogen may induce premature epiphyseal fusion and reduction of final height.

2. Other, more unusual causes of tall stature are GH excess (causing **acromegaly** and **gigantism**), hyperthyroidism, Marfan syndrome, and homocystinuria.

## STUDY QUESTIONS

**Directions:** Each of the numbered items or incomplete statements in this section is followed by answers or by completions of the statement. Select the **one** lettered answer or completion that is **best** in each case.

1. Autoimmunity is thought to play a pathogenetic role in which of the following conditions?

(A) Hypophosphatemic rickets
(B) Familial hypercholesterolemia
(C) Congenital hypothyroidism
(D) Insulin-dependent (type I) diabetes mellitus (IDDM)

2. Factors most likely to contribute to the development of diabetic ketoacidosis include all of the following EXCEPT

(A) overeating
(B) vomiting
(C) omission of insulin doses
(D) infection
(E) lack of patient education

3. All of the following conditions may lead to elevated total serum cholesterol levels EXCEPT

(A) LDL receptor deficiency
(B) pancreatitis
(C) acquired hypothyroidism
(D) high-fat diet
(E) diabetes

4. A 14-year-old child who presents with delayed skeletal maturation (bone age) may have any of the following disorders EXCEPT

(A) GH deficiency
(B) psychosocial deprivation
(C) hypothyroidism
(D) nonclassic (late-onset) 21-hydroxylase deficiency
(E) constitutional delay of puberty

5. All of the following may be manifestations of an insulin reaction (hypoglycemia) in an insulin-dependent diabetic patient EXCEPT

(A) loss of appetite
(B) sweating
(C) lethargy
(D) bizarre behavior
(E) slurred speech

6. All of the following are goals of newborn screening for congenital hypothyroidism EXCEPT

(A) to ensure normal linear growth
(B) to ensure normal intellectual function
(C) to facilitate genetic counseling
(D) to prevent sudden infant death syndrome

7. A newborn infant with ambiguous genitalia is found to have a 46,XX karyotype. All of the following are diagnostic possibilities EXCEPT

(A) 21-hydroxylase deficiency
(B) partial androgen resistance syndrome
(C) true hermaphroditism
(D) maternal virilizing tumor

8. A child with pheochromocytoma may present with all of the following signs and symptoms EXCEPT

(A) headache
(B) weight loss
(C) seizures
(D) sweating
(E) flushing

9. A 12-year-old boy is referred to his pediatrician by his teacher for poor attention span, deteriorating school performance, and frequent trips to the bathroom. By the pediatrician's records, the boy has lost 5 lb since his previous visit 6 months earlier. On physical examination, the boy's resting pulse is 110 beats/min, his blood pressure is 130/50, and his thyroid gland is about twice the normal size. The most likely diagnosis is

(A) Hashimoto's thyroiditis
(B) medullary carcinoma of the thyroid
(C) IDDM
(D) juvenile hypothyroidism
(E) thyrotoxicosis

| | | |
|---|---|---|
| 1-D | 4-D | 7-B |
| 2-A | 5-A | 8-E |
| 3-B | 6-D | 9-E |

10. A 5-year-old boy is discovered to have pubic hair during his prekindergarten physical examination. His mother says that recently he has been complaining of headaches. Additional findings on physical examination include height on the ninetieth percentile and acne. All of the following diagnostic studies are appropriate in this case EXCEPT

(A) serum testosterone measurement

(B) CT scanning of head

(C) serum HCG measurement

(D) smell testing to detect anosmia

(E) serum 17-hydroxyprogesterone measurement

11. A 15-month-old girl is brought to the emergency room because she is lethargic and may have had a "seizure." Her appetite has been decreased for 24 hours because of an intercurrent viral illness. Urinalysis reveals 3+ ketones, and blood chemistry evaluation reveals:

$[Na^+] = 140$ mEq/L
$[K^+] = 5.0$ mEq/L
$[Cl^-] = 100$ mEq/L
$[CO_2] = 19$ mEq/L
[glucose] = 31 mg/dl

Based on the history and initial laboratory evaluation of this child, what is the most appropriate course of action?

(A) Treat with intravenous glucose and admit to hospital for (diagnostic) 24-hour fast

(B) Treat with intravenous glucagon

(C) Perform oral glucose tolerance test

(D) Let the child eat and discharge from emergency room

(E) Obtain an EEG and begin treatment with phenobarbital

**Directions:** The group of items in this section consists of lettered options followed by a set of numbered items. For each item, select the **one** lettered option that is most closely associated with it. Each lettered option may be selected once, more than once, or not at all.

**Questions 12–16**

For each disorder, select the characteristic serum electrolyte pattern.

|   | $[Na^+]$ (mEq/L) | $[K^+]$ (mEq/L) | $[Cl^-]$ (mEq/L) | $[CO_2]$ (mEq/L) |
|---|---|---|---|---|
| (A) | 131 | 3.4 | 100 | 24 |
| (B) | 128 | 5.8 | 103 | 16 |
| (C) | 135 | 6.0 | 106 | 10 |
| (D) | 138 | 4.2 | 102 | 27 |
| (E) | 144 | 5.0 | 105 | 26 |

12. Diabetic ketoacidosis

13. Acute adrenal crisis

14. Diabetes insipidus

15. Psychogenic water drinking

16. Insulin shock

10-D        13-B        16-D
11-A        14-E
12-C        15-A

## ANSWERS AND EXPLANATIONS

**1. The answer is D** *[I A 1 a (2)]*.
Insulin-dependent (type I) diabetes mellitus (IDDM) is thought to have an autoimmune basis. Evidence for this is the presence of circulating islet cell antibodies in most newly diagnosed patients and the association of type I diabetes with other autoimmune disorders, such as Hashimoto's thyroiditis, Graves' disease, and Addison's disease. The other disorders listed in the question are not thought to be autoimmune in nature. Hypophosphatemic rickets is caused by an inherited defect in renal phosphate handling, familial hypercholesterolemia is caused by an inherited deficiency of low-density lipoprotein (LDL) receptors, and congenital hypothyroidism is caused by thyroid dysgenesis or defective thyroid hormone synthesis.

**2. The answer is A** *[I A 1 f (2)]*.
Central to the development of diabetic ketoacidosis is absolute or relative lack of insulin, most commonly due to omitted insulin doses. Inappropriate actions, such as withholding insulin during intercurrent illness—especially when vomiting—may play a role in an uninformed patient. Infection also is frequently associated with insulin resistance, which necessitates a compensatory increase in insulin dose to prevent ketoacidosis. Overeating may cause excessive hyperglycemia, but as long as the patient continues his usual insulin dose, there should be enough insulin present to suppress ketogenesis and subsequent ketoacidosis.

**3. The answer is B** *[II B]*.
Pancreatitis may be a complication of severe hypertriglyceridemia but, by itself, is not associated with hypercholesterolemia. Familial hypercholesterolemia is caused by a deficiency of LDL receptors. Individuals with familial hypercholesterolemia may be heterozygous (one defective gene for LDL receptor activity and, thus, half the normal number of LDL receptors) or homozygous (two defective genes for LDL receptor activity and, thus, an absence of LDL receptors). Hypothyroidism, diabetes, nephrotic syndrome, and liver disease are causes of secondary hypercholesterolemia. In some individuals, a high-fat diet induces hypercholesterolemia.

**4. The answer is D** *[V A 1 a (3)]*.
Children with nonclassic 21-hydroxylase deficiency have advanced skeletal maturation (i.e., bone age) in childhood due to the effect of adrenal androgen on bone maturation. Growth hormone (GH) deficiency and hypothyroidism cause marked retardation of skeletal maturation. Psychosocial deprivation may cause "functional" GH deficiency, which is reversible when the child is moved to a more nurturing environment. Children with constitutional delay of puberty have mild to moderate retardation of bone age secondary to prepubertal levels of gonadal steroids.

**5. The answer is A** *[I A 1 f (1) (a)]*.
IDDM is characterized by a loss of insulin secretion by pancreatic beta cells. With the loss of insulin—the major anabolic hormone—a catabolic state develops. When treating IDDM with insulin, there is a risk of relative insulin excess, with resultant hypoglycemia. Symptoms of hypoglycemia may be related to a sympathetic discharge and include sweating, tremulousness, and hunger (not loss of appetite). More severe symptoms (e.g., lethargy, bizarre behavior, slurred speech, seizures) are caused by glucose deprivation to the central nervous system (CNS).

**6. The answer is D** *[III B 1 f]*.
There is no known association of congenital hypothyroidism and sudden infant death syndrome. Children with congenital hypothyroidism diagnosed on clinical grounds usually manifest poor linear growth and weight gain and are developmentally delayed. With institution of thyroid hormone replacement, growth and weight gain improve, but there often is permanent neurodevelopmental impairment. With early diagnosis (usually by 4 weeks of age) through newborn screening, children with congenital hypothyroidism have neurologic function and intelligence comparable to their nonaffected siblings. Most affected children have a sporadic form of congenital hypothyroidism with no increased risk to subsequent offspring. Children with an enzymatic defect in thyroid hormone synthesis (dyshormonogenesis) generally have milder disease; however, there is a 25% chance of other siblings being similarly affected.

**7. The answer is B** *[VI A 2 a (2) (b)]*.
Infants with partial androgen resistance may have ambiguous genitalia, but the karyotype is 46,XY. These infants have testes and high levels of testosterone, which are incompletely effective in virilizing the ex-

ternal genitalia in a normal male pattern. The defect is at the level of the androgen receptor. Female infants with congenital adrenal hyperplasia due to 21-hydroxylase deficiency may exhibit a variable degree of masculinization of the external genitalia because of prenatal exposure to high levels of circulating adrenal androgens. Most infants with true hermaphroditism have a 46,XX karyotype. However, gonadal tissue includes both ovarian and testicular elements. The testicular androgens cause external virilization, leading to ambiguous genitalia. In a similar fashion, a maternal virilizing tumor may expose a female fetus to high levels of androgen.

**8. The answer is E** *[V B 1 a].*
The excessive production of catecholamines by a pheochromocytoma results in episodic or sustained hypertension, which usually is severe. Headache and seizures are symptoms typically related to hypertension and hypertensive encephalopathy. Sweating and weight loss are a result of a true hypermetabolic state caused by catecholamine excess. The usual appearance during a paroxysm is pallor; catecholamines do not cause flushing.

**9. The answer is E** *[III C 3].*
The 12-year-old boy described in the question has symptoms of thyrotoxicosis (Graves' disease), particularly weight loss, deterioration of behavior and school performance, and tachycardia. Medullary thyroid carcinoma presents as an asymptomatic nodule or mass in the neck. In children with juvenile hypothyroidism, school performance usually is not impaired, and clinical symptoms include lethargy and constipation. Hashimoto's thyroiditis generally presents as an asymptomatic goiter. Transient symptoms of thyrotoxicosis very rarely are present in Hashimoto's thyroiditis. IDDM would not account for thyromegaly, widened pulse pressure, and tachycardia.

**10. The answer is D** *[IV B 1 a (3); VI B 2].*
This 5-year-old boy presents with signs of precocious sexual development. The cause of his disorder could be congenital adrenal hyperplasia, gonadotropin-dependent precocious puberty, or, possibly, a CNS tumor secreting human chorionic gonadotropin (HCG). Smell testing for anosmia might be indicated for the evaluation of delayed puberty—because of the association of hypogonadotropic hypogonadism and anosmia (Kallmann syndrome)—but not in the evaluation of precocious puberty.

**11. The answer is A** *[I B 3 a].*
This child is hypoglycemic and ketonuric. The differential diagnosis includes idiopathic ketotic hypoglycemia, GH deficiency, and cortisol deficiency as well as some rare inborn errors of metabolism. After the acute episode is treated with intravenous glucose, the child should be fed and observed as she recovers from her intercurrent illness. She should then be admitted to the hospital for a 24-hour fast with frequent monitoring of blood glucose and urinary ketones. If she becomes hypoglycemic (blood glucose level < 40 mg/dl), blood should be obtained for measurement of electrolytes, cortisol, GH, and organic acids (blood and urine). If the patient's GH and cortisol levels are elevated (as they should be during the hypoglycemic stress) and she is not acidotic, the most likely diagnosis is idiopathic ketotic hypoglycemia. An oral glucose tolerance test is not an appropriate test for a child with hypoglycemia and ketonuria. In the presence of ketonuria, intravenous glucagon is unlikely to raise the blood sugar; therefore, it is not an appropriate treatment.

**12–16. The answers are: 12-C** *[I A 1 f (2) (c)],* **13-B** *[V A 2 b, c],* **14-E** *[IV B 1 b],* **15-A** *[IV B 1 e],* **16-D** *[I A 1 f (1)].*
Diabetic ketoacidosis results in an anion gap metabolic acidosis due to overproduction of strong organic ketoacids, thus lowering the serum carbon dioxide ($CO_2$) level. In the face of metabolic acidosis, potassium ($K^+$) is drawn out of cells, elevating the serum $K^+$ level, while total body $K^+$ actually is low due to urinary losses.

In acute adrenal crisis, lack of mineralocorticoid causes hyperkalemia due to urinary sodium ($Na^+$) wasting and $K^+$ retention. With increased renal excretion of bicarbonate ($HCO_3^-$), the patient also becomes acidotic.

The patient with diabetes insipidus loses water due to inability to produce a concentrated urine. This may result in hemoconcentration and a high-normal serum $Na^+$ level.

The effect of psychogenic water drinking is to cause dilutional hyponatremia.

In insulin-induced hypoglycemia (insulin shock), serum electrolyte levels are normal. This is helpful in distinguishing insulin shock from diabetic ketoacidosis in an unresponsive patient with IDDM.

# 17
# Neurologic Diseases
Barry S. Russman

## I. GENERAL PRINCIPLES OF PEDIATRIC NEUROLOGIC DIAGNOSIS

**A. History.** A well-performed history should emphasize whether the neurologic problem being analyzed is:

1. Focal or diffuse
2. Acute or insidious
3. Static or progressive

**B. Physical examination.** Special aspects of the pediatric neurologic examination include evaluation of the developmental reflexes (Table 17-1), measurement of head circumference, assessment of developmental milestones, and a search for birthmarks, which can signal a neurologic defect.

**C. Diagnostic studies.** Useful procedures, depending on the clinical problem, can include:

1. **Lumbar puncture and cerebrospinal fluid (CSF) examination** (e.g., for infectious, metabolic, and degenerative diseases)
2. **Electroencephalography [EEG]** (for epilepsy)
3. **Electromyography (EMG)** and nerve conduction studies (for neuromuscular diseases)
4. **Measurement of cortical evoked potentials** [for assessment of central nervous system (CNS) function]
5. **Radiographic studies**
   a. **Skull radiography** (e.g., for depressed skull fracture)
   b. **Computed tomography (CT) scan** (for anatomic problems)
   c. **Magnetic resonance imaging (MRI) scan** (for differentiation of white and gray matter)
   d. **Arteriography** (for vascular disease)
   e. **Positron emission tomography (PET) scan** (research tool for assessment of brain metabolism)
6. **Biopsies** of muscle, peripheral nerve, skin, liver, bone marrow, rectal mucosa, and, rarely, brain for evaluation of a degenerative disease)

## II. ALTERED STATES OF CONSCIOUSNESS.
When assessing a child's altered state of behavior or decreased responsiveness, the child's developmental age and how the child typically responds to various stimuli must be considered (determined by history).

**A. Definitions**

1. **Delirium** is an altered state of behavior. The patient appears to be fully alert; however, reactions to various stimuli (e.g., touch) are inappropriate.
2. **Coma** is a state of unarousable unconsciousness. A patient in deep coma may be unresponsive to painful stimuli. The patient's record should include a description of the stimulus used and the response observed. Inexact terms (e.g., "stupor," "lethargy," "semi-coma") are best avoided. The Glasgow coma scale is reliable (Table 17-2).

**Table 17-1.** Developmental Reflexes

| Reflex | Test Position | Stimulus | Response | Age at Onset | Age at Disappearance | Significance |
|---|---|---|---|---|---|---|
| Moro | Support head and shoulders 30° above horizontal | Allow head to drop to horizontal | Extension of upper extremities at shoulders and elbows | 28 weeks gestational age | 6 months | **Absence** suggests severe myopathy or severe CNS abnormality **Persistence** suggests CNS abnormality |
| Asymmetrical tonic neck | Supine with head in midline | Passive or active neck rotation to left or right | Extension of arm and leg on face side, with flexion of arm and leg on occiput side | 37 weeks gestational age | 6 months— never obligatory* | **If obligatory or persistent** suggests CNS pathology |
| Parachute | Support infant in vertical position | Sudden tip of upper body downward | Arms extend to prevent fall | 6–8 months | Persists | **Should be symmetrical** **If not developed at appropriate time** suggests CNS abnormality |

*An obligatory reflex is defined as a tonic neck posture that is maintained beyond 30 seconds after the head is turned.

**Table 17-2.** Glasgow Coma Scale

| Finding | Score* |
| --- | --- |
| **Best verbal response:** | |
| Oriented | 5 |
| Confused | 4 |
| Inappropriate words | 3 |
| Incomprehensible sounds | 2 |
| None | 1 |
| **Motor response:** | |
| Obeys commands | 5 |
| Able to localize pain | 4 |
| Flexion to pain | 3 |
| Extension to pain | 2 |
| None | 1 |
| **Eyes open:** | |
| Spontaneously | 4 |
| To speech | 3 |
| To pain | 2 |
| None | 1 |

*Scoring is as follows: 3–7 severe head injury; 8–11 moderate head injury; 12–14 mild head injury.

**B. Etiology.** Possible causes of altered consciousness and diagnostic clues include the following.

1. **Infection** may be suggested by an elevated temperature or a history of exposure to a person with an infectious disease. Nuchal rigidity suggests meningeal inflammation.

2. **Cerebrovascular disease** is suggested by the presence of a hemiparesis or nuchal rigidity without an elevated temperature.

3. **Trauma** may be suspected if skin bruises or middle ear hemorrhage is noted.

4. **Postictal state.** Occasionally, a state of decreased responsiveness will follow a convulsion or seizure that may or may not have been observed. An EEG is necessary to establish the diagnosis.

5. **Metabolic disorders.** Diabetes, for example, may be suggested by fruity odor in the urine or on the breath. Laboratory evaluation is necessary to establish a specific etiology.

6. **Poisoning** is one of the most common causes of an altered state of consciousness in a child (see also Ch 2 IX). The family should search the household to determine if the child has ingested anything suspicious, such as medications, paint that contains lead, cleaning supplies (in the case of a young child), or alcoholic beverages or drugs of abuse (in the case of a school-age child).

**C. Diagnosis**

1. **History.** The patient history must be obtained rapidly, usually while the child is being stabilized.

2. **Physical examination.** In addition to establishing the patient's standing on the Glasgow coma scale, special attention should be given to the following areas.
   a. **Eyes.** Pupil size and reaction to light may suggest the presence of a toxic substance or a brain stem injury. Decreased extraocular movements, as elicited by the "doll's eye" maneuver or caloric testing, will suggest brain stem damage. Papilledema suggests elevated intracranial pressure.
   b. **Motor status.** Spontaneous movements should be observed and carefully recorded. The presence of decorticate or decerebrate posturing or seizures should be specifically noted.
   c. **Respiratory pattern.** The rate of respiration as well as breathing abnormalities (e.g., Cheyne-Stokes respiration, central neurogenic hyperventilation, Biot's breathing) should be noted.

3. **Laboratory studies.** Tests to be ordered are determined by the history and physical examination.

a. **Blood** should be analyzed for metabolic abnormalities (e.g., hypoglycemia).

b. **Urine** can be analyzed for the presence of toxic substances, heavy metals, sugar, and acetone.

c. **CT scan** is best used for hemorrhage; **MRI scan** provides information about other intracranial lesions.

d. **EEG** can help to diagnose seizures as the cause of the coma (see V A 3 c).

e. **Lumbar puncture** should be performed if an infection is suspected.

### D. Therapy

1. **Supportive treatment** includes establishing an airway, maintaining hydration, and decreasing intracranial pressure. Hyperventilating the patients is the quickest way to lower intracranial pressure. Medications (e.g., mannitol, steroids) also are helpful.

2. **Specific treatment** depends on the etiology of the delirium or coma.

## III. MALFORMATIONS OF THE CNS

### A. Epidemiology

1. Approximately 3% of all infants have at least one minor CNS malformation.

2. About 40% of infants who die in the first year of life have one or more developmental abnormalities of the nervous system.

3. Fully 75% of fetal deaths are associated wth a major CNS malformation.

### B. Disorders of embryogenesis (induction disorders) occur during the first 4 weeks of fetal development.

1. **Posterior midline lesions** (also called **neural tube defects** or **dysraphia**) can range from complete failure of the brain to develop (**anencephaly**) to a clinically insignificant posterior defect of the vertebral bodies (**spina bifida occulta**). Neural tube defects occur because the neural groove fails to fuse completely during formation of the neural tube. These defects usually show a multifactorial inheritance pattern (see Ch 7 V B).

a. **Spina bifida cystica** is a herniation of the meninges (**meningocele**) or the meninges plus the spinal cord (**meningomyelocele**) through a vertebral defect, usually in the lumbar area.

(1) **Clinical features** depend on the level and severity of the lesion. Bladder and bowel sphincters may be affected. Distal orthopedic problems (e.g., club foot) are common. Cerebral deficits and seizures can develop as a result of secondary meningitis, hydrocephalus, or associated CNS anomalies.

(2) **Diagnosis.** When the diagnosis is suspected before birth, the α-fetoprotein (AFP) level in maternal serum and in amniotic fluid should be tested. Fetal ultrasonography also may establish an early diagnosis.

(3) **Therapy** begins with surgical closure of the defect to prevent infection. A multidisciplinary approach provides the best management of a patient with a severe lesion, since ongoing neurosurgical, orthopedic, urologic, and psychological care will be necessary.

(4) **Prognosis** for ambulation correlates with the level and severity of the defect.

b. **Arnold-Chiari malformation** is an elongation and protrusion of medullary and cerebellar tissue through the foramen magnum and into the cervical spinal cord. The condition often accompanies meningomyelocele.

(1) **Types.** Several types can occur. **Chiari type 1** is an isolated protrusion of the cerebellar tissue. **Chiari type 2** combines type 1 plus hydrocephalus, and **Chiari type 3** is a combination of these defects plus a cranium bifidum, with or without protrusion of cerebral tissue (encephalocele). Respiratory distress is the most common clinical sign of this abnormality.

(2) **Therapy** requires surgery to prevent compression of the neural tissue at the formen magnum. Shunting procedures may be necessary if the hydrocephalus is symptomatic.

c. **Other dysraphic states** can occur when embryonic nervous tissue comes in contact with the dermis.

**(1) Tethered cord** results when the filum terminale becomes entangled with fibrous and fatty tissue, preventing the normal upward migration of the spinal cord that occurs with age.

    **(a) Clinical features** develop as the child grows. Typically, a gait disturbance, caused by spasticity and weakness, develops during the third to sixth year of life.

    **(b) Therapy** consists of surgical release of the cord.

**(2) Diplomyelia and diastematomyelia** are, respectively, a duplication and a cleft in the spinal cord.

    **(a) Clinical features** of these lesions usually appear as the child grows.

    **(b) Therapy.** Prompt surgical treatment prevents further loss of function.

**(3) Syringomyelia** is a fluid-filled cavity or cyst (syrinx) in the cord. A decompression laminectomy or decompression of the syrinx itself can alter the otherwise relentless progression that causes loss of sensation and weakness below the level of the cyst.

**(4) Sacral dysgenesis** is seen in 1% of the offspring of diabetic mothers. The major neurologic disabilities are urinary incontinence and weakness of the lower extremities. Treatment is symptomatic.

**(5) Neurodermal sinus** usually does not cause a neurologic problem. However, exploration and closure are important, as the tract may extend from the skin into the spinal cord, leading to recurrent meningitis.

**2. Anterior midline defects (holoprosencephaly)** can cause hypoplasia of the hypothalamus and a single ventricle.

  **a. Clinical features.** Symptoms such as poor body temperature control, apnea, and severe psychomotor retardation suggest an anterior midline defect.

  **b. Diagnosis** is made by CT or MRI scan or ultrasonography.

**3. Developmental anomalies of the base of the skull**

  **a. Platybasia** is an upward displacement of the base of the skull, leading to narrowing of the foramen magnum.

    **(1) Clinical features** are due to compression of the cervical cord and include spasticity in the lower extremities, shooting pain in the arms, and weakness of the proximal arm muscles.

    **(2) Therapy** consists of surgical decompression.

  **b. Klippel-Feil syndrome** results from the absence or fusion of several cervical vertebral bodies. The symptoms are similar to those noted for platybasia. Commonly associated abnormalities include spina bifida, syringomyelia, sensorineural hearing loss, and congenital heart disease.

**C. Disorders of cellular migration and proliferation** usually occur for unknown reasons, although they have been associated with maternal ingestion of toxic substances (e.g., alcohol, phenytoin) during pregnancy as well as with chromosomal and other genetic abnormalities.

**1. Agenesis of the corpus callosum** can be diagnosed best by MRI scan. The ventricles are farther apart than normal. Clinical manifestations range from a seizure disorder and severe retardation to no symptoms at all.

**2. Microcephaly** (see also Ch 7 VI C 4) is, by definition, a head circumference more than 2 standard deviations below the norm; it most often occurs as a result of a small brain (**micrencephaly**), since the skull generally grows in response to brain growth.

  **a. Etiology.** Microcephaly occurs idiopathically, as a chromosomal anomaly, and as an autosomal recessive disorder. It has also been noted in patients with hypothyroidism, Hurler syndrome, or rickets and secondary to maternal irradiation during early pregnancy.

  **b. Differential diagnosis.** Skull radiographs help to assure that **craniosynostosis** (i.e., premature closure of the sutures) is not the cause of the microcephaly.

    **(1) Craniosynostosis** may occur alone or in association with other syndromes (e.g., Crouzon, Apert, Carpenter).

    **(2) Therapy.** Surgical intervention rarely is necessary to relieve pressure. Most often, surgery is performed for cosmetic reasons.

**3. Macrocephaly** (see also Ch 7 VI C 5) is a large head circumference. Either the brain is too large (**macrencephaly**) or a space-occupying lesion (including enlarged ventricles) is the cause.

  **a.** The most common cause of macrocephaly in infants is **hydrocephalus**.

  **b.** Macrocephaly can also be caused by several **inherited metabolic or chromosomal anomalies** and several leukodystrophies (e.g., Canavan's disease, Alexander's disease; see IX D 5 b, c). **Arachnoid cysts** can also cause an enlarging head circumference; they are best diagnosed by MRI scan.

4. **Hydranencephaly** is a severe necrosis of the cerebral cortex that occurs in utero, with subsequent accumulation of CSF. The etiology is still uncertain; a migration disorder and bilateral internal carotid artery occlusion are popular theories. Survival beyond the first year of life is uncommon.

**D. Hydrocephalus** is enlargement of the cerebral ventricles due to excessive accumulation of CSF. This relativley common condition is the most frequent cause of an enlarged head in neonates.

1. **Types. Noncommunicating (obstructive) hydrocephalus** is due to an obstruction of CSF flow within the ventricular system. **Communicating hydrocephalus** is due to a dysfunction in the absorption of CSF.

2. **Etiology.** Causes of hydrocephalus can be related to time of onset.
   a. Prenatally or during the first month of life, the common causes are intraventricular hemorrhage, infection, or congenital malformations (e.g., aqueductal stenosis).
   b. During the first few years of life, a brain tumor must be suspected if the patient presents with hydrocephalus. Also, an asymptomatic partial obstruction might manifest itself at this age.

3. **Clinical features.** Abnormal rate of head growth, irritability, lethargy, vomiting, and headache (in the older child) suggest this diagnosis. Obtaining head circumference measurements over time is more important than a one-time measurement.

4. **Diagnosis.** A CT or MRI scan can reliably diagnose hydrocephalus, as can ultrasonography if the anterior fontanelle is still open.

5. **Therapy** includes the use of dehydrating agents (e.g., mannitol, acetazolamide, furosemide), serial spinal taps, and shunting procedures.

6. **Prognosis**
   a. Arrested hydrocephalus designates the termination of the hydrocephalic condition, with subsequent return to normal intracranial pressure. However, the ventricles commonly remain enlarged.
   b. The child's future cognitive and motor functions are related to several factors, including the cause of the hydrocephalus, how rapidly it developed, the duration of asymptomatic hydrocephalus, the frequency of shunt infections, and the presence and type of associated malformations.

**E. Congenital defects of cranial nerves and related structures**

1. **Mobius syndrome** is characterized by facial diplegia and ophthalmoplegia. Lack of development of the cranial nerve nuclei in the brain stem is the main pathologic finding. No treatment is indicated other than possible cosmetic surgery.

2. **Sensorineural hearing loss** in many cases is the result of a congenital defect [see Ch 3 V A 1 b (2)].

**F. Cerebellar malformations** include **total agenesis of the vermis** and the **Dandy-Walker malformation** (i.e., cystic dilation of the fourth ventricle, with obstructive hydrocephalus secondary to a blockage or atresia of the foramen of Magendie and formen of Luschka). Shunt procedures invariably are required.

**IV. CEREBRAL PALSY** is a descriptive term that refers to a motor deficit due to a nonprogressive (static) lesion of the immature brain. The lesion or lesions may occur prenatally, perinatally, or postnatally.

**A. Etiology and risk factors.** The cause of cerebral palsy is unknown in approximately 70% of patients. Approximately 20% of cases can be correlated with risk factors, including prematurity, cerebral anoxia, and trauma. Specific causes include embryologic malformations and infection.

**B. Clinical features**

1. **Typical clinical patterns.** The classification system for cerebral palsy considers the number of limbs involved and the type of motor abnormality.
   a. **Anatomic classification**
      (1) **Diplegia.** The lower limbs are more affected than the upper limbs.
      (2) **Hemiplegia.** One side of the body is involved more than the other, and the arm usually is affected more than the leg.

**(3) Quadriplegia.** All four limbs are similarly affected.

**(4) Double hemiplegia.** Both sides of the body are affected, the arms more than the legs.

**(5) Paraplegia.** Both legs are affected; the arms are spared.

b. **Physiologic classification**

(1) **Spasticity** is an increase in muscle tone.

(2) **Dyskinesia** is a collective term for several movement disorders, including **chorea** (abrupt, jerky movements), **athetosis** (slow, writhing, continuous movements in the extremities), and **dystonia** (writhing movements leading to sustained, bizarre postures of the trunk and extremities).

(3) **Ataxia** is an incoordination of movement; it is commonly associated with hypotonia, at least during the first few years of life.

2. **Associated problems** include epilepsy, mental retardation, behavior problems, learning disabilities, and strabismus.

**C. Diagnosis**

1. **History.** The patient presents with a history of a motor delay that is nonprogressive.

2. **Physical examination.** Findings on physical examination place the lesion in the CNS and commonly include any or all of the following:

a. Hyperactive reflexes

b. Abnormal movements of chorea, athetosis, or dystonia

c. Abnormal absence or persistence of infantile reflexes (see Table 17-1)

3. **Differential diagnosis.** Distinguishing cerebral palsy from a progressive neurologic disorder may be difficult early on, as the infant is in the initial stages of developing skills and a loss of minimal skills may be impossible to determine. Screening tests are available for a number of the inherited metabolic disorders, which are the most likely causes of progressive disorders.

**D. Therapy.** Early on, physical therapy programs are usually indicated. When the patient reaches the toddler or school-age stage, orthopedic intervention (e.g., special shoes, braces, surgery) often is necessary. The treatment of associated problems (e.g., learning disabilities, seizures) is no different for cerebral palsy patients than for children who are impaired in other ways.

# V. PAROXYSMAL DISORDERS

**A. Seizures** represent abnormal neural discharges in the cerebral cortex. Seizures in children can be **acute (nonrecurring)** or **chronic (recurring)**. In the neonate (see Ch 5 V G 2), seizures most often are due to a birth injury or congenital defect. In infants and young children, the cause usually is an acute infection. In older children, idiopathic epilepsy is the typical cause of seizures.

1. **Acute, nonrecurring seizures**

a. **Febrile convulsions** are seizures that accompany febrile disorders (e.g., acute respiratory infections) in children usually between the ages of 6 months and 3 years; these seizures rarely occur after age 5 years. Febrile convulsions are the most common type of acute, nonrecurring seizures.

(1) **Clinical features and diagnosis.** The convulsions usually resemble the tonic-clonic convulsions of grand mal epilepsy. Favorable signs suggesting that a chronic seizure disorder will not follow febrile convulsions include a normal neurologic examination, a short-lived seizure, and the lack of a family history of epilepsy.

(2) **Therapy.** A simple febrile convulsion does not require treatment with an anticonvulsant drug. For recurrent febrile seizures, valproic acid and phenobarbital are effective. Phenytoin and carbamazepine are ineffective.

b. **Other causes of acute seizures** include toxic substances (e.g., drugs, household poisons), metabolic disturbances (e.g., hypoglycemia, tetany), and intracranial disorders (e.g., brain tumors, meningitis).

(1) **Diagnosis.** These disorders must be ruled out by a careful physical as well as neurologic examination.

(2) **Therapy.** These disorders usually do not require treatment with anticonvulsant medications. Rather, specific treatment of the underlying cause is indicated.

**2. Chronic, recurring seizures (epilepsy)**

**a. Definition.** Epilepsy is a disorder of the cerebral cortex characterized by recurring paroxysms of abnormal neuronal discharges that manifest as sudden changes in motor, sensory, or psychic function, with associated characteristic changes in the EEG. The seizure, or **ictus,** may present clinically as a convulsion, a minor motor movement, a sensation, or a momentary arrest of activity; consciousness usually, but not always, is affected.

**b. Etiology.** In most cases, no specific cause can be found (called **idiopathic, cryptogenic, primary,** or **essential epilepsy**). In about 20% of cases, a specific cause is identified (called **symptomatic, organic, secondary,** or **acquired epilepsy**). The many possible causes of epilepsy include:

**(1)** Inherited metabolic anomalies [e.g., phenylketonuria (PKU), degenerative diseases]

**(2)** Intracranial lesions (e.g., vascular or other congenital malformations, tumors)

**(3)** Trauma (e.g., birth injuries, anoxia)

**(4)** Infections or toxic substances (e.g., encephalitis, meningitis, lead poisoning)

**c. Classification.** Seizures are classified as partial or generalized, depending on the EEG findings.

**(1) Partial simple seizures** start focally, do not involve a loss of consciousness or awareness, and usually are motor. In **adversive seizures,** the patient's eyes and head turn away from the seizure focus.

**(2) Partial complex seizures (psychomotor** or **temporal lobe seizures)** start focally, may generalize, and are associated with a loss of awareness or consciousness. Changes in behavior or in affect may be subtle and difficult to identify as epileptic. During the seizure, repetitive purposeless acts are typical.

**(a)** In **adversive seizures,** the patient's eyes and head turn away from the seizure focus.

**(b)** In **jacksonian seizures,** motor symptoms begin locally (in the face, hand, or foot) and spread to other muscles; the seizure may become a generalized convulsion with loss of consciousness.

**(3) Generalized seizures**

**(a) Tonic-clonic seizures (grand mal)** are the classic epileptic convulsion. A brief tonic phase of generalized contractions is followed by a longer clonic phase of rhythmic convulsive spasms. Postictally, confusion and ataxia are followed by several hours of sleep. A prodromal phase of discomfort may precede the seizure by several hours. The seizure may begin with a sensory or motor aura (e.g., epigastric sensations, head movements) that indicates the cortical focus. The latter might be classified as a partial complex seizure with secondary generalization if the EEG shows focal discharges.

**(b) Absence seizures (petit mal)** typically consist of staring episodes lasting less than 10 or 20 seconds, which represent sudden, brief interruptions of consciousness. Absence attacks can occur many times a day and can be precipitated by hyperventilation or by flashing lights.

**(c) Myoclonic seizures** consist of sudden, shock-like movements of the extremities or trunk without loss of consciousness. They can throw an older child to the ground. Infantile spasms (infantile myoclonus), typically a sudden flexion of the arms and extension of the head, may occur hundreds of times daily. Myoclonic seizures are commonly due to metabolic or degenerative diseases, perinatal injuries, or encephalitis. The Lennox-Gastaut syndrome combines this seizure type with mental retardation.

**(d) Atonic and akinetic seizures** cause a sudden loss of muscle tone, so that the child slumps to the ground.

**d. Status epilepticus** is a succession of grand mal seizures that occur without the patient's regaining consciousness. It can occur spontaneously, but stopping anticonvulsant medication is the most common cause. Petit mal status, absence status, and other forms of epileptic status can occur as well.

**e. Diagnosis**

**(1) History.** The diagnosis of a seizure is established by observation of the event. Most commonly, the physician will not see the episode. A thorough history obtained from the observer is mandatory. The physical examination usually is normal.

**(2) EEG pattern.** The disorderly neuronal activity that induces seizures is reflected in the EEG pattern and helps to classify the patient's seizures. This in turn helps in choosing the appropriate medication (Table 17-3). As the EEG records the electrical activity from the top centimeter of the brain only, it is possible to have a seizure with a normal EEG.

**Table 17-3.** Anticonvulsant Medications

| Drug | Seizure Type | | Loading | Maintenance | Absorption | Half-life | Steady State | Therapeutic Level | Side Effects | Toxicity (Dose-related) |
|------|------|------|---------|-------------|------------|-----------|--------------|-------------------|--------------|-------------------------|
| | 1° | 2° | | | | | | | | |
| Phenobarbital | G | CP | 20 mg/kg | 5 mg/kg to age 2 years; 1–3 mg/kg thereafter | ~ 4 hr | 24–72 hr | May take 15 days | 20–40 µg/dl | Lethargy, irritability, hyperactivity (in ≥ 50%; subtle in 80%–100%); rash 1–3 weeks after starting treatment; liver failure (rare) | Lethargy |
| Primidone | G | CP | Never load | 5–10 mg/kg | 60–90 min | 12 hr | 3–5 days | 4–12 µg/ml | Similar to phenobarbital | Similar to phenobarbital |
| Phenytoin | G | CP | 10 mg/kg | 5 mg/kg | 4 hr | 24–36 hr | 7 days | 10–20 µg/dl | Rash 5–30 days after starting treatment; serum sickness; hepatic failure; decreased alertness | Ataxia, dysarthria, lymphadenopathy, encephalopathy |
| Carbamazepine | CP | G | Usually not necessary | 20–25 mg/kg | 30–90 min | 14 hr | 3 days | 6–12 µg/ml | Rash, leukopenia, aplastic anemia | Nausea, diplopia, ataxia |
| Ethosuximide | G(A) | … | Not necessary | 20–40 mg/kg | 1–4 hr | 30–60 hr | 5–7 days | 40–100 µg/ml | Rash, blood dyscrasia, lupus | Nausea, headache, hiccups |
| Valproic acid | … | … | Not necessary | 20–60 mg/kg | Rapid | 8–15 hr | 2 days | 50–100 µg/ml | Hepatotoxicity | Nausea, cramps, hair loss, weight gain, tremor |

1° = primary; 2° = secondary; G = generalized seizures; CP = complex partial seizures; A = absence seizures.

      **(a)** During simple or complex **partial seizures,** the EEG usually reflects the epileptogenic focus.

      **(b)** During **grand mal seizures,** the EEG shows numerous high-voltage spikes. The interictal EEG may show generalized paroxysmal multispike discharges or it may be normal.

      **(c)** During **petit mal seizures,** the EEG shows a spike and slow wave discharge at 3 cycles per second (cps). The background rhythms are normal.

      **(d)** During **myoclonic seizures,** the EEG usually is abnormal, showing multifocal spike activity at 2–4 cps. In infantile spasms, the EEG pattern shows a series of irregular high-voltage waves and spikes (hypsarrhythmia).

  **f. Therapy.** For the individual seizure, treatment consists of preventing injury and, when possible, treating the underlying cause.

    **(1) Counseling.** The child with epilepsy should lead as normal a life as possible. Physical and social activities should be encouraged. Family and teachers may need counseling to provide the needed psychological support.

    **(2) Anticonvulsant medication.** The choice of drug (see Table 17-3) is based on the seizure type and EEG findings. Blood levels are guidelines only: Some patients need lower drug doses, whereas others need and can tolerate higher doses. Medication must be increased slowly to avoid side effects (e.g., lethargy) and withdrawn slowly to avoid precipitating seizures.

    **(3) Diet.** A ketogenic diet is used for grand mal or petit mal seizures that are difficult to control with medication and is most effective in children age 2–5 years.

    **(4) Surgery.** When drug treatment is unsuccessful, surgical excision of the epileptic focus or corpus callostomy can be considered. Most patients who undergo surgery still require anticonvulsant medication.

  **g. Prognosis.** Anticonvulsant medication can control seizures in 35%–50% of patients. Adequate control is less likely when seizures begin early in life, occur frequently, are mixed in type, and are associated with mental retardation or an abnormal neurologic examination. If a patient is seizure-free for at least 2 years, discontinuing medication should be considered.

**B. Migraine** is characterized by recurrent attacks of headache, which usually is unilateral and throbbing and often is accompanied by neurologic disturbances and nausea. Migraine attacks may be precipitated by stress or by ingestion of certain foods or substances, such as chocolate, peanuts, tyramine (found in aged cheese, chicken liver, and beer), nitrites, and quinine.

  **1. Clinical features and diagnosis.** There are many variants of migraine.

    **a.** In **classic migraine,** the attack is preceded by an **aura** (flashing lights, scotomas) and a good sleep usually relieves the headache. The physical examination typically is negative. In approximately 75% of cases, a positive family history exists.

    **b.** In **common migraine,** an aura rarely is present. The headache tends to be diffuse rather than focal and is pounding in quality. Nausea usually is present.

    **c.** In **atypical forms,** there may be an aura.

      **(1)** Patients with **hemiplegic migraine** develop a transient neurologic deficit just before, or in association with, the headache. The neurologic deficit may consist of aphasia, hemiparesis, hemianopsia, or third nerve palsy.

      **(2)** Patients with **basilar artery migraine** have attacks resembling basilar artery occlusion, with confusion, vomiting, vertigo, and loss of vision. A positive family history of migraine helps to distinguish this form from vascular malformation, although the latter must always be considered.

  **2. Therapy.** Many drugs have been tried in the management of migraine, including vasoconstrictors (ergotamine), serotonin antagonists (cyproheptadine), drugs that prevent reuptake of norepinephrine (amitriptyline), prostaglandin inhibitors (aspirin, ibuprofen), membrane stabilizers (phenytoin), calcium channel blockers, and other agents (e.g., propranolol).

  **3. Prognosis** is extremely variable, and no helpful predictive factors have been found. The patient can go into remission for years, only to have the migraine return decades later.

**C. Sleep disorders**

  **1. Sleepwalking (somnambulism), sleeptalking,** and **night terrors** are common in children under age 5 years. These disorders occur in stage 4 (deep) sleep. There is no recollection of the event the following day. An EEG sometimes is necessary to rule out a seizure disorder. Diazepam may be helpful if the sleepwalking is a danger to the patient. Diazepam interferes with stage 4 sleep.

2. **Narcolepsy** is characterized by paroxysmal attacks of irrepressible sleep. This disorder usually is seen for the first time in adolescents, although it has been reported in younger children. Going from the alert state into rapid eye movement (REM) sleep over a short period of time, as recorded by an EEG, is diagnostic. Narcolepsy is treated with stimulant medication.

### D. Other paroxysmal disorders

1. **Syncope** (fainting, with loss of consciousness) occurs because of decreased blood flow in the posterior circulation of the brain. It is essentially a benign disorder and is treated by reassurance. Cardiac arrhythmias must be considered as a possible etiology.

2. **Breath-holding spells** occur between 3 months and 6 years of age. The child initially cries and then holds his breath, turns cyanotic, and becomes limp. Occasionally, the patient has a short-lived tonic seizure. This is a benign disorder; reassurance is the treatment.

## VI. TRAUMA

### A. Head trauma (see also Ch 2 III C 1; Ch 6 VI D 1)

1. **Clinical features**
   a. **Concussion** produces a transient loss of consciousness, with amnesia for the event but with no obvious pathologic cerebral changes.
      (1) **Diagnosis.** Neurologic examination is unremarkable except for the change in mental status. Nystagmus and a positive Babinski reflex may be present for several hours.
      (2) **Therapy** is symptomatic. Headache, dizziness, and poor attention span may persist for up to 1 year following the injury.
   b. **Contusion and laceration** of the brain can be the result of a depressed skull fracture, a penetrating injury, or a closed injury.
      (1) **Control of intracranial pressure is essential;** it increases because of brain swelling, bleeding, or both. The level of coma usually is deepest by the third to fifth day, when the cerebral swelling is at its maximum.
      (2) **Depressed skull fractures and penetrating injuries require surgery** as soon as the patient is stable, or at least within 24 hours of the injury, to minimize the possibility of meningitis. Penetrating injuries of the brain can be devastating, depending on the extent of damage caused by the missile.

2. **Complications**
   a. **Epidural hematoma** occurs within hours of the injury in an adult but may not develop for 1–2 days in a child. Tearing of the dural veins or the middle meningeal artery is responsible for this complication, which should be suspected when a patient's condition deteriorates. The diagnosis is established by CT scan. Surgical evacuation is necessary.
   b. **Subdural hematoma** can develop even more slowly than epidural hematoma. Especially in an infant less than 6–9 months of age, this problem might not develop for several weeks following the head injury. A common presenting sign is an enlarging head circumference; this, plus a change in feeding habits or in personality, heralds the onset of the problem. In the infant who still has an open anterior fontanelle, a subdural tap might be the only treatment necessary. If this is unsuccessful, surgical intervention is indicated.
   c. **Parenchymal hematoma** (blood clot within the brain) rarely requires surgical intervention. However, if swelling cannot be controlled by medical means, evacuation might be necessary.
   d. **Transtentorial herniation** may occur as a result of generalized cerebral edema or a space-occupying lesion. This complication is suspected with the observation of dilated pupils that are nonresponsive to light and the development of sixth nerve palsy. Rapid treatment with a dehydrating agent (e.g., mannitol) and hyperventilation often is necessary.
   e. **Recurrent meningitis** is a risk when the injury provides an entrance for bacteria. The cause is not always obvious. CSF rhinorrhea or otorrhea should be sought. The former may occur as a result of a cribriform plate fracture.
   f. **Arachnoid (leptomeningeal) cyst** typically occurs in a linear fracture. It can develop in children of any age but is more likely to occur in those younger than age 3 years. Onset

usually is several months following the injury. The patient's presenting feature is an enlarging head circumference. Excision of the cyst may be necessary.

3. **Prognosis**
   a. The duration of coma following head injury correlates with the extent of the future disability. Full cognitive and motor function cannot be expected if the coma lasts more than 1 week in an adolescent or adult, or 2–4 weeks in an infant or young child.
   b. A seizure at the time of the impact does not correlate with future epilepsy. On the other hand, coma lasting more than 24 hours does correlate with future epilepsy. A depressed skull fracture or a penetrating injury leads to a seizure disorder in 70%–80% of cases.
   c. Post-traumatic personality and learning problems tend to be exaggerations of the pretraumatic personality and cognitive skills.

B. **Spinal cord injuries**

1. **Clinical features.** The level of injury is determined by the lack of sensation below the level of the lesion. The absence of a normal wheal-and-flare response also may help to identify the level of the lesion.

2. **Diagnosis.** MRI scan is the most helpful procedure in determining whether a lesion is amenable to surgery.

3. **Therapy.** Once the patient's vital signs are stabilized and appropriate surgery is performed, the most immediate concern is the prevention of urinary retention. Catheterization of the bladder often is necessary.

4. **Prognosis.** The patient may be areflexic distal to the injury for several weeks. However, complete paralysis 5–10 days after the injury suggests permanency.

C. **Peripheral nerve injuries**

1. **Clinical features** include sensory loss as well as weakness and wasting of the muscles innervated by the affected nerves.

2. **Therapy** includes removal of the compressing force and reanastomosis of severed nerves, if possible, as well as minimizing complications, including contractures (with a physical therapy program) and causalgia (with medication).

3. **Prognosis** can be determined by EMG. The presence of reinnervation potentials augurs well for recovery.

## VII. CEREBROVASCULAR DISORDERS. Stroke is an uncommon cause of acute neurologic dysfunction in children.

A. **Vascular occlusion**

1. **Thrombosis.** Arterial thrombosis can occur as a result of cerebral arteritis, trauma, or a congenital vascular abnormality (e.g., carotid artery stenosis).
   a. **Moyamoya disease** is characterized by telangiectasias of the blood vessels, usually in the anterior circulation of the brain. Multiple strokes develop as a result of the vascular occlusion and insufficient collateral circulation.
   b. **Acute hemiplegia of childhood** usually occurs before age 3 years, often as a result of an internal carotid artery thrombosis. Associated focal or generalized seizures occur in 60% of patients.
      (1) **Differential diagnoses** include periarteritis nodosa, sickle cell anemia, Todd's paralysis (which occurs up to 24 hours following a focal seizure), and hemiplegic migraine. Todd's paralysis and hemiplegic migraine are distinguished by the patient's recovery without sequelae.
      (2) **Therapy** combines physical therapy for the motor deficit with the use of appropriate anticonvulsants for the seizures, which often are difficult to control. In children with seizures, mental retardation is likely.

2. **Embolism.** Cerebral embolism is seen in patients with cyanotic congenital heart disease (see Ch 11 IV).

**B. Hemorrhage.** Intraventricular hemorrhage in the neonate is discussed in Chapter 5 V G 3 e. Angiomas and other malformations of blood vessels are uncommon as causes of intracranial hemorrhage in children.

**C. Arteriovenous malformation (AVM)** is the most common of the brain angiomas. AVM rarely is hereditary.

**1. Clinical features**
   **a.** Seizure is the most common presentation. Rupture of an AVM causes sudden symptoms, which may include coma, nuchal rigidity, and hemiparesis or quadriparesis. The history may disclose past complaints of migraine-like headaches.
   **b. Malformation of the vein of Galen** usually does not present as a CNS hemorrhage. Rather, congestive heart failure may be the presenting problem in the newborn period, hydrocephalus at 6 months of age, and seizures at 18 months of age.

**2. Diagnosis** of AVM is established by a contrast CT scan or MRI scan. Arteriography is necessary to determine the extent of the malformation.

**3. Therapy.** Surgery is considered if the AVM is accessible. However, in nonoperable cases, 85% of the patients are alive at 5 years of age.

**VIII. DISEASES AFFECTING BOTH THE SKIN AND THE CNS.** Neurocutaneous disorders (**phakomatoses**) are disorders that have in common lesions of the skin, brain, and eyes. Most of these disorders are inherited.

**A. Neurofibromatosis** is an autosomal dominant disease with variable expression. There are two distinct forms of neurofibromatosis, although variant forms also exist. It is estimated that 1 in 3000 people have at least a very mild variety of this disease.

**1. Clinical features and diagnosis**
   **a. Neurofibromatosis-1 (NF-1; von Recklinghausen's disease).** The diagnosis of NF-1 is established by the presence of two or more of the following:
      **(1)** Six or more café au lait spots larger than 5 mm in greatest diameter in prepubertal individuals and larger than 15 mm in postpubertal individuals
      **(2)** Two or more neurofibromas of any type or one plexiform neurofibroma
      **(3)** Freckling in the axillary or inguinal region
      **(4)** Optic glioma
      **(5)** Two or more Lisch nodules
      **(6)** A distinctive osseous lesion (e.g., sphenoid dysplasia or thinning of long bone cortex with or without pseudoarthrosis)
      **(7)** A first-degree relative with NF-1 according to above criteria
   **b. Neurofibromatosis-2 (NF-2).** Diagnosis of NF-2 is established by the presence of:
      **(1)** Bilateral eighth nerve masses seen with appropriate imaging techniques, or
      **(2)** A first-degree relative with NF-2 and either unilateral eighth nerve mass or two of the following: neurofibroma, meningioma, glioma, schwannoma, or juvenile posterior subscapular lenticular opacity.
   **c. Important considerations.** Screening for visual change, hearing loss, and learning disabilities should be routine. A CT scan should be ordered if there is any clinical indication that a tumor may be present.

**2. Therapy and prognosis.** If tumors are confined to peripheral nerves only, a normal life span without deficits is very likely. Genetic counseling is indicated.

**B. Tuberous sclerosis (Bourneville's disease)** is an autosomal dominant disease of variable expression, which affects approximately 1 person in 30,000.

**1. Clinical features.** Tuberous sclerosis is characterized by the triad of skin lesions, seizures, and mental retardation.
   **a. Skin lesions** are seen by age 3 years in 40% of patients. The lesions include flat, hypopigmented "ash-leaf" spots (visible under a Wood's lamp), shagreen patches (unevenly thickened skin areas), and café au lait spots. During the second decade, angiokeratomas appear on the face. Retinal hamartomas are noted in 50% of patients.
   **b. Epilepsy** may begin early in life and may be difficult to control.

    **c. Mental retardation** may be slowly progressive. Periventricular tumors may occur, leading to hydrocephalus and, if large enough, causing the patient's death. **Autistic features** are noted in about 10%–15% of patients.

    **d. Cysts and malignant tumors** may develop in the heart, kidneys, pancreas, and peritoneal cavity.

  **2. Therapy and prognosis.** The various clinical problems are treated as they are in patients without tuberous sclerosis. Prognosis is related to the severity of the seizure disorder and the cognitive dysfunction.

**C. Sturge-Weber syndrome** is most likely a sporadic disease, although familial cases have been described.

  **1. Clinical features.** A port-wine stain (capillary hemangioma) occurs unilaterally in a trigeminal distribution (over the forehead and, often, the maxillary area); occasionally it is bilateral. Glaucoma develops later in 50% of patients. A seizure disorder is likely.

  **2. Therapy and prognosis.** Anticonvulsant therapy often is unsuccessful, and surgical removal of the damaged cortex is necessary. Prognosis is related to the ease of seizure control.

**D. von Hippel-Lindau disease** is an autosomal dominant disorder characterized by vascular tumors in the cerebellum and spinal cord. Associated retinal hemangiomas are seen in 50% of patients, and renal carcinoma is seen in 45%. The skin is not involved in this syndrome.

**E. Ataxia-telangiectasia (Louis-Bar syndrome)** is an autosomal recessive disease affecting the cerebellum, skin, and immune system.

  **1. Clinical features.** The ataxia typically develops during the first 5 years of life and must be distinguished from cerebral palsy and Friedreich's ataxia. The telangiectasias, most apparent on the conjunctiva and the ears, become prominent during the second 5 years of life. Lung infections, secondary to immunoglobulin A (IgA) deficiency, develop by about age 10 years, and malignant lymphomas begin to develop at approximately 15–20 years of age.

  **2. Therapy and prognosis.** Treatment is symptomatic. The disease is progressive, and death usually results from infection or malignancy.

## IX. DEGENERATIVE CNS DISEASES

**A. General approach to the patient with a degenerative CNS disease**

  **1. Clinical features.** Degenerative CNS diseases are characterized clinically by a deterioration of function over an extended period of time. Most of the diseases are genetic, and many have a metabolic basis. The clinical condition may start with seizures or with losses in motor, cognitive, or language skills. These losses may be subtle and difficult to recognize in the very young child.

  **2. Diagnosis**

    **a. History.** In evaluating the patient with a suspected neurodegenerative disease, a careful and probing history is necessary. An infant may show a lack of normal motor and social development and may have recurrent episodes of altered consciousness or unexplained vomiting. A toddler may show a loss of motor, cognitive, or social milestones. An older child may have problems with schoolwork. The presence of hepatosplenomegaly, retinitis, or a cherry-red spot on the retina are major clues.

    **b. Laboratory studies** may aid in the diagnosis of degenerative CNS diseases.

      **(1) Urine screening** should include:

        **(a)** Ferric chloride testing for PKU and maple syrup urine disease

        **(b)** Dinitrophenylhydrazine testing for PKU, maple syrup urine disease, and tyrosinosis

        **(c)** Benedict's solution testing for galactosemia and fructosemia

        **(d)** Nitroprusside testing for homocystinuria and hypermethioninemia

        **(e)** Cetrimonium bromide testing for mucopolysaccharidosis

      **(2) Blood screening** should include tests for fasting blood sugar, ammonium, lactate, and pyruvate levels; pH and carbon dioxide partial pressure ($P_{CO_2}$); and lysosomal enzymes.

**(3) Radiography** of the skull and vertebral bodies may be helpful.

**(4) Fibroblast evaluation.** Fibroblasts in skin and other tissues should be evaluated for microscopic abnormalities and missing enzymes.

**B. Degenerative diseases of the basal ganglia.** The major abnormalities noted in these diseases are **movement disorders** (e.g., tremor, chorea, athetosis, dystonia).

    **1. Wilson's disease (hepatolenticular degeneration;** see also Ch 10 IX F 2) is an autosomal recessive disorder due to a defect in copper metabolism, which causes copper to accumulate progressively in the liver, brain, cornea, kidney, and other tissues.

        **a. Clinical features.** An enlarged liver typically is the presenting symptom if the disease manifests in the first decade of life. The patient who presents in the second decade of life may show choreoathetoid movements. Hemolytic anemia may be present. A grayish hue surrounding the iris (**Kayser-Fleischer ring**) is seen on slit lamp examination in 75% of children who present in the first decade of life and in all children who have a neurologic defect.

        **b. Diagnosis.** A copper level of more than 250 μg/g of liver (dry weight) found on liver biopsy is diagnostic of this disorder. Total serum copper and serum ceruloplasmin levels usually are decreased. (Other causes of a low serum ceruloplasmin level include chronic active hepatitis and cirrhosis). The 24-hour urine copper excretion usually is increased.

        **c. Therapy.** The chelating agent D-penicillamine, if started early, can prevent the neurologic progression of this disease. Lifelong therapy is required.

    **2. Dystonia musculorum deformans** is a disorder that manifests as slow, twisting movements causing what appears to be a fixed deformity, only to disappear with relaxation. The movements involve the trunk, extremities, and head. The disorder may be dominant, recessive, or sporadic. The genetic dystonias tend to be progressive; the sporadic types are static as a rule.

        **a. Clinical features.** Intermittent or continuous muscle spasms are noted when the patient tries to move the muscles purposefully. The truncal muscles are affected initially in the dominant form and the extremity muscles in the recessive form. Sporadic dystonia may occur secondary to birth trauma or other trauma, exposure to toxic substances (e.g., lead), or vascular disease.

        **b. Diagnosis** is established by physical examination and, in the hereditary forms, by a positive family history. A CT or MRI scan is not helpful as no anatomic site has been identified.

        **c. Therapy.** Thalamotomy has been reported to alleviate the symptoms, possibly for up to 2 years. Clonazepam, trihexyphenidyl, and carbamazepine have provided moderate, but temporary, improvement in some patients.

    **3. Tourette syndrome** is an autosomal dominant disease with variable expression. It is characterized by bodily and vocal tics; the latter may progress to **coprolalia**.

        **a. Etiology.** The cause is unknown. Stimulant medications have been implicated in some patients [see Ch 3 III B 4 c (2)]. A family history can be found in about 35% of cases.

        **b. Clinical features.** The motor tics—involuntary, rapid movements—initially involve the face and then the neck. The tics commonly are exacerbated by anxiety. The onset is between 5 and 10 years of age, a time when many children display tics. If the problem lasts more than 1 year and involves different muscle groups at different times, a diagnosis of Tourette syndrome can be made. Obscene utterances are not necessary for the diagnosis.

        **c. Therapy.** Haloperidol is beneficial in approximately 50% of patients. Clonidine also has been found to be beneficial in possibly 60% of patients. Pimozide, a medication with significant side effects, is effective in 80% of patients.

        **d. Prognosis.** The problem persists for life, but prolonged remissions sometimes occur. Learning disabilities are seen in approximately 60%–70% of patients, and there is an understandably high incidence of emotional disturbances.

    **4. Benign hereditary (essential) tremor** is an autosomal dominant disorder with variable expression.

        **a. Clinical features.** The tremor consists of a rhythmic, oscillating movement of the distal muscles of the extremities. It does not worsen as the patient approaches a target. The major effect of the tremor is on performance of fine motor skills. The disorder is mildly progressive.

        **b. Diagnosis.** Essential tremor can be associated with many toxic, metabolic, and infectious disorders as well as hereditary CNS diseases. It is important to establish that a tremor is not a symptom of an underlying disorder.

        **c. Therapy** is indicated only if the tremor adversely affects functions such as handwriting. Propranolol has been successful in alleviating the tremor in some patients.

5. **Other pediatric basal ganglia disorders** include:
   a. **Hallervorden-Spatz syndrome** (progressive spasticity, dystonia, rigidity, and choreoathetosis, with iron deposits in the basal ganglia)
   b. The childhood form of **Huntington's chorea**
   c. **Lesch-Nyhan syndrome** (choreoathetosis, mental retardation, and self-mutilation, due to a defect in purine metabolism)
   d. **Fahr's disease** (calcification of the basal ganglia and cerebellum, possibly due to hypoparathyroidism)

C. **Degenerative diseases of the cerebellum, brain stem, and spinal cord.** These diseases often present as **gait ataxia**. Other signs and symptoms include disorders of eye movements, hearing loss, facial palsy, and swallowing difficulties. These and other features, including the pace at which the disease progresses, lead to a specific diagnosis.

   1. **Friedreich's ataxia,** an autosomal recessive disease, is the best understood of the genetic ataxias. The disease presents during the latter half of the first decade of life.
      a. **Clinical features.** Progressive ataxia is the presenting sign, with associated weakness and wasting of the distal muscles and, occasionally, spasticity. In addition, most patients have skeletal deformities (pes cavus, kyphoscoliosis), and a few show nystagmus or deafness. The electrocardiogram (ECG) becomes abnormal by age 20 years. Cardiomyopathy leading to congestive heart failure is the usual cause of death. Patients seldom live past age 30 years.
      b. **Diagnosis.** The Babinski sign is positive (cortical spinal dysfunction), and there is a loss of vibration and position sense with minimal loss of sensation of sharp pain (posterior column dysfunction). Nerve conduction velocities are mildly slowed and sensory conduction velocities are unobtainable.
      c. **Therapy.** A physical therapy program and appropriate orthopedic intervention can help patients with Friedreich's ataxia.

   2. **Other pediatric disorders of the cerebellum, brain stem, and spinal cord** include a varied group of hereditary cerebellar ataxias, dentate cerebellar ataxia, (Ramsay Hunt syndrome), familial spastic paraplegia, abetalipoproteinemia (Bassen-Kornzweig syndrome), and hypolipoproteinemia.

D. **Degenerative diseases of white matter.** These diseases commonly start with **spasticity** and **visual impairment**. Dementia and, occasionally, seizures appear as late manifestations. No treatment is available for this group of disorders. Many of these diseases were formerly classified as sudanophilic leukodystrophies. However, as specific etiologies have been determined, the older term is used less frequently.

   1. **Metachromatic leukodystrophy (sulfatide lipidosis)** is an autosomal recessive disease caused by a **deficiency of arylsulfatase A,** the enzyme that participates in the catabolism of myelin.
      a. **Clinical features.** Three forms of this disorder exist.
         (1) The most common—the **infantile form**—starts in the second year of life and presents initially as gait disturbance and spasticity and then as dementia. Unexplained bouts of fever and severe abdominal pain develop as well. This form is invariably fatal by age 5 or 6 years.
         (2) In the **juvenile form,** similar symptoms begin between ages 6 and 10 years.
         (3) In the **adult form,** dementia precedes the gait disturbance.
      b. **Diagnosis.** The presence of metachromatic granules in the urine suggests the diagnosis, and a deficiency of arylsulfatase A in the white cells establishes it.

   2. **Adrenoleukodystrophy** is an X-linked disease that usually develops in children 5–8 years old. The spastic gait disorder and dementia are accompanied by adrenal insufficiency. An MRI scan shows the degeneration of the white matter. Serum analysis shows an abnormal ratio of the C26–C22 fatty acids. The patients usually die within 2–5 years.

   3. **Rett syndrome** is a progressive disease presenting as dementia and ataxia in girls. Autistic behavior, microcephaly, and a peculiar wringing motion of the hands are hallmarks of this disease. No inheritance pattern and no enzymatic deficiency or other metabolic explanation has been identified.

   4. **Other diseases of white matter**
      a. **Pelizaeus-Merzbacher disease** is a slowly progressive X-linked disorder, which begins in infancy and clinically resembles cerebral palsy. Careful observation determines that the patient's problem is progressive.

**b. Canavan's disease** is a severe progressive autosomal recessive disorder with increasing macrocephaly, blindness, hypotonia, and spasticity.

**c. Alexander's disease** is a rare, apparently sporadic disorder characterized by macrocephaly and mental retardation.

**d. Krabbe's disease** (cerebroside lipidosis, globoid leukodystrophy) is a severe, progressive autosomal recessive disorder with diffuse lack of myelin, which causes rigidity, dysphagia, blindness, deafness, mental deterioration, quadriplegia, and death.

**E. Degenerative diseases affecting primarily gray matter.** Many of these diseases are **neuronal storage diseases,** in which a lipid (usually a ganglioside or other sphingolipid) accumulates in cerebral neurons. Patients with gray matter diseases typically present with **seizures** and **dementia**.

1. **Tay-Sachs disease,** an autosomal recessive disorder, is one of the best known of the gray matter diseases and the most common of the gangliosidoses. The neuronal accumulation of gangliosides is due to **hexosaminidase A deficiency**.

   **a. Clinical features.** Patients develop symptoms at age 3–10 months. A loss of alertness and excessive reaction to noise (**hyperacusis**) are the presenting complaints. Myoclonic and akinetic seizures follow 1–3 months later. Patients die by age 3 or 4 years.

   **b. Diagnosis.** A cherry-red spot on the macula is noted in 75% of cases. This spot, caused by deterioration of the retina, can sometimes be seen in other gray matter diseases (e.g., Niemann-Pick disease, generalized gangliosidosis). The absence of hexosaminidase A in white cells, serum, or other tissue establishes the diagnosis.

   **c. Therapy.** Replacement therapy with a modified form of glucocerebrosidase by intravenous infusion may now be offered to some patients with this disorder.

2. **Gaucher's disease** occurs in three forms: infantile, juvenile, and adult. In all types, a **deficiency of glucocerebrosidase** causes an accumulation of glucoceramide in various tissues.

   **a. Clinical features.** Hepatosplenomegaly is seen in all patients.

   (1) The **infantile form** is most severe, with delayed development and signs of bulbar palsy by age 6 months and death by age 1–2 years.

   (2) The **juvenile form** commonly starts with dementia in late childhood.

   (3) The **adult form** is without brain involvement.

   **b. Diagnosis** is suggested by the finding of large foam cells (Gaucher's cells) in the bone marrow and confirmed by enzyme analysis of white cells.

3. **Niemann-Pick disease** results from an accumulation of sphingomyelin in the reticuloendothelial system due to a **lack of sphingomyelinase**. There are at least five types, which vary in age at onset and rate of progression, and not all types show CNS involvement. All are autosomal recessive disorders associated with a limited life expectancy.

   **a. Clinical features.** Loss of alertness associated with an enlarged liver and spleen are the initial findings in the infantile form with CNS involvement. In juvenile types, neurologic symptoms begin as gait disturbances and learning difficulties.

   **b. Diagnosis** is suggested by the finding of vacuolated histiocytes (Niemann-Pick cells) in the bone marrow. An absence of sphingomyelinase in skin fibroblasts establishes the diagnosis.

4. **Other diseases affecting neurons** primarily include the following.

   **a. Neuronal ceroid lipofuscinoses** (a group of autosomal recessive disorders) are characterized by refractory seizures, loss of vision, ataxia, and dementia.

   **b. Generalized gangliosidosis** (a severe disorder, probably autosomal recessive) causes death before age 2 years.

   **c. Fabry's disease** (an X-linked glycolipid disorder) causes a burning, painful neuropathy, angiokeratomas, and renal and cardiac disorders; female carriers may show some symptoms.

   **d. Menkes kinky hair disease** (an X-linked defect in copper absorption) causes seizures, profound neurologic deficits, and death before age 2 years.

# X. DISORDERS OF THE MOTOR UNIT (NEUROMUSCULAR DISORDERS). Common to all patients with motor unit diseases are **weak muscles**. Most of the diseases in this category are progressive, and many are genetic.

**A. Anterior horn cell diseases.** These disorders cause muscle weakness and wasting. The proximal muscles are affected in the genetic forms (spinal muscular atrophies) and the distal muscles are affected in acquired diseases (e.g., poliomyelitis).

1. **Spinal muscular atrophies** are autosomal recessive diseases primarily, although rare autosomal dominant and X-linked types have been described. A similar disorder, amyotrophic lateral sclerosis, typically affects adults.
   a. **Clinical features**
      (1) In **Werdnig-Hoffman disease** (infantile spinal muscular atrophy, or **type I**), the weakness is apparent at birth or shortly thereafter.
      (2) In a second group of patients (**type II**), the muscle weakness may not appear until after age 4–8 months, when sitting skills have normally been developed.
      (3) In **Kugelberg-Welander disease** (juvenile spinal muscular atrophy, or **type III**), the onset of weakness occurs after walking has been established, in some cases not until adolescence.
   b. **Diagnosis** in all three types of spinal muscular atrophy is established by the history and physical examination in association with denervation in a muscle biopsy.
   c. **Therapy.** A physical therapy program is combined with appropriate orthopedic intervention.
   d. **Prognosis.** All patients with spinal muscular atrophy have progressive disease. Type I is often fatal before age 2 years. The prognosis is best for patients with type III disease; life expectancy may be "normal."

2. **Arthrogryposis multiplex congenita** is a nonprogressive disease characterized by muscle weakness and contractures of at least two joints. Although the clinical findings are present at birth, the condition seldom is familial.
   a. **Etiology.** A viral or toxic etiology primarily affecting the anterior horn cells is suspected in most cases. In others, a uterine problem (e.g., amniotic bands) is suspected.
   b. **Diagnosis** is established by physical examination.
   c. **Therapy and prognosis.** The extent of the contractures determines how disabled the patient will be and how amenable the problem will be to surgical correction.

B. **Peripheral neuropathies.** Trauma, infections, postinfectious states, toxins (e.g., lead), and genetic factors all may affect the axon, the myelin (via the Schwann cell), or both.

1. **Hereditary sensory and motor neuropathy (HSMN)** is the current nomenclature for a group of inherited neuropathies that are differentiated by electrophysiologic criteria and by the associated problems (e.g., ataxia, retinitis, deafness). The most common of this group is **Charcot-Marie-Tooth disease (peroneal muscular atrophy)**.
   a. **Clinical features.** In HSMN, weakness begins in the foot muscles starting in the first decade of life; eventually, the hand muscles are affected. Mild sensory loss may accompany the motor disability.
   b. **Diagnosis.** In most types of HSMN, the EMG demonstrates denervation, and nerve conduction times are delayed. Rarely is a nerve biopsy needed for diagnosis.
   c. **Therapy.** A rehabilitation program, including physical and occupational therapy, is indicated and should be devised by a knowledgeable physician, such as an orthopedist or a physiatrist. Vocational counseling also is important.
   d. **Prognosis.** Most diseases in this category are mild, and life expectancy is normal. However, some patients become significantly physically handicapped, becoming confined to a wheelchair by the fourth or fifth decade of life.

2. **Guillain-Barré syndrome** and other postinfectious, presumably autoimmune, neuropathies are discussed in XI E. **Peripheral nerve injuries** are discussed in VI C.

3. **Other peripheral neuropathies** are less common and include brachial and lumbar plexus neuropathies, hereditary sensory neuropathies, giant cell neuropathy, Leber's optic atrophy, and neuroaxonal dystrophy.

C. **Diseases of the neuromuscular junction—myasthenia gravis**

1. **Etiology.** Myasthenia gravis generally is a sporadic disease, although familial cases have been described. It is an autoimmune disease in which antibodies develop against the acetylcholine receptor protein at the motor end-plate.

2. **Clinical features**
   a. **Clinical forms.** The disease may present at different ages.
      (1) **Neonatal myasthenia.** One in seven mothers with myasthenia gravis transmits antibodies to the fetus transplacentally. The infant develops transient myasthenia, starting during the first week of life and lasting less than 2 months.

**(2) Congenital myasthenia.** Anti-acetylcholine antibodies are not detectable in the patient's serum in this form of myasthenia. Ptosis, usually the first symptom, is noted by age 2 years; swallowing difficulties and truncal weakness may follow.

**(3) Juvenile myasthenia.** This form is similar to the adult form, except it starts late in the first decade or in the second decade of life.

**b. Associated diseases,** including rheumatoid arthritis, thyroiditis, thymoma, and diabetes mellitus, occasionally may occur.

**3. Diagnosis.** Patients with myasthenia gravis show normal muscle strength after receiving 2–10 mg of edrophonium chloride; the involved muscles weaken 1–5 minutes later. Occasionally, a repetitive nerve stimulation test, causing rapid muscle fatigue, helps to establish the diagnosis.

**4. Therapy.** Pyridostigmine, an anticholinesterase agent, is helpful in more than 50% of patients. Immunosuppressant therapy with corticosteroids may be necessary. Plasmapheresis and thymectomy may benefit some patients.

**5. Prognosis.** If the muscle weakness of congenital or juvenile myasthenia remains limited to ocular muscles for more than 2 years, the progression of the disease is limited.

**D. Diseases of muscle.** Discussed here are the more common of the **hereditary myopathies** (see Chapter 8 V C for inflammatory myopathies). The classification of the hereditary muscle diseases is based on the clinical presentation and histology.

**1. Muscular dystrophies.** These progressive genetic diseases have similar histologic appearances and are differentiated by their clinical presentations.

**a. Duchenne (pseudohypertrophic) muscular dystrophy,** the most common, is an X-linked disease characterized by progressive muscle weakness seen first in the proximal muscles.

**(1) Clinical features.** Symptoms typically begin at 2–4 years of age. Independent walking may be delayed; affected children never run normally and never walk up stairs using alternating feet. The patients are wheelchair-bound by age 12 years and die, usually from congestive heart failure or pneumonia, before age 25 years.

**(2) Diagnosis**

**(a)** The muscle weakness may be difficult to detect on physical examination, as children younger than age 5 years have difficulty cooperating with a formal muscle evaluation. A positive Gowers' sign (Figure 17-1) indicates weakness of the lower back and pelvic girdle muscles.

**(b)** The serum creatine phosphokinase (CPK) level is 10–20 times normal.

**(c)** The EMG is consistent with a myopathy; muscle biopsy is consistent with a dystrophy.

**(d)** The missing gene and gene product have been identified recently. The **lack of dystrophin** (the gene product) in the external muscle membrane is considered to be diagnostic of Duchenne muscular dystrophy.

**(3) Therapy.** In addition to orthotic and orthopedic intervention, genetic counseling is extremely important. The latter is the reason that early diagnosis is so important. Steroid therapy may prolong ambulation.

**b. Other genetic muscular dystrophies** include:

**(1) Becker's dystrophy** (a later-appearing, more benign form that otherwise resembles Duchenne muscular dystrophy; dystrophin is quantitatively and/or qualitatively abnormal)

**(2) Landouzy-Dejerine dystrophy** (facioscapulohumeral)

**(3) Leyden-Möbius dystrophy** (limb-girdle, scapulohumeral); typically becomes clinically evident in the second decade of life)

**(4) Myotonic muscular dystrophies** (see X D 2)

**2. Myotonic muscle disorders.** Myotonia is the failure of voluntary muscles to relax after a contracture. The examiner can demonstrate myotonia by percussing the patient's tongue or thenar eminence.

**a. Myotonic muscular dystrophy (Steinert's disease)** is an autosomal dominant disorder that presents during the second decade of life. The patient initially complains of cramps or weakness. Cataracts and cardiac arrhythmias develop over the next 20 years in 60%–70% of the patients.

**b. Congenital myotonic muscular dystrophy** only occurs when the mother is the affected parent. It presents in the neonate as "floppiness" and a typical "fish-mouth" appearance. In

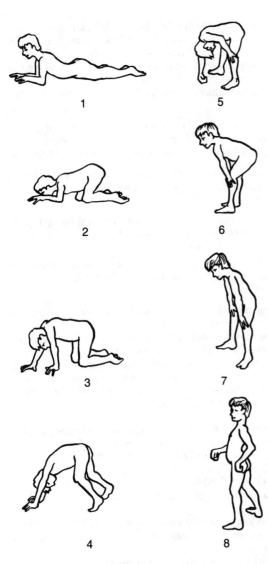

**Figure 17-1.** Gowers' sign. A patient with mild hip weakness uses this maneuver to arise from the floor. Rather than assuming a squatting position, the patient first pushes off the floor (*1, 2, 3*), forming an arch with buttocks at apex (*4*), then pushes against the knee with the non-floor hand (*5*), and then "walks" the hands up the legs (*6, 7*) to assume the standing position (*8*).

addition to the dystrophy, mental retardation is present. The patient gradually becomes stronger and usually starts to walk by about age 3 years. The diagnosis is established by examining the mother for evidence of the disorder.

    **c. Myotonia congenita (Thomsen's disease)** is an autosomal dominant disorder of delayed muscle relaxation. The patient experiences muscle cramps, which can be relieved with phenytoin. The disease is not progressive and is not associated with weakness. A recessive form exists with a later onset and with more severe myotonia.

  **3. Metabolic myopathies.** Several genetic abnormalities in carbohydrate or lipid metabolism cause identifiable myopathic syndromes; the underlying enzyme deficiencies have been elucidated in many of these disorders.

    **a. Glycogen storage diseases (GSDs;** see also Ch 7 III B d 2). **GSD type II** (Pompe's disease), **GSD type V** (McArdle's disease), and **GSD type VII** (Tarui's disease) affect the muscles. They can be diagnosed by finding glycogen inside the muscle cells or by ischemic exercise tests. Clinically, the patients complain of cramps.

    **b. Lipid storage myopathies,** including carnitine deficiency and carnitine palmityltransferase deficiency, are diagnosed by finding abnormal lipids in the muscle biopsy. Clinical findings include cramps, muscle weakness, and episodes of hepatic failure.

    **c. Myopathy with abnormal mitochondria** commonly presents as weakness and ophthalmoplegias in addition to CNS signs (e.g., dementia, intermittent coma).

    **d. Familial periodic paralysis** causes episodic muscle weakness in association with hypokalemia or hyperkalemia. Symptoms may start in the nursery or may not begin until the second decade of life. Acetazolamide may prevent or moderate attacks.

**4. Congenital myopathies.** Several disorders present as hypotonia in the newborn period and, therefore, must be considered in the differential diagnosis of the "floppy infant" syndrome. Specific disorders, usually named for the histologic findings, include **central core disease, nemaline myopathy** (rod disease), and **myotubular myopathy**.

    **a. Clinical features.** The congenital myopathies all are very similar. The patients are floppy at birth and have facial muscle weakness. Most of the diseases are static or improve with time. Scoliosis manifesting during the teenage years is common.

    **b. Diagnosis** is established by muscle biopsy, since these disorders differ histologically.

    **c. Therapy.** Respiratory support and nasogastric feeding may be necessary during the first few months of life. Later, orthopedic intervention, orthoses, and physical and occupational therapy may be required.

**XI. POSTINFECTIOUS, PRESUMED AUTOIMMUNE NEUROLOGIC DISORDERS** (see Ch 9 IV for acute CNS infections). The neurologic disorders discussed in this section are presumed to have an immunologic basis. Many are clearly preceded by an infectious (usually viral) disease, and the infectious agent is presumed to initiate a cell-mediated autoimmune reaction. In some diseases, the immune response occurs shortly after the original infection, and in other diseases, it does not occur until years later. In some of the disorders discussed here, no preceding infection has been identified, but clinicopathologic evidence strongly suggests an autoimmune, postinfectious etiology.

**A. Slow virus infections** are characterized by a lapse of months to years between the initial viral infection of the host and the appearance of a progressive CNS disease involving primarily dementia, seizures, and motor deficits.

    **1. Kuru,** a Samoan disease that was one of the first to be assigned a slow virus etiology, caused cerebellar degeneration leading to progressive ataxia and death. Establishing that ritual cannibalism was the source of the virus helped to put an end to the ritual and, thus, to the disease.

    **2. Subacute sclerosing panencephalitis (SSPE)** is caused by the measles virus or a measles-like virus that has been isolated from the brain.

        **a. Clinical features.** The disease starts 5–15 years after a natural measles infection or, uncommonly, after immunization with live measles vaccine. Changes in personality and other cognitive functions develop initially, followed by myoclonic seizures and, ultimately, by dementia and choreoathetoid movements. Death within 2 years of onset is the usual outcome, but the patient's condition may plateau and remain static for several years.

        **b. Diagnosis.** The EEG shows bursts of spike and slow wave activity, followed by suppression of the background rhythms. The measles antibody titer is elevated in both the CSF and the serum, differentiating SSPE from the hereditary lipidoses and from progressive rubella panencephalitis.

    **3. Progressive rubella panencephalitis** is a syndrome resembling SSPE that develops at age 10–20 years in some patients born with congenital rubella. The rubella antibody titer is elevated in both the CSF and the serum, and rubella virus can be recovered from brain tissue. The EEG does not show the pattern seen in SSPE.

**B. Acute disseminated (parainfectious) encephalomyelitis** occurs several days following certain viral infections (e.g., measles, chickenpox, and—rarely—influenza, rubella, or mumps) or following smallpox, rabies, or influenza vaccinations. A cell-mediated autoimmune reaction to myelin basic protein is the presumed etiology.

    **1. Clinical features and diagnosis.** The patient becomes irritable and lethargic, even comatose. The CSF commonly shows a slight increase in lymphocytes and an increase in protein.

    **2. Prognosis.** Many patients recover completely, but mental retardation, seizures, or even death can ensue.

    **3. Post-pertussis vaccination encephalopathy** is controversial and deserves special comment. Within hours to a few days after a pertussis vaccination, approximately 1 in 300,000 patients may develop encephalopathy, which, if not fatal, leaves the patient with mental retardation and a severe seizure disorder. Nevertheless, the argument for pertussis vaccination of infants is quite strong, as the complications of pertussis itself are more common in this age-group than are the reactions to the vaccine [see also Table 1-2]. Furthermore, recent research has suggested that the incidence of post-vaccine encephalopathy may be much lower than previously thought.

**C. Presumed autoimmune diseases affecting the cerebellum**

1. **Acute cerebellar ataxia** occurs in young children 1–2 weeks after a nonspecific respiratory infection. A brain tumor, intoxications, and an occult neuroblastoma must be excluded as causes. The disease is self-limited, with recovery occurring within 2 months.

2. **Myoclonic encephalopathy (Kinsbourne syndrome)** usually starts by age 6 months and causes irregular, rapid eye movements (**opsoclonus**) as well as polymyoclonus and ataxia. In some cases, the cause has been a neuroblastoma or a tumor of the brain stem or cerebellum. Adrenocorticotropic hormone (ACTH), usually needed for several years, has been helpful in suppressing the symptoms. Approximately half of the children who are afflicted are mildly retarded.

**D. Other presumed autoimmune postinfectious CNS diseases**

1. **Reye syndrome** (see Ch 10 IX G)

2. **Multiple sclerosis** currently is thought to be the result of an autoimmune reaction to an infectious agent that occurs in genetically susceptible persons. It is primarily a disease of young adults but has been diagnosed in children as young as age 2 years. A demyelinating disease noted for its exacerbations and remissions, multiple sclerosis in children manifests as ataxia, spasticity, and visual disturbances. MRI scan may help to establish the diagnosis.

3. **Diffuse cerebral sclerosis (Schilder's disease)** is a rare, acute, progressive demyelinating condition that histologically resembles multiple sclerosis. It occurs sporadically between age 5 and 12 years and has an unremitting, fatal outcome. The cause is not known but is presumed to be autoimmune or infectious.

4. **Transverse myelitis (transverse myelopathy)** is a presumed autoimmune disease that affects the spinal cord, causing sudden back pain followed by rapidly progressing weakness and loss of sensation below the level of the lesion. Loss of bladder and bowel function distinguishes this disorder from the Guillain-Barré syndrome; a space-occupying lesion is ruled out by CT or MRI scan.

**E. Presumed autoimmune, postinfectious diseases of peripheral nerves**

1. **Guillain-Barré syndrome,** the most common of these disorders in children, is a postinfectious demyelinating polyneuropathy. Lymphocytes sensitized to the basic protein of myelin have been identified in this disease, supporting the presumed autoimmune pathogenesis.
   a. **Clinical features**
      (1) Typically, 2 weeks after a viral infection or an immunization, weakness insidiously begins to develop in the distal muscles of the lower extremities, occasionally with accompanying paresthesias.
      (2) The weakness progresses upward and centrally over a period of 2–4 weeks, so that the diaphragm and the cranial nerve musculature may eventually become involved. A plateau lasting about 4 weeks then develops, followed by gradual recovery, which may take up to 1 year.
      (3) At the height of the clinical manifestations, the CSF shows an elevated protein level without an elevation in the cell count.
   b. **Therapy** is supportive, until the patient loses ambulation, at which time plasmaphoresis is indicated. Respiratory difficulties may require assisted respiration. Steroid therapy, plasmaphoresis, or intravenous gamma globulin is recommended for patients whose condition is chronically progressive (worsening 4–6 weeks after onset) or relapsing.
   c. **Prognosis.** Approximately 10%–15% of patients have residual deficits, such as weakness of the distal muscles of the feet, necessitating orthoses (e.g., special shoes, braces). Another 10% have a relapse, usually within the first year after recovery. Fatalities are rare, but can occur.

2. **Other presumably autoimmune, postinfectious neuropathies** include **Bell's palsy** (facial nerve palsy) and **sixth nerve palsy. Gradenigo syndrome** (sixth nerve palsy associated with pain in the distribution of the fifth cranial nerve) is secondary to osteomyelitis of the petrous ridge of the sphenoid bone. Brachial plexus neuropathies have been associated with influenza vaccination.

## STUDY QUESTIONS

**Directions:** Each of the numbered items or incomplete statements in this section is followed by answers or by completions of the statement. Select the **one** lettered answer or completion that is **best** in each case.

1. The anatomic site most affected by Werdnig-Hoffmann disease is the

(A) upper motor neuron
(B) anterior horn cell
(C) peripheral nerve
(D) neuromuscular junction
(E) muscle

2. The diagnosis of a concussion is established by which of the following findings?

(A) Pupillary constriction
(B) Nausea and vomiting
(C) Brief loss of consciousness and amnesia for the event
(D) A positive Babinski reflex

3. The diagnosis of cerebral palsy is established by which of the following findings on history and physical examination?

(A) Mental retardation
(B) Birth anoxia
(C) Epilepsy
(D) Motor dysfunction secondary to a brain lesion
(E) Choreoathetosis

4. Duchenne muscular dystrophy is associated with a lack of the protein dystrophin, which normally is found in

(A) nerve cells
(B) anterior horn cells
(C) the sacrotubular mechanism
(D) the muscle membrane
(E) the Z band

5. The diagnosis of epilepsy is made by

(A) abnormal EEG findings
(B) abnormal physical examination
(C) history of the event
(D) history of head trauma
(E) low Apgar scores at birth

6. Which of the following occurs during REM sleep?

(A) Sleepwalking
(B) Sleeptalking
(C) Night terrors
(D) Nightmares

7. Which of the following refers to slow, writhing, continuous movements in the extremities?

(A) Spasticity
(B) Athetosis
(C) Dystonia
(D) Ataxia
(E) Hypotonia

8. All of the following are characteristics of Rett syndrome EXCEPT

(A) autistic behavior
(B) microcephaly
(C) peculiar wringing motion of the hands
(D) autosomal recessive inheritance
(E) dementia

9. The EMG examination is NOT useful for the diagnosis of

(A) cerebral palsy
(B) spinal muscular atrophy
(C) Charcot-Marie-Tooth disease
(D) myasthenia gravis
(E) Duchenne muscular dystrophy

10. Common lesions seen in tuberous sclerosis include all of the following EXCEPT

(A) hypopigmented spots
(B) café au lait spots
(C) angiokeratomas
(D) retinal hamartomas
(E) glaucoma

| | | | |
|---|---|---|---|
| 1-B | 4-D | 7-B | 10-E |
| 2-C | 5-C | 8-D | |
| 3-D | 6-D | 9-A | |

11. All of the following statements about the Guillain-Barré syndrome are correct EXCEPT

(A) it is considered to be a postinfectious disease
(B) the CSF shows an elevated protein level without an increased cell count
(C) it affects the axons of the peripheral nerves
(D) relapses may occur
(E) it rarely is fatal

12. All of the following are disorders that involve basal ganglia dysfunction EXCEPT

(A) Wilson's disease
(B) dystonia musculorum deformans
(C) Tourette syndrome
(D) Huntington's chorea
(E) Friedreich's ataxia

13. All of the following statements about spina bifida cystica are true EXCEPT

(A) it often is associated with hydrocephalus
(B) it is fatal if not treated within 24 hours
(C) it may be diagnosed in utero with ultrasonography
(D) it can cause urologic problems
(E) it requires orthopedic management

**Directions:** Each item below contains four suggested answers of which **one or more** is correct. Choose the answer

  A   if **1, 2, and 3** are correct
  B   if **1 and 3** are correct
  C   if **2 and 4** are correct
  D   if **4** is correct
  E   if **1, 2, 3, and 4** are correct

14. A patient with basilar artery migraine might report which of the following features?

(1) Episodes of nausea and vomiting
(2) Attacks of dizziness
(3) Periodic loss of vision
(4) A family history of headaches

15. During the initial phases of a gray matter disease, which of the following symptoms would commonly be present?

(1) Spasticity
(2) Dementia
(3) Hepatosplenomegaly
(4) Seizures

16. Features that characterize many of the degenerative brain diseases include

(1) loss of motor function
(2) presence of seizures
(3) genetic inheritance
(4) metabolic pathogenesis

---

11-C    14-E
12-E    15-C
13-B    16-E

**Directions:** The group of items in this section consists of lettered options followed by a set of numbered items. For each item, select the **one** lettered option that is most closely associated with it. Each lettered option may be selected once, more than once, or not at all.

**Questions 17–20**

For each characteristic given below, select the birth defect with which it is most likely to be associated.

(A) Platybasia
(B) Syringomyelia
(C) Arnold-Chiari malformation
(D) Klippel-Feil syndrome
(E) Agenesis of corpus callosum

17. Fluid-filled cyst in the spinal cord
18. Hydrocephalus and meningomyelocele
19. Symptoms ranging from none to severe retardation
20. Sensorineural hearing loss and congenital heart defects

17-B        20-E
18-C
19-D

## ANSWERS AND EXPLANATIONS

**1. The answer is B** *[X A 1 a (1)]*.
Werdnig-Hoffmann disease and Kugelberg-Welander disease are spinal muscular atrophies—autosomal recessive diseases in which the proximal muscles become progressively weaker because of anterior horn cell deterioration. Poliomyelitis is a viral disease that preferentially strikes the anterior horn cell.

**2. The answer is C** *[VI A 1 a]*.
The diagnosis of a concussion following head trauma is established by virtue of a neurologic examination that is normal except for transient loss of consciousness and, often, amnesia for the event. A positive Babinski reflex (i.e., dorsiflexion of the toes), constricted pupils, nausea, and vomiting can all be associated with concussion but do not establish or rule out the diagnosis. If the patient is comatose for more than several minutes or has a neurologic deficit lasting more than 24 hours, other than the memory loss, a more serious lesion should be considered (e.g., cerebral contusion or laceration).

**3. The answer is D** *[IV C]*.
The diagnosis of cerebral palsy is established by determining with a history and physical examination that the patient's motor deficit is secondary to a nonprogressive brain lesion. Birth anoxia may be the etiology, and mental retardation and epilepsy are associated problems. Choreoathetosis is a movement abnormality found in many disorders, including cerebral palsy.

**4. The answer is D** *[X D 1 a (2) (d)]*.
Dystrophin, the gene product of the Duchenne gene, is part of the external muscle membrane. Dystrophin is believed to allow the influx and efflux of calcium, which is associated with muscle movement. The lack of dystrophin is considered to be diagnostic of Duchenne muscular dystrophy.

**5. The answer is C** *[V A 2 e]*.
Although abnormal findings on electroencephalography (EEG), low Apgar scores at birth, and a history of head trauma are associated with the presence of epilepsy, the diagnosis is not established by these entities. The diagnosis of epilepsy is established by a history of the abnormal behavior as described by a competent observer. A physical examination is carried out to determine a specific etiology of the seizure disorder.

**6. The answer is D** *[V C 1]*.
Sleepwalking, sleeptalking, and night terrors occur during stage 4 sleep. Nightmares occur during rapid eye movement (REM) sleep, and the patient should have recall of the specifics of the image developing during this particular disturbance. Night terrors can mimic convulsions. Occasionally, continuous night EEG recording with simultaneous videotaping can help resolve the diagnostic dilemma.

**7. The answer is B** *[IV B 1 b (2)]*.
Athetosis refers to slow, writhing, continuous movements in the extremities, which are seen in patients with cerebral palsy. Chorea, athetosis, spasticity, dystonia, ataxia, and hypotonia are physiologic classifications for the abnormal muscle tone or movement disorders commonly seen in children with cerebral palsy. When classifying a patient's disorder, both the anatomic location of the abnormality and the physiologic characteristic of the abnormality are considered.

**8. The answer is D** *[IX D 3]*.
The genetics of Rett syndrome has not yet been determined. Although thought to be a genetic syndrome, no inheritance pattern and no enzymatic deficiency or other metabolic explanation has been established for Rett syndrome. The other characteristics (autistic behavior, microcephaly, peculiar wringing motion of the hands, dementia) are common in patients with this disorder.

**9. The answer is A** *[I C 3; IV C 2]*.
Electromyography (EMG) usually is coupled with nerve conduction studies to delineate motor unit (neuromuscular) diseases, such as spinal muscular atrophy, peroneal muscular atrophy (Charcot-Marie-Tooth disease), myasthenia gravis, and Duchenne muscular dystrophy. The EMG examination is normal in patients with upper motor neuron lesions, such as cerebral palsy.

**10. The answer is E** *[VIII B 1 a]*.
Glaucoma is commonly seen in patients with Sturge-Weber syndrome, not tuberous sclerosis. Common findings in patients with tuberous sclerosis include flat, hypopigmented spots, shagreen patches, café au lait spots, angiokeratomas, and retinal hamartomas.

**11. The answer is C** *[XI E 1].*
The Guillain-Barré syndrome is a postinfectious disease that affects the myelin, not the axons, of peripheral nerves. Typically, the disease develops 2–4 weeks following what appears to be an insignificant viral illness. Death is extremely unusual, especially in children. A complete recovery occurs in about 75% of patients; about 10%–15% of patients will have residual deficits, and about 10% relapse, usually within the first year after recovery.

**12. The answer is E** *[IX C 1].*
The tremor of Friedreich's ataxia is secondary to a deterioration of the spinocerebellar tracts. Wilson's disease, dystonia musculorum deformans, Tourette syndrome, and Huntington's chorea are characterized by abnormalities of the basal ganglia (caudate nucleus, globus pallidus, putamen). In these conditions, the diagnosis is established by a physical examination in conjunction with a carefully obtained history. Computed tomography (CT) or magnetic resonance imaging (MRI) scans may or may not show an anatomic abnormality.

**13. The answer is B** *[III B 1 a].*
When a child is born with spina bifida cystica marked by either a meningomyelocele or a meningocele, early surgical closure of the defect is not necessary for survival, but it is indicated to prevent infection. Children with these defects commonly have hydrocephalus and require urologic care because the bladder is not under normal neurologic control and is prone to infection. Orthopedic care also is necessary, as kyphoscoliosis and hip dislocation are common complications.

**14. The answer is E (all)** *[V B 1 c (2)].*
The diagnosis of basilar artery migraine in children is difficult to establish. The symptoms include paroxysmal attacks of vomiting, vertigo, and loss of vision. However, without a family history of migraine, the diagnosis is difficult. A vascular malformation of the brain stem must be excluded, for example, in addition to possible gastrointestinal disease, before the diagnosis can be made.

**15. The answer is C (2, 4)** *[IX D, E].*
Patients with degenerative diseases of the gray matter typically present with seizures and dementia. Spasticity is a typical early sign in patients with degenerative diseases that affect the white matter, not the gray matter. Spasticity, when it develops in the course of a gray matter disease, is a late occurrence. Hepatosplenomegaly and a cherry-red spot on the retina are characteristic of some, but not all, gray matter diseases.

**16. The answer is E (all)** *[IX A 1, 2].*
Degenerative brain diseases are often characterized by one or more of all the features listed in the question. Some of these diseases may start with seizures, others with a motor loss, and still others with the onset of dementia. Almost all of these diseases are genetic, and, for most of them, a missing enzyme has been identified as being responsible for the pathology noted.

**17–20. The answers are: 17-B** *[III B 1 c (3)],* **18-C** *[III B 1 b],* **19-E** *[III C 1],* **20-D** *[III B 3 b].*
The disorders listed in the questions are developmental anomalies of the CNS. Syringomyelia is a cyst in the spinal cord, most commonly in the cervical or thoracic area. Patients present with loss of sensation to pinprick and cold, as the crossing fibers in the spinal cord are affected initially. Eventually, the corticospinal tract is involved, leading to spasticity of the lower extremities. Platybasia, an upward displacement at the base of the skull, eventually causes compression of the lower brain stem or upper part of the cervical cord; this also leads to spasticity of the extremities.

In the Arnold-Chiari malformation, downward displacement of the cerebellum and medulla leads to hydrocephalus. This anomaly commonly is associated with meningomyelocele.

Agenesis of the corpus callosum can be associated with no symptoms at all or with a variety of symptoms; suspicion of this problem is raised by the finding of orbital hypertelorism (widening of the orbital fissures).

Patients with Klippel-Feil syndrome, a defect of the cervical vertebrae, present with symptoms similar to those of platybasia. However, the Klippel-Feil syndrome is associated with other anomalies, including spina bifida, syringomyelia, sensorineural hearing loss, and congenital heart defects, requiring the examiner to evaluate the patient more completely.

# Comprehensive Exam

# Introduction

One of the least attractive aspects of pursuing an education is the necessity of being examined on what has been learned. Instructors do not like to prepare tests, and students do not like to take them.

However, students are required to take many examinations during their learning careers, and little if any time is spent acquainting them with the positive aspects of tests and with systematic and successful methods for approaching them. Students perceive tests as punitive and sometimes feel that they are merely opportunities for the instructor to discover what the student has forgotten or has never learned. Students need to view tests as opportunities to display their knowledge and to use them as tools for developing prescriptions for further study and learning.

A brief history and discussion of the National Board of Medical Examiners (NBME) examinations are presented in this introduction, along with ideas concerning psychological preparation for the examinations. Also presented are general considerations and test-taking tips as well as how practice exams can be used as educational tools. (The literature provided by the various examination boards contains detailed information concerning the construction and scoring of specific exams.)

## National Board of Medical Examiners Examinations

Before the various NBME exams were developed, each state attempted to license physicians through its own procedures. Differences between the quality and testing procedures of the various state examinations resulted in the refusal of some states to recognize the licensure of physicians licensed in other states. This made it difficult for physicians to move freely from one state to another and produced an uneven quality of medical care in the United States.

To remedy this situation, the various state medical boards decided they would be better served if an outside agency prepared standard exams to be given in all states, allowing each state to meet its own needs and have a common standard by which to judge the educational preparation of individuals applying for licensure.

One misconception concerning these outside agencies is that they are licensing authorities. This is not the case; they are examination boards only. The individual states retain the power to grant and revoke licenses. The examination boards are charged with designing and scoring valid and reliable tests. They are primarily concerned with providing the states with feedback on how examinees have performed and with making suggestions about the interpretation and usefulness of scores. The states use this information as partial fulfillment of qualifications upon which they grant licenses.

---

The author of this introduction, Michael J. O'Donnell, holds the positions of Assistant Professor of Psychiatry and Director of Biomedical Communications at the University of New Mexico School of Medicine, Albuquerque, New Mexico.

Students should remember that these exams are administered nationwide and, although the general medical information is similar, educational methodologies and faculty areas of expertise differ from institution to institution. It is unrealistic to expect that students will know all the material presented in the exams; they may face questions on the exams in areas that were only superficially covered in their classes. The testing authorities recognize this situation, and their scoring procedures take it into account.

## The Exams

The first exam was given in 1916. It was a combination of written, oral, and laboratory tests, and it was administered over a 5-day period. Admission to the exam required proof of completion of medical education and 1 year of internship

In 1922, the examination was changed to a new format and was divided into three parts. Part I, a 3-day essay exam, was given in the basic sciences after 2 years of medical school. Part II, a 2-day exam, was administered shortly before or after graduation, and Part III was taken at the end of the first postgraduate year. To pass both Part I and Part II, a score equalling 75% of the total points available was required.

In 1954, after a 3-year extensive study, the NBME adopted the multiple-choice format. To pass, a statistically computed score of 75 was required, which allowed comparison of test results from year to year. In 1971, this method was changed to one that held the mean constant at a computed score of 500, with a predetermined deviation from the mean to ascertain a passing or failing score. The 1971 changes permitted more sophisticated analysis of test results and allowed schools to compare among individual students within their respective institutions as well as among students nationwide. Feedback to students regarding performance included the reporting of pass or failure along with scores in each of the areas tested.

During the 1980s, the ever-changing field of medicine made it necessary for the NBME to examine once again its evaluation strategies. It was found necessary to develop questions in multidisciplinary areas such as gerontology, health promotion, immunology, and cell and molecular biology. In addition, it was decided that questions should test higher cognitive levels and reasoning skills.

To meet the new goals, many changes have been made in both the form and content of the examination. These changes include reduction in the number of questions to approximately 800 on Parts I and II to allow students more time on each question, with total testing time reduced on Part I from 13 to 12 hours and on Part II from 12.5 to 12 hours. The basic science disciplines are no longer allotted the same number of questions, which permits flexible weighing of the exam areas. Reporting of scores to schools include total scores for individuals and group mean scores for separate discipline areas. Only pass/fail designations and total scores are reported to examinees. There is no longer a provision for the reporting of individual subscores to either the examinees or medical schools. Finally, the question format used in the new exams, now referred to as Comprehensive (Comp) I and II, is predominately multiple-choice, best answer.

## The New Format

New question formats, designed specifically for Comp I, are constructed in an effort to test the student's grasp of the sciences basic to medicine in an integrated fashion. The questions are designed to be interdisciplinary. Many of these questions are presented as a vignette, or case study, followed by a series of multiple-choice, best-answer questions.

The scoring of this exam also is altered. Whereas, in the past, the exams were scored on a normal curve, the new exam has a predetermined standard, which must be met in order to pass. The exam no longer concentrates on the trivial; therefore, it has been concluded that there is a common base of information that all medical students should know in order to pass. It is anticipated that a major shift in the pass/fail rate for the nation is unlikely. In the past, the average student could only expect to feel comfortable with half the test and eventually would complete approximately 67% of the questions correctly, to achieve a mean score of 500. Although with the standard setting method it is likely that the mean score will change and become higher, it is unlikely that the pass/fail rates will differ significantly from those in the past. During the first testing in 1991, there will not be differential weighing of the questions. However, in the future, the NBME will be researching methods of weighing questions based on both the time it takes to answer questions vis à vis their difficulty and the perceived importance of the information. In addition, the NBME is attempting to design a method of delivering feedback to the student that will have considerable importance in discovering weaknesses and pinpointing areas for further study in the event that a retake is necessary.

Since many of the proposed changes were implemented in June 1991, specific information regarding actual standards, question emphasis, pass/fail rates, and so forth were unavailable at the time of publication. The publisher will update this section as information becomes available as we attempt to follow the evolution and changes that occur in the area of physician evaluation.

## Materials Needed for Test Preparation

In preparation for a test, many students collect far too much study material only to find that they simply do not have the time to go through all of it. They are defeated before they begin because either they cannot get through all the material, leaving areas unstudied, or they race through the material so quickly that they cannot benefit from the activity.

It is generally more efficient for the student to use materials already at hand; that is, class notes, one good outline to cover or strengthen areas not locally stressed and for quick review of the whole topic, and one good text as a reference for looking up complex material needing further explanation.

Also, many students attempt to memorize far too much information, rather than learning and understanding less material and then relying on that learned information to determine the answers to questions at the time of the examination. Relying too heavily on memorized material causes anxiety, and the more anxious students become during a test, the less learned knowledge they are likely to use.

## Positive Attitude

A positive attitude and a realistic approach are essential to successful test taking. If concentration is placed on the negative aspects of tests or on the potential for failure, anxiety increases and performance decreases. A negative attitude generally develops if the student concentrates on "I must pass" rather than on "I can pass." "What if I fail?" becomes the major factor motivating the student to **run from failure rather than toward success**. This results from placing too much emphasis on scores rather than understanding that scores have only slight relevance to future professional performance.

The score received is only one aspect of test performance. Test performance also indicates the student's ability to use information during evaluation procedures and reveals how this ability might be used in the future. For example, when a patient enters the physician's office with a problem, the physician begins by asking questions, searching for clues, and seeking diagnostic information. Hypotheses are then developed, which will include several potential causes for the problem. Weighing the probabilities, the physician will begin to discard those hypotheses with the least likelihood of being correct. Good differential diagnosis involves the ability to deal with uncertainty, to reduce potential causes to the smallest number, and to use all learned information in arriving at a conclusion.

This same thought process can and should be used in testing situations. It might be termed **paper-and-pencil differential diagnosis**. In each question with five alternatives, of which one is correct, there are four alternatives that are incorrect. If deductive reasoning is used, as in solving a clinical problem, the choices can be viewed as having possibilities of being correct. The elimination of wrong choices increases the odds that a student will be able to recognize the correct choice. Even if the correct choice does not become evident, the probability of guessing correctly increases. Just as differential diagnosis in a clinical setting can result in a correct diagnosis, eliminating incorrect choices on a test can result in choosing the correct answer.

Answering questions based on what is incorrect is difficult for many students since they have had nearly 20 years experience taking tests with the implied assertion that knowledge can be displayed only by knowing what is correct. It must be remembered, however, that students can display knowledge by knowing something is wrong, just as they can display it by knowing something is right. **Students should begin to think in the present as they expect themselves to think in the future.**

### Paper-and-Pencil Differential Diagnosis

The technique used to arrive at the answer to the following question is an example of the paper-and-pencil differential diagnosis approach.

> A recently diagnosed case of hypothyroidism in a 45-year-old man
> may result in which of the following conditions?
>
> **(A)** Thyrotoxicosis
> **(B)** Cretinism
> **(C)** Myxedema
> **(D)** Graves' disease
> **(E)** Hashimoto's thyroiditis

It is presumed that all of the choices presented in the question are plausible and partially correct. If the student begins by breaking the question into parts and trying to discover what the question is attempting to measure, it will be possible to answer the question correctly by using more than memorized charts concerning thyroid problems.

- The question may be testing if the student knows the difference between "hypo" and "hyper" conditions.
- The answer choices may include thyroid problems that are not "hypothyroid" problems.
- It is possible that one or more of the choices are "hypo" but are not "thyroid" problems, that they are some other endocrine problems.
- "Recently diagnosed in a 45-year-old man" indicates that the correct answer is not a congenital childhood problem.
- "May result in" as opposed to "resulting from" suggests that the choices might include a problem that **causes** hypothyroidism rather than **results from** hypothyroidism, as stated.

By applying this kind of reasoning, the student can see that choice **A**, thyroid toxicosis, which is a disorder resulting from an overactive thyroid gland ("hyper") must be eliminated. Another piece of knowledge, that is, Graves' disease is thyroid toxicosis, eliminates choice **D**. Choice **B**, cretinism, is indeed hypothyroidism, but it is a childhood disorder. Therefore, **B** is eliminated. Choice **E** is an inflammation of the thyroid gland—here the clue is the suffix "itis." The reasoning is that thyroiditis, being an inflammation, may **cause** a thyroid problem, perhaps even a hypothyroid problem, but there is no reason for the reverse to be true. Myxedema, choice **C**, is the only choice left and the obvious correct answer.

## Preparing for Board Examinations

1. **Study for yourself.** Although some of the material may seem irrelevant, the more you learn now, the less you will have to learn later. Also, do not let the fear of the test rob you of an important part of your education. If you study to learn, the task is less distasteful than studying solely to pass a test.

2. **Review all areas.** You should not be selective by studying perceived weak areas and ignoring perceived strong areas. This is probably the last time you will have the time and the motivation to review **all** of the basic sciences.

3. **Attempt to understand, not just memorize, the material.** Ask yourself: To whom does the material apply? When does it apply? Where does it apply? How does it apply? Understanding the connections among these points allows for longer retention and aids in those situations when guessing strategies may be needed.

4. **Try to anticipate questions that might appear on the test.** Ask yourself how you might construct a question on a specific topic.

5. **Give yourself a couple days of rest before the test.** Studying up to the last moment will increase your anxiety and cause potential confusion.

## Taking Board Examinations

1. In the case of NBME exams, be sure to **pace yourself** to use time optimally. Each booklet is designed to take 2 hours. You should check to be sure that you are halfway through the booklet at the end of the first hour. You should use all your allotted time; if you finish too early, you probably did so by moving too quickly through the test.

2. **Read each question and all the alternatives carefully** before you begin to make decisions. Remember the questions contain clues, as do the answer choices. As a physician, you would not make a clinical decision without a complete examination of all the data; the same holds true for answering test questions.

3. **Read the directions for each question set carefully.** You would be amazed at how many students make mistakes in tests simply because they have not paid close attention to the directions.

4. It is not advisable to leave blanks with the intention of coming back to answer the questions later. Because of the way board examinations are constructed, you probably will not pick up any new information that will help you when you come back, and the chances of getting numerically off on your answer sheet are greater than your chances of benefiting by skipping around. If you feel that you must come back to a question, mark the best choice and place a note in the margin. Generally speaking, it is best not to change answers once you have made a decision, unless you have learned new information. Your intuitive reaction and first response are correct more often than changes made out of frustration or anxiety. **Never turn in an answer sheet with blanks.** Scores are based on the number that you get correct; you are not penalized with incorrect choices.

5. **Do not try to answer the questions on a stimulus–response basis.** It generally will not work. Use all of your learned knowledge.

6. **Do not let anxiety destroy your confidence.** If you have prepared conscientiously, you know enough to pass. Use all that you have learned.

7. **Do not try to determine how well you are doing as you proceed.** You will not be able to make an objective assessment, and your anxiety will increase.

8. **Do not expect a feeling of mastery** or anything close to what you are accustomed. Remember, this is a nationally administered exam, not a mastery test.

9. **Do not become frustrated or angry** about what appear to be bad or difficult questions. You simply do not know the answers; you cannot know everything.

### Specific Test-Taking Strategies

Read the entire question carefully, regardless of format. Test questions have multiple parts. Concentrate on picking out the pertinent key words that might help you begin to problem solve. Words such as "always," "all," "never," "mostly," "primarily," and so forth play significant roles. In all types of questions, distractors with terms such as "always" or "never" most often are incorrect. Adjectives and adverbs can completely change the meaning of questions—pay close attention to them. Also, medical prefixes and suffixes (e.g., "hypo-," "hyper-," "-ectomy," "-itis") are sometimes at the root of the question. The knowledge and application of everyday English grammar often is the key to dissecting questions.

### Multiple-Choice Questions

Read the question and the choices carefully to become familiar with the data as given. Remember, in multiple-choice questions there is one correct answer and there are four distractors, or incorrect answers. (Distractors are plausible and possibly correct or they would not be called distractors.) They are generally correct for part of the question but not for the entire question. Dissecting the question into parts aids in discerning these distractors.

If the correct answer is not immediately evident, begin eliminating the distractors. (Many students feel that they must always start at option A and make a decision before they move to B, thus forcing decisions they are not ready to make.) Your first decisions should be made on those choices you feel the most confident about.

Compare the choices to each part of the question. **To be wrong,** a choice needs to be incorrect for only part of the question. **To be correct,** it must be **totally** correct. If you believe a choice is partially incorrect, tentatively eliminate that choice. Make notes next to the choices regarding tentative decisions. One method is to place a minus sign next to the choices you are certain are incorrect and a plus sign next to those that potentially are correct. Finally, place a zero next to any choice you do not understand or need to come back to for further inspection. Do not feel that you must make final decisions until you have examined all choices carefully.

When you have eliminated as many choices as you can, decide which of those that are left has the highest probability of being correct. Remember to use paper-and-pencil differential diagnosis. Above all, be honest with yourself. If you do not know the answer, eliminate as many choices as possible and choose reasonably.

### Vignette-Based Questions

Vignette-based questions are nothing more than normal multiple-choice questions that use the same case, or grouped information, for setting the problem. The NBME has been researching question types that would test the student's grasp of the integrated medical basic sciences in a more cognitively complex fashion than can be accomplished with traditional testing formats. These questions allow the testing of information that is more medically relevant than memorized terminology.

It is important to realize that several questions, although grouped together and referring to one situation or vignette, are independent questions; that is, they are able to stand alone. Your inability to answer one question in a group should have no bearing on your ability to answer subsequent questions.

These are multiple-choice questions, and just as is done with the single best answer questions, you should use the paper-and-pencil differential diagnosis, as was described earlier.

## Single Best Answer—Matching Sets

Single best answer—matching sets consist of a list of words or statements followed by several numbered items or statements. Be sure to pay attention to whether the choices can be used more than once, only once, or not at all. Consider each choice individually and carefully. Begin with those with which you are the most familiar. It is important always to break the statements and words into parts, as with all other question formats. **If a choice is only partially correct, then it is incorrect.**

## Guessing

Nothing takes the place of a firm knowledge base, but with little information to work with, even after playing paper-and-pencil differential diagnosis, you may find it necessary to guess the correct answer. A few simple rules can help increase your guessing accuracy. Always guess consistently if you have no idea what is correct; that is, after eliminating all that you can, make the choice that agrees with your intuition or choose the option closest to the top of the list that has not been eliminated as a potential answer.

When guessing at questions that present with choices in numerical form, you will often find the choices listed in an ascending or descending order. It is generally not wise to guess the first or last alternative, since these are usually extreme values and are most likely incorrect.

## Using the Comprehensive Exam to Learn

All too often, students do not take full advantage of practice exams. There is a tendency to complete the exam, score it, look up the correct answers to those questions missed, and then forget the entire thing.

In fact, great educational benefits can be derived if students would spend more time using practice tests as learning tools. As mentioned earlier, incorrect choices in test questions are plausible and partially correct or they would not fulfill their purpose as distractors. This means that it is just as beneficial to look up the incorrect choices as the correct choices to discover specifically why they are incorrect. In this way, it is possible to learn better test-taking skills as the subtlety of question construction is uncovered.

Additionally, it is advisable to go back and attempt to restructure each question to see if all the choices can be made correct by modifying the question. By doing this, four times as much will be learned. By all means, look up the right answer and explanation. Then, focus on each of the other choices and ask yourself under what conditions they might be correct? For example, the entire thrust of the sample question concerning hypothyroidism could be altered by changing the first few words to read:

> "Hyperthyroidism recently discovered in . . . ."
> "Hypothyroidism prenatally occurring in . . . ."
> "Hypothyroidism resulting from . . . ."

This question can be used to learn and understand thyroid problems in general, not only to memorize answers to specific questions.

In the Comprehensive Exam that follows, every effort has been made to simulate the types of questions and the degree of question difficulty in the various licensure and qualifying exams (i.e., NBME Comp I and FLEX). While taking this exam, the student should attempt to create the testing conditions that might be experienced during actual testing situations.

## Summary

Ideally, examinations are designed to determine how much information students have learned and how that information is used in the successful completion of the examination. Students will be successful if these suggestions are followed:

- Develop a positive attitude and maintain that attitude.
- Be realistic in determining the amount of material you attempt to master and in the score you hope to obtain.
- Read the directions for each type of question and the questions themselves closely and follow the directions carefully.
- Guess intelligently and consistently when guessing strategies must be used.
- Bring the paper-and-pencil differential diagnosis approach to each question in the examination.
- Use the test as an opportunity to display your knowledge and as a tool for developing prescriptions for further study and learning.

NBME examinations are not easy. They may be almost impossible for those who have unrealistic expectations or for those who allow misinformation concerning the exams to produce anxiety out of proportion to the task at hand. They are manageable if they are approached with a positive attitude and with consistent use of all the information the student has learned.

Michael J. O'Donnell

# QUESTIONS

**Directions:** Each of the numbered items or incomplete statements in this section is followed by answers or by completions of the statement. Select the **one** lettered answer or completion that is **best** in each case.

1. Asphyxia is a common occurrence in the perinatal period. During an episode of mild asphyxia, the $Po_2$ is highest in the

(A) brain
(B) gastrointestinal tract
(C) kidney
(D) liver
(E) skeletal muscle

2. Which of the following coagulopathies is associated with a prolonged bleeding time?

(A) Hemophilia A
(B) Christmas disease
(C) von Willebrand's disease
(D) Vitamin K deficiency
(E) Liver disease

3. Which of the following bacteria is a common cause of infective endocarditis in adults but a rare cause of this infection in children?

(A) Enterococcus
(B) *Staphylococcus aureus*
(C) *Staphylococcus epidermidis*
(D) Viridans streptococcus (α-hemolytic streptococcus)

4. Which of the following diseases represents a slow virus infection?

(A) Varicella
(B) Papovavirus encephalitis
(C) Subacute sclerosing panencephalitis
(D) Rubella

5. Occasionally, early adolescent girls with familial tall stature may be treated to reduce predicted adult stature. This treatment usually consists of which one of the following agents?

(A) Glucocorticoid
(B) Thyroid hormone
(C) Estrogen
(D) Gn-RH agonist
(E) Progesterone

6. Proper management of a child with an absolute neutrophil count (ANC) of $100/mm^3$ would be

(A) the start of broad-spectrum intravenous antibiotics after blood cultures are obtained
(B) careful physical examination and chest x-ray; close observation pending results of blood cultures
(C) granulocyte transfusion
(D) nutritional support with oral iron and intramuscular injection of vitamin $B_{12}$

7. Physiologic jaundice in term newborns is best characterized by

(A) the onset of clinical jaundice by 12 hours of age
(B) persistence of clinical jaundice for at least 1 week
(C) equal elevation of direct and indirect serum bilirubin values
(D) a decrease in serum bilirubin level following discontinuation of breast-feeding
(E) a rise in serum bilirubin concentration of less than 5 mg/dl/day

8. Which of the following statements regarding Hirschsprung's disease is true?

(A) The presence of ganglion cells on a suction rectal biopsy is diagnostic
(B) A barium enema may show a transition zone between affected and normal bowel
(C) Balloon distension of the rectum results in reflex relaxation of the internal rectal sphincter
(D) Medical therapy recently has been shown to be a reasonable alternative to surgery

| | | |
|---|---|---|
| 1-A | 4-C | 7-E |
| 2-C | 5-C | 8-B |
| 3-A | 6-A | |

9. A 4-month-old child is seen in the emergency room for fever and irritability. A lumbar puncture is performed and the CSF analysis reveals a red cell count of 10, a white cell count of 1050, a protein level of 50 mg/d, a glucose level of 40 mg/dl, and a Gram stain that shows numerous white cells but no bacteria. The most appropriate therapy is

(A) observation in the hospital without antibiotics
(B) intravenous ampicillin and gentamicin
(C) intravenous ceftriaxone
(D) intravenous oxacillin and gentamicin
(E) intravenous ampicillin

10. A 2-year-old girl is brought to the emergency room, having choked while eating a hot dog 10 minutes earlier. She has been coughing intermittently and has a very hoarse voice since the acute episode. The first step to be taken in the emergency room is to

(A) insert fingers into the child's mouth to locate and remove the foreign body
(B) apply five back blows followed by five chest thrusts
(C) apply three abdominal thrusts (Heimlich maneuver)
(D) obtain vital signs and assess respiratory status
(E) obtain x-rays of the chest and neck

11. A 16-year-old female complains of a malodorous vaginal discharge that began 3 days earlier. Microscopic evaluation of a sample of the discharge in normal saline reveals numerous moving organisms, each with a posterior flagellum. The most likely etiology of this vaginal discharge is

(A) *Candida albicans*
(B) *Phthirus pubis*
(C) *Gardnerella vaginalis*
(D) *Neisseria gonorrhoeae*
(E) *Trichomonas vaginalis*

12. A 5-year-old child presents with coarse facial features, hepatosplenomegaly, and progressive loss of developmental milestones. In considering this clinical picture, the most likely cause is

(A) mucopolysaccharidosis
(B) carbohydrate metabolism disorder
(C) amino aciduria
(D) urea cycle enzyme deficiency
(E) hereditary fructose intolerance

13. A 16-year-old girl who had mononucleosis at age 13 goes to a walk-in clinic complaining of chronic fatigue. The physician at the clinic draws antibodies to the Epstein-Barr virus. The girl then takes the test results to her family physician to be interpreted. What pattern is consistent with previous mononucleosis?

| | VCA-IgM | VCA-IgG | EA | EBNA |
|---|---|---|---|---|
| (A) | − | − | − | − |
| (B) | + | − | + | − |
| (C) | − | + | − | + |
| (D) | + | + | − | + |
| (E) | − | − | − | + |

VCA = Epstein-Barr viral capsid antigen; EA = Epstein-Barr virus–induced antigen; EBNA = Epstein-Barr nuclear antigen.

14. A 4-month-old boy develops a temperature of 101° F and is irritable for 2 hours after immunization with DTP vaccine. What is the appropriate procedure when this boy is seen at 6 months of age?

(A) Defer immunization with the pertussis vaccine and, instead, administer diphtheria and tetanus toxoid vaccine
(B) Defer immunization with the pertussis vaccine and, instead, administer tetanus toxoid and reduced-dose diphtheria toxoid vaccine
(C) Administer half the usual dose (i.e., split dose) of the DTP vaccine
(D) Defer all immunizations until the infant is 12 months old
(E) Administer the DTP vaccine with instructions for fever control

15. A 10-year-old Bangaladesh refugee presents with migrating joint pain. Which of the following findings would suggest the diagnosis of acute rheumatic fever in this patient?

(A) Swollen finger joints
(B) Urticarial rash
(C) Elevated erythrocyte sedimentation rate
(D) Severe anemia
(E) Elevated antistreptolysin O titer

---

9-C        12-A        15-E
10-D       13-D
11-E       14-E

16. A full-term, 2-day-old boy develops petechiae and is found to have a platelet count of 2000/mm³. The child is otherwise healthy and has no other abnormal physical findings. The mother's platelet count is normal. The most likely diagnosis is

(A) maternal autoimmune thrombocytopenia
(B) isoimmune thrombocytopenia
(C) sepsis
(D) congenital infection
(E) DIC

17. In late summer, a 2-year-old boy presents with a 2-day history of painful, ulcerative lesions of the mouth and a 1-day history of fever to a temperature of 103° F. He refuses to eat. On physical examination he is irritable, has a temperature of 102° F, and has numerous erythematous, ulcerative lesions on the buccal mucosa, gums, and tongue. The most likely diagnosis is

(A) herpangina
(B) aphthous stomatitis
(C) candidal gingivostomatitis
(D) herpetic gingivostomatitis
(E) necrotizing ulcerative gingivitis

18. A 15-year-old male is brought to the emergency room by his parents for evaluation of a suicide attempt. The most likely precipitating event leading to the suicide attempt was

(A) breakup with a girlfriend
(B) failing in school
(C) being dropped from the soccer team
(D) loss of a close friend
(E) conflict with parents

19. A patient with newly diagnosed ANLL who presents with neutropenia and a temperature of 40° C should be managed by

(A) prompt institution of chemotherapy because the fever is most likely due to leukemia
(B) prompt procurement of cultures and initiation of broad-spectrum parenteral antibiotics
(C) administration of granulocyte transfusions to correct the neutropenia
(D) extensive search for an underlying infection and withholding antibiotics until one is found
(E) vigorous antipyretic therapy with aspirin to lower the temperature

20. A 12-year-old boy presents with an erythematous, sandpaper-like rash, a temperature of 103° F, and an infected laceration of the leg. A rapid streptococcal test done on the purulent discharge is positive for group A β-hemolytic streptococcus. The most likely diagnosis is

(A) rheumatic fever
(B) scarlet fever
(C) erysipelas
(D) impetigo
(E) erythema infectiosum

21. A 5-year-old boy with insulin-dependent diabetes on a single morning dose of insulin has begun to have nightly enuresis. His fasting blood glucose level generally is 200–250 mg/dl, and his blood glucose level before supper generally is 75–150 mg/dl. The most likely cause of this patient's enuresis is

(A) glucosuria from under-insulinization overnight
(B) stress of chronic disease
(C) urinary tract infection
(D) Somogyi phenomenon
(E) hypoglycemia

22. The mother of a 2-year-old boy is concerned about the child's speech. He began speaking single words at 12 months of age and now has a speaking vocabulary of at least 20–30 words. He even is combining words into simple sentences. However, for the past month he has begun to repeat words while speaking, which results in an uneven speech pattern. His complete history and physical examination are otherwise normal. Based on this information, what is the most appropriate management plan?

(A) Refer the child for a hearing evaluation
(B) Refer the child for a speech and language evaluation
(C) Recommend a language-oriented preschool program
(D) Encourage the mother to correct the child's speech gently
(E) Reassure the mother and observe the child during later visits

| | | |
|---|---|---|
| 16-B | 19-B | 22-E |
| 17-D | 20-B | |
| 18-E | 21-A | |

23. A 2-day-old infant is cyanotic but does not have respiratory difficulty. Physical examination reveals a right ventricular heave, a single $S_2$, no murmur, and normal pulses. Chest x-ray shows mild cardiomegaly and mildly increased pulmonary blood flow. The ECG is normal. These findings are consistent with a diagnosis of

(A) pulmonary atresia with ventricular septal defect
(B) pulmonary atresia with intact ventricular septum
(C) L-transposition of the great arteries without intracardiac abnormalities
(D) D-transposition of the great arteries without intracardiac abnormalities
(E) ventricular septal defect

24. A mother requests advice about how to deal with her 16-year-old son. This past weekend her son came home 3 hours after his curfew. This was the first time he did not call to say he would be late. The mother states that she was so worried waiting for him to come home that it took all her energy not to yell at him when he walked through the door. The most appropriate recommendation to give this mother would be to tell her to

(A) ground her son for a weekend
(B) tell her son how she feels and take away his phone privileges temporarily
(C) share her feelings and negotiate with her son about the consequences of his being late again without calling
(D) feel relieved that nothing happened and not make an issue of it

25. A 7-year-old boy with leukemia in remission develops a fever, vesicular rash, and cough. A Tzanck test is positive, and a chest x-ray shows a small left lower lobe infiltrate. The boy's mother is uncertain whether he has had chickenpox in the past. What is the most appropriate initial course of action?

(A) Administer herpes zoster immune globulin
(B) Administer antibiotics based on Gram stain from bronchoscopic washings
(C) Administer intravenous acyclovir and ceftriaxone
(D) Admit to the hospital and observe closely

26. A previously healthy 4-year-old boy is brought to a clinic with an acute onset of petechiae and purpura. His hemoglobin, white blood cell count, and differential count are normal. The most likely diagnosis is

(A) ALL
(B) ITP
(C) aplastic anemia
(D) hemophilia A
(E) Diamond-Blackfan syndrome

27. A 7-year-old boy with T cell ALL in bone marrow remission presents with headache, vomiting, stiff neck, and papilledema. He has no other abnormalities on physical examination. The most likely diagnosis is

(A) meningeal relapse
(B) adverse reaction to cranial irradiation
(C) bacterial meningitis
(D) superior vena cava syndrome
(E) intracranial hemorrhage

28. A 17-year-old female presents in the emergency room with lower abdominal pain. On pelvic examination, significant cervical motion tenderness is found. The most likely diagnosis is

(A) cystitis
(B) appendicitis
(C) vaginitis
(D) pelvic inflammatory disease
(E) inflammatory bowel disease

29. An 11-year-old boy complains of photophobia, stringy mucous discharge, and itching and tearing of the eyes. Examination shows some corneal damage and eosinophilia in the exudate. The most likely cause of this patient's symptoms is

(A) blepharitis
(B) allergic conjunctivitis
(C) vernal conjunctivitis
(D) atopic keratoconjunctivitis

| | | |
|---|---|---|
| 23-D | 26-B | 29-C |
| 24-C | 26-A | |
| 25-C | 28-D | |

30. A 6-year-old child presents with headaches, fever, and pain over the left maxillary sinus. A sinus x-ray shows an air-fluid level in the left maxillary sinus. The two most likely bacterial causes of this illness are

(A) *Streptococcus pyogenes* and *Staphylococcus aureus*
(B) *Hemophilus influenzae* and *S. aureus*
(C) *H. influenzae* and *Streptococcus pneumoniae*
(D) *S. pyogenes* and *S. pneumoniae*
(E) *Branhamella catarrhalis* and anaerobic bacteria

31. A full-term male infant is noted to have circumoral cyanosis and twitching of his left hand at 12 hours of age. On physical examination, he is found to have absent pupillary response to light and a small penis. The most likely diagnosis is

(A) hypocalcemia
(B) hypoglycemia
(C) congenital hypothyroidism
(D) congenital heart disease
(E) idiopathic epilepsy

32. A 14-year-old female is evaluated for irregular menstrual cycles. Menarche began 6 months ago, and menses occur every other month. The bleedings last 3–4 days and are not associated with significant dysmenorrhea. No other symptoms are noted. On physical examination, she is found to be stage 4 in both breast and pubic hair development. The next step in the evaluation should be

(A) pelvic examination
(B) thyroid function testing
(C) pelvic ultrasound
(D) reassurance about irregular menses
(E) liver function testing

33. A mother complains that her 7-year-old child seems to be allergic to milk. The best approach to the diagnosis of this child's possible food allergy is

(A) skin testing
(B) sublingual food testing
(C) cytotoxicity testing
(D) oral challenge testing
(E) RAST

34. A child with chronic diarrhea, failure to thrive, and bulky, foul-smelling stools, presents with a bleeding diathesis. Platelet count is normal, but both PTT and PT are abnormally prolonged. The most appropriate therapy for correcting the underlying cause of bleeding in this child is

(A) fresh frozen plasma
(B) cryoprecipitate
(C) vitamin K
(D) whole blood transfusion
(E) platelet infusion

35. A 10-year-old girl presents with a 2-day history of fever and a 4-cm warm, tender, and fluctuant left anterior cervical lymph node. The most likely diagnosis is

(A) Hodgkin's disease
(B) ALL
(C) histiocytosis X
(D) acute bacterial lymphadenitis
(E) metastatic neuroblastoma

36. An 18-month-old girl is brought to a pediatrician by her parents, who say she has had a fever of 104° F and refused to walk since she awoke that morning. The pediatrician obtains a hip x-ray, which reveals a subtle widening of the left hip joint space. The most appropriate initial course of action is

(A) close observation in the hospital or at home if the parents are reliable
(B) intravenous ceftriaxone
(C) surgical drainage of the hip joint
(D) intravenous oxacillin

37. A 6-year-old boy returns from a visit to a farm with an attack of hives from playing with the barn cats. The principal therapeutic modality in the management of this child's urticaria is

(A) application of cold packs
(B) corticosteroids
(C) β-adrenergic blocking agents
(D) atropine
(E) antihistamines

| | | |
|---|---|---|
| 30-C | 33-D | 36-C |
| 31-B | 34-C | 37-E |
| 32-D | 35-D | |

38. A 6-month-old boy in otherwise good health is found to be anemic. His reticulocyte count is 0.1% and his MCV is high. The most likely diagnosis is

(A) Fanconi's anemia
(B) Diamond-Blackfan syndrome
(C) aplastic anemia
(D) autoimmune hemolytic anemia
(E) sickle cell anemia

39. Common causes of hydrocephalus in the first month of life include all of the following EXCEPT

(A) intraventricular hemorrhage
(B) brain tumor
(C) meningitis
(D) aqueductal stenosis
(E) Arnold-Chiari deformity

40. Renal biopsy is the definitive procedure for histologic diagnosis of renal disease. All of the following statements about renal biopsy are true EXCEPT

(A) renal biopsy generally is performed as a closed procedure using a biopsy needle inserted percutaneously
(B) the presence of a single kidney should preclude a closed renal biopsy
(C) tissue obtained from a needle biopsy may be examined by light, immunofluorescent, and electron microscopy
(D) complications of renal biopsy include bleeding, infection, and failure to obtain enough tissue
(E) serial renal biopsies are used in chronic renal insufficiency to monitor the progression to end-stage renal failure

41. Injuries that have a high association with child abuse include all of the following EXCEPT

(A) cigarette burns
(B) distal tibial fracture
(C) scald burns of the buttocks
(D) spiral fracture of the femur
(E) retinal hemorrhage

42. Anorexia nervosa is characterized by all of the following features EXCEPT

(A) weight loss of at least 15% of original body weight
(B) onset in early childhood
(C) missing two consecutive menstrual cycles
(D) a disturbed body image
(E) a high predominance in girls

43. Hypophosphatemia is likely to be associated with all of the following disorders EXCEPT

(A) hyperparathyroidism
(B) vitamin D–dependent rickets
(C) chronic renal failure
(D) rickets of prematurity

44. Frequent complications of cystic fibrosis include all of the following EXCEPT

(A) cor pulmonale
(B) nasal polyposis
(C) digital clubbing
(D) mental retardation
(E) hemoptysis

45. All of the following statements about epileptic seizures are true EXCEPT

(A) seizures are caused by abnormal neuronal discharges in the cerebral cortex
(B) the nature of a partial seizure reflects the site of its cortical origin
(C) focal motor seizures can spread to adjacent muscle groups
(D) absence seizures are a type of complex partial seizure
(E) an aura can be either sensory or motor

46. All of the following statements concerning hyaline membrane disease are true EXCEPT

(A) the clinical symptoms include tachypnea, grunting, nasal flaring, chest retraction, and cyanosis
(B) the infant begins to improve by 24 hours of life
(C) therapy may include oxygen and positive pressure ventilation
(D) preeclampsia and prolonged rupture of the fetal membranes are associated with accelerated lung maturation
(E) the chest x-ray has a uniform ground-glass appearance with air bronchograms

| | | |
|---|---|---|
| 38-B | 41-B | 44-D |
| 39-B | 42-B | 45-D |
| 40-E | 43-C | 46-B |

47. True statements regarding the edematous child with acute nephrotic syndrome include all of the following EXCEPT

(A) the child should be aggressively treated with fluid restriction and loop diuretics
(B) the child is at increased risk for bacterial infections
(C) the child may have decreased intravascular volume despite the increase in total body water
(D) the degree of edema generally correlates inversely with the serum protein concentration

48. Which of the following statements about hypovolemic shock is FALSE?

(A) Tachycardia, prolonged capillary refill, and hypotension are early clinical findings
(B) The principal therapeutic intervention is re-establishment of circulating volume by crystalloid or colloid infusion
(C) Hormonal response to hypovolemia leads to decreased urine output and increased cardiac contractility
(D) Inotropic support is used only when a prolonged shock state has caused myocardial damage

49. A child who was perfectly alert one day is comatose the next day. All of the following are possible causes of coma in this child EXCEPT

(A) a brain tumor
(B) a convulsion
(C) an infection
(D) excessive medication

50. Signs and symptoms of early neonatal sepsis include all of the following EXCEPT

(A) neutropenia
(B) apnea
(C) unexplained respiratory distress
(D) lethargy
(E) anemia

51. Which of the following statements regarding IVP is FALSE?

(A) Allergic reactions, including anaphylaxis, can follow injection of contrast material
(B) IVP is inferior to radionuclide renal scanning for anatomic delineation of the kidney and ureters
(C) IVP may precipitate acute renal failure
(D) Radiation exposure is greater with IVP than with radionuclide renal scanning
(E) The presence of a single kidney on IVP does not exclude the possibility of a contralateral nonfunctioning kidney

52. All of the following studies should be included in the workup of an adolescent with chronic liver disease EXCEPT

(A) hepatitis A serology
(B) hepatitis B serology
(C) ophthalmologic examination
(D) antinuclear and antismooth muscle antibody serology

53. Reasons that a newborn does not gain weight during the first week of life may include all of the following EXCEPT

(A) extracellular water loss occurs
(B) use of phototherapy for hyperbilirubinemia
(C) caloric intake is suboptimal
(D) basal metabolism decreases
(E) preterm birth

54. All of the following are problems commonly associated with cerebral palsy EXCEPT

(A) epilepsy
(B) mental retardation
(C) blindness
(D) emotional problems
(E) strabismus

55. Which of the following is NOT a parameter used to assess renal tubular function?

(A) The ability of the kidney to acidify the urine
(B) The ability of the kidney to excrete a water load
(C) The endogenous creatinine clearance
(D) The presence of urinary amino acids
(E) The tubular reabsorption of phosphate (TRP)

| | | |
|---|---|---|
| 47-A | 50-E | 53-D |
| 48-A | 51-B | 54-C |
| 49-A | 52-A | 55-C |

56. Signs and symptoms of severe perinatal asphyxia include all of the following EXCEPT

(A) coma
(B) acute tubular necrosis
(C) necrotizing enterocolitis
(D) hemolytic anemia
(E) seizures

57. All of the following are developmental reflexes EXCEPT

(A) Moro reflex
(B) tonic neck reflex
(C) superficial abdominal reflex
(D) rooting reflex
(E) parachute reflex

58. Renal function in the newborn is limited in several important ways, including all of the following EXCEPT the ability to

(A) maximally acidify the urine during acidosis
(B) maximally concentrate the urine to an osmolality of 1200 mOsm/kg if fluid intake is limited
(C) conserve sodium if sodium intake is severely limited
(D) dilute the urine to an osmolality of less than 100 mOsm/kg
(E) rapidly excrete a water load because of a much diminished GFR

59. All of the following statements concerning diaphragmatic hernia are true EXCEPT

(A) the defect usually is on the right
(B) bilateral lung hypoplasia may occur in moderate to severe cases
(C) severe respiratory distress, cyanosis, and dyspnea are apparent shortly after birth
(D) pulmonary hypertension is a common complication
(E) bag-mask ventilation may cause respiratory compromise

60. A 7-year-old girl is brought to the emergency room because of hematemesis. Her mother states that the child had complained of epigastric pain and had eaten very little the previous day. That morning she vomited several times, and at noon she vomited a large amount of coffee ground–like material. On the way to the hospital, the child became dizzy and upon arrival was carried into the examining room by her father. All of the following measures should be taken immediately in the emergency room EXCEPT

(A) insertion of a large-bore intravenous catheter for administration of fluid
(B) blood sampling to determine the hematocrit and blood type
(C) upper endoscopy to determine the site and cause of bleeding
(D) insertion of a nasogastric tube
(E) questioning of the parents for further medical history

61. A 15-year-old male says that his friend has asked him to try some amphetamines. He has heard that using "uppers" can be fun. All of the following are hazards of amphetamines EXCEPT

(A) depression
(B) arrhythmias
(C) hypertension
(D) irritation of the nasal mucosa
(E) psychosis

62. A 14-year-old girl is taken to her pediatrician because she has not begun to menstruate. On physical examination, she is noted to be in less than the fifth percentile for height and weight. She has no breast development. The remainder of the history and physical examination are normal. Possible conditions responsible for this patient's presentation include all of the following EXCEPT

(A) Turner syndrome
(B) 21-hydroxylase deficiency
(C) hypothyroidism
(D) constitutional delay of growth and puberty
(E) anorexia nervosa

56-D    59-A    62-B
57-C    60-C
58-D    61-B

63. A 16-year-old girl complains of frequent abdominal pain during the last 6 months. The pain is usually periumbilical, often exacerbated by eating, and frequently associated with nausea. All of the following conditions would be included in the differential diagnosis EXCEPT

(A) lactose intolerance
(B) peptic ulcer disease
(C) irritable bowel syndrome
(D) chronic pancreatitis
(E) Meckel's diverticulum

64. An 18-year-old female comes in for her first sports physical. She denies ever being sexually active, and her menstrual cycles are regular and without significant dysmenorrhea. A review of systems does not yield any positive findings. All of the following laboratory studies would be useful in this evaluation EXCEPT

(A) hematocrit and hemoglobin
(B) urinalysis
(C) skin test for tuberculosis
(D) Pap smear
(E) rubella titers

65. A 10-year-old boy presents with chest pain and dyspnea on exertion. Family history reveals that his mother died of a "cardiac problem." On physical examination, the boy is found to have a biferious pulse and a murmur of left ventricular outflow obstruction that increases with a Valsalva maneuver. The ECG shows left ventricular hypertrophy and ST segment changes, and the echocardiogram is diagnostic for hypertrophic cardiomyopathy. Appropriate therapeutic measures include all of the following EXCEPT

(A) calcium channel blockers
(B) β-adrenergic blockers
(C) antiarrhythmic agents
(D) digoxin
(E) restriction from competitive sports

66. Because of severe asphyxia at birth, an infant has been placed on life support, and there is little chance of a good long-term outcome. It is appropriate for the physician to do all of the following in an effort to determine whether to continue life support EXCEPT

(A) discuss the situation with both parents at the same time
(B) refrain from indicating a preference for or against treatment
(C) involve the parents in all phases of decision making
(D) consult with the hospital's ethics committee to clarify the issues involved
(E) discuss frankly with the parents the possibility of the death of the infant

67. A boy presents with indications of mental retardation. All of the following evaluations are indicated for this patient EXCEPT

(A) chromosome analysis
(B) fragile X study
(C) urinalysis for amino aciduria
(D) serum AFP testing
(E) pedigree analysis

68. A full-term, 3-day-old infant suddenly becomes irritable, vomits several times, and passes two bloody stools. Physical examination is unremarkable. Laboratory findings include a hematocrit of 50% and a white cell count of 15,000/mm$^3$ (30% neutrophils, 50% leukocytes, 5% monocytes, and 15% eosinophils). All of the following measures are appropriate in the management of this infant EXCEPT

(A) abdominal x-ray to evaluate for malrotation with volvulus
(B) sigmoidoscopy and rectal biopsy to evaluate for allergic enterocolitis
(C) dietary restriction of lactose for possible lactose malabsorption
(D) stool culture to exclude infection
(E) careful review of the infant's diet history

---

63-E        66-B
64-D        67-D
65-D        68-C

69. A 4-month-old infant presents with severe lethargy, multiple ecchymoses, and obvious malnutrition. No fever is noted. Physical examination reveals a bulging anterior fontanelle, and laboratory evaluation reveals a hematocrit of 20%, platelet count of 300,000, PT of 30 seconds (control = 11.5–13 seconds), and PTT of more than 100 seconds (control = 28–35 seconds). The differential diagnosis should include all of the following EXCEPT

(A) child abuse
(B) hemophilia A
(C) cystic fibrosis
(D) sepsis
(E) liver failure

70. Physical examination of a 2-month-old infant reveals a funnel-shaped chest deformity and a harsh noise during inspiration. The differential diagnosis of stridor in this infant would include all of the following EXCEPT

(A) bronchogenic cyst
(B) laryngeal web
(C) vocal cord paralysis
(D) subglottic hemangioma
(E) laryngomalacia

71. A healthy-appearing, short boy does not show signs of puberty by age 14. Which of the following conditions is NOT a likely cause of this clinical picture?

(A) Inflammatory bowel disease
(B) Constitutional growth delay
(C) Hypogonadotropic hypogonadism
(D) Klinefelter syndrome
(E) Prolactin-secreting adenoma

72. A 10-year-old boy is referred to a pediatrician with a 6-month history of fatigue, anorexia, and deterioration of school performance and a 2-week history of scleral icterus. Serum evaluation reveals a total bilirubin level of 4.2 mg/dl, direct bilirubin level of 2.6 mg/dl, AST level of 240 U/L, and ALT level of 180 U/L. Physical findings that would strongly suggest chronic liver disease in this patient include all of the following EXCEPT

(A) digital clubbing
(B) splenomegaly
(C) lymphadenopathy
(D) multiple telangiectasias on the face, trunk, and extremities

73. A developmentally delayed 10-month-old boy is referred to a pediatrician for evaluation of small size for age, unusual facial features, abnormal palmar creases, and a heart defect. The likely etiologies for this infant's condition include all of the following EXCEPT

(A) a sporadic syndrome
(B) a single gene abnormality
(C) a chromosome anomaly
(D) an inborn error of metabolism
(E) a teratogenic exposure

74. A 12-year-old boy is seen in the emergency ward because of scleral icterus. Questioning reveals that he has had a low-grade fever, malaise, and anorexia for several weeks. His liver is enlarged and tender, and his spleen is palpable. The serum ALT level is 700 U/L, and the total bilirubin level is 6 mg/dl. Serum findings consistent with hepatitis virus as the single cause of acute hepatitis include the presence of all of the following EXCEPT

(A) IgM antibodies to hepatitis A
(B) IgG antibodies to hepatitis A
(C) antibodies to HBcAg
(D) HbsAg

75. A 6-year-old boy is shorter than all of his classmates. Diagnostic testing supports a diagnosis of idiopathic isolated GH deficiency. All of the following are expected clinical findings in this patient EXCEPT

(A) normal body proportions
(B) a growth velocity of 3 cm/yr
(C) mild truncal obesity
(D) hypertension
(E) delayed skeletal maturation

---

69-B          72-C          75-D
70-A          73-D
71-D          74-B

76. A 17-year-old female says she has been raped by her stepfather. All of the following statements about rape are correct EXCEPT

(A) contact of the male genitalia with the labia majora is insufficient evidence for rape
(B) ejaculation is not necessary for an act to be rape
(C) before examination, it is important to establish that there has been no change in the vaginal environment since the rape (e.g., by bathing or douching)
(D) evaluation for sexually transmitted disease and pregnancy should be performed

77. An 8-year-old girl has a 6-week history of vomiting, weight loss, and abdominal pain. Endoscopic evaluation of the upper gastrointestinal tract reveals antral gastritis, and biopsy reveals gram-positive bacteria on inflamed areas of gastric tissue. The management of this patient is likely to include all of the following measures EXCEPT

(A) stool culture
(B) $H_2$-blocker therapy
(C) bismuth suspension therapy
(D) antibiotic therapy

**Questions 78–80**

A 6-year-old girl with asthma is brought to the emergency room with wheezing and shortness of breath. Arterial blood gas analysis reveals the following:

pH $= 7.49$
$P_{CO_2} = 32$ mm Hg
$P_{O_2} = 68$ mm Hg
base excess $= +2$

78. These arterial blood gas data indicate the presence of which of the following acid-base disorders?

(A) Respiratory acidosis
(B) Respiratory alkalosis
(C) Metabolic acidosis
(D) Metabolic alkalosis

79. Initial treatment of this child should include all of the following measures EXCEPT

(A) administration of oxygen
(B) inhaled bronchodilator therapy
(C) frequent clinical reassessment
(D) chest physical therapy

Despite initial improvement with therapy, the child suddenly becomes cyanotic and experiences increased respiratory distress. Repeat arterial blood gas analysis reveals the following:

pH $= 7.28$
$P_{CO_2} = 52$ mm Hg
$P_{O_2} = 48$ mm Hg
base excess $= -1$

80. These arterial blood gas data indicate the presence of which of the following acid-base disorders?

(A) Respiratory acidosis
(B) Respiratory alkalosis
(C) Metabolic acidosis
(D) Metabolic alkalosis

**Questions 81–83**

An infant is seated on her mother's lap in the examining room. She sits well with support, grasps a rattle, and puts it in her mouth. When placed on the examining table, she promptly rolls over from front to back. She smiles spontaneously and laughs and squeals with delight.

81. This child's age is most likely

(A) 2 months
(B) 4 months
(C) 6 months
(D) 8 months
(E) 10 months

82. During this health maintenance visit, anticipatory guidance may include all of the following developmental issues EXCEPT

(A) synchrony
(B) attachment
(C) temperament
(D) motor skills
(E) autonomy/independence

83. During the physical examination of this infant, special attention should be given to all of the following areas EXCEPT

(A) chest
(B) hips
(C) skin
(D) back
(E) head

| 76-A | 79-D | 82-E |
|------|------|------|
| 77-A | 80-A | 83-D |
| 78-B | 81-B |      |

**Questions 84–85**

A 4-year-old girl has complained of intermittent, severe abdominal pain for 2 weeks. She now has a purpuric and petechial rash on her buttocks and ankles and complains of joint pain. She is afebrile and appears clinically well.

84. Of the following possible diagnoses, the most likely explanation is

(A) Kawasaki disease
(B) meningococcemia
(C) juvenile rheumatoid arthritis
(D) Henoch-Schönlein purpura
(E) hemolytic-uremic syndrome

85. All of the following findings are compatible with this child's condition EXCEPT

(A) very low C3
(B) hematuria and proteinuria on urinalysis
(C) hypertension
(D) prominent IgA deposition in the glomeruli on renal biopsy
(E) normal BUN and creatinine

**Questions 86–88**

A 12-year-old boy is hit by a car while riding his bicycle without a helmet. Upon arrival at a pediatric trauma center, he is unconscious, apneic, hypotensive, and tachycardic.

86. Priorities for care in the first 10 minutes after arrival include all of the following EXCEPT

(A) intubation or tracheotomy
(B) establishment of large-bore vascular access
(C) stabilization of the cervical spine until cervical x-ray series has been performed
(D) head and abdominal CT scans
(E) infusion of isotonic crystalloid, colloid, or blood

87. After initial treatment, stabilization, and assessment, severe cerebral edema is diagnosed, without other significant injuries. Which of the following modalities of therapy will be LEAST effective in controlling this patient's increased intracranial pressure?

(A) Administration of mannitol
(B) Hyperventilation
(C) Removal of CSF by ventriculostomy
(D) Pentobarbital infusion
(E) Fluid restriction

88. Despite aggressive management, the patient deteriorates and cerebral death is diagnosed. Which of the following statements is true in this case?

(A) Brain death can be documented if the patient has a Glasgow coma score of 3
(B) Brain death can be documented without an isoelectric EEG
(C) A four-vessel cerebral angiogram must be performed before the diagnosis of cerebral death is made
(D) Use of barbiturate medications will not affect the ability to diagnose brain death
(E) Decerebrate posturing is compatible with a diagnosis of brain death

**Questions 89–90**

A 3-year-old boy is seen in the emergency ward at 3 A.M. for an ear infection. The physician notices multiple bruises over the child's body. Some are red, some are yellow, and others are brown. The parents claim no knowledge of the origin of the child's bruises.

89. All of the following are appropriate steps in the initial evaluation of this child EXCEPT

(A) a review of the child's past medical history
(B) a detailed physical examination
(C) coagulation studies
(D) a CT scan of the head
(E) a discussion with the child about his bruises

| | |
|---|---|
| 84-D | 87-C |
| 85-A | 88-B |
| 86-D | 89-D |

90. If the examining physician suspects child abuse, the next most appropriate step is to

(A) refer the family to a mental health agency
(B) retain the child in the emergency ward until morning to see a social worker
(C) admit the child to the hospital
(D) discharge the child with an early morning appointment for the pediatric clinic

**Questions 91–93**

A 2-year-old boy presents with bilateral proptosis and periorbital ecchymoses, a large right flank mass, and lower back and right arm pain. Evaluation demonstrates moderate anemia, a large right suprarenal mass displacing the right kidney inferiorly and laterally, clumps of primitive cells in the bone marrow, and bone scan showing increased activity in the right humerus, left and right orbits, and L1–L3 vertebrae.

91. The most likely diagnosis is

(A) histiocytosis X
(B) rhabdomyosarcoma
(C) neuroblastoma
(D) Wilms' tumor
(E) lymphoblastic lymphoma

92. Laboratory features that may be associated with this disease include all of the following EXCEPT

(A) increased urinary VMA excretion
(B) amplification of c-*myc* oncogene in the involved cells
(C) elevation of serum ferritin
(D) translocation (9;22) in the involved cells
(E) leukoerythroblastic peripheral blood smear

The patient develops increased back pain and is unable to walk. Neurologic examination reveals decreased strength in the lower extremities.

93. Management of this patient should begin with

(A) analgesic therapy for bone metastases with a nonsteroidal anti-inflammatory agent
(B) lumbar puncture
(C) imaging studies to evaluate the dorsolumbar epidural space
(D) careful, serial neurologic examinations
(E) physical therapy to decrease lumbar muscle spasm and increase strength of lower extremity muscles

**Questions 94–95**

A 2-year-old boy is found to have an elevated blood lead level as part of routine screening at his well-child care examination. He is not anemic, his physical examination is normal, and he is developing normally.

94. Which of the following statements about this case is correct?

(A) It is unusual to have an elevated blood lead level without clinical findings
(B) Immediate chelation therapy is indicated to prevent neurologic damage
(C) A CaEDTA challenge test may help to determine the need for therapy
(D) The child's family should move from their current home immediately to prevent further lead exposure

95. Which of the following is NOT a potential source of lead in this case?

(A) Eating paint chips
(B) Exposure to household dust
(C) Eating backyard soil
(D) Sucking on a lead pencil point
(E) Drinking orange juice stored in a ceramic pitcher

**Questions 96–98**

An 18-month-old boy is brought to his pediatrician because his mother is concerned about speech delay. He is saying "mama" and "dada" but no other words. He has been healthy since birth.

96. Evaluation of this child should begin with

(A) physical examination
(B) chromosome analysis
(C) hearing evaluation
(D) developmental testing
(E) CT scan of the head

97. Which part of this child's history does NOT hold clues to the reason for his language delay?

(A) Prenatal history
(B) Delivery history
(C) Allergy history
(D) Motor development history
(E) Family history

| | | |
|---|---|---|
| 90-C | 93-C | 96-A |
| 91-C | 94-C | 97-C |
| 92-D | 95-D | |

98. Possible explanations for this child's language delay include all of the following EXCEPT

(A) genetic deafness due to a single gene defect
(B) multiple chest x-rays of the mother during pregnancy
(C) prenatal rubella exposure
(D) fragile X syndrome
(E) normal child who is slow to start speaking

## Questions 99–100

During a health maintenance visit, the mother of a 12-year-old boy mentions that she and her husband are concerned about their son's reluctance to try out for the local swim team. Despite the boy's ability to compete effectively, he becomes upset whenever his parents raise the topic. His physical examination is entirely normal, although he is prepubertal. A review of the boy's early health records reveals concerns with past behavior (his parents were initially reluctant to leave him with sitters because of his difficulties with separation; he adapts slowly to new situations such as school and camp).

99. Anticipatory guidance in this case should consider each of the following developmental issues EXCEPT

(A) gender identity
(B) temperament
(C) puberty
(D) autonomy/independence
(E) peer interaction

100. On the basis of this information, which of the following is the most developmentally appropriate advice to offer the boy's parents?

(A) Ask about the possibility of the boy competing with a younger group of children
(B) Allow the boy to make up his own mind about trying out for the team
(C) Request that the boy's friends encourage him to try out for the team
(D) Urge the boy to attend the tryout sessions
(E) Arrange for mental health counseling for the boy

## Questions 101–102

A previously healthy 8-month-old boy with a 4-day history of diarrhea, poor intake, and little urine output presents with irritability, dry mucous membranes, decreased skin turgor, tachycardia, tachypnea, cool extremities, and capillary refill of 2 seconds.

101. Which of the following measures is NOT appropriate in the management of this infant?

(A) Obtain stool, urine, and blood cultures
(B) Obtain blood for electrolytes and cell counts and urine for electrolytes and urinalysis
(C) Obtain an IVP to exclude urinary tract obstruction with infection
(D) Administer normal saline (20 ml/kg over 30 minutes) and continuously assess cardiovascular status
(E) Discontinue oral feeding and give all fluids parenterally for 24 hours

102. Laboratory studies reveal that the infant has a hemoglobin of 5.6 g/dl, a platelet count of 50,000, and a serum creatinine of 1.3 mg/dl. The most likely diagnosis is

(A) viral gastroenteritis with dehydration and bone marrow depression
(B) gastrointestinal hemorrhage and hypovolemia
(C) chronic renal insufficiency with acute gastroenteritis
(D) hemolytic-uremic syndrome
(E) HIV illness

98-B       101-C
99-A       102-D
100-B

**Questions 103–104**

A 2-month-old girl is rushed to the emergency department. Her father is hysterical and does not speak English. The child is cyanotic, breathes with gasping respirations, and has a heart rate of 40.

103. Which of the following diagnoses most accurately describes the physiologic status of this patient?

(A) Respiratory failure
(B) Respiratory distress
(C) Shock
(D) Cardiopulmonary failure
(E) Cardiopulmonary arrest

104. The first intervention should be

(A) intraosseous cannulation
(B) synchronized cardioversion
(C) chest compressions
(D) bag-mask ventilation with 100% oxygen

**Questions 105–106**

An 8-year-old boy with a 6-year history of steroid-responsive nephrotic syndrome has increasingly frequent relapses and is relapsing on significant doses of alternate-day prednisone. He is cushingoid and grossly obese, his growth velocity has slowed, and he has a small cataract. His creatinine clearance and urinalysis are normal.

105. What should be the next step in the treatment of this child?

(A) Discontinue the prednisone and manage subsequent edema with diuretics
(B) Increase the dose of prednisone and administer it daily to achieve a more permanent remission
(C) Begin a course of an alkylating agent (cyclophosphamide or chlorambucil) to achieve a long-term remission
(D) Assume the relapsing course is due to an occult chronic infection and administer broad-spectrum antibiotics
(E) Treat with cyclosporine

106. If a renal biopsy is performed, the most likely histologic picture would be compatible with

(A) focal glomerulosclerosis
(B) minimal change disease
(C) IgA nephropathy
(D) tubulointerstitial nephritis
(E) membranoproliferative glomerulonephritis

**Directions:** Each group of items in this section consists of lettered options followed by a set of numbered items. For each item, select the **one** lettered option that is most closely associated with it. Each lettered option may be selected once, more than once, or not at all.

**Questions 107–111**

Match each laboratory test listed below with the immune deficiency disorder it is most useful for diagnosing.

(A) Leukocyte adhesion defect
(B) Bruton's disease
(C) DiGeorge anomaly
(D) Wiskott-Aldrich syndrome
(E) Chronic granulomatous disease

107. Platelet count and morphology

108. Measurement of serum calcium level

109. Quantitation of serum immunoglobulins

110. Flow cytometry

111. Nitroblue tetrazolium test

103-D 106-B 109-B
104-D 107-D 110-A
105-C 108-C 111-E

## Questions 112–113

Match each statement below with the form of muscular dystrophy it best describes.

(A) Pseudohypertrophic (Duchenne) muscular dystrophy
(B) Congenital myotonic muscular dystrophy
(C) Fascioscapulohumeral (Landouzy-Dejerine) muscular dystrophy
(D) Limb-girdle (Leyden-Möbius) muscular dystrophy

112. An X-linked disorder of progressive muscular weakness that begins at about age 3 years

113. A recessive disorder of muscular weakness that begins in the second decade of life

## Questions 114–119

For each statement about childhood injuries listed below, select the associated type of injury.

(A) Motor vehicular injury
(B) Falls
(C) Burns
(D) Drowning
(E) Choking

114. The leading cause of death between 6 months and 19 years of age

115. The highest mortality to morbidity ratio of all major injuries

116. The most common cause of injury-related death in the first year of life

117. The type of injury most frequently associated with child abuse

118. The most common type of injury resulting in an emergency ward visit

119. An often unrecognized method of suicide in adolescents

## Questions 120–123

Match each pathophysiologic feature described below with the congenital cardiac defect it best characterizes.

(A) Hypoplastic left-heart syndrome
(B) Persistent truncus arteriosus
(C) Tricuspid atresia
(D) Pulmonary atresia with ventricular septal defect
(E) Critical aortic stenosis

120. An obligatory right-to-left atrial shunt

121. Symptoms primarily related to pulmonary resistance and size of the pulmonary arteries

122. Ductus-dependent systemic flow with an obligatory left-to-right atrial shunt

123. Ductus-dependent pulmonary flow with an obligatory right-to-left ventricular shunt

## Questions 124–128

For each developmental issue listed below, select the behavior pattern with which it is associated.

(A) Synchrony
(B) Temperament
(C) Attachment
(D) Autonomy/independence
(E) State organization

124. The markedly irregular sleeping and feeding schedules of a 3-week-old infant

125. The night awakening and night crying of an 8-month-old infant

126. The temper tantrum of a 15-month-old toddler who is not allowed to climb on a chair

127. A 2-year-old toddler's resistance to toilet training

128. The quiet, subdued classroom behavior of a "slow-to-warm-up" child in early September

| | | | | | |
|---|---|---|---|---|---|
| 112-A | 115-D | 118-B | 121-B | 124-E | 127-D |
| 113-D | 116-E | 119-A | 122-A | 125-C | 128-B |
| 114-A | 117-C | 120-C | 123-D | 126-D | |

## Questions 129–132

For each malignancy listed below, select the laboratory finding with which it is most likely to be associated.

(A) Elevated serum AFP level
(B) Elevated urinary excretion of HVA
(C) Malignant cells with deletion of the long arm of chromosome 13
(D) Positive serology for HIV
(E) TdT cells in the CSF

129. Retinoblastoma

130. Burkitt's lymphoma

131. Hepatoblastoma

132. Lymphoblastic lymphoma

## Questions 133–137

Match each of the following descriptions with the appropriate physical sign of pulmonary disease.

(A) Crackles
(B) Grunting
(C) Nasal flaring
(D) Stridor
(E) Wheezing

133. A sign of increased airway resistance

134. A sign of laryngeal or tracheal obstruction

135. A sound produced by partial airway obstruction

136. An inspiratory sound produced by opening of airways that closed on the previous breath

137. A sign of loss of lung volume

## Questions 138–142

Match each indication for drugs used in the treatment of inflammatory bowel disease with the appropriate agent.

(A) Prednisone
(B) Sulfasalazine
(C) 6-Mercaptopurine
(D) Loperamide
(E) Metronidazole

138. Treatment of perirectal Crohn's disease

139. Facilitation of the reduction of corticosteroid dosage in severe Crohn's disease

140. Treatment of mild to moderate colonic inflammation

141. Treatment of the extraintestinal manifestations of inflammatory bowel disease

142. Alleviation of cramping and diminution of diarrhea in patients with inflammatory bowel disease

## Questions 143–146

For each pregnant patient described below, select the optimal first test to offer the patient for prenatal diagnosis.

(A) Level II (specialized) fetal ultrasound
(B) Amniocentesis or CVS
(C) Maternal serum AFP
(D) Fetoscopy

143. A 27-year-old woman in her eighteenth week of pregnancy; both the patient and her husband are heterozygous for the sickle cell gene

144. A 25-year-old woman who is married to her first cousin

145. A 29-year-old woman who previously had a child with microcephaly

146. A 22-year-old woman in her tenth week of pregnancy whose husband is a carrier of a familial balanced translocation

| 129-C | 132-E | 135-E | 138-E | 141-A | 144-C |
| 130-D | 133-C | 136-A | 139-C | 142-D | 145-A |
| 131-A | 134-D | 137-B | 140-B | 143-B | 146-B |

**Questions 147–150**

Match each case described below with the appropriate level of mental retardation.

(A) Mild
(B) Moderate
(C) Severe
(D) Profound

147. A 7-year-old girl is referred from a school administrator because of academic problems. Her parents and peer group never noticed any developmental delays, but upon school entry her reading skills were significantly behind others and she had made limited academic progress. She has friends and relates well to others. Psychoeducational evaluation suggests mental retardation.

148. A 9-year-old boy has severe motor handicaps. He is unable to talk, has no other communication skills, and has no self-care skills.

149. A 10-year-old girl has entry-level kindergarten skills. Her academic program focuses on daily living activities.

150. An 8-year-old boy has limited communication skills. Although he requires continuous supervision by his parents and teachers, he is capable of washing his face and brushing his teeth.

**Questions 151–154**

The parents of a 4-month-old girl phone the pediatrician's office complaining that their daughter has a persistent diaper rash. The rash has been present for a week and has not responded to frequent diaper changes, exposing the diaper area to air, or an over-the-counter cream. Because of the rash's persistence, the parents are instructed to bring their daughter to the office for examination. For each characteristic appearance below, select the corresponding variety of diaper dermatitis.

(A) Candidal
(B) Infantile seborrheic
(C) Generic
(D) Intertrigo

151. White or yellow exudate involving the deep skin folds

152. Satellite lesions and bright red erosions involving the deep skin folds

153. Dry wrinkled skin and erythema that spares the skin folds

154. Erythema and satellite lesions that also involve the face, scalp, and flexural areas

**Questions 155–159**

Match each disorder listed below with the type of immune dysfunction that most likely underlies it.

(A) B cell deficiency
(B) T cell deficiency
(C) T cell deficiency and B cell abnormalities
(D) Complement component deficiency
(E) Complement inhibitor deficiency

155. Recurrent *Mycobacterium* infections

156. Hereditary angioedema

157. AIDS

158. Recurrent *Giardia* infections

159. Recurrent *Neisseria* infections

| 147-A | 150-C | 153-C | 156-E | 159-D |
|-------|-------|-------|-------|-------|
| 148-D | 151-D | 154-B | 157-C |       |
| 149-B | 152-A | 155-B | 158-A |       |

**Questions 160–164**

Match each congenital cardiac defect listed below with the chest x-ray finding that is most suggestive of that deformity.

(A) "Snowman" sign
(B) Egg-shaped heart
(C) "3" sign
(D) Convex left heart border
(E) Boot-shaped heart

160. Coarctation of the aorta

161. Tetralogy of Fallot

162. D-Transposition of the great arteries

163. L-Transposition of the great arteries

164. Total anomalous pulmonary venous return

**Questions 165–167**

Match each of the statements below with the neurocutaneous disorder it best describes.

(A) Neurofibromatosis
(B) Tuberous sclerosis
(C) Sturge-Weber syndrome
(D) von Hippel-Lindau disease
(E) Ataxia-telangiectasia

165. Café au lait spots are one of the hallmarks of this disease

166. The triad of adenoma sebaceum, seizures, and mental retardation characterizes this disease

167. Periventricular tumors occur within the brain in this disease

## ANSWERS AND EXPLANATIONS

**1. The answer is A** *[Ch 5 II A 2].*
During periods of hypoxia or mild asphyxia, there is a redistribution of blood flow to the vital organs, including the brain, heart, and adrenal glands. In order for this to occur, blood flow to other organs, such as the kidney and gastrointestinal tract, is sacrificed. The increased blood flow to the vital organs compensates for the lower oxygen concentration of the blood and, thus, allows a constant delivery of oxygen to these tissues. This compensatory mechanism operates during periods of normal blood pressure but fails if the neonate becomes extremely hypotensive.

**2. The answer is C** *[Ch 14 VI D 1 c (3)].*
The factor VIII complex consists of both the factor VIII procoagulant molecule and the von Willebrand factor, which is necessary for normal platelet adhesion. In von Willebrand's disease, there is a deficiency of both components of the factor VIII complex, leading to abnormalities in the intrinsic coagulation pathway as well as in platelet function. In classic hemophilia (hemophilia A), only the factor VIII procoagulant molecule is defective, and, therefore, only the intrinsic coagulation pathway is affected. Likewise, Christmas disease (hemophilia B, factor IX deficiency), vitamin K deficiency, and liver disease (deficiency of any coagulation factor except factor VIII) affect only the coagulation cascade.

**3. The answer is A** *[Ch 9 VIII A 1 c].*
Enterococcus, which is a common cause of infective endocarditis in adults, is a very rare cause of endocarditis in children. The reasons for this are unknown. Viridans streptococcus causes many cases of endocarditis in children and adults but has decreased in importance since the introduction of antimicrobial therapy. *Staphylococcus aureus* and *Staphylococcus epidermidis* have become progressively more important causes of infective endocarditis in patients of all ages, especially hospitalized patients.

**4. The answer is C** *[Ch 17 XI A 2].*
A slow virus disease shows a lapse of months to years, rather than a few days, between the initial viral infection and the appearance of the clinical disorder. Subacute sclerosing panencephalitis (SSPE) is an encephalitis caused by the measles virus or a very similar virus. Other slow virus diseases include progressive rubella panencephalitis (PRP), which occurs years later in persons born with congenital rubella, and Kuru (now extinct), which occurred as a result of cannibalism in Samoa.

**5. The answer is C** *[Ch 16 VIII C].*
High-dose estrogen treatment may induce premature epiphyseal fusion and a reduction of final adult stature. The growth-suppressing effects of corticosteroids are accompanied by severe side effects. Thyroid hormone promotes linear growth in prepubertal children. Gonadotropin-releasing hormone (Gn-RH) agonists will initially stimulate gonadotropin release. However, continued administration will actually suppress gonadotropin, making Gn-RH agonists useful in treating precocious puberty. Progesterone has no role in accelerating skeletal maturation.

**6. The answer is A** *[Ch 14 V B 1 a].*
A child with an absolute neutrophil count (ANC) of 100/mm³ is severely neutropenic and is at risk of death from overwhelming septicemia. Since most signs of infection (e.g., pulmonary infiltration, pyuria) depend on the presence of neutrophils, serious infection may be present in such a patient without producing characteristic physical, radiologic, or laboratory findings. Thus, broad-spectrum intravenous antibiotics (to treat a variety of possible infections) must be started promptly after cultures are obtained. Deferring such treatment until culture results are available may result in overwhelming septicemia and death. Granulocyte transfusions usually are not beneficial in these patients because of the short survival time of the cells in the bloodstream (the plasma half-life is approximately 7 hours). Iron and vitamin $B_{12}$ are treatments for different types of anemia and are of no therapeutic value in neutropenia.

**7. The answer is E** *[Ch 1 V F 4 a].*
Physiologic jaundice in term newborns is characterized by the appearance of clinical jaundice after 24 hours, an increase in bilirubin concentration of less than 5 mg/dl/day, total serum bilirubin concentrations of less than 13 mg/dl, direct serum bilirubin levels of less than 1.5–2 mg/dl, and the resolution of jaundice by the age of 1 week. Jaundice related to breast-feeding is termed breast-feeding jaundice, which typically responds to temporary discontinuation of breast-feeding.

**8. The answer is B** *[Ch 10 VIII E 3 c].*
Hirschsprung's disease results from a failure of ganglion cell precursors to complete their migration into the distal bowel. The junction between normal proximal bowel and abnormal distal bowel is most frequently in the rectosigmoid. The usual diagnostic tests include barium enema, rectal manometry, and rectal biopsy. The barium enema may demonstrate a change in bowel caliber between the dilated normal

colon and the contracted aganglionic colon. Rectal manometry fails to demonstrate the normal relaxation to the internal sphincter on balloon distension of the rectum. If a suction rectal biopsy shows ganglion cells, Hirschsprung's disease is ruled out. If none are seen, a full-thickness biopsy is indicated. Surgery remains the only acceptable therapy for Hirschsprung's disease.

### 9. The answer is C *[Ch 9 IV A 4–5]*.
This infant has bacterial meningitis, a serious, common infection in infants and children. Early, nonspecific signs include fever and irritability. Examination of the cerebrospinal fluid (CSF) typically reveals an increased white cell count, an increased protein level, and a decreased glucose level. Gram stain and culture often are positive for bacteria. In infants and children, the most common causes of bacterial meningitis are *Hemophilus influenzae* type b, *Streptococcus pneumoniae,* and *Neisseria meningitidis.* Antibiotic therapy must be directed at the common causative organisms and, therefore, may be cefotaxime, ceftriaxone, or ampicillin and chloramphenicol.

### 10. The answer is D *[Ch 2 VI C]*.
The cardinal rule in foreign body aspiration is if a child is alert and has a spontaneous cough, no attempt to dislodge the presumed foreign body should be made initially. Rapid and careful assessment of the patient's status, including vital signs, is mandatory. Chest or neck x-rays may be useful in this case but only after assessment and initial observation. Insertion of the fingers into the mouth to remove a foreign body is not recommended, since it may lodge the object more firmly in the airway. The Heimlich maneuver, which is preferred over back blows and chest thrusts in children who are older than 1 year, should not be employed as a first step in a conscious, breathing patient.

### 11. The answer is E *[Ch 4 IV A 1 k, B 2]*.
*Trichomonas vaginalis* is a flagellate protozoa that is easily identified in a fresh sample of vaginal discharge because of its characteristic motility. If the vaginal discharge sample sits too long before being examined under a microscope, the protozoa will die and look like slightly enlarged white cells. *Phthirus pubis* (crab lice) can cause significant pubic itching but not a vaginal discharge. The other organisms (*Candida albicans, Gardnerella vaginalis, Neisseria gonorrhoeae*) are either yeast or bacteria, which are not diagnosed by their motility but by their structure or by culture.

### 12. The answer is A *[Ch 7 III B 3 e]*.
Mucopolysaccharidoses are a group of disorders caused by an inability to catabolize the molecules that make up intracellular substance. Therefore, mucopolysaccharides accumulate in skin (causing coarse features), internal organs (causing hepatosplenomegaly), and the brain (causing progressive intellectual impairment). Disorders of carbohydrate metabolism, amino acid metabolism, and the urea cycle and hereditary fructose intolerance are not associated with storage of metabolites.

### 13. The answer is D *[Ch 9 V H 3 c]*.
Laboratory confirmation of infectious mononucleosis consists of positive serologic findings. Patients with this infection produce antibodies to various specific antigens, including Epstein-Barr viral capsid antigen (VCA), Epstein-Barr nuclear antigen (EBNA), and Epstein-Barr virus–induced early antigen (EA). Antibodies to VCA [initially immunoglobulin M (IgM) followed by IgG] peak in the second or third week of illness and persist for life. Antibodies to EA appear early in the course of the illness and disappear after 2–6 months. Antibodies to EBNA appear 3–6 months after the onset of the infection and probably persist for life. Thus, a patient who had infectious mononucleosis 3 years earlier would be expected to show positive results for VCA-IgM, VCA-IgG, and EBNA. EA should be negative.

### 14. The answer is E *[Ch 1 Table 1-2]*.
A prior severe reaction to a vaccine is a contraindication to repeat administration. Severe reactions may be either local (consisting of marked edema, induration, erythema, and pain) or systemic (including high fever, extreme irritability, and seizures). Low-grade fever and brief fussiness are considered to be mild reactions and are not contraindications to repeat administration. If the child developed a high fever and had a prolonged period of fussiness, administration of the diphtheria and tetanus toxoid vaccine with elimination of the pertussis component would be a reasonable approach at the age of 6 months. Split doses should never be used, as their efficacy is uncertain.

### 15. The answer is E *[Ch 8 V A 4, 5]*.
There is no single clinical or laboratory finding that characterizes rheumatic fever. An elevated antistreptolysin O titer would suggest this diagnosis, but further evaluation would be needed to prove rheumatic fever. Fingers almost never are involved in rheumatic fever, in contrast to digital involvement in

rheumatoid arthritis. An elevated erythrocyte sedimentation rate and anemia are nonspecific findings. The rash of rheumatic fever (erythema marginatum) is not at all like hives (urticaria).

**16. The answer is B** *[Ch 14 VI C 1 c (2)].*
In immune-mediated thrombocytopenia in the newborn, maternal antibody is formed against antigen on the mother's platelets (maternal autoimmune thrombocytopenia) or on the fetus' platelets (isoimmune thrombocytopenia). In maternal autoimmune thrombocytopenia, the mother usually is thrombocytopenic (unless she has been previously splenectomized). Septic infants and those with disseminated intravascular coagulation (DIC) usually appear ill. Infants with congenital infections usually have other abnormal physical findings, including low birth weight, hepatomegaly, splenomegaly, and jaundice. Hemophilia A is a coagulopathy; the platelet count is not affected.

**17. The answer is D** *[Ch 9 V C 3].*
This patient most likely has herpetic gingivostomatitis, the most common type of gingivostomatitis in children. Herpetic gingivostomatitis is characterized by painful, erythematous, edematous, and ulcerative lesions that occur on the buccal mucosa, gums, and, occasionally, the hard palate and tongue. There usually is a fever, which may be quite high. Herpetic gingivostomatitis may be so severe that a child refuses to eat or drink. Although herpangina occurs during the summer and is associated with fever, the oral lesions of herpangina are located in the posterior pharynx. The oral lesions of aphthous stomatitis may appear anywhere on the oral mucosa but are localized as a single shallow ulcer or a small cluster of ulcers and are not associated with fever. Candidal gingivostomatitis can cause widespread oral involvement, as in this child, but the lesions are grayish white, usually are not associated with fever, and are uncommon after 3 months of age. Necrotizing ulcerative gingivitis consists of necrosis and ulceration of the interdental papillae.

**18. The answer is E** *[Ch 4 VI B 2 b (3)].*
Suicide attempts frequently are triggered by a precipitating event, most commonly a conflict with parents. Identifying this event can help in the planning of appropriate support for the adolescent. At the same time, there should be an investigation into the adolescent's background history, which usually is filled with other episodes of stress or depression that can contribute to the development of suicidal ideation.

**19. The answer is B** *[Ch 15 II A 5 a (2)].*
Prompt treatment of the febrile, neutropenic patient with acute nonlymphocytic leukemia (ANLL) is essential and lifesaving. Appropriate cultures should be obtained to identify the responsible microorganism, but extensive evaluation in lieu of treatment places the patient in jeopardy of overwhelming sepsis. Since fever most likely is due to infection rather than leukemia, institution of antibiotic therapy takes precedence over antileukemic therapy, which can begin once antibiotic treatment has commenced. Granulocyte transfusions are not indicated at this point but may be considered if the patient's infection does not respond to antibiotics. Vigorous antipyretic therapy should certainly not be the initial approach. Should antipyretics be needed subsequently for comfort, aspirin, which interferes with platelet function, must be specifically avoided in the patient who is potentially thrombocytopenic as well as neutropenic.

**20. The answer is B** *[Ch 9 VII F 1–2].*
The most likely diagnosis in this 12-year-old boy is scarlet fever. Scarlet fever is an acute illness characterized by fever, an erythematous rash, and—in most cases—pharyngitis. Scarlet fever is caused by infection with group A streptococcal strains that produce erythrogenic toxin. Although the disease most often is associated with pharyngeal infection, it may rarely follow streptococcal infection at other sites (e.g., cellulitis, impetigo). The cutaneous manifestations of other streptococcal infections such as erysipelas, rheumatic fever, and impetigo are quite different. Erythema infectiosum is caused by a parvovirus.

**21. The answer is A** *[Ch 16 I A 1 e].*
The development of enuresis in this child not previously enuretic is most likely related to hyperglycemia and resultant increased urine volume due to osmotic diuresis. During the day, this may present as increased frequency of urination (polyuria). At night, in some children, it presents as bedwetting (enuresis). Most children require a split-dose (every 12 hours) of insulin to maintain good glycemic control. Emotional stress of chronic disease is an unlikely cause of enuresis. A urinary tract infection typically presents as other signs and symptoms, such as unexplained fever and abdominal complaints. If an evening dosage of insulin is too high, hypoglycemia (without obvious signs or symptoms) may occur during sleep, resulting in the release of counter-regulatory hormones and an elevated blood sugar in the morning. These events, termed the Somogyi phenomenon, are unlikely to cause enuresis. Hypoglycemia may be associated with early morning lethargy, pallor, sweating, and a seizure. Enuresis is not a feature.

**22. The answer is E** *[Ch 1 VII F 4].*
One or two years after learning to speak, many children develop an intermittent difficulty in producing a smooth flow of speech. Such normal speech disfluency is typically characterized by the repetition of whole words and phrases and, thus, differs from stuttering. Normal disfluency spontaneously resolves between age 2 and 5 years and requires no treatment.

**23. The answer is D** *[Ch 11 IV K 3–4].*
The findings in this 2-day-old infant are characteristic of D-transposition of the great arteries with intact ventricular septum. Pulmonary blood flow is diminished in pulmonary atresia with intact ventricular septum and in pulmonary atresia with ventricular septal defect. Physiologically, the circulation is normal in L-transposition of the great arteries. A heart murmur would be audible in a patient with ventricular septal defect.

**24. The answer is C** *[Ch 4 II B 2].*
Parents need to involve their teenage children in decision making. It is essential for the teen to understand how the parent feels, yet it is also very important for the teen to be responsible for his actions. Grounding the adolescent for a weekend and taking away his phone privileges are not only arbitrary punishments arrived at without discussion, but they also isolate the teen from his peer support group. Peers are very important in mid-adolescence. Not dealing with the behavior will give the teen the message that he does not need to be accountable for his actions at all times.

**25. The answer is C** *[Ch 9 VII E 4 b].*
Immunocompromised children who have not had varicella and who are exposed to the disease are at increased risk for such complications as meningoencephalitis, pneumonia, and hepatitis. The mortality rate in such cases is approximately 20%. Because of this danger, immunocompromised children (e.g., those with leukemia) should receive herpes zoster immune globulin upon exposure (no later than 72 hours) and be closely observed. Those who develop signs of disseminated varicella or herpes zoster should be treated with vidarabine or acyclovir. Because there is evidence of possible bacterial pneumonia, antibiotic therapy also should be provided for this patient.

**26. The answer is B** *[Ch 14 VI C 1 b (1)].*
Idiopathic thrombocytopenic purpura (ITP) may occur after a mild viral illness or an immunization and typically presents abruptly as bleeding of the skin and mucous membranes. Acute lymphocytic leukemia (ALL) and aplastic anemia usually are associated with a more insidious onset than ITP and with abnormalities in the hemoglobin concentration, white blood cell count, and differential count. Hemophilia A, since it is a congenital disorder, usually presents earlier in life and usually the bleeding is in the muscles and joints. Diamond-Blackfan syndrome is a disorder of red blood cell production.

**27. The answer is A** *[Ch 15 I D 7; II B 5 b].*
Meningeal leukemia is common in T cell ALL. Meningeal relapse, which produces increased intracranial pressure, can occur in some patients with T cell ALL even if they have received prophylactic therapy to the central nervous system. Cranial irradiation does not cause increased intracranial pressure. Acute bacterial meningitis can produce this symptom, but it would be rare in a leukemic child. Superior vena cava obstruction from a mediastinal mass is a possible but less common cause of increased intracranial pressure in a patient with T cell ALL and should be associated with facial plethora and signs of airway compromise. Intracranial hemorrhage may produce similar symptoms but would be uncommon, especially in a patient in remission who is unlikely to be severely thrombocytopenic and at risk for intracranial hemorrhage.

**28. The answer is D** *[Ch 4 IV D].*
A hallmark of pelvic inflammatory disease (PID) is significant cervical motion tenderness. Cystitis can occur with dysuria that usually begins at the start of urination and with abdominal pain independent of cervical motion tenderness. Vaginitis may involve some cervical tenderness but not abdominal pain. Appendicitis and inflammatory bowel disease present with abdominal pain but not with cervical motion tenderness.

**29. The answer is C** *[Ch 8 IV D 2].*
Photophobia, a stringy mucous discharge, itching, and lacrimation are symptoms of vernal conjunctivitis, a bilateral conjunctival disease occurring primarily in preadolescent boys. The discharge contains many eosinophils, which are the hallmark of this disease. Both IgE- and IgG-mediated mechanisms probably play a role in the pathogenesis of vernal conjunctivitis. Granulation (cobblestoning) develops in the upper lids in vernal conjunctivitis, and this may result in corneal damage, ulceration, and corneal scarring. Scarring is not seen in patients with allergic conjunctivitis.

**30. The answer is C** *[Ch 9 V B 3].*
The finding of an air-fluid level on sinus x-ray is strong evidence of acute sinusitis in this 6-year-old child. Sinusitis is inflammation of the mucous membrane lining the paranasal sinuses, which may be acute or chronic. Common features in children older than 5 years include fever, facial pain, and headache. The predominant microorganisms in acute sinusitis are *Streptococcus pneumoniae,* unencapsulated strains of *Hemophilus influenzae,* and *Branhamella catarrhalis.*

**31. The answer is B** *[Ch 16 I B 2 b (2)].*
The cyanosis and focal seizures in this infant are due to hypoglycemia related to congenital hypopituitarism. The physical findings of microphallus and lack of light response suggest the syndrome of septo-optic dysplasia, which frequently is associated with deficiency of growth hormone (GH), adrenocorticotropic hormone (ACTH), thyroid-stimulating hormone (TSH), and arginine vasopressin [antidiuretic hormone (ADH)]. Hypoglycemia should be anticipated in infants with these findings. Low cortisol and GH levels during hypoglycemia confirm the diagnosis of congenital hypopituitarism. Hypoglycemia resolves with appropriate hormone replacement. Hypocalcemia is a cause of neonatal seizures but would not explain the other findings. Seizures are not characteristic of congenital hypothyroidism. Congenital heart disease may result in cyanosis but would not explain the other findings. Idiopathic epilepsy is an unlikely etiology for neonatal seizures and would similarly not account for the other findings.

**32. The answer is D** *[Ch 4 III A].*
The menstrual cycle may not be regular during the first 2 years after menarche. Once appropriate pubertal development is documented and no other symptoms are noted, the patient can be reassured that the menstrual irregularity is not abnormal and that the cycles will become more regular with time. A menstrual calendar can facilitate keeping a record of these cycles, and a follow-up visit can be scheduled for 6 months later.

**33. The answer is D** *[Ch 8 IV G 3].*
The diagnosis of food allergy is best made by oral challenge testing with the food in some disguised form, followed by observations for signs and symptoms of allergy. Radioallergosorbent testing (RAST) or intracutaneous skin testing often can be misleading in food allergies. For example, a patient with atopic dermatitis may show multiple positive skin tests, yet food challenge testing may demonstrate that only a few specific foods actually are a problem. Sublingual food testing and cytotoxicity testing are unproven and are of little or no diagnostic value.

**34. The answer is C** *[Ch 14 VI D 3 b].*
This child appears to have a malabsorption syndrome, which would interfere with absorption of fat-soluble vitamins (e.g., vitamin K). Vitamin K deficiency affects coagulation factors involved in both the extrinsic and intrinsic pathways of coagulation; thus, both the partial thromboplastin time (PTT) and prothrombin time (PT) would be prolonged. Fresh frozen plasma or whole blood transfusion would temporarily correct the coagulopathy, but it is not a specific treatment and would unnecessarily expose the child to the risk of blood-borne viruses. Cryoprecipitate is used to treat severe cases of hemophilia A. Hemophilia A is a congenital disorder not associated with malabsorption syndrome; only the PTT is prolonged since factor VIII deficiency only affects the intrinsic pathway. Platelet infusion is not indicated in a child with a normal platelet count and will not treat a deficiency of clotting factors.

**35. The answer is D** *[Ch 15 I D 4 a].*
Fever and signs of suppuration strongly suggest an acute bacterial infection. Hodgkin's disease, ALL, histiocytosis X, and metastatic neuroblastoma may be associated with fever and adenopathy; however, their onset would not be as acute as that seen with acute bacterial lymphadenitis, and suppuration would be an unlikely presenting problem. Furthermore, histiocytosis X in this age-group is much more likely to involve the bones than the lymph nodes, and metastatic neuroblastoma is uncommon in children of this age.

**36. The answer is C** *[Ch 9 IX B 3 a, 4 b].*
This patient most likely has septic arthritis of the hip. Signs and symptoms associated with septic arthritis of the hip often are subtle and may be limited to a limp or refusal to walk. X-ray frequently shows widening of the joint space. Septic arthritis of the hip requires immediate surgical drainage, because the blood supply to the femoral head may be compromised, causing permanent destruction to the joint. Drainage may be performed by needle aspiration or surgical excision. Gram stain and culture of the synovial fluid should be obtained and appropriate antibiotic therapy begun.

**37. The answer is E** *[Ch 8 IV F 2 a].*
The principal therapeutic modality in the management of urticaria and angioedema is oral administration of an antihistamine. It may be necessary to change from one antihistamine to another to optimize therapy. Corticosteroids should only be used in patients with severe, unrelenting urticaria or angioedema. Neither β-adrenergic blocking agents nor atropine is indicated. In fact, β blockers are contraindicated since they may promote the release of mediators from mast cells by decreasing intracellular levels of cyclic adenosine 3′,5′-monophosphate (cAMP).

**38. The answer is B** *[Ch 14 III D 2 a].*
Diamond-Blackfan syndrome is hypoproliferative macrocytic anemia [i.e., anemia characterized by a high mean corpuscular volume (MCV)], which presents early in life. Fanconi's anemia, which also may be macrocytic and hypoproliferative, usually does not present in the first year of life and usually is associated with neutropenia, thrombocytopenia, or both. Autoimmune hemolytic anemia generally is associated with an elevated reticulocyte count. Sickle cell anemia generally does not produce severe anemia at this early an age.

**39. The answer is B** *[Ch 17 III D 2].*
The common causes of hydrocephalus in infants are intraventricular hemorrhage, infection, and congenital malformations (e.g., aqueductal stenosis, Arnold-Chiari deformity). Brain tumors rarely occur in the first year of life, and, if present at this age, they are most likely to be supratentorial. When tumors occur infratentorially, hydrocephalus may be part of the presenting picture.

**40. The answer is E** *[Ch 13 I B 6].*
Renal biopsy is indicated for the diagnosis of renal disease, to help direct therapy and to provide prognostic information. Once the diagnosis of a progressive renal disease is established, repeat biopsies rarely are indicated. Progression of chronic renal failure is best followed by tests such as creatinine clearance and may frequently be predicted by plotting the reciprocal of the serum creatinine against time. All of the other statements in the question correctly describe the features of and indications for renal biopsy.

**41. The answer is B** *[Ch 2 I E 1 d].*
Distal tibial fractures are not unusual at any age and have not specifically been linked to child abuse, although when associated with other fractures or recurrent injuries, the possibility of abuse must be considered. Cigarette burns, scald burns of the buttocks, spiral fracture of the femur, and retinal hemorrhage all are unlikely to occur "accidentally." It is extremely unlikely that a child would burn his buttocks without burning other parts of his body, such as his legs. Retinal hemorrhages occur almost exclusively as part of the "shaken baby syndrome." Cigarette burns, especially when multiple, usually are inflicted. Spiral femur fractures are suspect, especially when the history is not consistent with that injury.

**42. The answer is B** *[Ch 4 VI D 1 a].*
Onset of anorexia nervosa is bimodal, usually occurring in either early adolescence (age 11–14 years) or late adolescence (age 17–20 years). A later onset of the disease is associated with a poor prognosis. The severity of the illness seems to be associated with the degree of body image disturbance (i.e., the greater the disturbance, the more severe the disease), and the greater the body image disturbance, the greater the denial of the illness. Associated endocrine abnormalities exist secondary to starvation. At least two consecutive menstrual cycles are missed in postmenarchal females.

**43. The answer is C** *[Ch 13 X D 3 b; Ch 16 VII A, B].*
Chronic renal failure results in phosphorus retention and hyperphosphatemia. Hyperparathyroidism is associated with an increase in serum calcium and a decrease in serum phosphorus secondary to the effects of increased parathyroid hormone (PTH) levels (i.e., increased mobilization of calcium and phosphorus from bone and decreased renal tubular reabsorption of phosphorus). Vitamin D–dependent rickets causes secondary hyperparathyroidism, with similar effects on the renal handling of phosphorus. Rickets of prematurity is thought to be caused by inadequate mineral (calcium and phosphorus) in the diet for adequate skeletal mineralization. In the face of a low serum phosphorus, there is renal conservation of phosphorus.

**44. The answer is D** *[Ch 12 IV C].*
Mental retardation is not associated with cystic fibrosis. In fact, most children with cystic fibrosis are of above-average intelligence. Failure to thrive, cor pulmonale, nasal polyposis, digital clubbing, and hemoptysis all are frequent complications of cystic fibrosis.

**45. The answer is D** *[Ch 17 V A 2 c (3) (b)].*
Absence seizures (also called petit mal) are a type of generalized seizure. These frequent, brief lapses of

consciousness may be mistaken for absentmindedness by parents and teachers. Epileptic seizures are presumed to be caused by an abnormal firing of cerebral neurons. The site of the discharging neurons in the brain determines the nature of the seizure—generalized or localized (partial), sensory or motor. The spread of these abnormal discharges from their origin to neighboring neurons is clearly evident in jacksonian seizures. These focal motor seizures typically begin in one hand or foot and "march" up the extremity. The aura that initiates grand mal convulsions in some patients seems to be the focal manifestation of the initial abnormal discharge, which then spreads to cause a generalized convulsion. Depending on the site of the initial firing, the aura can be sensory or motor.

**46. The answer is B** *[Ch 5 V A 1 b (3), 2 f].*
The clinical signs of hyaline membrane disease reflect the pathophysiology that leads to poor lung compliance and hypoxia, namely surfactant deficiency. The chest x-ray reflects diffuse microatelectasis. Therapy includes oxygen to correct hypoxia and positive pressure ventilation to open collapsed alveoli. Preeclampsia and prolonged rupture of the fetal membranes, as well as maternal steroid administration, will accelerate fetal lung maturation. Preterm infants from such affected pregnancies have a decreased incidence of hyaline membrane disease. The disease worsens for the first 48–72 hours and then slowly improves over the following few days.

**47. The answer is A** *[Ch 13 III B 4 c].*
In nephrotic syndrome, the intravascular volume is decreased because the acutely lowered oncotic pressure causes movement of water to the interstitial space. Therefore, aggressive use of either diuretic agents or fluid restriction is not sensible and is potentially dangerous. Salt restriction, on the other hand, does help to limit the severity of edema. In the acute phase, the lower the serum protein concentration, the greater the amount of edema, although there are other variables, such as salt intake, which modify it. The edematous child is at an increased risk for infections, in part because the massive urinary loss of serum proteins includes immunoglobulins and other immunoregulatory proteins and also because edema fluid is an excellent culture medium and impairs white blood cell chemotaxis.

**48. The answer is A** *[Ch 6 IV B 2].*
Hypovolemic shock is the result of decreased circulating volume. The body attempts to maintain blood pressure and perfusion of vital organs by raising systemic vascular resistance, decreasing urine output, and increasing heart rate and contractility. This is accomplished by secretion of ADH, aldosterone, renin, angiotensin, and catecholamines. Because young children can raise their systemic vascular resistance and heart rate to a very high degree, blood pressure does not fall until quite late, after 40% of circulating volume has been lost. In contrast, cardiac output falls after loss of only 15%–20% of circulating volume. The principal mode of therapy is restoration of circulating volume by infusion of isotonic crystalloid or colloid. Inotropic infusion is required only for patients who have sustained myocardial damage secondary to prolonged hypoperfusion.

**49. The answer is A** *[Ch 17 II B].*
Infection, medication overdose, or a convulsion can produce a coma over a very short period of time, usually less than 6 hours. Brain tumors develop slowly over weeks or months. The child with a brain tumor might develop delirium but will not go into a coma acutely.

**50. The answer is E** *[Ch 5 V F 2 d].*
Sepsis in the newborn is associated with such signs and symptoms as abnormal white blood cell count, unstable body temperature, respiratory distress, apnea, and lethargy. Neutropenia suggests that the infection is overwhelming and that neutrophils are being consumed at a high rate. This often is associated with depletion of the neutrophil storage pool in the bone marrow and a high mortality rate. Apnea and respiratory distress are associated with viral as well as bacterial infections. Group B β-hemolytic streptococcus is the most common bacterial cause of unexplained respiratory distress in the newborn. As in older children, lethargy is a nonspecific but important symptom of infection in the newborn. Although anemia may be associated with infection, it is not a feature of early neonatal sepsis.

**51. The answer is B** *[Ch 13 I B 5 b, d].*
Intravenous pyelography (IVP) is the standard anatomic renal imaging procedure; in comparison, radionuclide renal scanning offers relatively poor structural delineation. Although IVP permits good visualization of the kidneys and upper urinary tract, this diagnostic test is not without risks. The intravenous injection of contrast material may cause allergic reactions and acute renal failure. Renal failure is more likely to occur in children with preexisting renal disease or with intravascular volume depletion and in those who are receiving potentially nephrotoxic agents (e.g., aminoglycoside antibiotics). In children

with a markedly diminished glomerular filtration rate (GFR), the contrast material may not be excreted rapidly enough to allow visualization of the kidneys. A standard IVP exposes the child to approximately 10 times the gonadal radiation dose of a radionuclide renal scan. Visualization of renal tissue on IVP requires the presence of reasonably normal GFR and tubular concentrating capacity. Thus, a nonfunctioning kidney will not be seen in IVP. Because of the diminished GFR and concentrating capacity in the newborn kidney, IVP is of limited value in this age-group.

**52. The answer is A** *[Ch 10 IX E].*
Hepatitis A has not been associated with chronic hepatitis in children. Hepatitis B, however, is a cause of chronic persistent or chronic active hepatitis or cirrhosis and should be sought in any adolescent with chronic liver disease. An ophthalmologic exam using a slit lamp to look for Kayser-Fleischer rings may provide the first clue to the diagnosis of Wilson's disease. Antinuclear and antismooth muscle antibodies are commonly found in autoimmune chronic active hepatitis in adolescent and young adult females.

**53. The answer is D** *[Ch 5 IV A 1, B 2].*
During the first week of life, the extracellular water space contracts, causing a large decrease in body water. The resulting weight loss, as a percentage of birth weight, decreases with the increasing gestational age of the newborn. Prematurely born infants have a thin epithelium, which results in increased transdermal water loss. Phototherapy for hyperbilirubinemia increases insensible water loss (water loss through evaporation); this may lead to a severe decrease in body water and weight if fluids are not replaced properly. Newborns do not feed vigorously during the first few days of life; therefore, caloric intake is not adequate to support growth (weight gain). Basal metabolism does not decrease during this time; in fact, caloric requirements increase due to such factors as cold stress and increased activity.

**54. The answer is C** *[Ch 17 IV B 2].*
Rarely is blindness a complication of cerebral palsy. However, strabismus occurs in approximately 40% of patients with cerebral palsy, mental retardation or learning disabilities in approximately 40%–50%, behavior problems in at least 20%, and epilepsy in approximately 30%.

**55. The answer is C** *[Ch 13 I B 2 a (2)].*
The creatinine clearance is a measure of glomerular function, not renal tubular function. Creatinine is an ideal substance for estimating GFR since it is produced at a constant rate, is freely filtered by the kidney, is not metabolized, is not eliminated elsewhere, is easily measured, and is not reabsorbed by the tubules. There is a small amount of tubular secretion of creatinine but not enough to invalidate creatinine clearance as a test of glomerular function.

The renal response to an acid load is to acidify the urine through the tubular secretion of hydrogen ion, which is then excreted as titratable acid and ammonium. The urine pH should be less than 5.4 in response to an acid load that would otherwise cause systemic acidosis.

The kidney's ability to dilute the urine is a tubular function that depends on the reabsorption of solute in excess of water. This occurs in the ascending loop and the cortical diluting segment of the distal nephron. A severely depressed GFR will slow the kidney's ability to excrete a water load but will not prevent it.

The renal handling of amino acids includes filtration by the glomerulus and almost total reabsorption by the proximal tubules. Thus, the presence of aminoaciduria suggests proximal tubular dysfunction.

Phosphate is filtered by the glomerulus and normally is reabsorbed almost completely (> 85%) by the tubules. Therefore, excessive phosphaturia usually reflects tubular dysfunction, although such factors as PTH, vitamin D, and dietary phosphate play a role in renal phosphate handling.

**56. The answer is D** *[Ch 5 II B 3].*
The effects of perinatal asphyxia may reflect multiorgan involvement, including hypoxic cardiomyopathy, acute tubular necrosis, necrotizing enterocolitis, seizures, intracranial hemorrhage, and intravascular coagulopathy. Prenatal hemolytic anemia may contribute to the process of birth asphyxia but is not a result, sign, or symptom of birth asphyxia.

**57. The answer is C** *[Ch 17 I B; Table 1-4].*
The superficial abdominal reflex, characterized by muscular contraction with stroking of the skin, may be demonstrated at any age and is not a developmental reflex. The other reflexes are developmental. The Moro, tonic neck, and rooting reflexes are present at birth; the parachute reflex does not develop until about age 10 months.

**58. The answer is D** *[Ch 13 II B 4].*
The kidney of a newborn is limited in most renal functions. However, it is capable of maximally diluting

the urine. On the other hand, renal concentrating and acidifying mechanisms are not fully developed at birth. Sodium handling also is impaired at birth with respect to both excreting a sodium load and conserving it when sodium-deprived. The normal GFR in the newborn is approximately 5 ml/min and, therefore, limits the speed with which an exogenously administered water load can be excreted.

**59. The answer is A** *[Ch 5 V A 2 d].*
In diaphragmatic hernia, the defect almost always is on the left, allowing the abdominal contents (which may include—in addition to the small bowel—the stomach and parts of the liver and spleen) to enter the chest. This results in compression of the left lung and shift of the mediastinal structures. In moderate and severe situations, the shift of the mediastinal structures causes compression and hypoplasia of the contralateral lung as well. Respiratory distress, cyanosis, and dyspnea are noted in the affected newborn shortly after birth. For unknown reasons, pulmonary hypertension almost always is present. This causes right-to-left shunting of blood and contributes to the infant's hypoxia. The infant should be ventilated through an endotracheal tube as bag-mask ventilation results in distension of the bowels with air and further compression of the lungs. A nasogastric tube should be inserted to remove air from the gastrointestinal tract.

**60. The answer is C** *[Ch 10 IV].*
When a patient presents with signs of significant gastrointestinal blood loss, the first priority is to stabilize the patient. Although upper endoscopy may help to direct therapy by documenting a specific lesion, it is contraindicated until the patient is stabilized. All vital signs should be checked and a brief physical examination performed. A large-bore intravenous catheter should be inserted to obtain blood for testing and to allow fluid resuscitation. While these procedures are being performed, further medical history should be obtained. It is particularly important to determine whether there is a previous history of gastrointestinal bleeding, a bleeding tendency, underlying liver disease or other chronic illness, recent ingestion of drugs known to induce bleeding (e.g., aspirin), or a family history of gastrointestinal bleeding. A nasogastric tube should be inserted to determine whether there is an upper gastrointestinal tract source of bleeding and, if so, to assess the magnitude of blood loss.

**61. The answer is D** *[Ch 4 VII F].*
Amphetamines are ingested and not snorted and, hence, do not cause irritation of the nasal mucosa. Amphetamines can lead to psychosis and, when the effects subside, can cause depression. Stimulants can also result in significant cardiovascular impairments, such as arrhythmias and hypertension.

**62. The answer is B** *[Ch 16 V A 1 a (2)].*
All of the conditions noted in the question, except 21-hydroxylase deficiency, may present as short stature and delayed puberty. 21-Hydroxylase deficiency may present as signs of virilization with accelerated growth in childhood secondary to excessive adrenal androgens. Girls with Turner syndrome may not have the physical stigmata associated with the syndrome. Likewise, physical findings in acquired hypothyroidism may be quite subtle. Although Turner syndrome and hypothyroidism should be considered, the most likely diagnosis is constitutional delay of growth and development. A history of weight loss, compulsive exercise, and abnormal eating behavior might indicate anorexia nervosa.

**63. The answer is E** *[Ch 3 VI C 1; Ch 10 VII A 3 a (2)].*
A Meckel's diverticulum is associated with pain only on rare occasions. If the diverticulum acts as a lead point in an intussusception, acute, severe pain is observed. Rarely, diverticulitis may occur and may also lead to abdominal pain. Lactose intolerance, peptic ulcer disease, irritable bowel syndrome, and chronic pancreatitis all may be associated with chronic postprandial abdominal pain.

**64. The answer is D** *[Ch 4 II D].*
A Pap smear is not necessary unless the teen is sexually active. Laboratory studies such as a hemoglobin, urinalysis, skin test for tuberculosis, and rubella titers should be performed on an initial visit as a screening. Repeat physical examination need only include a recheck of the hematocrit and other studies as indicated by presenting symptoms.

**65. The answer is D** *[Ch 11 VI B 2 e].*
In hypertrophic cardiomyopathy, therapy is aimed at preventing fatal arrhythmias and at decreasing stiffness of the left ventricle with negative inotropic medications (e.g., calcium channel blockers, β-adrenergic blockers). Since systolic function is well preserved, an inotropic agent such as digoxin may be harmful, since it may increase outflow obstruction. Because of the risk of sudden death with exertion, these patients should be excluded from participating in competitive sports.

**66. The answer is B** *[Ch 5 VI C, D].*
Physician participation in the decision-making process is appropriate. To make a decision, the parents must have accurate and timely information. So, the appropriate actions are to assess the situation, keep the parents informed, make recommendations regarding treatment, and involve the parents in decisions. If the relative costs and benefits of the situation are not entirely clear or if the parents do not agree with the proposed treatment, the hospital's ethics committee should be consulted. Proper support for the parents of a dying infant includes discussing the issue with both parents at the same time and speaking openly about the possibility of the infant's death.

**67. The answer is D** *[Ch 7 I F 1; VI D 1].*
Mental retardation can be associated with chromosome abnormalities, including the fragile X syndrome, metabolic disorders, and heritable syndromes. Serum α-fetoprotein (AFP) testing is used only for prenatal screening or screening for cancer.

**68. The answer is C** *[Ch 10 V B 2 b].*
It is important not to confuse lactose malabsorption and cow's milk protein sensitivity. Lactose malabsorption itself never is associated with passage of bloody stools; however, cow's milk protein intolerance may result in bloody stools associated with colonic injury. Any infant with vomiting and bloody stools should be evaluated for intestinal ischemia (e.g., volvulus), bacterial infection, and possible allergic bowel disease. Although eosinophilia may accompany allergic enterocolitis, it is not always present; occasionally, intestinal tissue may reveal eosinophilic infiltration. A careful diet history should be obtained, and protein (from cow's milk or soy) should be restricted.

**69. The answer is B** *[Ch 14 VI D 1 b].*
The clinical and laboratory findings in this infant suggest an intracranial bleed associated with a severe coagulopathy. Hemophilia A is associated only with factor VIII deficiency and an abnormal PTT and, thus, is not a likely cause of the coagulopathy in this patient. This infant has an abnormal PT and PTT, suggesting deficiency in clotting factors of both the intrinsic and extrinsic systems. The clotting factor deficiency may be the result of increased consumption (e.g., due to sepsis) or decreased production (e.g., due to unavailability of vitamin K or to liver failure). Infants with cystic fibrosis may have severe fat malabsorption leading to malnutrition and deficiency of fat-soluble vitamins (A, D, E, K). Child abuse should be suspected in any infant with bruising or poor nutrition.

**70. The answer is A** *[Ch 12 I C 2 c (3); VII D].*
A bronchogenic cyst usually is found in the mediastinum and would not produce signs of stridor. Upper airway obstruction at the level of the larynx causes inspiratory stridor and may cause a pectus excavatum chest deformity. Laryngomalacia is the most common cause of stridor in infancy and usually resolves by age 12 months. Direct examination of the larynx and trachea by flexible bronchoscopy can determine if stridor is caused by other disorders of the larynx, such as vocal cord paralysis, laryngeal web, or subglottic hemangioma.

**71. The answer is D** *[Ch 7 IV C 2; Ch 16 VI B 1 b (2) (a)].*
Boys with Klinefelter syndrome usually are of average or tall stature. Puberty begins at the usual age and secondary sex characteristics are acquired. However, gynecomastia frequently is present, and the testes are small and firm. Adolescents with chronic disease (e.g., inflammatory bowel disease, chronic renal failure) may present with few outward signs except for slow growth and delayed puberty. Idiopathic constitutional delay of growth is the most common cause of this clinical picture. Frequently, there is a family history of a similar growth pattern in older siblings or parents. It may be difficult to distinguish between constitutional delay of puberty and hypogonadotropic hypogonadism, unless there are associated features, such as anosmia (Kallmann syndrome). Prolactinoma is a rare cause of delayed or arrested puberty and, in the male, may produce few other symptoms until the tumor size causes visual or other neurologic complaints.

**72. The answer is C** *[Ch 10 IX E 1 c, 2 c].*
The history, clinical features, and elevated serum aminotransferase levels in this patient suggest chronic liver disease. To support this diagnosis, the physical examination should reveal findings consistent with cirrhosis (i.e., physical evidence of portal hypertension), such as splenomegaly, ascites, and gastrointestinal blood loss due to varices (esophageal, gastric, or colonic). Digital clubbing and telangiectasias of the face, trunk, and extremities also are seen in the setting of cirrhosis. These findings are thought to be related to cutaneous vascular anomalies, including arteriovenous communication and capillary proliferation. Lymphadenopathy is not a specific finding for chronic liver disease.

**73. The answer is D** *[Ch 7 I D 2, 3; VI C 2].*
When several dysmorphic, functional, and structural abnormalities are seen together, they often form a syndrome (a recognizable pattern of malformations). Syndromes may be sporadic or may be caused by a single gene or chromosome abnormality. Teratogenic agents also can cause a recognizable pattern of anomalies. All of these possibilities should be investigated through the use of family history analysis and chromosome analysis. With very few exceptions, syndromes of dysmorphic features and malformations are not associated with inborn errors of metabolism (although developmental delay, alone, can be seen in such disorders).

**74. The answer is B** *[Ch 10 IX C 1].*
Hepatitis B surface antigen (HBsAg) is positive in virtually all patients with acute viral hepatitis B if the serum sample is obtained early in the course of the illness. The antibody to heptatitis B core antigen (HBcAg) is the first antibody formed in uncomplicated acute hepatitis B and, in fact, may be the only marker of infection if HBsAg has already disappeared. The presence of IgM anti-HBcAg suggests active infection, while the IgG antibody indicates past infection. The same advantage is gained by fractionating hepatitis A antibodies, with hepatitis A antibodies of the IgM class indicating acute hepatitis A and those of the IgG class indicating past infection.

**75. The answer is D** *[Ch 16 IV A 1 b; V A 3 b].*
Idiopathic GH deficiency accounts for most cases of GH deficiency. Typical features include short stature, slow growth velocity (< 5 cm/yr in older children), mild truncal adiposity, and delayed skeletal maturation. Body proportions are normal, in contrast to the immature proportions seen in congenital hypothyroidism. Hypertension is not associated with idiopathic GH deficiency, although it is a common feature of Cushing syndrome, another cause of slow growth during childhood.

**76. The answer is A** *[Ch 4 VI E 1].*
Rupture of the hymen, vaginal penetration, or ejaculation is not necessary for the diagnosis of rape to be made; it is sufficient if there was contact of the male genitalia with the labia majora. For the evaluation of rape to be accurate, the vaginal environment should not have changed by bathing or douching since the rape. Women who are raped may also acquire sexually transmitted disease or become pregnant after the event.

**77. The answer is A** *[Ch 10 III B].*
Increasing evidence links *Helicobacter pylori* with gastritis in both children and adults. The organism generally is identified by careful examination and, occasionally, by culture of gastric biopsy specimens. Stool cultures are not helpful in the diagnosis, since the inflammatory process usually is limited to the stomach and duodenum. Therapy with $H_2$-blockers, bismuth suspensions, and antibiotics usually is necessary.

**78–80. The answers are: 78-B** *[Ch 12 III E; Ch 13 VIII D 1],* **79-D** *[Ch 12 III G],* **80-A** *[Ch 13 VIII C 1].*
Patients with acute asthma initially hyperventilate, lowering their carbon dioxide tension ($P_{CO_2}$) and causing an acute respiratory alkalosis. Characteristic arterial blood findings in respiratory alkalosis include pH exceeding 7.45 and $P_{CO_2}$ less than 35 mm Hg. The initial blood gas analysis of patients with acute asthma also commonly shows mild hypoxemia.

The treatment of choice for acute wheezing in asthmatic children is inhaled $\beta_2$-adrenergic bronchodilator therapy. Oxygen also should be provided, since most patients are hypoxemic due to ventilation: perfusion mismatching. Frequent clinical reassessment is necessary; peak expiratory flow measurements are helpful to document the severity of airway obstruction, and inhaled bronchodilator treatments can be given up to 3 times every 20 minutes. Chest physical therapy may cause increased bronchospasm in patients with acute asthma and, thus, would not be indicated in the acute treatment of such patients.

With increased severity of airway obstruction, asthma patients may develop acute respiratory acidosis subsequent to hypoventilation. Characteristic arterial blood findings in respiratory acidosis include pH less than 7.35 and $P_{CO_2}$ exceeding 45 mm Hg. If a patient with severe acute asthma has significant hypoxemia, metabolic acidosis (secondary to lactic acid production from anaerobic metabolism) may complicate the respiratory acidosis. Intubation and mechanical ventilation may be necessary in severe acute asthma.

**81–83. The answers are: 81-B** *[Ch 1 V D 3–6],* **82-E** *[Ch 1 V B 6],* **83-D** *[Ch 1 V C].*
While the timing of acquiring skills varies widely among normal infants, by 4 months of age, many infants can roll over, sit with support, grasp objects and place them in their mouth, smile responsively, and squeal.

Although several developmental issues exist in early infancy (e.g., synchrony, attachment, temperament, motor skills), the struggle for autonomy and independence typically does not emerge until the second year of life. During early infancy, synchrony is characterized by the reciprocal nature of parent-infant interaction and the evolution of mutual awareness and expectations. By age 2–3 months, attachment becomes the main affective agenda. The infant's behavioral style becomes increasingly evident. By age 4–6 months, the infant's increasing mobility becomes evident.

Physical examination during early infancy should include special emphasis on the infant's general appearance, skin, head and neck, chest, abdomen, genitalia, hips, and nervous system. Examination of the back for scoliosis does not assume special significance until school-age years.

Cardiac auscultation during early infancy may reveal functional murmurs or murmurs of various disorders. Examination of the hips may reveal congenital dislocation, even if the newborn examination was normal. Common skin disorders include infantile atopic dermatitis or seborrheic dermatitis. The anterior fontanelle is palpable for 1–2 years, whereas the posterior fontanelle usually closes by the second month of life.

### 84–85. The answers are: 84-D, 85-A *[Ch 13 IV G]*.
This child's clinical presentation is very characteristic of Henoch-Schönlein purpura. Kawasaki disease usually is associated with fever and a different rash. A child with meningococcemia would appear sicker, and the rash would be rapidly progressive and diffuse. The rash of juvenile rheumatoid arthritis also is diffuse and not purpuric or petechial. Hemolytic-uremic syndrome usually is not associated with rash or joint pain.

Henoch-Schönlein purpura often is associated with renal involvement, which most commonly is mild with urine abnormalities (hematuria, proteinuria) and normal renal function. Elevated blood pressure may occur with or without nephritis. IgA is found in the kidney and in other affected tissues. Henoch-Schönlein purpura is not associated with complement activation and depletion.

### 86–88. The answers are: 86-D *[Ch 6 VI B, C]*, 87-C *[Ch 6 V A 4]*, 88-B *[Ch 6 V B 1–4]*.
Initial priorities in the treatment of the severely traumatized patient include assurance of airway, breathing, and circulatory sufficiency. The cervical spine should be protected until it has been certified as uninjured. Hypotension is treated by isotonic crystalloid, colloid, or blood infusions. While this child may benefit from the diagnostic power of head and abdominal computed tomography (CT) scans, these should not be performed until hypoxia and hypotension have been treated.

Ventriculostomy is unlikely to be helpful in controlling intracranial pressure, because the ventricles are quite small due to compression by the interstitial fluid and compensatory shunting of CSF into the spinal canal. Mannitol, hyperventilation, and pentobarbital may be beneficial in controlling increased intracranial pressure in this setting. Mild dehydration from fluid restriction may contribute to vasoconstriction of the cerebral vasculature, which will help to control cerebral blood flow in the absence of autoregulation.

Brain death is complete and irreversible failure of cortical and brain stem function. In children older than age 1 year, with a known etiology for their neurologic status, brain death may be diagnosed on physical findings alone. The Glasgow coma score is a prognostic score and does not assess cranial nerve functions (e.g., pupillary response). Four-vessel angiography is highly sensitive but very invasive; it is not required for the determination of brain death. Decerebrate posturing indicates some function, although abnormal, of the brain stem. Electroencephalogram (EEG) and physical examinations for determination of brain death are not reliable in the presence of coma-producing levels of barbiturates.

### 89–90. The answers are: 89-D *[Ch 3 VIII D]*, 90-C *[Ch 3 VIII E]*.
A CT scan is necessary only if the child's history or physical examination suggests the possibility of head injury. Since the child is alert and neurologic examination is normal, there is no indication of such injury. The past medical history is important in determining whether there have been other suspicious injuries. The physical examination is necessary to document the extent of injuries. Coagulation studies rule out a coagulopathy as an explanation for the child's bruises. A developmentally appropriate, nonthreatening discussion with the child about the bruises is indicated also.

Children in whom abuse is suspected should be hospitalized, and the appropriate child protective agency must be notified. If the child is sent home, there is the distinct possibility that the family will not return for follow-up, and there is a strong risk of repeated injury to the child. If the child is left unsupervised in the emergency ward, the family may become anxious and leave, taking the child with them against medical advice.

### 91–93. The answers are: 91-C *[Ch 15 V B 1 a, 2 b]*, 92-D *[Ch 15 II D 1 a]*, 93-C *[Ch 15 V B 1 d]*.
This is a typical presentation of stage IV neuroblastoma, with the primary tumor arising from the right adrenal medulla and metastasizing to bone marrow, cortical bone, and the retro-orbital tissues. Histio-

cytosis X may have a somewhat similar presentation and involve multiple bones, but it generally involves one rather than both orbits; the right flank mass and tumor clumps in the marrow of this patient also are not characteristic of histiocytosis X. Rhabdomyosarcoma may arise in the orbit but usually is unilateral; the tumor also rarely is associated with systemic metastases at initial diagnosis. Wilms' tumor would produce a right renal rather than suprarenal mass and would metastasize to the lungs rather than to bone and bone marrow. Lymphoblastic lymphoma usually arises in the anterior mediastinum or peripheral nodes. Even if it were to present with widespread dissemination, abdominal rather than thoracic disease would be unusual and lymphoblasts rather than tumor clumps would be seen in the marrow.

The Philadelphia chromosome contains translocation (9;22) and is seen in adult chronic myelogenous leukemia (CML), not neuroblastoma. Increased urinary excretion of catecholamine metabolites (e.g., vanillylmandelic acid) is common in neuroblastoma. In many cases of neuroblastoma, the cells demonstrate amplification of the c-*myc* oncogene and elevated levels of ferritin are detected in serum. The presence of either or both of these findings often worsens the prognosis for neuroblastoma patients. Patients with marrow metastases from neuroblastoma often have leukoerythroblastic changes demonstrable on peripheral blood smear.

The development of back pain, inability to walk, and decreased lower extremity strength indicate a medically emergent situation in which the tumor has grown posteriorly through the intervertebral foramina into the epidural space. In this location, the tumor can compress the spinal cord and produce irreversible damage from ischemia to the cord. Prompt evaluation with a magnetic resonance imaging (MRI) or CT scan is needed to detect the tumor in the epidural space. Lumbar puncture would not be useful unless it were combined with myelography to detect the encroachment on the cord. Institution of analgesic therapy or physical therapy would be inappropriate in this situation, as would be serial neurologic examinations. Speed in establishing a diagnosis and in preventing permanent cord damage is critical.

### 94–95. The answers are: 94-C, 95-D [Ch 2 IX E 5].
In cases of asymptomatic lead poisoning, an ethylenediaminetetraacetic acid (CaEDTA) chelation challenge test may help determine the total body burden of lead. Excretion of a significant amount of chelated lead in urine would indicate the need for a complete course of chelation therapy. Most cases of lead poisoning in children are asymptomatic. Current thinking is that chelation should be performed only when clinical symptoms are present, toxic levels of lead are present, or CaEDTA challenge is positive. Elevated lead levels are toxic to the developing neurologic system; therefore, lead toxicity is a problem throughout childhood. Before the child's family is advised to seek new housing, assessment of the home as a source of lead should be performed.

Contrary to its name, the core of a lead pencil is graphite, which is nontoxic. Paint chips, household dust, and backyard soil can be contaminated with lead. Glazed ceramic containers that have been fired at low temperatures, most of which are imported from other countries, also can be contaminated with lead.

### 96–98. The answers are: 96-A [Ch 3 IV B 5; Ch 7 VI C 2], 97-C [Ch 7 I D 3 e; II; VI C 2], 98-B [Ch 7 II D].
The first step in the evaluation of this 18-month-old child should be physical examination for evidence of neurologic problems, dysmorphic features, growth deficiency, microcephaly, macrocephaly, or hearing impairment. Chromosome analysis, hearing evaluation, developmental testing, and CT scan of the head all may be appropriate in the further evaluation of developmental delay, depending on the findings on physical examination and history.

Allergic disorders are unlikely causes of developmental delay, and allergy history would not provide significant clues to the reason for language delay in this child. However, prenatal infections or teratogenic exposures, perinatal anoxia, and family history of mental retardation or speech delay all could explain the language delay in this child. Concomitant delay of motor development would suggest a generalized process.

Diagnostic radiation, such as chest x-ray, falls far below the threshold for teratogenic effect in a fetus. Fetal rubella exposure can cause deafness as well as mental retardation, cataracts, and congenital heart defects. Fragile X syndrome is a common cause of mental retardation in boys; speech and language function usually are affected most by this disorder. Deafness may present as speech delay. Finally, some normal children may begin to speak late, without having hearing loss or mental retardation.

### 99–100. The answers are: 99-A [Ch 1 VII B 8 g; VIII B 5], 100-B [Ch 1 VIII B 5].
At 12 years of age, important developmental issues to consider during anticipatory guidance include autonomy/independence, temperament, peer interaction, and puberty. The concept of gender as fixed and stable emerges around 4–5 years of age and is unlikely to be a major issue at age 12 years for most children.

The drive for autonomy typically is characterized by the child's strong desire to assume increasing responsibility for his own actions and resist parental suggestions and limit setting. A further manifestation of this drive for independence is the transferring of allegiance from the family to a peer group. A relative delay compared to peers in the onset of the physical changes of puberty may cause concern on the part of the child or parents. The consistency of a child's "slow-to-warm-up" temperament or behavioral style should suggest his likely response to a new situation.

During the school-age years, allowing the child to assume increasing responsibility for his actions may lessen family conflict and promote autonomy and positive self-regard. Competing with younger children would be unacceptable, as it would be likely to lead to segregation among peers at a time when allegiance to a peer group is normal and important. Parental attempts to coerce the boy into participation, either directly or indirectly through friends, would likely be met with resistance. Neither the boy's "slow-to-warm-up" temperament nor his stage-related behavior indicates the need for a mental health referral, although pediatric counseling for parents and child is indicated.

**101–102. The answers are: 101-C** *[Ch 13 I B 5 b; VII B 5]*, **102-D** *[Ch 13 IX C]*.
This infant has signs of significant dehydration and should receive prompt parenteral fluid resuscitation. Appropriate bloodwork and cultures also should be performed. Urine electrolytes can be useful in a child with oliguria. It is reasonable to discontinue oral fluids in a severely dehydrated child with diarrhea and to administer maintenance and deficit fluids intravenously. An IVP is not appropriate in the management of this infant. There is no reason to suspect urinary tract obstruction, and injection of radiocontrast agents in a dehydrated patient can precipitate renal failure.

A hemoglobin of 5.6 mg/dl, platelet count of 50,000, and serum creatinine of 1.3 mg/dl suggest that this infant has hemolytic-uremic syndrome. Hemolytic-uremic syndrome most commonly follows a gastrointestinal illness and is associated with hemolytic anemia, thrombocytopenia, and acute renal failure. The degree of anemia and renal insufficiency in this infant (a creatinine of 1.3 mg/dl is 3–4 times what is normal for an 8-month-old child) would not be expected with viral gastroenteritis. Gastrointestinal hemorrhage severe enough to drop the hemoglobin to 5.6 g/dl would have been apparent, and chronic renal disease with an acute superimposed illness would not have such severe anemia or the thrombocytopenia. Examination of the peripheral red cell smear would be helpful and would show a microangiopathic appearance in hemolytic-uremic syndrome. Human immunodeficiency virus (HIV)-associated infection can cause acute or chronic diarrheal illness, but such severe hematologic involvement and renal disease is unlikely to occur in an 8-month-old infant.

**103–104. The answers are: 103-D** *[Ch 6 II C 1 c]*, **104-D** *[Ch 6 II C 2]*.
Cardiopulmonary failure is characterized by agonal respirations and bradycardia. It may arise from respiratory failure or from shock and is quickly followed by cardiac arrest if intervention is not appropriate. Cyanosis is a late and inconstant sign of respiratory failure. The acute onset of respiratory distress (e.g., from foreign body aspiration) may be accompanied by cyanosis.

The first intervention in the patient with cardiopulmonary failure is to provide adequate ventilation. If vital signs improve with bag-mask ventilation or subsequent intubation, respiratory failure was the source of the condition. Transition to a shock state after ventilation implies circulatory compromise as the etiology. Subsequent interventions are guided by the reassessment following ventilation.

**105–106. The answers are: 105-C, 106-B** *[Ch 13 III B]*.
This child appears to have developed steroid dependence (i.e., inability to discontinue steroids) as well as serious side effects of steroid treatment. The use of an alkylating agent is indicated in an attempt to treat the child's nephrotic syndrome effectively without reliance on steroids. Although infections frequently trigger relapses and must be considered, empiric use of antibiotics is not warranted. Cyclosporine does not appear to be capable of inducing long-term remissions. Diuretics do have a role in controlling the edema of chronic nephrotic states, but they do not induce remissions or prevent relapse.

The course of this child's nephrotic syndrome is not unusual for minimal change disease. The normal renal function and urinalysis support this diagnosis. While the other glomerulopathies may occasionally respond to steroids and masquerade as minimal change disease, they occur less frequently and, thus, are less likely to be found on renal biopsy.

**107–111. The answers are: 107-D, 108-C, 109-B, 110-A, 111-E** *[Ch 8 Tables 8-1, 8-2, 8-3, 8-4]*.
Many of the immune deficiency disorders can be diagnosed by a single blood test. For example, Wiskott-Aldrich syndrome is a triad of recurrent infections, eczema, and thrombocytopenia. Examination of the peripheral blood smear will show small and defective platelets that are markedly decreased in number.

DiGeorge anomaly is an embryologic defect of the third and fourth pharyngeal pouches, in which the parathyroid glands and thymus fail to develop. A decreased serum calcium level combined with characteristic facial abnormalities help to make the diagnosis of DiGeorge anomaly.

Patients with Bruton's disease have agammaglobulinemia. Quantitation of serum immunoglobulins will show an absence of IgG, IgA, and IgM.

Patients with leukocyte adhesion deficiency have defective expression of a leukocyte adherence molecule (e.g., CD11, CD18) on their cell surface. Flow cytometry, with specific monoclonal antibodies to these cell surface glycoproteins, can be used to make the diagnosis of this disorder.

Chronic granulomatous disease is a group of disorders characterized by an inability of neutrophils and macrophages to kill organisms after ingesting them. The important laboratory test for the diagnosis of this disorder is the nitroblue tetrazolium dye (NBT) test, in which the dye fails to become reduced (change to purple) during the process of phagocytosis.

**112–113. The answers are: 112-A, 113-D** *[Ch 17 X D 1 a, b (3)].*
Muscular dystrophies are progressive genetic diseases that have similar appearances on muscle biopsy. The specific diagnosis is based on an accurate history and physical examination.

Pseudohypertrophic (Duchenne) muscular dystrophy is an X-linked disease that typically appears at age 2–4 years. The muscle weakness may be difficult to detect on physical examination in children younger than 5 years. However, most affected children are wheelchair-bound by age 12.

Limb-girdle (Leyden-Möbius) muscular dystrophy is a recessive disease that typically becomes clinically apparent in the second decade of life. Muscular weakness involves the pelvic girdle, and the rate of progression is variable. Fascioscapulohumeral (Landouzy-Dejerine) muscular dystrophy may begin in the first decade of life and typically has facial and shoulder girdle weakness. Congenital myotonic muscular dystrophy is characterized by "floppiness" and a typical "fish-mouth" appearance during the neonatal period.

**114–119. The answers are: 114-A** *[Ch 2 II A]*, **115-D** *[Ch 2 IV A 3]*, **116-E** *[Ch 2 VI A]*, **117-C** *[Ch 2 I E 1 d]*, **118-B** *[Ch 2 III]*, **119-A** *[Ch 2 I E 2].*
Children between 6 months and 19 years of age are more likely to die from injuries involving motor vehicles than from any other cause. A reported case of drowning is more likely to result in death than an incident of any other childhood injury. This high mortality to morbidity ratio may be influenced by the many minor incidents of drowning that go unreported. Choking is the most common cause of injury-related death in the first year of life, while burns—most often scald burns to the buttocks and cigarette burns—are the type of injury most frequently associated with child abuse. Falls result in more emergency room visits than any other injuries, and single-passenger automobile accidents often are overlooked as a possible cause of suicide among adolescents.

**120–123. The answers are: 120-C** *[Ch 11 IV E 2 a (2)]*, **121-B** *[Ch 11 IV G 2]*, **122-A** *[Ch 11 IV E 1 a (2)]*, **123-D** *[Ch 11 IV E 2 b (2)].*
A right-to-left atrial shunt is obligatory only in tricuspid atresia and in pulmonary atresia with intact ventricular septum. In pulmonary atresia with ventricular septal defect, a right-to-left ventricular shunt is obligatory.

In persistent truncus arteriosus, conotruncal septation does not proceed normally, resulting in a single arterial trunk arising from the heart. Symptoms of this anomaly are dependent on the status of pulmonary blood flow and, thus, are directly related to the size of the pulmonary arteries and the pulmonary vascular resistance.

In hypoplastic left-heart syndrome with aortic or mitral atresia, there is no forward flow across the left side of the heart; consequently, pulmonary venous return must traverse the atrial septum from left to right. In critical aortic stenosis, systemic flow may be ductus dependent; however, a left-to-right atrial shunt is not obligatory, although it may be present.

In pulmonary atresia with ventricular septal defect, pulmonary blood flow is ductus dependent, with an obligatory right-to-left ventricular shunt. In tricuspid atresia, adequate pulmonary blood flow may be maintained by atrial septal defect.

**124–128. The answers are: 124-E** *[Ch 1 V B 6 a]*, **125-C** *[Ch 1 VI B 7 a, F 1]*, **126-D** *[Ch 1 VI B 7 c, F 2]*, **127-D** *[Ch 1 VI B 4; VII B 8 a]*, **128-B** *[Ch 1 VII B 8, C].*
The state organization of the newborn is characterized by "predictable unpredictability." Thus, irregular feeding and sleeping schedules are to be expected. By the age of 2 months, the infant's demands should become more regular.

Night awakening reflects the continuing importance of attachment. Reinforcing the awakening by holding or feeding the infant should be avoided. The behavior will resolve normally within several weeks if parents provide only brief, positive interaction and lovingly, but firmly, indicate that the child must sleep.

By 15–18 months of age, a child's negativism and resistant behavior dramatically reflect the struggle for autonomy, typified by temper tantrums. The child continually explores the limits of the environment, while remaining dependent on adults. Distracting the child or ignoring his behavior (having first ensured his safety) is a reasonable approach to temper tantrums. Toilet training can also provide a forum for the struggle for independence. Toilet training is most successful when it is child-oriented. Attempts at toilet training should, therefore, be deferred until the child's negativism and resistant behavior subside.

The consistency of a child's style of behavior, or temperament, is predictive of the child's responses to certain situations. Slow adjustment to new situations, people, and places is typical of the "slow-to-warm-up" child. Entering school may pose particular difficulties for this child until she becomes more comfortable upon repeated exposure.

**129–132. The answers are: 129-C** *[Ch 15 I C 1 a (4) (a)]*, **130-D** *[Ch 15 I C 2 b (2)]*, **131-A** *[Ch 15 X B]*, **132-E** *[Ch 15 II B 2 a (2); III B 2 a]*.
The malignant cells of patients with retinoblastoma are thought to have lost constitutional heterozygosity for genetic material on the long arm of chromosome 13. This loss sometimes produces a visible deletion of part of the genetic material in this area, which is thought to be the location of either a suppressor gene or an antioncogene that limits retinoblast proliferation. Individuals homozygous for absence of this genetic material in their retinoblasts will develop tumors. If the first genetic defect is carried in the patient's germ cells and the second genetic defect on the other chromosome 13 develops postnatally within one or more retinoblasts, the patient has the hereditary form of retinoblastoma. If the defects in both chromosomes 13 occur postnatally in a retinoblast, the patient has the sporadic form of retinoblastoma.

Patients infected with HIV develop a progressive immunodeficiency that renders them incapable of mounting a T cell response to control B cell proliferation induced by Epstein-Barr virus or other B cell mitogens. If one of the proliferating B cells undergoes a chromosomal translocation that transforms it into a malignant cell, a B cell lymphoma (e.g., Burkitt's lymphoma) will develop.

Almost all hepatoblastomas synthesize $\alpha$-fetoprotein (AFP), which is present in elevated amounts in the patient's serum. Serum AFP level is a useful marker for response to treatment and tumor recurrence. Successful therapy is associated with a fall to normal levels, and recurrence is heralded by an increased level.

Terminal deoxyribonucleotidyl transferase (TdT) is an enzyme that is expressed in primitive lymphoid cells of the early pre–B cell, pre–B cell, and T cell phenotypes. TdT is involved in the process of immunoglobulin and T cell receptor gene rearrangements and is one of the enzymes that contributes to the great diversity of these rearrangements. Lymphoblastic lymphoma is a primitive lymphoid neoplasm whose cells generally are of T cell lineage, express a T cell–associated antigen, and contain TdT. Lymphoblastic lymphoma may spread to the central nervous system (CNS), where it usually produces diffuse meningeal seeding. The cells in the CSF are positive for TdT, which can help in their identification as malignant lymphoid cells.

**133–137. The answers are: 133-C, 134-D, 135-E, 136-A, 137-B** *[Ch 12 I C 2 b, c]*.
Flaring of the nostrils is a sign of dyspnea from increased airway resistance. It is a useful indication of respiratory distress in infants.

Stridor is a harsh sound, heard primarily on inspiration. It is produced by laryngeal or tracheal obstruction. The most common cause of stridor in infants is laryngomalacia.

Wheezing is produced by airflow through a narrowed airway. Most often wheezing is due to asthma, but it can occur in many respiratory disorders.

Crackles are produced by the opening of small airways that closed on the previous breath. They are heard primarily during inspiration.

Grunting is a sign of a loss of lung volume. It is seen in infants with respiratory distress syndrome and pulmonary edema. Grunting also may be noted in children with pleuritic chest pain.

**138–142. The answers are: 138-E, 139-C, 140-B, 141-A, 142-D** *[Ch 10 VI G 1]*.
Metronidazole, when used chronically, has been shown to facilitate healing of perirectal fistulae, although this problem generally recurs when the drug is stopped. Administration of 6-mercaptopurine, a toxic antimetabolite, may allow for reduction of steroid dosage but generally does not permit steroid discontinuation. Sulfasalazine is effective in treating mild to moderate colonic inflammation, and it also has prophylactic value in ulcerative colitis; it does not prevent recurrent disease in Crohn's colitis. Prednisone generally is the most efficacious therapy in inflammatory bowel disease, particularly in treating extraintestinal complications. Loperamide decreases intestinal electrolyte secretion and reduces stool volume, concomitantly decreasing cramps.

**143–146. The answers are: 143-B** *[Ch 7 I F 3 c (6)]*, **144-C** *[Ch 7 I E 3 c, F 1 a; V B 4 a]*, **145-A** *[Ch 7 I F 2 b]*, **146-B** *[Ch 7 I F 3 c (5)]*.
Amniocentesis is a procedure performed as early as 16 weeks gestation for various analyses of amniotic fluid, including the study of specific cell or fluid biochemical or DNA markers. Chorionic villus sampling (CVS) is performed at 8–11 weeks gestation and can provide fetal cells for biochemical or DNA analysis;

amniotic fluid is not available by this technique. Sickle cell disease is an autosomal recessive disorder for which a DNA probe is available. When both parents are heterozygotes, their child has a 25% chance of being affected. Amniocentesis and CVS provide material containing fetal DNA that can be analyzed for the sickle cell gene.

Consanguineous matings increase the risk for multifactorial disorders as well as autosomal recessive disorders. Among the most common multifactorial birth defects are neural tube defects. Maternal serum AFP testing is a low-risk screening tool for neural tube defects, which cause increased levels of maternal serum AFP. If the value is increased, level II ultrasound and amniocentesis can be offered for further evaluation.

Microcephaly can be genetic and may be diagnosed in utero where accurate head measurements can be obtained by ultrasound, since norms exist for head size at each gestational age.

A familial balanced translocation predisposes the couple to having chromosomally unbalanced and, therefore, abnormal offspring. Amniocentesis or CVS allows determination of fetal chromosome constitution.

**147–150. The answers are: 147-A, 148-D, 149-B, 150-C** *[Ch 3 IV B 3].*
Children with mild retardation rarely are identified prior to school entry. While they can acquire reading and writing skills, they have increasing difficulty in school as academic demands increase.

Children with profound retardation have little or no self-care or communication skills and often have associated medical problems.

Children with moderate retardation are capable of some limited academic achievement. Their academic program typically focuses on self-care skills. They require some supervision or support and ultimately are capable of employment in a sheltered setting.

Children with severe retardation may learn some language, but the communication skills will be very limited. These children can be trained to perform elementary health habits. Because they are not able to distinguish between safety and danger, they require constant supervision.

**151–154. The answers are: 151-D, 152-A, 153-C, 154-B** *[Ch 1 V F 2].*
Both candidal and intertrigo dermatitis involve the deep skin folds. Intertrigo is characterized by moderate erythema and a white or yellow exudate. Candidal diaper rash has bright red erosions that spread peripherally by satellite lesions to involve the genitalia, lower abdomen, thighs, and buttocks.

The most common variety of diaper rash is termed generic diaper dermatitis. This rash is characterized by erythema involving the lower abdomen, anteromedial thighs, scrotum, and labia. The rash usually spares the deep skin folds and produces dryness and wrinkling of the skin.

Infantile seborrheic dermatitis often begins in the diaper area and appears as a beefy red, sharply circumscribed rash with satellite lesions. The rash frequently spreads to other areas of the body. Common sites of the involvement include the flexural creases, cheeks, scalp, and extremities.

**155–159. The answers are: 155-B** *[Ch 8 II D 1]*, **156-E** *[Ch 8 II A 5]*, **157-C** *[Ch 8 II E 3]*, **158-A** *[Ch 8 II C 1]*, **159-D** *[Ch 8 II A 3].*
Recurrent infections caused by intracellular pathogens (e.g., mycobacteria) are associated with T cell immune deficiencies. This is seen in patients with acquired immune deficiency syndrome (AIDS), who have a marked T cell deficiency and often have *Mycobacterium avium-intracellulare* infections.

Hereditary angioedema is associated with a deficiency of C1 esterase inhibitor, one of the plasma inhibitors of the complement system.

AIDS is caused by a retrovirus infection that produces a profound deficiency of T cell immunity and, particularly in children, B cell abnormalities. The B cell defects appear to be secondary to the T cell deficiency, although further information is needed to clarify this. Children with AIDS suffer from a variety of opportunistic infections.

Recurrent infections with the parasite *Giardia lamblia* usually are associated with B cell or antibody deficiencies and, thus, are seen in patients with common variable hypogammaglobulinemia or IgA deficiency. Giardiasis causes chronic diarrhea and malabsorption.

Recurrent infections with *Neisseria* usually are associated with deficiency of late complement components (C5, C6, C7, C8).

**160–164. The answers are: 160-C** *[Ch 11 IV I 4 b (1)]*, **161-E** *[Ch 11 IV F 4 b (1)]*, **162-B** *[Ch 11 IV K 4 b (1)]*, **163-D** *[Ch 11 IV L 4 b (1) (a)]*, **164-A** *[Ch 11 IV M 1 d (2) (a)].*
The chest x-ray sometimes gives clues to the diagnosis of congenital heart defects. In coarctation of the aorta, the "3" sign is produced by soft tissue densities consisting of the aortic knob and the dilated descending aorta. In tetralogy of Fallot, the apex of the heart is upturned and the base is convex where the

pulmonary artery would have been, producing a boot-shaped contour. In D-transposition of the great arteries, the anterior-posterior arrangement of the great arteries produces a narrow base so that the heart resembles an egg on its side. In L-transposition of the great arteries, the ascending aorta produces convexity of the left heart border as it emerges from the right ventricle on the left side of the heart. In supracardiac total anomalous venous return, the cardinal veins above the heart produce a double shadow resembling a snowman or figure 8 as they drain into the superior vena cava.

**165–167. The answers are: 165-A, 166-B, 167-D** *[Ch 17 VIII A 1 a, B 1].*
Neurofibromatosis-1 (von Recklinghausen's disease) is diagnosed by the presence of two or more characteristics of the disease, one of which is the presence of six or more café au lait spots (measuring > 5 mm in diameter in prepubertal individuals and > 15 mm in diameter in postpubertal individuals). The spots are most commonly found in the crease areas or over the trunk.

The presence of epilepsy in association with mental retardation and a variety of skin lesions is characteristic of tuberous sclerosis. In addition, "tubers" (i.e., nonmalignant tumors) are found in the walls of the ventricles. These can enlarge, obstructing the flow of cerebrospinal fluid (CSF) and causing hydrocephalus.

von Hippel-Lindau disease is characterized by vascular tumors in the cerebellum and spinal cord. Ataxia-telangiectasia is a progressive ataxic syndrome. The telangiectasias usually do not develop until after age 5 years, making it difficult to diagnose ataxia-telangiectasia early on. Sturge-Weber syndrome is characterized by a port-wine stain over the face and by epilepsy; in addition, the leptomeninges may show abnormal vasculature. This tends not to be a progressive disease, but the epilepsy can be difficult to control.

# Index

**Note:** (t) after a page number denotes a table; an italicized page number denotes a figure; Q denotes a question; and E denotes an explanation.